AF556818

IMMUNOLOGY OF LIVER TRANSPLANTATION

EDITED BY

James Neuberger

The Liver and Hepatobiliary Unit, Queen Elizabeth Hospital, Birmingham, UK

AND

David Adams

Experimental Immunology Branch, National Cancer Institute, Bethesda, Maryland, USA

Edward Arnold

A division of Hodder & Stoughton

LONDON BOSTON MELBOURNE AUCKLAND

First published in Great Britain 1993

Distributed in the Americas by Little, Brown and Company
34 Beacon Road, Boston, MA 02108

British Library Cataloguing in Publication Data

Neuberger, James
Immunology of Liver Transplantation
I. Title II. Adams, David
616.3

ISBN 0-340-55310-3

Typeset in 10/11pt Linotron Times by Rowland Phototypesetting Limited, Bury St Edmunds, Suffolk.
Printed and bound in Great Britain for Edward Arnold, a division of Hodder and Stoughton Limited, Mill Road, Dunton Green, Sevenoaks, Kent TN13 2YA by Butler and Tanner Limited, Frome, Somerset.

Contents

List of Contributors

David H Adams, Experimental Immunology Branch, National Cancer Institute, National Institutes of Health, Bethesda, Maryland 20897, USA

Arne Akbar, Department of Clinical Immunology, Royal Free Hospital, London

Nancy Ascher, Professor of Surgery, University of California, Department of Surgery, Division of Liver Transplantation, San Francisco, CA 94143, USA

Reuben C Ayres, Liver Unit, Queen Elizabeth Hospital, Edgbaston, Birmingham

David Burnett, Department of Immunology, University of Birmingham and Lung Immunobiochemical Research Laboratory, B4 6NH

T D H Cairns, Department of Transplant Immunology, Oxford Transplant Centre, Churchill Hospital, Oxford

A Chousleb, Professor of Surgery, Universidad Nacional Antonoma de Mexico, Mexico City

Charles A Dinarello, Department of Medicine, New England Medical Center, 750 Washington Street, Boston MA 02111, USA

Olivier Farges, Unité de Chirurgie Hépatobiliaire et Digestive, Hôpital Paul Brousse, Villejuif, France

Ronald G Gill, Barbara Davis Center for Childhood Diabetes, University of Colorado Health Sciences Center, 4200 East 9th Avenue, Box B-140, Denver, CO80262, USA

L Hao, Barbara Davis Center for Childhood Diabetes, University of Colorado Health Sciences Center, 4200 East 9th Avenue, Box B-140, Denver, CO80262, USA

C J Hawkey, Department of Therapeutics, University Hospital, Nottingham

Stefan G Hubscher, Department of Pathology, University of Birmingham

N Hudson, Department of Therapeutics, University Hospital, Nottingham

R Jenkins, Department of Surgery, New England Deaconess Hospital and Harvard Medical School, Boston, Massachusetts, USA

N Kamada, Department of Experimental Surgery, National Children's Medical Research Centre, Taishido, Setagaya-ku, Tokyo, Japan

Saija Koskimies, Tissue Typing Laboratory, Finnish Red Cross Blood Transfusion Service, Helsinki, Finland

Kevin J Lafferty, Barbara Davis Center for Childhood Diabetes, University of Colorado Health Sciences Center, 4200 East 9th Avenue, Box B-140, Denver, CO80262, USA

Peter Lane, Basel Institute for Immunology, Grenzacherstrasse 487, CH-4005 Basel, Switzerland

Irmeli Lautenschlager, Transplantation Laboratory, Fourth Department of Surgery, University of Helsinki, Finland

Fiona McConnell, Basel Institute for Immunology, Grenzacherstrasse 487, CH-4005 Basel, Switzerland

James M Neuberger, The Liver and Hepatobiliary Unit, Queen Elizabeth Hospital, Edgbaston, Birmingham B15 2TH

John G O'Grady, Consultant Hepatologist, St James University Hospital, Leeds, LS9 7TF

L H Toledo-Pereyra, Michigan Transplant Institute, 1631 Gull Road, Suite 110, Kalamazoo, Michigan 49001, USA

J Lopez Ranger, Hospital Regional Ignacio Zaragoza, ISSTE, and Universidad Nacional Autonoma de Mexico, Mexico City

Mary A Ritter, Department of Immunology, Royal Postgraduate Medical School, London

S C Robson, MRC Liver Research Centre, Department of Medicine, University of Cape Town, South Africa

Robert Rothlein, Boehringer Ingelheim Pharmaceutical Inc., Ridgefield, CT 06877, USA

Mike Salmon, Department of Rheumatology, The Medical School, Birmingham University, Birmingham, B15 2TT

Linda A Scharschmidt, Boehringer Ingelheim Pharmaceutical Inc., Ridgefield, CT 06877, USA

Gustav Steinhoff, Klinik für Abdominal und Transplantationschirurgie, Medizinische Hochschule Hannover, Postfach 610180, D-300 Hannover 61, Germany

Sheena Sutherland, Virology Laboratory, Dulwich, and King's College Hospital, Denmark Hill, London

C Trey, Department of Medicine, New England Deaconess Hospital and Harvard Medical School, Boston, Massachusetts, USA

G Trey, Department of Medicine and Gastroenterology, Baylor College of Medicine, Houston, Texas, USA

K I Welsh, Department of Transplant Immunology, Oxford Transplant Centre, Churchill Hospital, Oxford

D J G White, Department of Surgery, Addenbrooke's Hospital, Hills Road, Cambridge

Roger Williams, Institute of Liver Studies, King's College Hospital, Denmark Hill, London

Kathryn J Wood, Nuffield Department of Surgery, University of Oxford, John Radcliffe Hospital, Oxford

R Xavier, Hospital Regional Ignacio Zaragoza, ISSTE, and Universidad Nacional Autonoma de Mexico, Mexico City

Introduction

The idea for a book on the immunology of liver transplantation was first suggested by the late Professor Ralph Wright of Southampton University who identified a gap between the clinical transplanters and the immunologists on whose work so many of the advances are dependent. In trying to provide that bridge, we have been fortunate in gaining the support of so many contributors, both scientists and clinicians, from all parts of the world.

In drawing up the format of the book, we realised early on that it would be necessary to make rather arbitrary and artificial divisions. The book has been divided into three sections: the first section deals primarily with some of the immunological factors which are involved in transplantation (liver allograft rejection). It is not intended to be a mini text book of immunology, but to convey some of the scientific concepts underlying transplantation immunology. The middle section is concerned primarily with mechanisms of allograft rejection, and the final section concentrates on clinical issues. We have tried hard to ensure that no major areas are omitted and realise that some aspects are covered more than once. We realise, too, that it is very rare for any volume of this kind to be read through from cover to cover and, therefore, we have tried to ensure that each chapter is complete in itself which means a degree of reiteration is inevitable. We are also aware that some aspects are controversial and different views on the same topic are expressed in different chapters.

Neither of us realised the difficulties and the amount of work involved in drawing together contributors from so many different countries. Neither did we appreciate the enjoyment of such an undertaking. We extend our thanks to all the contributors and to them must go the credit for any success of this volume. There are a number of other people who must be thanked for their work: in particular Michelle Calcutt at The Queen Elizabeth Hospital for doing so much to coordinate the secretarial side of things, and to Geoff Nuttall, Diana Waha and Diane Leadbetter-Conway at Edward Arnold for all their editorial work.

The interest in this volume has encouraged the publishers to publish companion volumes in the fields of renal, heart and other solid organ transplantation. In this very rapidly advancing field, it is likely that certain aspects of the contributions may well be overtaken by new developments, but this volume will, we hope, outline the basis on which these new developments can be assessed.

James Neuberger
David Adams

SECTION I

Aspects of the Immune System

1

T lymphocytes

M Ritter

Introduction

Adaptive immune responses are dependent upon the action of two separate antigen-specific cell lineages – T lymphocytes and B lymphocytes. This dichotomy within the lymphocyte population was first recognised in the early 1960s when it was shown that 'cell mediated' immune responses were dependent upon an intact thymus. Thus, in experimentally thymectomised animals and in congenitally athymic patients, there is a characteristic inability to reject a graft of foreign tissue and to mount a delayed type hypersensitivity reaction; there is also a marked peripheral lymphopaenia.[1,2] Complementary experiments in the avian system demonstrated that a second population of lymphocytes was responsible for 'antibody-mediated' immune responses, and that these cells are dependent upon the presence of a second major lymphoid organ – the bursa of Fabricius.[3] Mammals lack this organ, and it was later realised that the mammalian foetal liver and adult bone marrow serve an equivalent function in the production of B lymphocytes.[4]

These crucial discoveries gave rise to an entire field of scientific endeavour from which we have now gained a good understanding of many related processes including the development of lymphocyte populations, the generation and selection of the antigen-receptor repertoire, the specific recognition of antigen by lymphocytes, the signals required for lymphocyte activation, and the characteristics and functional capabilities of different lymphocyte subsets. These scientific advances were made possible by successive advances in methodology, amongst the most notable of which were the production of monoclonal antibodies, cell labelling techniques, T cell cloning, recombinant DNA technology and the development of transgenic animals.

This chapter will review current understanding of the development, characteristics and functional properties of human T lymphocytes. However, since a considerable amount of information has come from studies in experimental animals, some reference will be made to other mammalian systems when necessary.

The development of T lymphocytes

The haemopoietic stem cell

T lymphocytes derive ultimately from the same pluripotent haemopoietic stem cell as do all other blood cells (Figure 1.1). This stem cell develops within the bone marrow where, under the influence of specific microenvironmental niches, it can give rise to all major haemopoietic lineages (erythrocyte, granulocyte, monocyte and B lymphocyte) with the exception of T lymphocytes.[5] For T lymphopoiesis, the stem cell/lymphoid progenitor must leave the bone marrow and migrate through the vascular system to the thymus where the microenvironment provides the signals required for T lymphocyte development (Figure 1.2).[6,7]

The thymus

The organ is composed of two major lobes surrounded by a connective tissue capsule. Each lobe is subdivided into many pseudolobules by connective tissue septa which push deep into the organ, bringing with them an extensive vascular and neuronal supply.[8,9]

Three major zones can be recognised within the thymus: the outer subcapsule, the cortex and the central medulla. The organ is composed of large

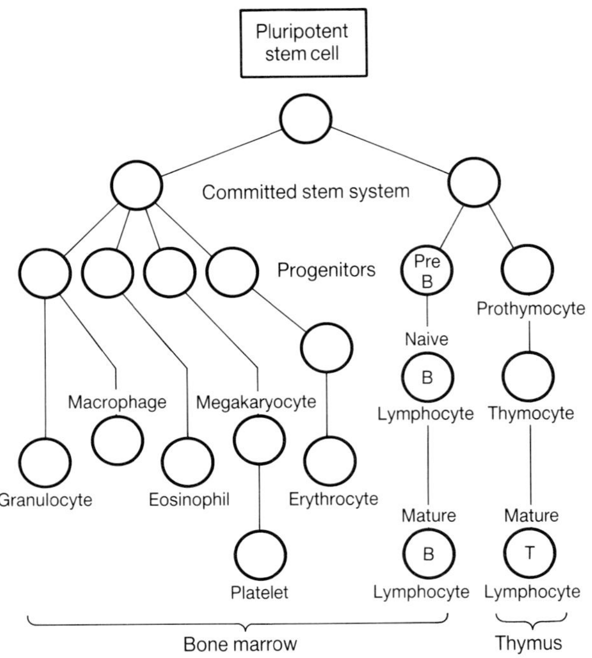

Fig. 1.1 Diagrammatic summary of haemopoiesis

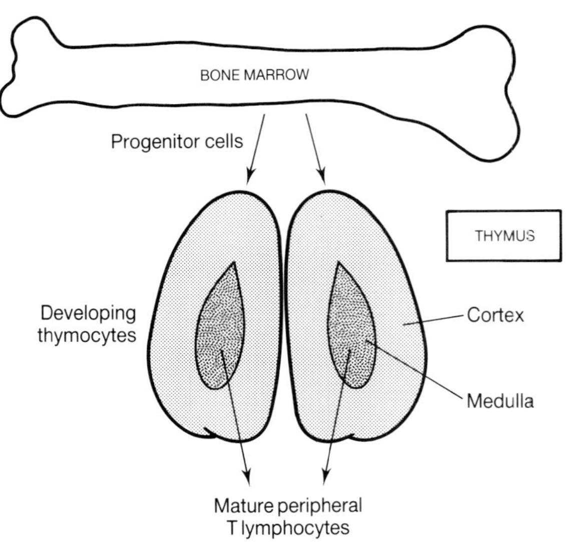

Fig. 1.2 T lymphocyte development takes place within the thymus micro environment.

numbers of developing lymphocytes (thymocytes) held in a framework of stromal cells.

The least mature thymocytes (prothymocytes) are large blast-like cells located in the subcapsular zone; these represent approximately 5% of total thymic lymphocytes. The majority of thymocytes (approximately 80–85%) are mostly small immature lymphocytes found in the cortex. The remaining 10–15% constitute the mature medullary T lymphocyte population.

Thymic stromal cells mainly comprise epithelial cells, macrophages and dendritic cells, and are important in creating the unique microenvironment that is required for T cell development. Moreover, stromal cells in the different thymic zones show characteristic differences in their morphology, cell surface molecules and secretory products, giving support to the idea that there are many different microenvironmental niches within the thymus, each responsible for the induction of a discrete phase of T lymphopoiesis.[9]

The thymus is well supplied by blood vessels that enter the organ at the cortical-medullary junction and which give rise to capillary networks in both cortex and medulla. Although bloodborne molecules are known to have access to the thymic medulla, the cortex was for a long time thought to be isolated by a 'blood–thymic barrier' maintained by the cortical capillary endothelial cells and basement membrane. However, it has recently been shown that extrathymic macromolecules can gain entry to the cortex via the outer capsule which contains fenestrated capillaries.[10] This has important implications for the induction of tolerance to non-thymic self-antigens (see section on 'Negative selection').

Intrathymic T cell development

Thymocyte development involves several distinct components; these include cell migration, proliferation, generation and selection of the antigen-receptor repertoire, phenotypic and functional maturation.[9,11]

Migration

The bone marrow-derived bloodborne progenitor cell enters the thymus in the cortical-medullary region. From here it migrates to the subcapsular zone where it starts its development. As development proceeds the thymocytes follow a centripetal pathway of migration, first to the cortex where many of the major stages of differentiation and selection take place, and then to the medulla where, as mature T cells, they are ready to migrate out to the periphery to join the recirculating lymphocyte pool.

Proliferation

Cell proliferation is an early and important event in T cell development. A single progenitor cell can give rise to sufficient offspring to populate an entire thymic lobe with the normal spectrum of cell subpopulations.[12] In numerical terms, a newborn mouse thymus, which contains between 2 to 5×10^8 cells *in toto*, generates approximately 0.5×10^8 new cells each day, although up to 95% of these are destined to die within the organ (see section on 'Negative selection').[13,14]

Phenotype maturation

T cell development is characterised by the sequential acquisition and loss of many cell surface and some intracellular molecules.[9] Extensive cell labelling studies using monoclonal antibodies in immunocytochemical and flow cytometric techniques have been performed with one, two, three and sometimes four colour detection systems. This has led to the identification of many phenotypically distinct thymocyte populations, and in combination with cell separation and transfer techniques, has led to a concensus on the precursor-product interrelationships between these different cell subsets (Figure 1.3). (Details of the CD classification of molecules defined by monoclonal antibodies are given in the Appendix.)

The earliest progenitor cell that is found in the thymus bears the pan T cell glycoprotein CD7 and the adhesion molecule CD44, the latter probably reflecting the recent migratory activity of the cell. These prothymocytes also express the nuclear enzyme TdT [terminal deoxynucleotidyl transferase] which plays an important role in the generation of T cell receptor diversity[15] (see section on 'The T cell repertoire'). The more mature prothymocytes are characterised by surface expression of CD8 (the immature CD8+ 'single positive' thymocytes).

Following extensive proliferation, prothymocytes give rise to cortical thymocytes that express both CD4 and CD8 cell surface molecules (CD4+ 8+ 'double positive' thymocytes). Several other cell surface molecules also appear during cortical thymocyte maturation; these include CD1, CD2 and CD5. Most importantly, it is at this stage that the cells start to express their cell surface receptor for antigen [TCR] and the associated CD3 complex (see section on 'The T cell receptor for antigen'), a process that reflects an underlying sequence of genetic rearrangement events in the TCR gene loci (see section on 'The T cell repertoire). Thus these developing cortical double positive thymocytes first produce cytoplasmic TCR beta chain and CD3 molecules.[15] Later, when they have the capability also to produce the TCR alpha chain, they express complete TCR alpha beta heterodimers on the cell surface in association with surface CD3. The cell surface expression of a complete TCR and the CD3 complex is interdependent and therefore coordinated. A minority of thymocytes carry an alternative heterodimeric TCR structure that is composed of a gamma and delta chain. This TCR is also tightly linked to CD3.

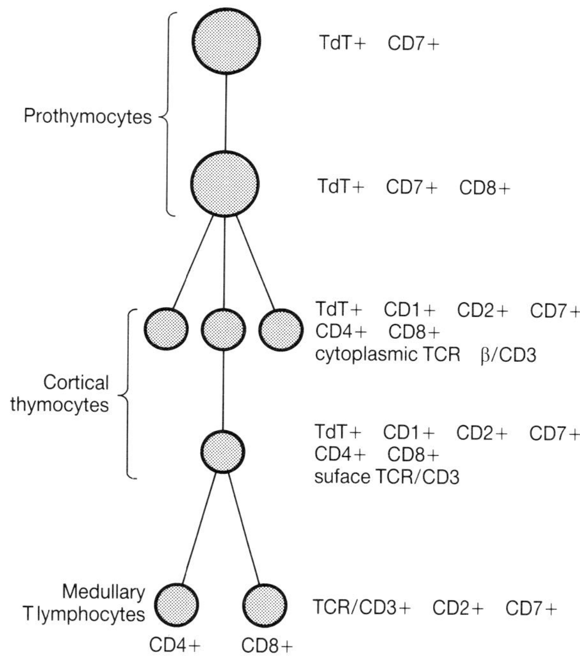

Fig. 1.3 Intrathymic T lymphocyte development.

The majority of double positive cortical thymocytes are thought to die intrathymically as a result of stringent repertoire selection. The minority that survive give rise to the mature single positive CD4+ or CD8+ medullary thymocytes.

The T cell receptor repertoire

Generation

Two of the most critical events in intrathymic T lymphocyte development are the generation and subsequent selection of the T cell antigen receptor repertoire. Prothymocyte proliferation furnishes the thymus with a large number of cells within

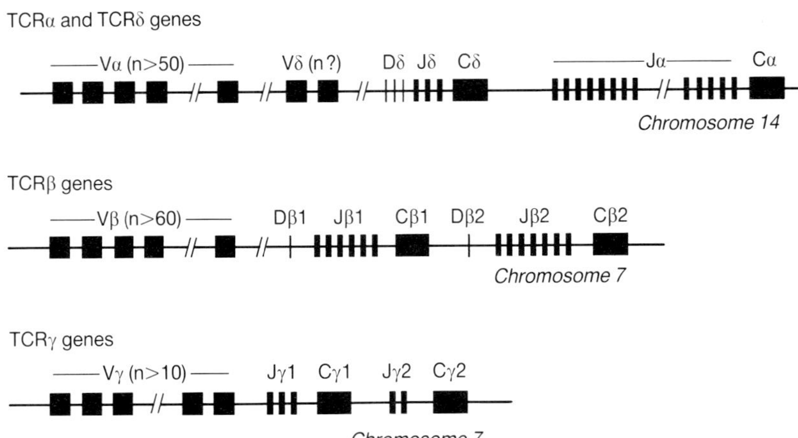

Fig. 1.4 Organisation of human T cell receptor gene loci.

which random genetic rearrangements can create an enormous diversity of TCR-bearing thymocytes, each cell being characterised by its own unique TCR. Each TCR protein chain is encoded within a complex genetic locus. The generation of TCR diversity is based upon the somatic recombination of multiple germline genetic elements within these loci.[9,16,17]

The beta and gamma loci are quite separate from each other on chromosome 7, while the delta locus is nested within the alpha locus on chromosome[14] (Figure 1.4). In the alpha and gamma loci there are two sets of rearranging genes, the V (variable) and J (joining) genes, while the beta and delta loci contain V, J and additional D (diversity) genes that can recombine. Gene rearrangement within these TCR loci follows very much the same rules as those used by the immunoglobulin loci. For example, a developing alpha beta T cell will first join one of its 2 D beta genes to one of 13 J beta genes, by removing all intervening DNA under the action of the DNA recombinase enzyme system. Similarly, the cell can then juxtapose this newly created DJ combination to any one of its V beta genes (estimated to be at least 60 in number). These genetic rearrangements are guided by palindromic heptomer and nonamer sequences, according to the 12 base pair (12bp) and 23 base pair (23bp) spacer rule, followed by B cells.[16,17] However, unlike the situation in B cells where D genes are flanked by 23bp spacers on both 5' and 3' sides ensuring VDJ joining, in T cells the D beta genes are flanked by a 5' 23bp and a 3' 12bp thus permitting direct VJ and VDDJ joins in addition to the regular VDJ combination. In theory this is likely to enhance the possibilities for TCR diversity although how frequently these combinations actually occur is unclear. Additional variation is created at the joins between the various genetic elements by variation in the exact point at which two genes will join (junctional inaccuracies) and by *de novo* addition of nucleotides at the site of the join (new, or N, sequences), catalyzed by the enzyme TdT which requires no second strand DNA template. These rearranged VD and VDJ genes encode the variable domain of each TCR polypeptide chain, while non-rearranging C genes encode the constant domain of each chain (the structure of the TCR is discussed in the section on 'The T cell receptor for antigen').

Similar recombinatorial events occur within the other TCR genetic loci leading to VDJ (delta locus) and VJ (alpha and gamma loci) joining. Additional diversity is created by the fact that within the alpha/delta locus, the V delta genes can associate with either the D delta or J alpha, and can thus contribute to either delta or alpha TCR genes. For the human alpha beta TCR the potential diversity that can be created by these mechanisms has been estimated to be of the order of 2.75×10^{10}.[16,17] For the gamma delta TCR this appears to be more limited, at approximately 4×10^5.

Allelic exclusion acts for T cells as it does for B cells. Thus a successful rearrangement in a locus will block further rearrangement not only within that locus, but also within the equivalent locus on the homologous chromosome. The factors that govern whether a cell uses a gamma delta or an alpha beta TCR are unknown. Gamma delta TCR-bearing T cells are the first to appear in ontogeny; however, in the adult, only 5% of T cells use this TCR (see section on 'Gamma-delta T cells').

Selection

TCR diversity is created at random. T cells must therefore pass through stringent selection systems before they are permitted to leave the thymus and join the peripheral lymphocyte pool.[9,18] Firstly, some randomly created TCR may be strongly self-reactive. Cells bearing these must be deleted from the system in order to avoid autoimmune phenomena – a process termed 'negative selection'. Secondly, the way in which T cells recognise antigen in association with a self-MHC molecule (MHC restriction; see section on 'T cell activation') imposes further constraints upon the repertoire, such that only those T cells whose TCR can interact with self-MHC are selected to survive through all stages of intrathymic development. This process is termed positive selection.

Positive selection

T cells recognise antigen in the form of a peptide that is associated with a self-MHC molecule, either class I or class II (MHC restriction). It was therefore proposed that a necessary step in the creation of a functional TCR repertoire must be the positive selection of those T cells whose TCR could recognise a self-MHC molecule. The corollary to this would be that all those TCR that could not interact with self-MHC would be ignored or deleted. The original demonstration of the phenomenon of MHC restriction also highlighted the importance of the thymus in this aspect of T cell 'education'.[19] Recent experiments employing mice that are transgenic for an alpha beta TCR of known specificity have provided data in support of this proposal, and have elucidated some of the processes that are involved.[18]

Elegant studies of thymocyte development in mice carrying a transgenic TCR with specificity for the H-Y male antigen in association with an MHC class I molecule [H-2D^b] have shown that in female mice, where the restricting element (the class I molecule) but not the specific antigen is present, the T cells that develop and mature are almost all channelled into the mature CD8+ single positive medullary population (Figure 1.5). Conversely, for transgenic mice carrying an MHC class II restricted TCR, development is skewed towards the mature CD4+ single positive subset (Figure 1.6). Positive selection thus appears to consist of two main elements; a signal for survival within the thymus, and a maturation signal that determines the ultimate phenotype of the mature T cell. Survival depends upon an interaction between the TCR on the surface of a developing double positive thymocyte and self-MHC molecules on the surrounding cortical epithelium.[20] Phenotype development involves the retention of either CD4 or CD8 (and associated loss of CD8 or CD4 respectively), and is determined by the class of MHC molecule with which the TCR interacts. Thus, after intrathymic development and positive selection, emerging T cells are either CD4+ and MHC class II restricted or CD8+ and MHC class I restricted.

Negative selection

A second phase of intrathymic selection is designed to delete those developing T cells that, after random rearrangement of TCR genes, have created a TCR with specificity for a self-antigen. The deletion of such self-reactive thymocytes is initiated by interaction between the autoreactive T cell and an auto-antigen-MHC complex on the surface of an antigen presenting cell (APC). The APCs involved in this 'negative selection' are of bone marrow origin and likely to be the dendritic cells (and perhaps also macrophages) that are located at the cortical-medullary junction and in the medulla of the thymus.[21]

The mechanism whereby self-reactive thymocytes are deleted appears to be one of suicide. Engagement of the T cell's TCR with its specific antigen+MHC complex induces apoptosis in the T cell; endogenous endonucleases are produced which cleave the thymocyte DNA into oligomeric fragments, leading to cell death within a few hours.[22]

It is easy to imagine how negative selection can account for tolerance to any self-antigen that is expressed in the thymus, but what of peripheral self-antigens? Until recently it was thought that the thymus was inaccessible to non-thymic antigens due to the blood–thymus barrier. However, it is now known that macromolecules can enter both medullary and cortical regions, such that the developing thymocytes and thymic stromal cells are bathed in peripheral antigens.[10,23] Thus intra-

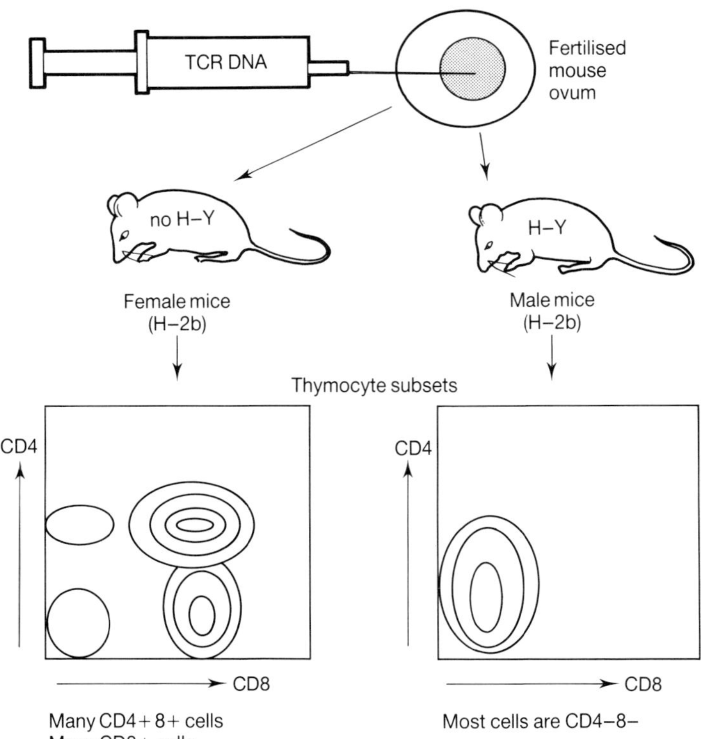

Fig. 1.5 Diagrammatic summary of experimental studies on positive and negative selection in mice expressing transgenic anti-H-Y T cell receptors*.

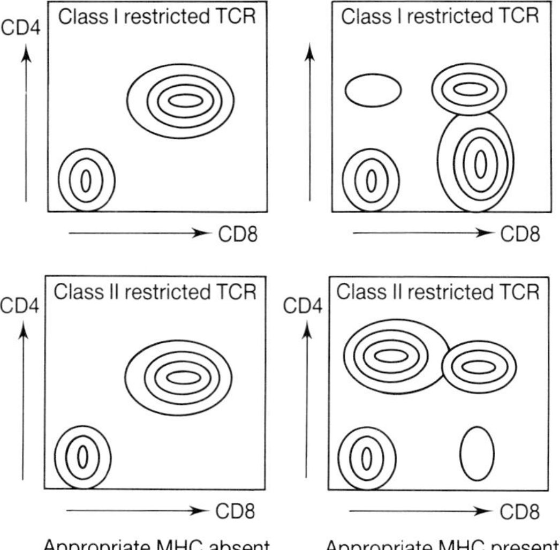

Fig. 1.6 Positive selection of thymocytes. Maturation of T cells requires interaction of the TCR with either MHC class I or class II molecules. This interaction also determines the ultimate phenotype of the T cell (MHC class I, CD8; MHC class II, CD4).

thymic selection can probably account for most self-tolerance. However, two further mechanisms, anergy and suppression, have been shown to act in the periphery and may provide a critical 'back-up' in maintaining self-tolerance. These will be discussed later in this chapter (section on 'T suppressor cells').

Sequence of selective events

For the majority of developing thymocytes selection occurs at the CD4+CD8+ double positive stage as soon as the cells have started to express their TCR (TCR low and TCR intermediate stages), with positive selection usually preceding negative selection (Figure 1.7).[9]

Positive selection is critically dependent upon interaction with the cortical epithelium and its timing is therefore controlled by the physical location of the developing T cell within the thymus. In contrast, negative selection can act on a wider developmental range of thymocytes (usually

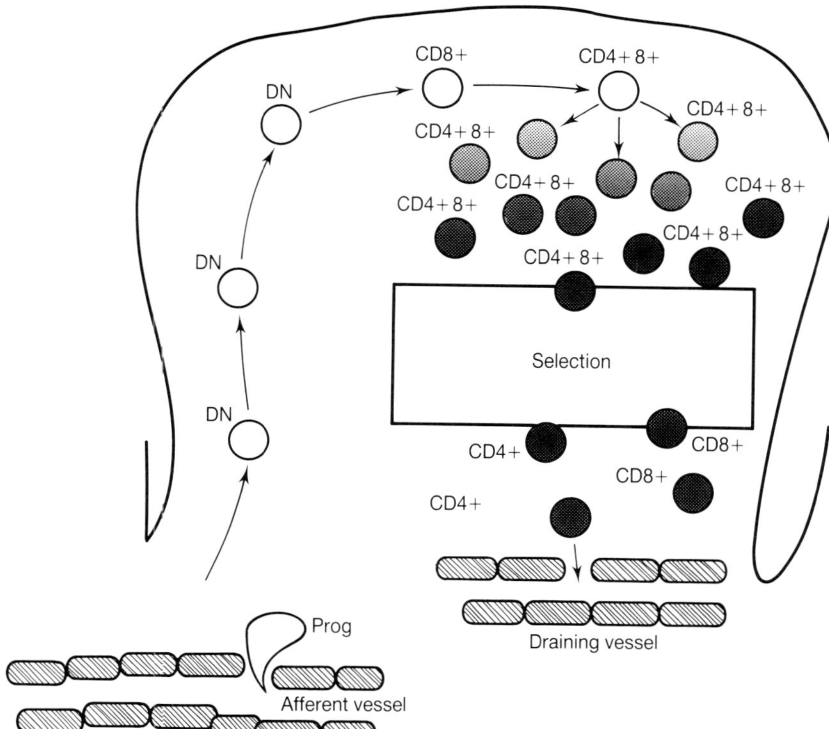

Fig. 1.7 Summary of intrathymic T cell development. Prog = progenitor cell: DN = double negative (CD4-, CD8-) thymocyte.

double positives, but also double negatives and single positives in some experimental situations), and can be induced by interaction with any professional APC.

As a result of all these developmental and selective processes, the thymus supplies the periphery with a population of functionally mature CD4+ and CD8+ T cells that are self-MHC restricted and which are not autoreactive (summarised in Figure 1.7). This process of T lymphopoiesis is most active during the foetal period and the first few years of post-natal life. However, even in old age (80 years) when the thymus is drastically reduced (termed involution) in size, the tissue that does remain appears quite normal in both its lymphocyte and stromal cell composition.[8,24] The thymus is therefore probably active in 'topping up' the peripheral T cell pool throughout life.

Finally, the thymus may undergo acute involution in response to external stress, as during an acute infection.[8] Unlike age-associated involution where there is a balanced and progressive reduction in all areas of the thymus, acute involution involves the rapid loss of almost all cortical thymocytes (by apoptosis) but leaves other areas of the thymus unaffected.[25] Acute involution is thought to be a defence mechanism whereby the generation of new T cells is 'shut down' until the pathogenic organism has been cleared by the mature cells of the peripheral pool. This may be essential in preventing the development of tolerance to pathogen-derived antigens that may reach the thymus in significant amounts during the height of the infection. Subsequently, the thymus quickly regenerates and T lymphopoiesis resumes.

Certain immunosuppressive regimes can also induce thymic involution. Corticosteroids induce an acute reversible involution of the cortex, comparable to that seen during acute infection, and resulting in a shutdown of intrathymic T cell development. In contrast, therapy with cyclosporin A and FK506 has a quite different effect, leading to almost total loss of the thymic medulla (both lymphoid and stromal cell populations) whilst leaving the cortex apparently unimpaired.[26,27,28] Functional studies in experimental animals have revealed T cell development is blocked at the CD4+ and CD8+ stage and that deletion of auto-reactive T cells (negative selection) does not occur during cyclosporin A treatment, thus increasing the likelihood of auto-immune phenomena.[29] These defects may result from the direct effect of cyclosporin A on developing T cells in the thymus, although the drug is also thought to influence thymic epithelium and dendritic cells.[27] It is not known whether similar effects occur in the human thymus.

The T cell receptor for antigen

The hunt for the TCR was a long one, hampered by the absence of a plentiful source of soluble receptor comparable to that provided by serum and myeloma immunoglobulin for B cell receptor studies. Success was finally achieved by two experimental approaches. In the first, monoclonal antibodies were raised to cloned T cells. Those reagents that were specific for a single clone were selected, following the argument that the only surface molecule that would distinguish one T cell clone from another would be its receptor for antigen. This approach revealed that the TCR was a heterodimer composed of two disulphide-linked polypeptide chains of approximately 45 KDa and 40 KDa molecular weight, termed alpha and beta respectively.[30]

Other studies employed molecular genetic techniques, and were designed to identify genes that were separate from but shared certain characteristics with those that encoded the heavy and light chains of immunoglobulin – multiple germline genes that rearranged during T cell development and whose product is only expressed by cells of the T lineage. In this way, two genetic loci were identified and sequenced. However, although one of these clearly encoded the beta chain, the other did not match the known structure of the alpha chain.[31,32] This second gene was therefore named gamma. Subsequent studies at both DNA and protein level revealed the presence of four genes and four corresponding polypeptide chains: alpha, beta, gamma and delta.[33,34,35] These associate to give two separate classes of TCR, the alpha beta (termed TCR2) and gamma delta (termed TCR1).

The structure of both TCRs are strongly homologous, and both clearly belong to the immunoglobulin superfamily (Figure 1.8).[16,36,37] Each TCR chain is a transmembrane polypeptide with two external domains. Each domain has an Ig-like structure with intrachain disulphide bond and beta pleated sheet folding pattern. The membrane proximal domain is constant in structure while the membrane distal domain is highly variable. Variability is concentrated in three major hypervariable regions, or CDR (complementary determining regions), which lie exposed at the ends of the beta

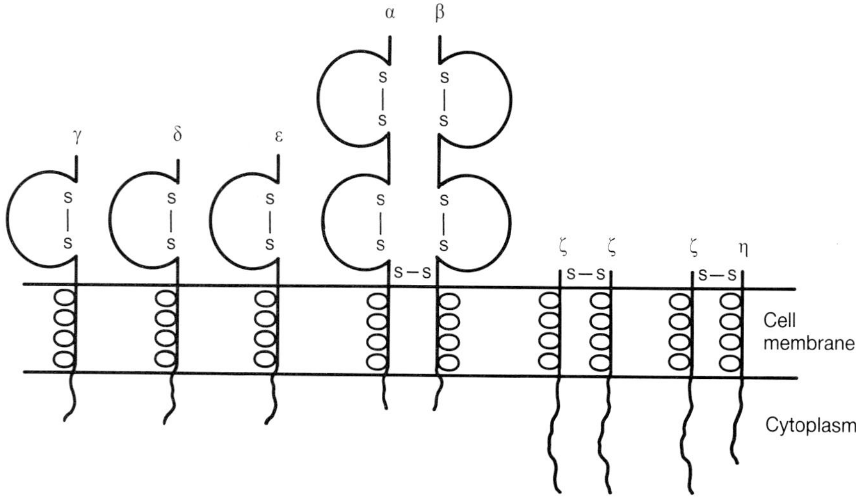

Fig. 1.8 The structure of the alpha/beta T cell receptor and associated gamma, delta, epsilon, zeta and eta chains of the CD3 complex. S-S = disulphide bond.

pleated sheets in a way comparable to that seen for the immunoglobulin molecule. CDR1 and 2 are encoded within the V genes, whereas CDR3 is formed around the VJ (alpha and gamma) and VDJ (beta and delta) joining regions. When the TCR interacts with the antigen+MHC complex, CDR1 and 2 are thought to be involved in binding to MHC while CDR3 binds predominantly to the peptide antigen lying in the groove on the surface of the MHC molecule (see section on 'T cell activation').

Alpha beta and gamma delta TCR are very similar in their overall structure, although the loss of a cysteine in the C gamma 2 domain prevents the formation of a gamma-delta intrachain disulphide bond when this constant domain is used.[35]

Cell surface TCR is always closely associated with a group of small polypeptide molecules collectively referred to as the CD3 complex.[16,37,38] The closeness of this association has been demonstrated by cell surface co-capping, using either anti-CD3 or anti-TCR antibodies, and by co-immunoprecipitation of TCR/CD3 from detergent lysates of T cell membranes, using anti-CD3 antibodies.

The CD3 complex is composed of four polypeptide chains: gamma, delta, epsilon and zeta. A fifth chain, eta, has been identified in the mouse. The gamma, delta and epsilon chains are three distinct transmembrane polypeptides of 20 to 25 KDa molecular weight whose portion that is external to the cell membrane shows strong homology to an Ig domain. They therefore belong to the Ig superfamily.[36,37] The 21 KDa zeta and 16 KDa eta are not members of this family.[39] They have less than ten amino acids external to the cell membrane, while the major part of the molecule is transmembrane and cytoplasmic. Zeta and eta chains are linked by disulphide bonds between their extracellular portions to form zeta-zeta homodimers and, for a minority of molecules in the mouse, zeta-eta heterodimers. These small chains are involved in signal transduction, and show strong homology with the gamma chain of the high affinity Fc receptor for IgE (FcR epsilon I) and IgG [FcR II].[40,41] In addition, the zeta chain is essential for transportation of the TCR/CD3 complex to the cell surface. The exact mechanism underlying this observation is unclear, although non-covalent binding of zeta to the beta chain of the TCR is known to be a prerequisite. Moreover, although TCR alpha and beta chains and CD3 gamma, delta and epsilon are produced intracellularly in excess amounts, the level of zeta is limiting, thus providing a means whereby it can regulate surface expression.

T cell activation

T cells can only be activated by antigen that is present on a cell surface. The underlying significance of this probably lies in the fact that T cell effector mechanisms are all designed to destroy cellular targets. Thus for a T cell to mount a response to a soluble target antigen that it cannot clear from the body would at best be a waste of metabolic energy and at worst could lead to inflammatory side effects. It is therefore probably for these reasons that during evolution the immune system developed the use of MHC products as 'guiding' molecules, directing T cell immunity to a cell surface – hence the phenomenon of MHC restriction.[19]

The interaction between TCR and antigen+MHC complex

T cell activation is initiated by the interaction between the TCR and its specific antigen+MHC on a target cell/antigen presenting cell (Figures 1.9 and 1.10).[16,42,43] The antigen is presented as a small peptide fragment that has been processed by the target cell and which has then bound in the groove on the MHC molecule (Figure 1.11).[44] In general, the peptides that are presented on MHC class I are derived from endogenous molecules that have been produced within the presenting cell, and as such will be either self-proteins or molecules encoded by the genome of a virus that is infecting the presenting cell. In contrast, MHC class II presented peptides are usually derived from exogenous proteins that have been endocytosed by the APC.[45,46]

This TCR+antigen+MHC interaction is stabilised by additional molecular interactions.[47,48,49,50] For CD4+ T cells, the CD4 molecule binds to a non-polymorphic site on the beta 2 domain of the class II molecules involved in the TCR+antigen+MHC complex (CD4 may also bind to MHC class II molecules that are not involved in the specific TCR/antigen interaction; see Figure 1.11). For CD8+ T cells, the CD8 molecule interacts in a similar way with the alpha 3 domain MHC class I on the target cell. However, in ad-

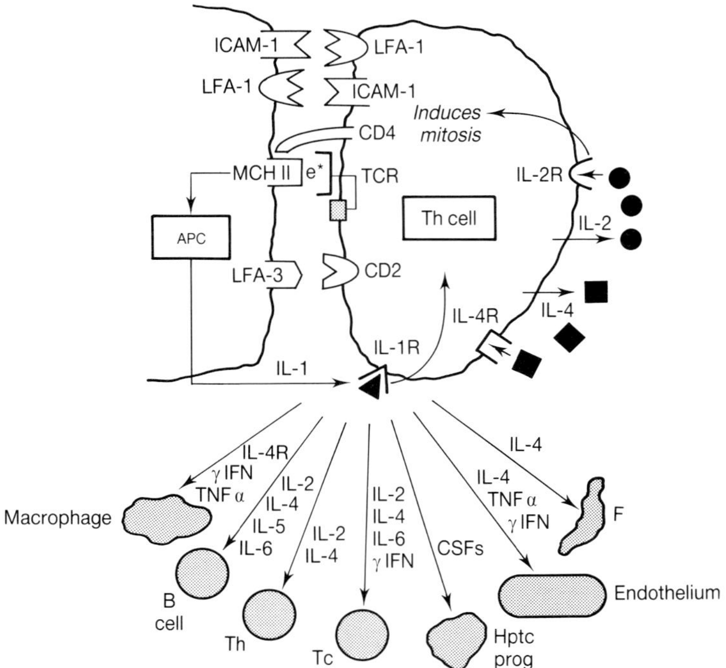

Fig. 1.9 Activation and function of CD4+ T helper cells. ICAM-2 (not shown) has a similar distribution to ICAM-1.

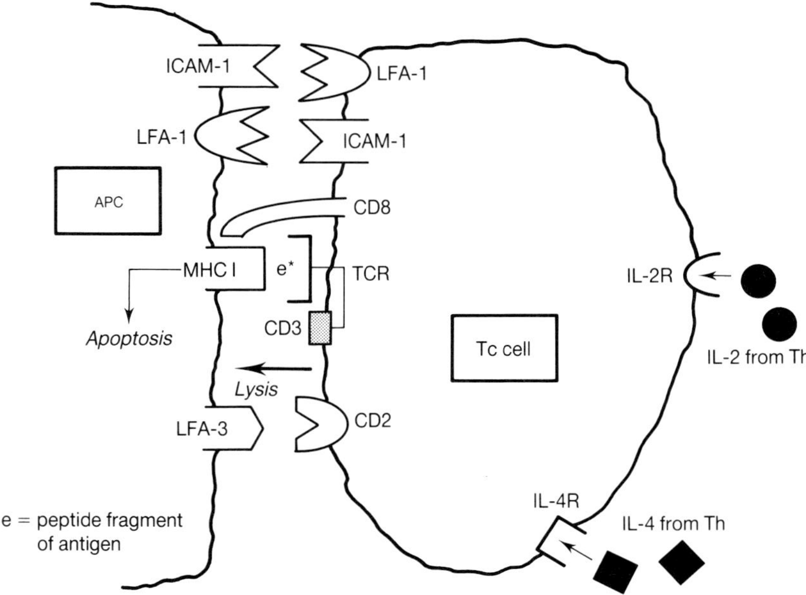

Fig. 1.10 Activation and function of CD8+ T cytotoxic cells. ICAM-2 (not shown) has a similar distribution to ICAM-1.

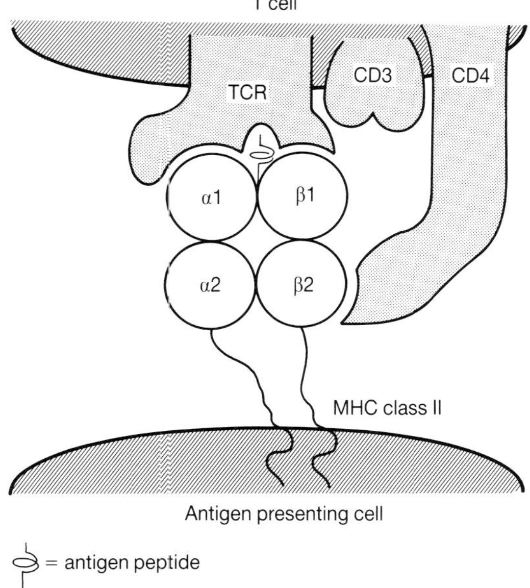

Fig. 1.11 Role of accessory molecules in T cell recognition (CD4+ T cell; antigenic peptide presented by MHC class II).

dition to enhancing the affinity of interaction between the T cell and its target, CD4 and CD8 are also involved in signal transduction, as described below. The binding of T cell and target is additionally enhanced by the interaction of T cell CD2 with LFA-3 (CD58) on the target, and by adhesion of LFA-1 (CD11a/CD18) to ICAM-1 (CD54) and ICAM-2.[47] This latter interaction is bi-directional since LFA-1, ICAM-1 and ICAM-2 are present on both the T cell and its target/presenting cell. Interaction between T cells and antigen presenting B cells is further enhanced by binding of CD28 on the T cell with the B cell restricted antigen B7/BB-1.[51] Interestingly, the majority of these molecules (CD2, CD4, CD8, CD28, MHC class I, MHC class II, LFA-3, ICAM-1 and ICAM-2) are all members of the Ig superfamily. Such diversification of a basic molecular motif (Ig domain) probably represents successive evolutionary adaptions that led to enhancement of the immune response. The expression of most of these adhesion molecules on T cells and their targets is upregulated following T cell activation. For some (for example, the VLA antigens), their affinity for their target molecule is also increased.[47]

Second signals

Engagement of the TCR/CD3 complex with antigen+MHC (or an artificial ligand such as antibody to the TCR or CD3) is necessary but not sufficient for the activation of an immune response. All T cells require a second signal, although the exact nature of this signal differs according to the function of the responding T cell. T cells fall into two major functional categories, the helper T cells [Th] that secrete cytokines and the cytotoxic T cells [Tc] that lyse their targets. The majority of the Th are CD4+ and respond to exogenous antigen+MHC class II, presented to them by a specialised antigen presenting cell (such as dendritic cells, macrophages or B cells). In contrast, the majority of Tc are CD8+ and recognise endogenous antigen in the context of MHC class I on the target cell. Since MHC class I molecules are present on all nucleated cells, the limiting factor in this type of response is the distribution of the specific endogenous antigen rather than that of the cells that bear the restriction element. Whatever the function of the T cell, the second signal is provided by one or more soluble molecules (cytokines). The combined effect of signal 1 (via the TCR) and signal 2 (cytokine) leads to activation of the T cell and results in two main responses: proliferation (via autocrine and/or paracrine pathways) to generate a large clone of T cells with specificity for the stimulating antigen+MHC complex; and maturation of these clonal cells to give a majority effector population (cytotoxic or cytokine secreting) and a minority memory population ready to initiate a secondary or subsequent response on re-encounter with the specific antigen. The events leading to and following activation differ for Th and Tc.

The second signal required for activation of Th is the cytokine interleukin-1 (IL-1) which is secreted by the antigen presenting cell. Thus the Th cell will receive both signal 1 (via TCR/CD3) and signal 2 (IL-1) from the cell that presents it with antigen.[52] Other cytokines such as IL-6 and TNF may also act as second signals, and may qualitatively affect the outcome of activation.

Tc cells also require two main signals. Signal 1 comprises the interaction between the TCR and antigen+MHC on the target cell. Signal 2 is provided by the Th cells and consists of IL-2 together with other cytokines such as IL-4, IL-6 and gamma interferon.[53] These lead to the proliferation and maturation of the cytotoxic T cell.

Signal transduction

The link between external stimuli (Signals 1 and 2) and the functional effect of these stimuli (e.g. proliferation, cytokine production, cytotoxicity) is provided by a series of transmembrane and intracellular events collectively termed 'signal transduction' or 'second messenger' systems. Several distinct second messenger systems have been identified in mammalian cells. These include the cyclic AMP pathway, the phosphoinositol pathway, cell surface molecules whose cytoplasmic tails are either tyrosine kinases or are associated with a tyrosine kinase, and the recently described glycophosphatidylinositol pathway involving myristic acid derivatives.[54–58] Ultimately, all systems activate a series of protein kinases. These enzymes catalyse the addition of a phosphate group to a wide variety of intracellular proteins. The majority of kinases phosphorylate a serine residue on the target protein; a minority phosphorylate tyrosine (the tyrosine kinases) and it is these that appear to be particularly involved in cell proliferation. The precise functional effect of phosphorylation is not clear, although resultant conformational changes are thought either to activate or inhibit the phosphorylated protein's function. The exact range of target proteins available for phosphorylation is determined by the phenotype/lineage of the cell itself. Ultimately, some of these altered target proteins will be DNA-binding molecules that enter the cell nucleus and regulate either DNA replication (for cell proliferation) or transcription of selected genes (for example, for production of cytokines or upregulation of cell surface cytokine receptors and adhesion molecules). A control mechanism is provided by a second set of intracellular enzymes, the phosphatases, which remove the phosphate groups, thus cancelling the kinase-mediated signal. Interestingly, the cell surface leucocyte common antigen (CD45) has been shown to possess phosphatase activity in its cytoplasmic tail.[59]

Th cells

The role of different second messenger systems in T cell activation has been best studied for the Th subset. Signal 1, provided by engagement of the TCR by antigen+MHC, is transduced via the phosphoinositol pathway. In this system, receptor occupancy leads (possibly via a series of G proteins) to the activation of the membrane enzyme phospholipase C. This cleaves the membrane phospholipid phosphatidyl 4,5-bisphosphate (PIP2), resulting in two breakdown products, membrane associated diacyl glycerol [DAG] and cytoplasmic inositol 1,4,5-trisphosphate (IP3). DAG activates membrane protein kinase C (PKC); this in turn activates a membrane ion channel, leading to a rise in intracellular pH. Under these conditions a series of pH-sensitive kinases is activated and it is at least some of their phosphorylated protein targets which are thought to exert an influence on the T cell's DNA.

IP3 forms a second arm to the phosphoinositol pathway. This intracellular messenger activates the release of calcium (Ca^{++}) from intracellular stores. This calcium binds to calmodulin which in turn activates the calmodulin-sensitive intracellular protein kinases. These catalyse the phosphorylation of many substrate proteins, many of which are also thought to act within the T cell nucleus. Other intracellular molecules are also the targets of serine phosphorylation. The gamma, and to a lesser extent epsilon, chains of CD3 become serine phosphorylated during T cell activation, although the functional significance of this is not known. There is also some 'cross-talk' within the inositol pathway since an increase in Ca^{++} can lead to enhanced PKC activity.

The role of these two arms of the phosphoinositol pathway in T cell activation has been studied experimentally using phorbol esters and calcium ionophore to activate the DAG and IP3 systems respectively. Thus, signal transduction via *both* IP3 and DAG is required for proliferation and IL-2 secretion, whereas *either* IP3 *or* DAG is sufficient for the production and cell surface expression of the IL-2 receptor.

An additional mechanism involved in Th activation is the phosphorylation of tyrosine.[56] Although no lymphocyte growth factor receptor has yet been shown to possess a cytoplasmic domain with tyrosine kinase activity, several tyrosine kinases have been identified within lymphoid cells. The most relevant of these is p56-lck. This 56 KDa tyrosine kinase is expressed at high levels only in mature T cells and its expression is regulated during T cell activation. It is therefore thought to be the most likely candidate for the tyrosine kinase that is responsible for the phosphorylation of the CD3 zeta chain – an event that is crucial to T cell activation. Interestingly, p56-lck is physically associated with CD4 and CD8 (according to the phenotype of the cell) on the inner side of the plasma membrane. This supports the view that CD4 and CD8 are not simply adhesion molecules, but are also involved in the membrane events that lead to T cell activation. Under resting conditions the TCR/CD3 complex may be quite separate from CD4/p56-lck (or CD8/p56-lck), but binding of antigen+MHC to the TCR/CD3 leads to an interaction between CD4 (or CD8) and the same MHC molecule; this brings p56-lck sufficiently close to the CD3 zeta chain for tyrosine phosphorylation to occur.

However, this cannot be the full story since Th cell activation also requires signal 2 (IL-1). At present there is little information on the precise second messenger systems used by cytokines, although the hydrolysis of plasma membrane myristic acid may be important (demonstrated for IL-2 and IL-4 in B cells).[55]

Tc cells

The activation of cytotoxic T cells involves clonal proliferation and development of cytotoxic capability. The signal transduction processes involved in this activation have been the subject of relatively few studies, although data indicate that the mechanisms are similar to those seen in Th cells. Thus stimulation via antigen+MHC (signal 1) requires both DAG and IP3 arms of the phosphoinositol pathway, although the addition of IL-2 is required to activate the Tc cell. Thus, as with Th cells, the cytokines appear to use a different pathway, perhaps via products of the glycophosphatidlysositol pathway. The CD8-associated p56-lck is again likely to be responsible for CD3 zeta phosphorylation following antigen+MHC/TCR and CD8/MHC interactions, and hence be involved in transmission of signal 1.

Effector functions of mature T cells

There are essentially two main classes of effector T cell, the CD4+ (and a minority of CD8+) cytokine secreting cells and the CD8+ (and a minority of CD4+) cytotoxic cells, although different subtypes of function exist within these two T cell categories (See Figures 1.9 and 1.10).[60] Additional T cell subsets, in particular suppressor T cells (Ts) and delayed type hypersensitivity T cells, are sometimes given separate identities.

T helper cells

T helper cells have been described as the 'conductors of the immunological orchestra', since the cytokines that they secrete are essential for the growth and maturation of both cytotoxic T cells and of B lymphocytes and plasma cells (see Figure 1.9).[61,62,63] In experimental murine systems there appear to be two separate Th subpopulations: Th2 which 'help' B cells via the secretion of IL-2 and IL-4, and Th1 which 'help' T cells via IL-2 and gamma interferon.[64]

However, no such dichotomy has been defined in the human system, and it seems likely that it is the conditions under which a Th cell is stimulated that define the spectrum of cytokines that it will secrete.[65] Moreover, the very considerable overlap of cytokine requirements by T and B cells (e.g. IL-2, IL-4 and gamma interferon are used by both lineages) makes a rigid division of the helper population difficult to justify. Cytokines are critical to cytotoxic T cell activation and function. IL-2 and IL-4 act as paracrine stimulators of proliferation, while IL-2, IL-4 and gamma interferon are required for the maturation of full cytotoxic function. Although some B cell immunity is T-independent, the majority of B responses require T cell help. IL-2 and IL-4 are again required as growth factors, while IL-4, IL-5, IL-6 and gamma interferon are important maturation factors and are required for immunoglobulin class switching and secretion.[66,67]

Two further effects of CD4+ cytokine secreting T cells have been recognised. An inflammatory response (classically defined as delayed type hypersensitivity) is mediated via cytokines such as IL-2, IL-4, gamma interferon, TNF, and perhaps other chemotactic and activation factors (see Figure 1.9).[65,68–72] These act on other cell types such as endothelium and macrophages, leading to increased endothelial adhesiveness, increased vascular permeability, attraction and activation of accessory cells such as macrophages and neutrophils, and recruitment of additional antigen specific T lymphocytes. The IL-2 stimulates autocrine proliferation of the CD4+ T cell. In addition, when IL-2 is produced at very high levels it will also induce paracrine proliferation of other activated T cells, many of which may not be specific for the eliciting antigen. IL-2 may also enhance the secretion of other cytokines, the most important of these being gamma interferon and TNF. In the afferent phase of the response, gamma interferon enhances/induces the expression of MHC class II molecules on antigen presenting cells such as macrophages and vascular endothelium, thus increasing their antigen presenting ability.

Gamma interferon, together with TNF and IL-4, induces enhanced expression of several adhesion molecules (e.g. VCAM-1, ELAM) on endothelial cells, thereby increasing their adhesiveness for leucocytes and so enhancing their migration into the inflammatory site.[47] These recruited leucocytes then become functionally activated, the major feature of this being the activation of macrophages by gamma interferon. Finally, the target antigen is destroyed by the activated accessory cells via phagocytosis (macrophages and neutrophils) and the secretion of extracellular proteases and collagenase (neutrophils) (described in detail in Chapter 3). Although traditionally associated with hypersensitivity, this type of response has a genuine adaptive function in the destruction and clearance of intracellular pathogens whose host cell is a class II positive APC (usually a macrophage) and is the major defence mechanism against intracellular bacteria such as *Listeria monocytogenes* and *Mycobacteria spp*. In addition, this type of CD4+ T cell-mediated immunity is also involved in some stages of graft rejection.

Finally, CD4+ T cells are responsible for the production and secretion of many of the colony stimulating factors that are required for bone marrow haemopoiesis (for example, GM-CSF) (see Figure 1.9).[73] It is probably significant that all myeloid and B lymphoid progenitors in the bone marrow pass through an MHC class II+ stage. This MHC expression may be crucial to their interaction with CD4+ T cells and the subsequent production of the necessary colony stimulating factors. T cells are also known to secrete soluble factors that stimulate osteoclasts (osteoclast stimulating factor) and fibroblasts (such as IL-4) and are therefore probably involved in wound repair.

The simplest scheme within which to accommodate these many and varied actions of T cells would therefore seem to be one where they are all considered to belong to a single group of CD4+ cytokine secreting cells. The final cytokines secreted would be determined by the situation in which the T cell is activated.

Cytotoxic T cells

The Tc that emerge from the thymus are not able to lyse target cells, and are frequently referred to as cytotoxic T cell precursors (CTLp). Activation and maturation of CTLp to CTL involves two signals – antigen+MHC and cytokines. Since the majority of Tc are CD8+, presentation of antigenic peptides (signal 1) takes place on MHC class I molecules (see Figure 1.10). Signal 2 (cytokines) is provided by Th cells. IL-2 stimulates limited proliferation, while IL-2, IL-4, IL-6, TNF and gamma interferon are involved in the maturation of CTLp to CTL (Figure 1.12).

Following activation, the Tc is ready to kill any antigen specific target that it encounters, requiring only antigen+MHC to be triggered to lyse the target. Each Tc at this stage is capable of killing several targets, one after the other. Target cell destruction follows three main stages: conjugate formation between the CTL and its target; activation of killing mechanisms in the CTL by recognition of antigen+MHC on the target; and finally, target cell death (see Figure 1.12).[74–77] Recognition of a target cell of CTL and conjugate formation between the two cells involves interaction of the CTL's TCR with antigen+MHC on the target, together with several interactions between adhesion molecules (CD2-LFA3; LFA1-ICAM1;

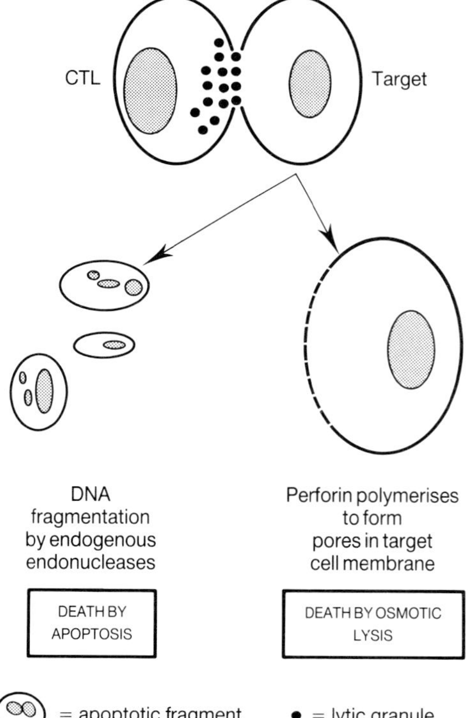

Fig. 1.12 Cytotoxic T cell effector mechanisms.

LFA1-ICAM2). During this process, CTL and target cell come very close together and form many interdigitations of their surface membranes. Cytoplasmic granules are formed within the Tc and move towards the interface between Tc and target. The content of granules are then exocytosed by the Tc, cross the gap separating the two cells and bind to the target cell membrane. The major effector molecule within these granules is 'perforin', which shows strong structural and functional homology with C9 (the ninth component of the complement cascade). This is secreted as a monomer, but then, under the influence of extracellular calcium, it polymerises in the target cell membrane. As with C9, polymerisation of perforin leads to the formation of membrane pores and the osmotic lysis of the target cell. Other molecules have been identified with Tc granules, but their function is currently unknown. Typically, the Tc will then dissociate from the target and is capable of repeating the lytic process with a new target cell. A single activated Tc has been estimated to have the ability to kill at least ten separate target cells.

Some studies have suggested that target cell death may not always be via perforin mediated lysis. Experiments using virus infected lymphoma cells as targets have demonstrated target cell death by apoptosis whereby a secreted toxin from the Tc activates target cell endonucleases which cleave DNA into small fragments and leads to cell death (see Figure 1.12). Whether this form of suicide (as opposed to perforin mediated murder) is a frequent response to attack by a Tc under normal physiological conditions is not known. These two mechanisms of cell death are quite separate and can occur independently of each other.

The adaptive function of the Tc component of the immune system is the control of virus infections via the lysis/apoptosis of virus infected self cells. In addition, Tc produce gamma interferon which has antiviral activity. Tc killing mechanisms are also important, together with CD4+ cytokine producing cells, in transplant rejection.

T suppressor cells

Ts have been the subject of debate for many years with protagonists ranging from those who believe Ts to be an entirely separate T cell subpopulation to those who dispute their existence altogether. Some of the most convincing data on the suppression of T cell responses by other T cells come from work in the field of transplantation immunology, where the rejection of tissue and organ allografts can be suppressed by the transfer of 'suppressor' lymphocytes.

These experiments clearly demonstrate the difference between this active suppression, requiring the presence of specific Ts, and anergy, where individual cells are unable to mount an immune response as a result of their own previous, abortive, encounter with antigen (such as lack of signal 2 during activation).[78–82]

Despite the ability to demonstrate suppression as a function, the identity of the T cells that mediate it has remained elusive. Thus, although adoptive transfer experiments indicate that the majority of Ts are CD8+, some are clearly CD4+. Recent experiments suggest that it may be possible to distinguish between CD8+ Ts and Tc by the presence (Tc) or absence (Ts) of the CD28 cell surface molecule. However, such phenotypic differences could reflect a temporary activation/functional state rather than separate T cell lineages.

T cell suppression is antigen specific. Hence, in an organ allograft, the target antigen must be either the allo-antigen itself or the idiotypes of the T cell receptors of the T cells that are mediating graft rejection. The latter is supported by observations that Ts can act by inhibiting the proliferation of autologous cells to an allo-antigenic stimulus. Thus the signal 1 for a Ts may be provided by self-MHC+peptide, where the peptide is derived from the idiotypic portion of the responding T cell's own TCR. The mechanism of inhibition by these cells is unclear, but could be via direct cytotoxicity or inhibitory cytokines.

Gamma delta T cells

T cells whose heterodimeric TCR is composed of gamma and delta chains (TCR1) are the first to appear during thymic ontogeny, although after birth and in adult life they form the minority (<5%) of thymocytes and peripheral blood T cells.[35] They are characteristically CD8+ (as in mucosal surfaces such as the gut) or CD4−, CD8− double negative, and although some gamma delta T cell clones have been shown to be MHC restricted, others appear not to be. These non-MHC restricted TCR1+ T cells may instead use one of the non-polymorphic MHC class I-like

2

B lymphocytes

P Lane and F McConnell

Introduction

Vigorous and rapid rejection of foreign transplanted organs is the hallmark of an intact normal immune response. Therapeutic intervention in transplantation medicine is directed at suppressing immune reaction: the consequences of getting the balance of immunosuppression wrong are on the one hand infection and on the other rejection. Immunosuppression in its current form is a rather blunt tool which might be refined by a more detailed understanding of the molecular mechanisms of immune responses.

T cells clearly play a key role in orchestrating immune responses, with regard to both clonal expansion and differentiation of effector cells; their role is discussed elsewhere in this volume. This chapter will try to give an overview of the other antigen specific immune cell, the B cell, considered in the context of a regulated system, as well as at the individual cell level.

The role of antibody in rejection processes is often forgotten because it is overshadowed by the pivotal part that T cells play. However, the destructive potential of preformed antibody is evinced by the rapid rejection of transplanted organs bearing mismatched ABO blood group antigens. It is worth remembering that each millilitre of human serum contains of the order of 4×10^{16} molecules of IgG antibody. Given that an average adult has about 10^{12} lymphocytes, it is clear that a foreign cell is much more likely to bind to an antibody molecule than meet an immune cell. Preformed specific antibody has the virtue that it can then specifically recruit a wide variety of effector cells such as neutrophils, macrophages and so-called killer cells, which are dependent on antibody for target recognition. Antibody is therefore extremely effective at immune surveillance and this explains its importance in protective immunity.

Understanding tissue rejection requires a basic knowledge of the progression of an immune response against a foreign antigen. There is a primary phase of initiation, where clonal expansion takes place, followed by differentiation of members of the activated clones of lymphocytes to produce effector cells. Therapeutic intervention directed against the initiation of immune responses should be a more effective way of suppressing graft rejection without interfering with defence against previously encountered infective antigens.

This review will deal initially with the basic structure of lymphoid tissue and the general kinetics of lymphocyte populations. This will be put in the context of an immune response to a protein antigen which is most representative of the sequence of events leading to rejection of a foreign protein graft.

The specific pathways of recirculation of lymphocytes, the microenvironments in which they proliferate, differentiate or die, are regulated at least in part by the proteins which they express on their surfaces. Mutual recognition of surface molecules between cells forms the basis of the complexity and heterogeneity in lymphocyte responses. Although the elucidation of these interactions is by no means complete, some general concepts are beginning to emerge, which serve to form a useful framework for the understanding of the molecular mechanisms involved. These will be discussed in the second part of this review. Finally there is a brief summary with particular emphasis on how immune responses might be selectively targeted in the future.

CD8– cytolytic T lymphocytes. *Nature* 1989; **341,** 447–450.

84. Triebel F, Hercend T. Subpopulations of human peripheral T gamma delta lymphocytes. *Immunol Today* 1989; **10,** 186–188.
85. Kaufman SHE. Heat shock proteins and the immune response. *Immunol Today* 1990; **11,** 129–136.
86. Born W, Happ MP, Dallas A *et al.* Recognition of heat shock proteins and gamma-delta cell function. *Immunol Today* 1990; **11,** 40–43.
87. De Graeff-Meeder ER, van der Zee R, Rijkers GT *et al.* Recognition of human 60 KD heat shock protein by mononuclear cells from patient with juvenile chronic arthritis. *Lancet* 1991; **337,** 1368–1372.
88. Beverley P. Immunological memory in T cells. *Current Topics in Immunol* 1991; **3,** 355–360.
89. Sanders ME, Makgoba MW, Sharrow SO *et al.* Human memory T lymphocytes express increased levels of three cell adhesion molecules (LFA-3, CD2 and LFA-1) and three other molecules (UCHL1, CDW29 and Pgp-1) and have enhanced IFN-gamma production. *J Immunol* 1988; **140,** 1401–1407.
90. Mackay CR. T cell memory: the connection between function, phenotype and migration pathways. *Immunol Today* 1991; **12,** 189–192.

2

B lymphocytes

P Lane and F McConnell

Introduction

Vigorous and rapid rejection of foreign transplanted organs is the hallmark of an intact normal immune response. Therapeutic intervention in transplantation medicine is directed at suppressing immune reaction: the consequences of getting the balance of immunosuppression wrong are on the one hand infection and on the other rejection. Immunosuppression in its current form is a rather blunt tool which might be refined by a more detailed understanding of the molecular mechanisms of immune responses.

T cells clearly play a key role in orchestrating immune responses, with regard to both clonal expansion and differentiation of effector cells; their role is discussed elsewhere in this volume. This chapter will try to give an overview of the other antigen specific immune cell, the B cell, considered in the context of a regulated system, as well as at the individual cell level.

The role of antibody in rejection processes is often forgotten because it is overshadowed by the pivotal part that T cells play. However, the destructive potential of preformed antibody is evinced by the rapid rejection of transplanted organs bearing mismatched ABO blood group antigens. It is worth remembering that each millilitre of human serum contains of the order of 4×10^{16} molecules of IgG antibody. Given that an average adult has about 10^{12} lymphocytes, it is clear that a foreign cell is much more likely to bind to an antibody molecule than meet an immune cell. Preformed specific antibody has the virtue that it can then specifically recruit a wide variety of effector cells such as neutrophils, macrophages and so-called killer cells, which are dependent on antibody for target recognition. Antibody is therefore extremely effective at immune surveillance and this explains its importance in protective immunity.

Understanding tissue rejection requires a basic knowledge of the progression of an immune response against a foreign antigen. There is a primary phase of initiation, where clonal expansion takes place, followed by differentiation of members of the activated clones of lymphocytes to produce effector cells. Therapeutic intervention directed against the initiation of immune responses should be a more effective way of suppressing graft rejection without interfering with defence against previously encountered infective antigens.

This review will deal initially with the basic structure of lymphoid tissue and the general kinetics of lymphocyte populations. This will be put in the context of an immune response to a protein antigen which is most representative of the sequence of events leading to rejection of a foreign protein graft.

The specific pathways of recirculation of lymphocytes, the microenvironments in which they proliferate, differentiate or die, are regulated at least in part by the proteins which they express on their surfaces. Mutual recognition of surface molecules between cells forms the basis of the complexity and heterogeneity in lymphocyte responses. Although the elucidation of these interactions is by no means complete, some general concepts are beginning to emerge, which serve to form a useful framework for the understanding of the molecular mechanisms involved. These will be discussed in the second part of this review. Finally there is a brief summary with particular emphasis on how immune responses might be selectively targeted in the future.

Overview of lymphocyte physiology

Organisation of lymphoid tissue

The primary lymphoid organs are the bone marrow, thymus, spleen, lymph nodes and mucosal-associated lymphoid tissue, e.g. tonsils and Peyer's patches in the gut. These organs are connected together by the blood and the lymphatics, as shown schematically in Figure 2.1.

Primary B and T lymphopoiesis

Both B and T lymphocytes are generated from precursors arising in primary lymphoid organs. After birth, such precursors develop mainly within the microenvironment of the bone marrow, while in neonatal life, foetal liver and spleen are the important organs of lymphogenesis.

T cell precursors migrate to the thymus where expansion and selection of T cells occur. Using the mouse as a paradigm, roughly 50 million new potential T cells are produced in the infant thymus daily. This represents about 20% of the total number of peripheral T cells. However, it has been estimated that only about 1–2% of the daily production actually survive to leave the thymus and populate the periphery.[1] Elegant experiments using genetically manipulated mice have shown that rigorous selection operates. T cells with high affinity for self-antigens are deleted, although there is also positive selection for T cells bearing receptors with some affinity for self.[2]

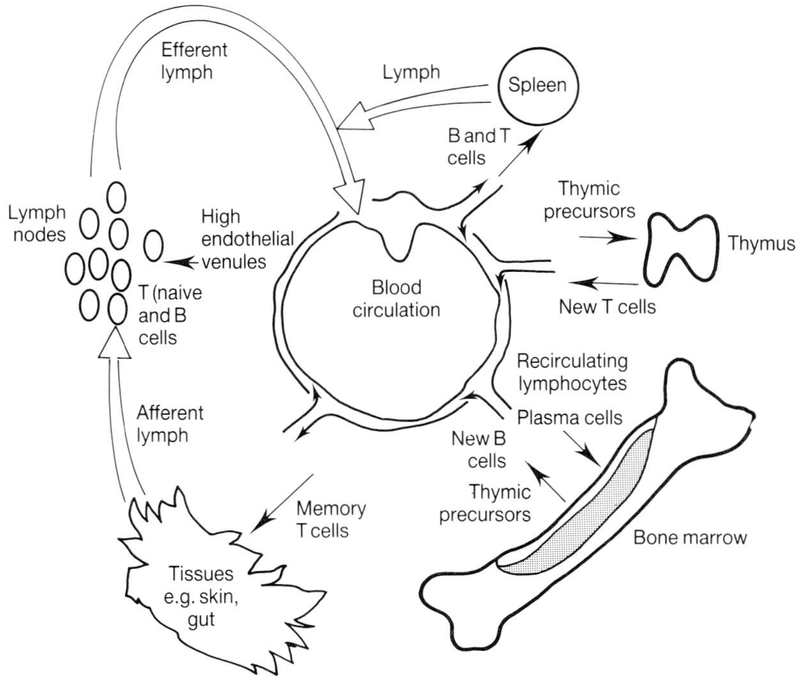

Fig. 2.1 Organisation of lymphoid tissue in the adult human. This diagram does not show lymphocyte recirculation between blood and mucosal associated lymphoid tissue. Lymphocyte precursors are generated in the bone marrow. T cell precursors proliferate and mature after migration to the thymus via the blood. Naive B cells are produced in the bone marrow and migrate via the blood to the spleen and lymph nodes. The majority of newly formed lymphocytes have a short life span (a few days) unless they are selected by antigen.

Mature peripheral lymphocytes continuously recirculate. Most of them enter lymph nodes via high endothelial venules and return to the bloodstream via efferent lymphatics. A proportion of T cells with a 'memory' phenotype migrate into tissues like the skin and gut, and enter lymph nodes via afferent lymphatics. Interdigitating dendritic cells migrate from the bone marrow into tissues and also enter lymph nodes via the afferent lymphatics. In the spleen, cells enter directly from the bloodstream and leave via the efferent lymphatics.

New B cells are produced principally on the bone marrow on adults. Like T cells, in the mouse some 50 million new B cells are formed each day,[3] again representing about 20% of the peripheral B cell pool. Unlike T cells, which undergo selection in the thymus, most new B cells leave the bone marrow and migrate into the periphery,[4] where many have a short lifespan and are not normally incorporated as permanent members of the peripheral B cell pool. During antigen driven immune responses, however, new B cells can be recruited as longer term occupants of the periphery.[5] Furthermore, in circumstances where the peripheral pool of lymphocytes has been depleted, for example by radiation or cytotoxic drugs, new B cells can fill up the space created.[4]

Kinetics of lymphocytes in mature lymphoid organs

In the periphery in the absence of an antigenic stimulus, most mature T and B lymphocytes turn over slowly, with an intermitotic lifespan of weeks rather than days.[4,6] Most B and T cells undergo continuous recirculation between blood and lymph.[7] They enter lymph nodes through specialised vessel which have high endothelial venules (modified post capillary venules). B cells migrate through the the T cell areas to the B cell areas which are located within follicular structures (Figure 2.2a), whereas T cells migrate to the interfollicular areas of lymph node. Recent experiments have shown that T cells have distinct recirculating pathways: so called 'memory' T cells migrate through tissues (e.g. skin and gut) into the afferent lymphatics of secondary lymphoid organs

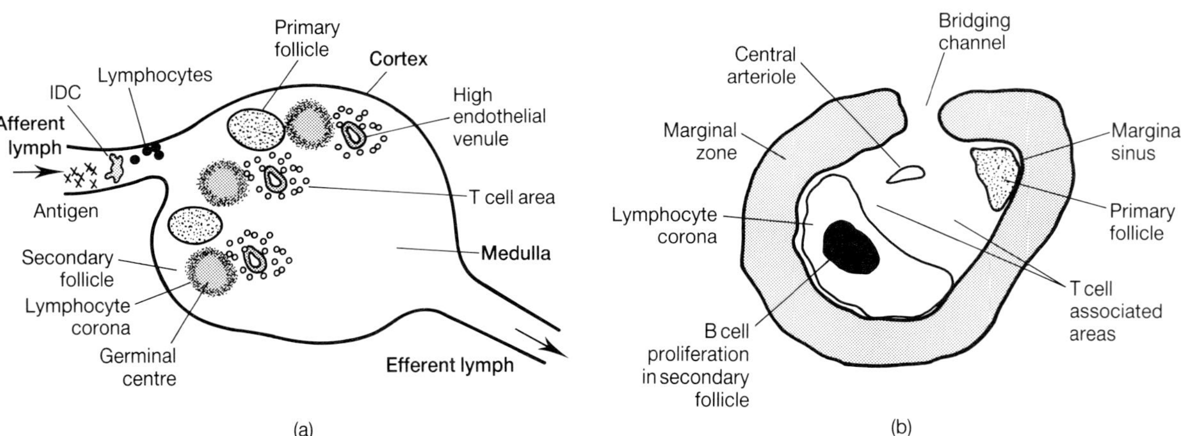

Fig. 2.2 Arrangement of lymphocytes in peripheral lymphoid organs. (a) *Lymph node* A lymph node has afferent and efferent lymphatics and blood supply. There is a cortex and a medulla. B cells are principally located within follicular structures which have follicular dendritic cells (FDCs). Follicles which have not been stimulated by antigen are primary follicles, while germinal centres are secondary follicles. A few T cells of memory phenotype are located within secondary follicles. T cells are in the interfollicular and paracortical areas, in contact with interdigitating dendritic cells (IDCs).

Lymphocytes enter lymph nodes from the bloodstream through high endothelial venules. B cells traverse through the T cell areas to the B cell areas; T cells migrate to interdigitating cells.

The afferent lymphatics are connected to the efferent lymphatics by a network of sinuses in the interfollicular areas. Afferent lymph contains IDCs and T cells with a memory phenotype. Antigen also enters lymph nodes here. The interaction of IDCs, T cells, B cells and antigen in the interfollicular areas initiates primary immune responses.

Resting and activated lymphocytes leave the lymph node in the efferent lymphatics. Many B cells activated in primary immune responses differentiate locally to plasma cells in the medullary region. In established responses, plasma cell precursors migrate to the bone marrow, which is the principal antibody forming organ in the adult. (b) *Spleen* Lymphocytes and antigen presenting cells enter via the bloodstream which terminates in a large sinus in the marginal zone. The spleen has a second major B cell area in the marginal zone. The B cells here are different from other follicular B cells: they do not recirculate, they have a distinct phenotype and many are memory B cells.

Activated B cells migrate into the red pulp through bridging channels in the white (lymphocyte) pulp. They differentiate into plasma cells locally, or re-enter the bloodstream with the efferent lymph.

and the T cell areas.[8] In contrast, 'naive' T cells enter lymph nodes via high endothelial venules. Although follicles and the paracortex broadly subdivide the B and T cell areas, there are some T cells (memory phenotype) within B cell follicles, and some B cells trafficking through the T cell areas. After a period within the lymph node, lymphocytes continue to circulate through efferent lymphatics, eventually entering the thoracic duct and hence returning to the bloodstream.

In the bloodstream the spleen is the predominant lymphatic organ, and at any one time 25% of all lymphocytes are located here. The arrangement of lymphoid tissue differs slightly between spleen and lymph node (Figure 2.2b). Antigens and lymphocytes enter the spleen via the bloodstream which terminates in a large low pressure blood sinus called the marginal sinus. From here they migrate to the T and B cell areas. Unlike a lymph node, there is a large B cell pool of nonrecirculating B cells in the marginal zones of the spleen. The importance of this B cell compartment will be discussed later. Lymphocytes leave the spleen in the efferent lymphatics and re-enter the blood via the thoracic duct. The majority of new bone marrow B cells migrate to the spleen and probably die there unless they are selected by antigen.

The normal peripheral pool of lymphocytes maintains a constant size, suggesting that there is some way that the immune system regulates its overall number. The most likely means of regulation is by positive signals from accessory cells which lymphocytes encounter as they migrate through lymphoid organs. Because access to these sites is limited, so is the overall number of lymphocytes. The molecules responsible for this counting process have not been identified. An intriguing insight is provided by follicular B cell lymphoma, where the counting process is dysregulated and neoplastic B cells accumulate. A genetic translocation has been identified in patients with this disorder which places the *bcl-2* oncogene adjacent to the immunoglobulin enhancer,[9] leading to increased production of the *Bcl-2* protein.[10] A causal relationship between overproduction of the *Bcl-2* protein and the disease has been established by overexpressing the *bcl-2* gene in transgenic mice[11] which subsequently develop the symptoms of follicular lymphoma. B lymphocytes in the *bcl-2* transgenic mice accumulate in large numbers, and also have increased survival in culture. In normal B lymphocytes, the expression of the protein produced by the *bcl-2* gene is increased by stimulating B cells through the surface antigen CD40 (see Table 2.2).[12] Stimulation through CD40 using monoclonal antibodies has been associated with prolonged survival of B cells in culture.[13] The natural ligand and cellular source of the CD40 antigen are yet to be discovered. However, it remains a potential candidate for the regulation of B cell numbers.

Professional antigen presenting cells

Interdigitating cells (IDCs) in the T cells areas

Class II antigens are expressed on B cells, macrophages, activated epithelium, activated T cells and interdigitating dendritic cells (IDCs) (see Figure 2.3a). Of all these cell types, IDCs are by far the most potent antigen presenting cells for T cells. They are bone marrow derived cells implicated in the initiation of primary immune responses.[14,15,16] IDCs are derived from bone marrow precursors, migrating into tissues via the bloodstream and entering lymphatic tissue via the afferent lymph. They enter the spleen directly from the bloodstream. IDCs are found in the T cell dependent areas of spleen and lymph node, where they cluster with T cells in an antigen independent manner. They turn over rapidly within a few days and are replaced.

IDCs are very efficient antigen presenting cells. They take up both soluble and particulate material by pinocytosis. Degraded peptide fragments from fluid phase proteins then become associated with MHC class II molecules which are expressed at high density on the surface of IDCs. As a consequence of their antigen presenting capabilities, IDCs are potent stimulators of mixed lymphocyte reactions, and are thought to be the important cells in grafts which initiate the rejection process in the host. Experiments in animals have shown that depleting transplanted organs of passenger IDCs markedly increases survival in the recipient.[17] In addition to activating T cells through the T cell receptor, IDCs seem particularly good at providing the 'second signal' required to trigger T cells.[18] The efficiency of IDCs in presenting to T cells is in part attributable to their high surface expression of class II molecules, but it is also

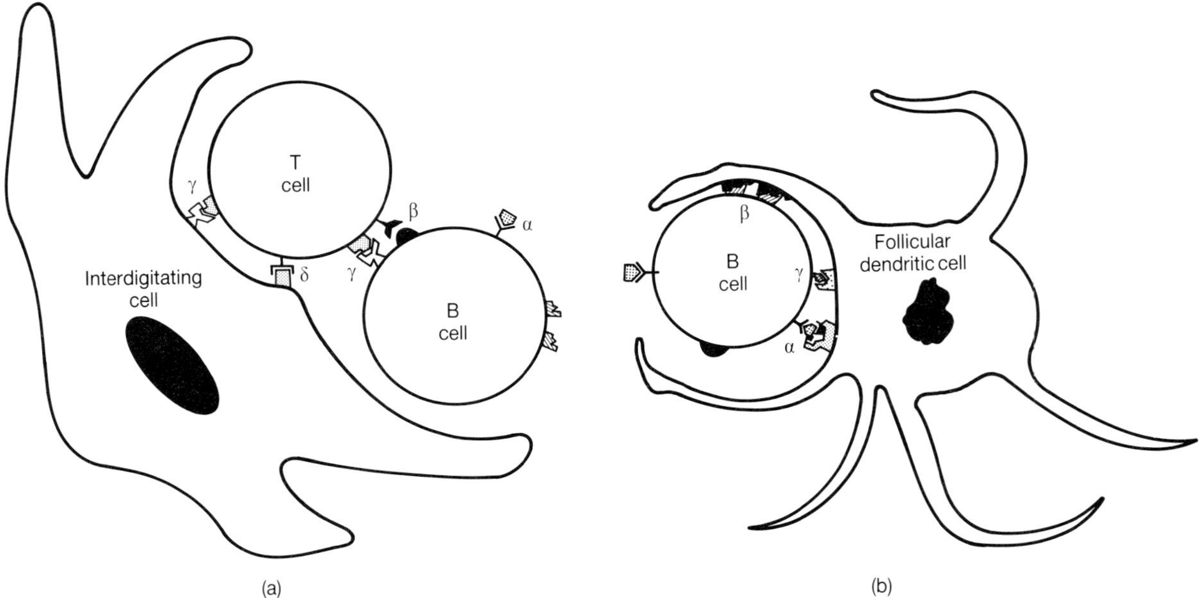

Fig. 2.3 Schematic representation of cellular and molecular interactions of B cells with the principal antigen presenting cells – FDCs and IDCs. (a) Interactions between interdigitating dendritic cells, B cells and T cells in the T zones of lymph node and spleen. B cells can take up specific antigen by their immunoglobulin receptors (α) and present it to T cells in the form of peptide associated with class II molecules (β). IDCs can also present antigen directly to T cells using class II. Interactions between pairs of adhesion molecules (γ) stabilise the cell–cell contact and possibly play an active part in signal transduction. Co-stimulatory signals may also be delivered through other molecules (δ) such as BB-1/B7 which is expressed on antigen presenting cells and also activated B cells. BB-1/B7 provides critical co-stimulatory signals for T cells through their surface CD28 molecules. (b) Interactions between activated B cells and follicular dendritic cells. B cells are stimulated by antigen retained in the form of immune complexes on FDCs (α). This interaction may be stabilised by the binding of ligand–receptor pairs of adhesion molecules (β). Accessory signals (γ) may preferentially induce differentiation, e.g. CD23 may induce germinal centre B cells to differentiate to plasma cells.

likely that there are other molecules on their surface that provide second signals to T cells.

Both newly formed and mature B cells migrate to the T cell dependent areas,[19] where their localisation is antigen specific, and associated with both T cells and IDCs simultaneously. A detailed phenotypic study has recently been made of human tonsillar IDCs.[20] In addition to their strong expression of class II molecules, they have epitopes recognised by some CD4 mAbs. They also express the B cell associated antigen CD40 (see Table 2.2).

Follicular dendritic cells (FDCs) in B cell follicles

The principal antigen presenting cell for B cells is the follicular dendritic cell (FDC) (see Figure 2.3b). Antibody responses to exogenous antigens are associated with B cell proliferation in lymphoid follicles. Native antigen is retained on FDCs in immunogenic form for some length of time, perhaps the lifetime of an individual.[21,22,23] There is evidence that the continued presence of antigen is required both for the maintenance of immunological memory and for sustained antibody responses.[24]

FDCs are non-phagocytic specialised antigen presenting cells of uncertain origin.[25] Characterisation of purified human FDCs has shown they have a distinct phenotype,[26,27] displaying a mixture of myeloid and B cell markers, together with many non-lineage specific adhesion molecules. Activated B cells have been shown to bind to FDCs, and this binding is dependent on interactions between pairs of adhesion molecules in addition to antigen.[28] In keeping with their role in localising immune complexes, FDCs are well endowed with complement receptors of all three types which are involved in the localisation of antigens which continue to stimulate B cells.[24,29]

The ontogeny of an immune response to a protein antigen

Challenge by a previously unencountered foreign protein – a primary B cell response

In the absence of immunisation, infection or transplantation, lymphocytes continue to recirculate between blood, lymph and their home base in the T cell areas associated with IDCs or on FDCs in association with B follicles. The majority of physiological antigens are infectious agents, and many of these, like transplanted organs, bear foreign proteins. It is assumed that when these foreign proteins are present in sufficient quantity, they compete with self proteins for uptake by pinocytosis into IDCs which are continuously circulating through tissues on their way to lymph nodes via the afferent lymphatics. IDCs bearing ingested protein fragments derived from foreign tissue then enter the T cell area of lymph node or spleen. Peptide fragments derived from both foreign and self proteins become associated with class II molecules of IDCs cells, and complexes are presented on the surface to T cells which are constantly passing through this area as they recirculate. T cells which recognise foreign peptide fragments presented on IDCs are stimulated to divide. During transplantation, it appears that donor dendritic cells potently stimulate a T cell response in the host, especially when there is an incompatibility between MHC class II molecules.[17] They either stimulate T cells directly within the graft or migrate to draining lymph nodes. The reason foreign dendritic cells are such potent stimulators of T cells is probably because the set of peptides which bind each MHC haplotype is different. Most peptide fragments presented by the foreign IDCs are in fact self proteins as these are most abundant in the serum. Because T cells in the host will not previously have encountered the particular self peptides presented on foreign MHC, many of them will be stimulated by foreign dendritic cells.

IDCs have no specific receptors for antigen uptake, and consequently host proteins compete with foreign antigens to be presented by IDCs. Therefore, the load of foreign antigen is in most cases substantial before enough gets taken up by IDCs in order to prime T cells. Because B cells have clonally distributed antigen specific receptors, they have the potential to concentrate antigen for which they are specific and present it to T cells. This has been shown for B cells[30] but at present it remains a contentious issue whether B cells alone can prime T cells in primary immune responses.[31,32] B cells migrate through the T cell areas and it is conceivable that they are involved in bringing antigen into a three way association between IDCs and T cells. At any rate the consequence of these priming events leads to the proliferation of T cells in the T cell area.[33]

Although the exact timing of T and B cell priming is not clear, it is likely that the initial site of B cell activation in T cell dependent antibody responses is also within the T cell areas.[4,34] The subsequent sequence of events depends on whether B cells are 'naive' or 'memory' cells. Unprimed B cells which have not previously seen antigen are first activated in the T cell areas, then migrate into B cell follicles. The cognate interaction between B and T cells leads to mutual stimulation of both cells which is partly dependent on antigen specific signal transduction and partly dependent on recognition of other adhesion receptors.[35,36] Interleukins, especially IL-4 secreted by T cells, induce such activated B cells to increase the expression of certain molecules, in particular CD23 (see Table 2.2). Initial activation of B cells in the T cell areas is associated with some specific antibody formation, and immune complexes of antigen and antibody become localised on FDCs in the B cell follicles. Activated B cells migrate into follicles where they proliferate very rapidly within these structures to form 'germinal centres'. The purpose of these germinal centres is twofold: clonal expansion of antigen specific cells, and also the selection from amongst these of mutants which bear high affinity receptors for antigen.[29]

B cells are distinct from other somatic cells in that mutation, occurring at a high rate within the variable region of the immunoglobulin genes, is induced during antibody responses to protein antigens.[37] The mechanism for this process is unknown, but the environment of the germinal centre allows first the mutation process to occur as antigen specific B cells expand, and subsequently selection of high affinity B cells by antigen on FDCs.

The progeny of successful B cells (those surviving the selection process) migrate out of follicles and differentiate into memory B cells and plasma cells, which produce specific antibodies. The molecular mechanisms which lead to this dichotomy of differentiation are still poorly characterised. However, there seem to be two distinct types of FDCs which differ in their expression of sets of surface markers. It has been suggested that one phenotype is associated with differentiation to immunoglobulin secretion, and one with differentiation to memory cells.[38] That is, the pathway of B cell differentiation may be dictated by the local microenvironment.

Plasma cells produced in primary immune responses differentiate locally in the medulla of lymph node and red pulp of spleen. Memory B cells, formed from the germinal centre reaction, can and do enter the recirculating pool of lymphocytes. This ensures that challenge with antigen at sites remote from the site of primary immunisation leads to a memory response. The spleen is unusual in that a substantial number of memory B cells become incorporated into the marginal zone B cell compartment. These B cells do not recirculate, and have a different phenotype from follicular B cells.[39,40] The spleen is atypical amongst lymphoid organs in that antigen enters via the bloodstream. The local anatomy is such that the site where antigens first encounter lymphocytes is within the marginal zone, with the consequence that memory cells can readily be activated by a repeated antigenic challenge.

Rechallenge with a protein antigen – a secondary B cell response

The response of B lymphocytes during secondary immune responses is quite different to that seen following primary immunisation. Whereas antigen specific B lymphocytes in primary responses proliferate extensively in follicles, during secondary responses, memory B cells proliferate in the T cell areas.[4,41] The process of activation by antigen seems to lead to changes in the B cell which allow it to migrate to the T cell areas. It is not known whether this involves down-regulation of adhesion receptors, or perhaps a change in the affinity of the receptors which normally keep marginal zone B cells in place.

Activated marginal zone B cells seem particularly effective at eliciting T cell help, with the result that extensive B cell proliferation occurs. The progeny of this proliferation give rise to a cohort of antibody producing plasma cells which migrate to the bone marrow. Some of the rapidly dividing cells give rise to a fresh wave of memory B cells which return to the marginal zone, ready for subsequent rechallenge.

Why are primary and memory B cell responses different?

The most important conclusion to be drawn from a comparison of primary and secondary responses is that they can be distinguished, not simply by intrinsic differences between the cells, but also because the two cell types migrate to and proliferate at different sites. An obvious mechanism for these differences in behaviour would be the direction of cells on the basis of their surface phenotype. How this regulates function at the individual cell level will be discussed in the next section. Table 2.1 illustrates some of the phenotypic differences between naive and mature B cells, and also the important molecules with which they interact on FDCs and IDCs. Table 2.2 summarises briefly the function of these molecules.

Molecular basis for the different patterns of proliferation and migration within the various B cell compartments

An overview of signal transdution in lymphocytes

At the risk of oversimplification, cells receive signals, usually via surface receptors, which lead to one of a number of effects, e.g. division, differentiation (e.g. secretion) or even death. In addition to the above, cells are also regulated by the cells which they contact. Lymphocytes have an additional level of complexity in that they are not static, so need to express molecules allowing and/or causing them to recirculate. All these processes are regulated by the interaction of surface receptors with complementary sets of molecules on interacting cells.

Signal transduction in cells mediates the conversion of information received at the cell surface into an appropriate intracellular response. The process of signal transduction in lymphocytes is not comprehensively understood, but the basic mechanism of antigen specific signal transduction has been established.[42,43,44] Recent data have shown that in B lymphocytes, antigen specific receptors are linked to intracellular protein tyrosine kinases.[45,46,47] Upon engagement of the receptor, these tyrosine kinases are activated by autophosphorylation on tyrosine residues, and subsequently tyrosine phosphorylates many protein

Table 2.1 Phenotype of B cells at different stages of their development and antigen presenting IDCs and FDCs

	Lineage associated markers		**Adhesion molecules**		**Activation antigens**	
Naive B cell	CD19	+ve	CD44	weak	CD23	+++
	CD20	+ve	LFA-1	weak	CD40	++
	CD21	−ve	VLA-4	?	CD44	+++
	CD22	−ve			LFA-1	++
	CD23	−ve			VLA-4	?
	CD39	−ve			CD39	−ve
	IgM	+ve				
	IgD	−ve				
Follicular B cell	CD19	+	CD44		CD23	+++
	CD20	+	LFA-1		CD40	++
	CD21	+			CD44	+++
	CD22	+			LFA-1	++
	CD23	weak			VLA-4	?
	CD39	+ve			CD39	−ve
	IgM	+ve				
	IgD	+ve				
Marginal zone B cells (memory)	CD19	+	CD44		B7/BB1	?
	CD20	+	LFA-1			
	CD21	+++	VLA-4?			
	CD22	+++				
	CD23	−ve				
	CD39	+ve				
	IgM	+++				
	IgD	−ve				
Interdigitating dendritic cells (IDCs)	Class II	+++	ICAM-1			
	CD4	+	LFA-3			
	CD40	+				
	BB1/B7	++?				
Follicular dendritic cells (FDCs)	All C3 complement receptors		ICAM-1			
	CD21		VCAM-1			
	CD23	(some)				

substrates, including phospholipase C, generating a cascade of secondary signals.[48] The consequences of this cascade of events depend on the state of differentiation of the cell. For example, an active signal in an immature lymphocyte may lead to death rather than proliferation or differentiation. A simple view of signal transduction is shown in Figure 2.4.

One of the puzzles of lymphocyte biology is how the different patterns of migration and proliferation of lymphocytes *in vivo* can be regulated if lymphocytes share a common method of signal transduction. One obvious way in which heterogeneity in responses might be regulated is if other molecules on the surface of cells modulated signal transduction through the antigen specific receptor. Differential expression of these sets of molecules might then regulate their sensitivity to antigen and the microenvironment in which they proliferated. At the last international workshop, 78 different clusters of differentiation antigens (CD) have been identified on cells of the haemopoietic lineage[49] and already several new clusters have been identified. Not all of these markers are found on lymphocytes. However, it is clear that both B and T lymphocytes at different stages of their development express different membrane markers. Table 2.1 illustrates phenotypic differences between naive and mature B cells, FDCs and IDCs. This list is not comprehensive, but illustrates how diversity in responses might occur. The way in which B cell associated molecules might regulate their function has been reviewed recently.[40]

Table 2.2 Summary of the structure and function of the CD antigens discussed in this chapter

CD antigen	Other name	Structure	Function
CD11a	α-chain LFA-1	Forms heterodimer with CD18 integrin	Adhesion ligand ICAM-1/2
CD18	β-chain LFA-1	Forms heterodimer with CD18 integrin	Adhesion ligand ICAM-1/2
CD19	None	Ig superfamily	Unknown
CD20	None	Multiple trans-membrane domains	?Ca^{++} channel
CD21	C3d receptor	Complement family	Ligand C3d
CD22	None	Ig superfamily	?B cell adhesion
CD23	Low affinity IgE R	Motif for binding integrins	Unknown
CD28	None	Ig superfamily homodimer	Co-stimulation for T cells
CD29	VLA-4 β chain	Integrin	Adhesion ligand VCAM-1
CD39	None	Unknown	?
CD40	None	Tumour necrosis factor receptor superfamily	B cell proliferation and survival
CD44	Pgp-1	Adhesion	Ligand hyaluronic acid in the extracellular matrix ? other ligands
CD49d	α-chain VLA-4	Integrin	Adhesion ligand VCAM-1
CD54	ICAM-1	Ig superfamily	Adhesion ligand LFA-1
CD58	LFA-3	Ig superfamily	Adhesion ligand CD2 on T cells
	VCAM-1	Ig superfamily	Adhesion ligand VLA-4
	BB1/B7	Ig superfamily	Co-stimulation of T cells via ligand CD28

Role of adhesion receptors in augmenting antigen specific signal transduction

When lymphocytes interact with antigen presenting cells, several other co-receptors are engaged besides antigen specific receptors. This is diagramatically illustrated in Figure 2.3. Until quite recently these pairs of adhesion molecules were thought simply to stabilise the cellular interactions, whereas signal transduction occurred through the antigen receptor alone. This view may be too simple, since it now appears that engagement of co-receptors between cells can considerably augment antigen specific signal transduction.[40,50] The finding that pairs of accessory molecules can signal generates a paradox, because it would suggest that signalling might occur in the absence of an antigen specific stimulus. Elegant experiments using purified adhesion proteins have shown that the affinity of the adhesion receptors LFA-1 (CD11 (α-chain), CD18 (β-chain)) and ICAM-1 (CD54) for each other is regulated by signal transduction through the antigen specific receptor.[51] Given that the initial signal is antigen specific, positive signalling through the pair of adhesion receptors would only occur following the rise in the affinity of the interaction between pairs of adhesion molecules. This now seems also to be true for other pairs of receptors. Positive feedback and augmentation of the initial response through pairs of molecules would lead to an appropriate response if both interacting cells expressed the complementary sets of adhesion molecules. In support for this active role in signalling, during interactions between antigen specific B cells and T cells, ICAM-1 and LFA-1 can be shown to be actively involved in the signalling process (Lane, unpublished observations). In contrast, an antigen specific signal in the absence of the appropriate co-receptors would not give

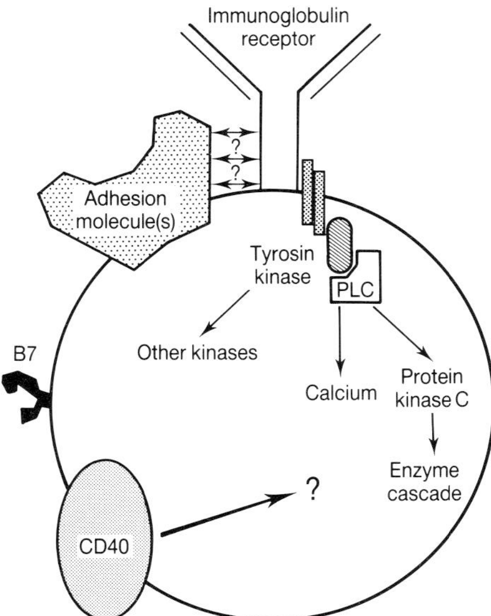

Fig. 2.4 Simplified view of signal transduction in human B cells. The immunoglobulin receptor is linked by a protein complex to cellular protein tyrosine kinases. Many different tyrosine kinases are expressed in lymphocytes, and other surface molecules may be linked to signal transducing pathways in this way. Tyrosine kinase activation leads to a cascade of intracellular events including phospholipase C–γ activation and concomitant mobilisation of protein kinase C and intracellular calcium release. Several other cellular kinases are also activated by tyrosine kinases. This enzyme cascade eventually leads to gene transcription and proliferation or differentiation events. Adhesion molecules may augment signal transduction through the antigen specific pathway.

The mechanism of activation of B cells through the CD40 molecule is unknown. Finally, the expression of antigens such as BB-1/B7 induces T cells to secrete lymphokines which activate B cells indirectly.

the appropriate signal for the cell to divide or differentiate. The attractive feature of this system is that the interaction is regulated by specificity for antigen, but whether a cell gets a strong enough signal to commit it to a pathway of differentiation will depend on the set of accessory molecules which it expresses. In this way particular microenvironments and accessory cell interactions could foster proliferation of particular sets of lymphocytes.

Role of CD28/B7 interaction in priming immune responses

Clearly not all accessory cell interactions are regulated by the antigen specific receptor. The molecule defined by the CD40 antigen does not involve the immunoglobulin receptor, but perhaps plays an important role in regulating lifespan and proliferative capacity. With regard to transplantation, a recently described pair of coreceptors may play a critical role in the induction of rejection. The CD28 protein molecule is a homodimer expressed on the majority of CD4 positive lymphocytes, and about half of CD8 positive cells.[52] Its ligand is on activated B cells[53] and also thymic stromal cells[54] and is identified by two monoclonal antibodies as the BB1/B7 antigen. Recent data suggest BB1/B7 is more widely expressed, and present on all cells capable of presenting antigen. Stimulation through CD28 strongly augments resting T cell proliferation induced by stimulation through the T cell receptor, and this may be mediated by stabilisation of mRNA for T cell derived lymphokines.[55] It does not seem to exert its effect by modifying signal transduction through the T cell receptor, but it has the properties of the second signal first proposed to exist by Lederberg.[56] Monoclonal antibodies which block the interaction of CD28 on T cells with B7/BB1 block the T cell proliferation induced by mismatched lymphocytes.[57] If this is proved to be generally true for other antigen presenting cells, it would be an excellent molecule to selectively block in transplanted tissue. This is at the heart of the problem of graft rejection for, as has been discussed, passenger dendritic cells in grafted tissue are the most potent stimulators of host immune responses,[17] and their elimination leads to enhanced survival of transplanted grafts. It is not clear whether their potent immunogenicity is related to the expression of the antigen B7/BB1.

Conclusion

This chapter has tried to give an overview of the organisation of peripheral lymphoid tissue, and specifically to give a picture of the sequence of events which follow injection of a foreign protein. We have speculated on the molecular events which regulate lymphocyte proliferation at different sites during the course of immune responses and summarised some of the major phenotypic differences between lymphocytes and antigen presenting cells. One of the basic conclusions to be drawn from this review is that primary immune responses are different from memory responses at least in part because of phenotypic differences in the expression of surface molecules. This implies that it might be possible to selectively interfere with one type of response. Clearly this could have important consequences for graft rejection where it is necessary to suppress a primary response but preserve host immunity to previously encountered antigens. Selectively identifying molecules which are involved in the priming process but do not interfere with memory responses might lead to the solution of the rejection/infection problem.

References

1. Egerton M, Scollay R, Shortman K. Kinetics of mature T-cell development in the thymus. *Proc Nat Acad Sci USA* 1990; **87,** 2579–2582.
2. Von Boehmer H, Kisielow P. Self-nonself discrimination by T cells. *Science* 1990; **248,** 1369–1373.
3. Opstelten D, Osmond D. Pre-B cells in mouse bone marrow: immunofluorescence stathmokinetic studies of proliferation of cytoplasmic m-chain-bearing cells in normal mice. *J Immunol* 1983; **131,** 2635–2640.
4. MacLennan IC, Oldfield S, Liu Y-J, Lane PJL. Regulation of B cell populations. *Cell Immunol* 1989; **79,** 37–57.
5. Gray D, MacLennan ICM, Lane PJL. Virgin B cell recruitment and the lifespan of memory clones during antibody responses to 2,4-dinitrophenyl-hemocyanin. *Eur J Immunol* 1986; **16,** 641–648.
6. Sprent J, Basten A. Circulating T and B cells of the mouse II. Lifespan. *Cell Immunol* 1973; **7,** 40–59.
7. Gowans JL, Knight EJ. The route of recirculation of lymphocytes in the rat. *Proc Roy Soc London (Biol)* 1964; **159,** 257.
8. Mackay CR, Marston WL, Dudler L. Naive and memory B cells show distinct pathways of lymphocyte recirculation. *J Exp Med* 1991; **171,** 801–817.
9. Tsujimoto Y, Cossman J, Jaffe E, Croce CM. Involvement of the bcl-2 gene in human follicular lymphoma. *Science* 1985; **228,** 1440–1443
10. Hockenbery D, Nunez G, Milliman C, Schreiber RD, Korsmeyer SJ. Bcl-2 is an inner mitochondrial membrane protein that blocks programmed cell death. *Nature* 1990; **348,** 334–336.
11. McDonnell TJ, Deane N, Platt FM *et al.* bcl-2-immunoglobulin transgenic mice demonstrate extended B cell survival and follicular lymphoproliferation. *Cell* 1989; **57,** 79–88.
12. Liu Y-J, Joshua DE, Williams GT, Smith CA, Gordon J, MacLennan ICM. Mechanism of antigen-driven-selection in germinal centres. *Nature* 1989; **342,** 929–931.
13. Banchereau J, De PP, Valle A, Garcia E, Rousset F. Long-term human B cell lines dependent on interleukin-4 and antibody to CD40. *Science* 1991; **251,** 70–72.
14. Steinman RM, Nussenzweig MC. Dendritic cells: features and functions. *Immunol Rev* 1980; **53,** 127–147.
15. Inaba K, Steinman RM, van Voorthis WC, Muramatsu S. Dendritic cells are critical accessory cells for thymus-dependent antibody responses in mouse and man. *Proc Nat Acad Sc USA* 1983; **80,** 6041–6045.
16. Inaba K, Witmer M, Steinman R. Clustering of dendritic cells, helper T lymphocytes, and histocompatible B cells during primary antibody responses *in vitro*. *J Exp Med* 1984; **160,** 858–876.
17. Lechler RI, Batchelor JR. Restoration of immunogenicity to passenger cell-depleted kidney allografts by the addition of donor strain dendritic cells. *J Exp Med* 1982; **155,** 31–41.
18. Mueller DL, Jenkins MK, Schwartz RH. Clonal expansion versus functional clonal inactivation: a costimulatory signalling pathway determines the outcome of T cell antigen receptor occupancy. *Ann Rev Immunol* 1989; **7,** 445–480.
19. Lortan J, Roobottom C, Oldfield S, MacLennan I. Newly-produced virgin B cells migrate to secondary lymphoid organs but their capacity to enter follicles is restricted. *Eur J Immunol* 1987; **17,** 1311–1316.
20. Hart DNJ, McKenzie JL. Isolation and characterisation of human tonsil dendritic cells. *J Exp Med* 1988; **168,** 157–170.
21. Tew J, Mandel T. The maintenance and regulation of serum antibody levels: Evidence indicating a role for antigen retained in lymphoid follicles. *J Immunol* 1978; **120,** 1063–1069.
22. Klaus G, Humphrey JH, Kunkl A, Dongworth DW. The follicular dendritic cell: its role in antigen presentation in the generation of immunological memory. *Immunol Rev* 1980; **53,** 3–28.
23. Szakal AK, Kosco MH, Tew JG. Microanatomy of lymphoid tissue during humoral immune responses: structure function relationships. *Ann Rev Immunol* 1989; **7,** 91–109.
24. Gray D, Skarvall H. B cell memory is shortlived in the absence of antigen. *Nature* 1988; **336,** 70–73.
25. Humphrey JH, Sundaram V. Origin and turnover of follicular dendritic cells and marginal zone macrophages in the mouse spleen. *Adv Exp Med Biol* 1985; **186,** 167–170.
26. Johnson GD, Hardie DL, Ling NR, MacLennan ICM. Human follicular dendritic cells (FDC): a study with monoclonal antibodies (MoAb). *Clin Exp Immunol* 1986; **64,** 205–213.
27. Schriever F, Freedman AS, Freeman G *et al.* Isolated follicular dendritic cells display a unique antigenic phenotype. *J Exp Med* 1989; **169,** 2043–2058.

28. Freedman AS, Munro JM, Rice GE *et al.* Adhesion of human B cells to germinal centers in vitro involves VLA-4 and ICAM-110. *Science* 1990; **249,** 1030–1033.
29. MacLennan IC, Gray D. Antigen-driven selection of virgin and memory B cells. *Immunol Rev* 1986; **91,** 61–85.
30. Lanzavecchia A. Antigen-specific interaction between T and B cells. *Nature* 1985; **314,** 537–539.
31. Ron Y, Sprent J. T cell priming in vivo: a major role for B cells in presenting antigen to T cells in lymph nodes. *J Immunol* 1987; **138,** 2848–2856.
32. Lassila O, Vainio O, Matzinger P. Can B cells turn on virgin T cells? *Nature* 1988; **334,** 253–255.
33. Ford WL. Lymphocyte migration and immune responses. *Prog Allergy* 1975; **19,** 1–59.
34. Jacob J, Kassir R, Kelsoe G. In situ studies of the primary immune response to (4-hydroxy-3-nitrophenyl) acetyl. l. The architecture and dynamics of responding cell populations. *J Exp Med* 1991; **173,** 1165–1176.
35. Hirohata S, Jelinek DF, Lipsky PE. T cell-dependent activation of B cell proliferation and differentiation by immobilised monoclonal antibodies to CD3. *J Immunol* 1988; **140,** 3726–3744.
36. Wacholtz MC, Patel SS, Lipsky PE. Leukocyte function-associated antigen 1 is an activation molecule for human T cells. *J Exp Med* 1989; **170,** 431–448.
37. Berek C, Milstein C. The dynamic nature of the antibody repertoire. *Immunol Rev* 1988; **105,** 5–26.
38. Liu YJ, Cairns JA, Holder MJ *et al.* Recombinant 25-kDa CD23 and interleukin 1α promote the survival of germinal center B cells: evidence for bifurcation in the development of centrocytes rescued from apoptosis. *Eur J Immunol* 1991; **21,** 1107–1114.
39. MacLennan ICM, Gray D, Kumararatne DS, Bazin H. The lymphocytes of the splenic marginal zones: a distinct B cell lineage. *Immunol Today* 1982; **3,** 305–307.
40. Clark EA, Lane PJL. Regulation of human B cell activation and adhesion. *Ann Rev Immunol* 1991; **95,** 97–127.
41. Liu Y-J, Oldfield S, MacLennan I. Memory B cells in T cell-dependent antibody responses colonise the splenic marginal zones. *Eur J Immunol* 1988; **18,** 355–362.
42. Imboden J, Weiss A. The T-cell antigen receptor regulates sustained increases in cytoplasmic free Ca^{2+} through extracellular Ca^{2+} influx and ongoing intracellular Ca^{2+} mobilisation. *Biochem J* 1987; **247,** 695–700.
43. Cambier JC, Ransom JT. Molecular mechanisms of transmembrane signalling in B lymphocytes. *Ann Rev Immunol* 1987; **5,** 175–199.
44. Lane PJL, Valentine MA, Barrett T, McConnell F, Meier KE, Clark EA. Surface molecules and signal transduction events in human B cells. In: *Receptors and Signal Transduction in Regulation of Lymphocyte Function*, Cambier JC (ed). 1990. American Society for Microbiology, Washington DC.
45. Gold MR, Law DA, DeFranco AL. Stimulation of protein tyrosine phosphorylation by the B-lymphocyte antigen receptor. *Nature* 1990; **345,** 810–813.
46. Lane PJL, Ledbetter JA, McConnell FM *et al.* The role of tyrosine phosphorylation in signal transduction through surface immunoglobulin in human B cells: inhibition of tyrosine phosphorylation prevents intracellular calcium release. *J Immunol* 1991; **146,** 715–722.
47. Yamanashi Y, Kakiuchi T, Mizuguchi J, Yamamoto T, Toyoshima K. Association of B cell antigen receptor with protein tyrosine kinase. *Science* 1991; **251,** 192–194.
48. Ullrich A, Schlessinger J. Signal transduction by receptors with tyrosine kinase activity. *Cell* 1990; **61,** 203–212.
49. Knapp W, Rieber P, Dörken B, Schmidt RE, Stein H, Borne AEG. Towards a better definition of human leucocyte surface molecules. *Immunol Today* 1989; **10,** 253–258.
50. Van Seventer GA, Shimizu Y, Shaw S. Roles of multiple accessory molecules in T-cell activation: bilateral interplay of adhesion and costimulation. *Curr Opinions Immunol* 1991; **3** (3): 294–303.
51. Dustin ML, Springer TA. T-cell receptor cross-linking transiently stimulates adhesiveness through LFA-1. *Nature* 1989; **341,** 619–624.
52. June CH, Ledbetter JA, Linsley PS, Thompson CB. Role of the CD28 receptor in T-cell activation. *Immunol Today* 1990; **11,** 211–216.
53. Freedman AS, Freeman G, Horowitz JC, Daley J, Nadler LM. B7, A B cell-restricted antigen that identifies preactivated B cells. *J Immunol* 1987; **139,** 3260–3267.
54. Turka LA, Ledbetter JA, Lee K, June CH, Thompson CB. CD28 is an inducible T cell surface antigen that transduces a proliferative signal in CD3+ mature thymocytes. *J Immunol* 1990; **144,** 1646–1653.
55. Thompson CB, Lindsten T, Ledbetter JA *et al.* CD28 activation pathway regulates the production of multiple T-cell-derived lymphokines/cytokines. *Proc Nat Acad Sci USA* 1989; **86,** 1333–1337.
56. Lederberg J. Genes and antibodies. *Science* 1959; **129,** 1649–1653.
57. Koulova L, Clark EA, Shu G, Dupont B. The CD28 ligand B7/BB1 provides costimulatory signal for alloactivation of CD4+ T cells. *J Exp Med* 1991; **173,** 759–762.

3

Other effector cells

D Burnett

Introduction

Alloreactive lymphocytes are considered to be the cells that initiate the process of allograft rejection but histological evidence has shown that the cell infiltrates of rejecting liver transplants also contain substantial numbers of other 'inflammatory' cells (Figure 3.1) including neutrophils, monocytes and eosinophils.[1–6] The contribution of these cells to the rejection process is not yet known. Nevertheless, during rejection bile is chemotactic for monocytes and neutrophils,[7] blood neutrophils are 'activated'[8] and the potentially cytotoxic cationic protein of eosinophils has been detected in portal tracts.[9] These preliminary observations suggest that future studies will implicate further a role for these, and possibly other non-lymphocytic cells, in the tissue damage associated with allograft rejection.

The purpose of this chapter is to review some of the functions and characteristics of non-lymphocytic 'effector' cells that may be involved in the process of liver allograft rejection. These cells will be defined as non-lymphocytic cells of haemopoietic origin that may contribute to inflammatory processes. The types of cells to be considered therefore include monocytes/macrophages, platelets and granulocytes – eosinophils, basophils, mast cells and neutrophils. These cells may be resident in the tissues or recruited to sites of inflammation and are recognised as important elements in the regulation of inflammation, particularly in the elimination of pathogens. There is also considerable evidence to suggest that they contribute to, or are responsible for, the pathological damage associated with diseases in many organ systems. It is impossible to cover the complete biology of all these cells in one chapter, but selected aspects of their origins, recruitment from the blood to tissues and functions will be covered with an emphasis on the properties with potential for pathological tissue damage. Finally, there is the question of the ultimate fate of these cells.

Morphology, origins and differentiation

Mast cells

Mast cells are classically associated with atopic reactions and are found in their greatest numbers at mucosal surfaces although they are also present in most other tissues including the liver. These cells contain many granules, which comprise over half the cell contents. Mast cells vary in size (10–20 μm diameter) and shape, but can be identified in tissues by using probes that detect the specific constituents of the mast cell granule (Figure 3.2). For instance, astra blue[10] is a simple histochemical stain and the presence of the mast cell protease, tryptase, can be identified by immunocytochemistry.[11,12] Whereas tryptase is present in all or most mast cells, some also contain another serine protease, chymase. Mast cells are classified as MC_{TC} (those containing tryptase and chymase) or MC_{T} (those containing tryptase only).[12,13] This is more than an arbitrary distinction since, although each subset is found in most tissues, they respond differently to stimulating agents (see below) and there are differences in the proportions found at different sites; MC_{TC} cells predominate in skin whereas the MC_{T} subset is found in the lung.[13] Furthermore, the subset phenotype appears to be determined by differentiating factors within the tissues.

It has been suggested[13] that mast cells may share their early differentiation phase, from bone

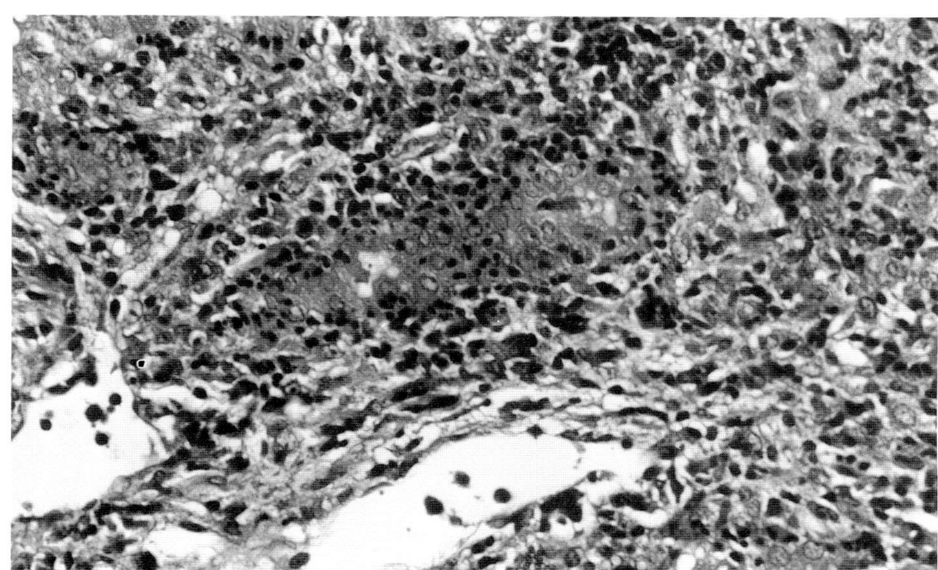

Fig. 3.1 Tissue section of a portal tract during acute liver allograft rejection, showing a mixed inflammatory cell infiltrate. There is an infiltrate of predominantly neutrophils within the interlobular bile duct (reproduced by kind permission of Dr S. Hubscher).

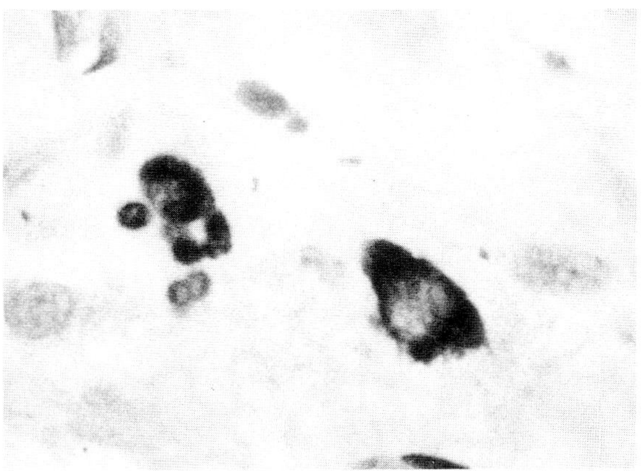

Fig. 3.2 Tissue mast cells indentified by staining with astra blue (reproduced by kind permission of Dr J. Crocker).

marrow stem cell precursors, with monocytes/macrophages, rather than granulocyte precursors partly because they can synthesise cytokines.[14] It is now clear that many cell types, including granulocytes and non-leucocytic cells such as endothelium, fibroblasts and epithelium,[15] have the potential to produce cytokines. Cytokine production is not therefore a characteristic that can be used to establish cell origins. It is not yet clear what factors are involved in human mast cell differentiation. On entering the tissues from the blood, committed mast cell progenitors differentiate into immature cells which, under the influence of unknown factors, become mature mast cells of either MC_{TC} or MC_T phenotype. The maturation of the MC_T cells appears to be dependent on a factor derived from T lymphocytes, which in rodents has been identified as interleukin-3 (IL-3)[16] but its identity in humans remains to be established. Thus terminal differentiation, which determines the phenotype, behaviour and granule contents of mast cells, is controlled by local conditions in the tissues in which they reside. This is in contrast to neutrophils, which are mature before recruitment to tissues and whose granule contents are synthesised exclusively at the promyelocytic and myelocytic stages of differentiation within the bone marrow.[17]

Basophils

Basophils are often described as the bloodborne form of the mast cell. Although basophils and mast cells have some features in common, they also differ in ways which suggest they are distinct cell types.[18] Basophils, which stain with basic dyes, have granules which, like mast cells, contain histamine and have high affinity receptors for IgE. Basophils, however, are thought to be terminally differentiated before leaving the bone marrow, contain different mediators to mast cells and behave differently to cell activators.[13,18] *In vitro* studies suggest that IL-3 and GMCSF are involved in the sequential selection of basophils from stem cells that may also have the potential to mature to mast cells.[18,19]

Eosinophils

Eosinophils are granulocytes of similar size to neutrophils, with usually bilobed nuclei and three distinct types of cytoplasmic granule. The cells can be identified in tissues by their morphological appearance and by staining with acid dyes such as eosin (Figure 3.3). Eosinophils are phagocytic and have the capacity to kill bacteria but their major role is thought to be associated with the non-phagocytic killing and elimination of larger multicellular parasites such as helminths.[20,21] These cells are thought to contribute to pathological tissue damage, classically during late phase atopic reactions, through the release of cytotoxic granule proteins.[22] Most eosinophils are resident in the tissues, particularly at mucosal sites, which they enter after circulating in the blood for between eight and 24 hours.[23] Their life span in the tissues is uncertain, estimates ranging from two days[23] to several weeks.[24] Eosinophil production in the bone marrow appears to be controlled by several cytokines. It appears that early progenitors are stimulated by IL-3, interleukin-5 (IL-5) and granulocyte macrophage colony stimulating factor (GMCSF), with later differentiation being controlled specifically by IL-5.[24,25]

Neutrophils

Neutrophils, characterised by multilobed nuclei (hence 'polymorphonuclear leucocyte') and cytoplasmic granules are the most abundant white cells in the body, normally totalling some 6×10^{11} in the circulation. They are an important component of the body's defences against micro-organisms, as evinced by the recurrent infections seen in subjects with the various deficiencies of neutrophil functions.[26] As with other leucocytes,

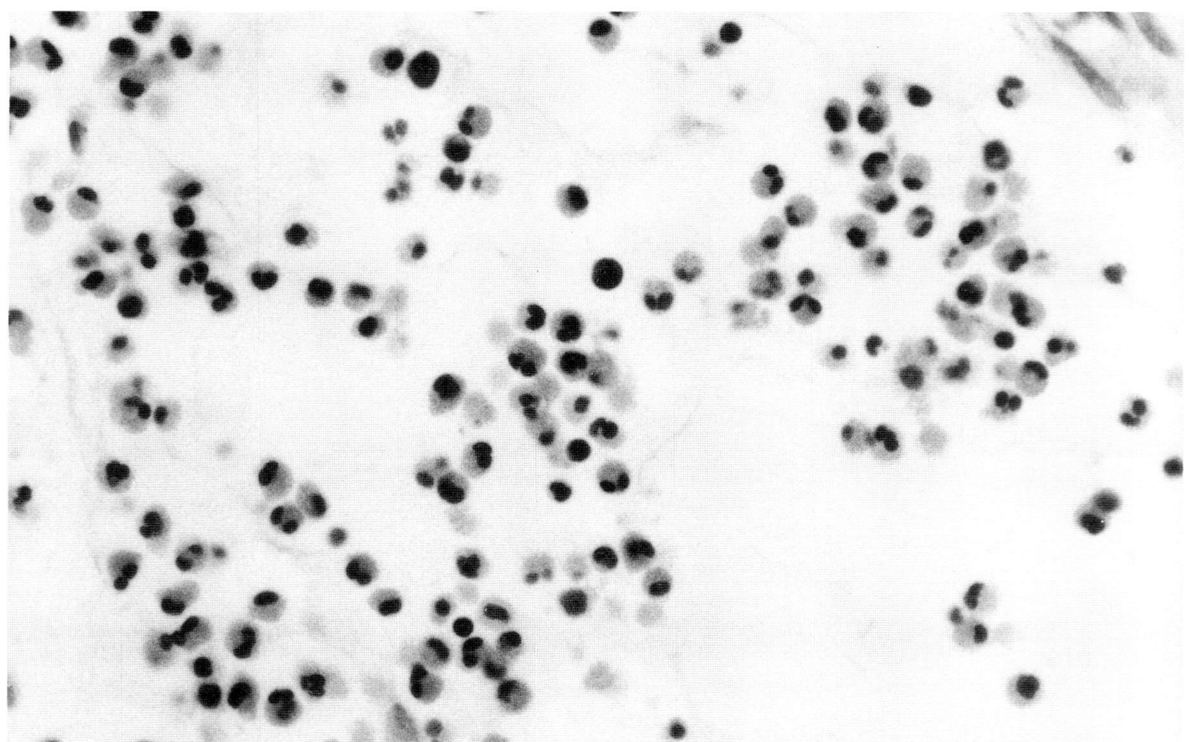

Fig. 3.3 Tissue eosinophils stained with vital new red (reproduced by kind permission of Dr J. Crocker).

the factors controlling differentiation are not well understood although GMCSF and granulocyte colony stimulating factor appear to be involved in the granulopoiesis of these cells.[27] Neutrophils derive from stem cells through several recognised stages of maturation[17] (Figure 3.4), the first being the myeloblast, a large cell with an oval nucleus and no cytoplasmic granules. This cell matures further to the promyelocyte in which the primary or azurophil granules and their protein constituents (see below) are produced. A second population of granules (specific granules) are produced at the next, myelocytic, stage of differentiation and cell division results in all cells containing a complement of granules. Cell proliferation and synthesis of granule products ceases by the next stage, the metamyelocyte, and the cell proceeds via the 'band' stage to a mature neutrophil with a multilobed nucleus (see Figure 3.6). This differentiation process takes about two weeks and the mature cells remain in the marrow for about two days before entering the blood where their half-life is 6–8 hours. About half of the neutrophils in the circulation are 'marginated' but these cells can be mobilised rapidly[28] which, together with increased granulopoiesis and release from the bone marrow,[29] can quickly expand the population of available mature cells during episodes of infection and inflammation. After recruitment to tissue sites of inflammation, neutrophils are thought to survive a further one or two days only.

Monocytes/macrophages

Monocytes and macrophages represent an extremely heterogeneous family of leucocyte. The blood monocyte is a large, round cell with a 'horseshoe' shaped nucleus but tissue macrophages represent a wide variety of morphological features. Monocytes at different stages of differentiation, and the macrophages which they derive, also demonstrate differences in staining for intracellular enzymes, surface molecules, secreted products and functional qualities.[30]

The differentiation of monocytes within the bone marrow, as with neutrophils, is characterised by distinct stages. After maturing from a granulocyte/macrophage colony forming unit, elements called monoblasts develop through promonocytes to mature monocytes which remain in the marrow for up to one day before entering the blood. These cells circulate for up to three days but if recruited to tissue sites may live for many months. *In vitro* studies suggest that a major factor in monocyte differentiation is the protein macrophage colony stimulating factor (MCSF),[31] also known as CSF-1 although other factors, in-

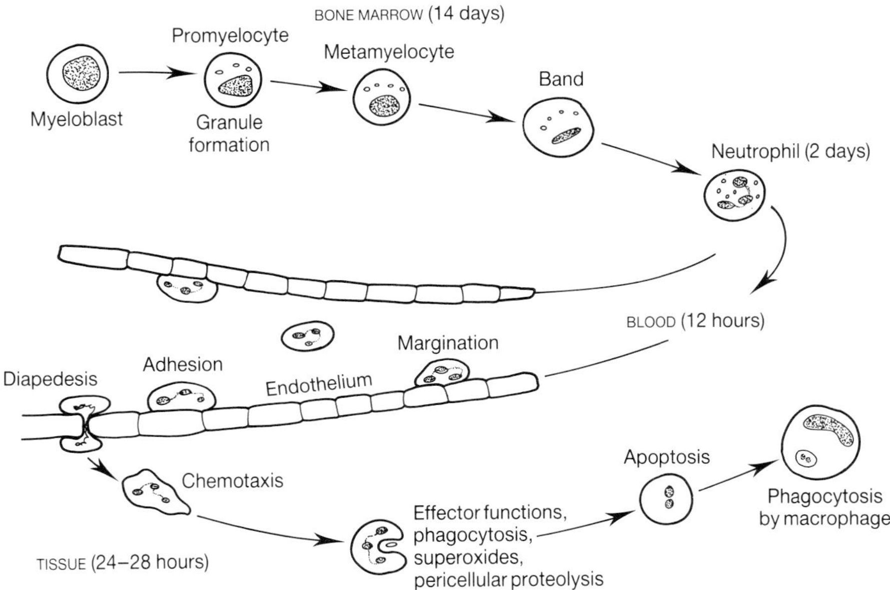

Fig. 3.4 The life of a neutrophil. Schematic representation of the events leading from differentiation in the bone marrow to recruitment to inflamed tissue and ultimate death.

cluding interferon-γ and interleukin-4 (IL-4) also have this potential.[30] Blood monocytes maintained in culture medium including serum do mature into cells with some characteristics of macrophages.[30] It is not clear whether this differentiation is due to specific factors present in the supporting media or an inevitable consequence of cell ageing. Nevertheless, the heterogeneity of tissue macrophages indicates that these cells must also be influenced by factors that are produced at the tissue site and specifically alter the phenotype of the macrophage. There has been debate whether tissue macrophages retain the potential to replicate but there is evidence to suggest that alveolar macrophages[32] and Kupffer cells[33] have this capability. Macrophages have several roles, particularly associated with host defence including antigen presentation, phagocytosis, microbial killing, recruitment and activation of other cells, and in the resolution of inflammation. These roles are reflected in their behaviour and the huge range of products synthesised and released by these cells.[34,35]

Platelets

Platelets are heterogeneous elements, varying in size, morphology and staining characteristics but, in general, are represented by essentially rod-shaped anucleate cells about 5 μm long. Despite having no nucleus, the platelet is a metabolising and secreting cell, having mitochondria, and is able to synthesise proteins.[36] The platelet contains a 'canalicular' system of interconnecting channels and vesicles throughout the cytoplasm and connected to the surface of the cell. Platelets absorb proteins, including plasma proteins, and it is likely they are located within these canaliculi, which also might be a route through which substances such as granule contents are secreted from the cell. Although platelets are not motile cells, they do contain contractile proteins such as myosin and actin.[36]

Platelets are derived from megakaryocytes, which differentiate from stem cells through several recognised stages. The first defined stage is the megakaryoblast, a nucleated cell of about 20 μm diameter. These differentiate, with granule synthesis, to larger (20–80 μm) promegakaryocytes, leading to megakaryocytes 40–150 μm diameter. This differentiation process takes about five days. Each megakaryocyte results in about 4000 platelets, which are derived from cytoplasmic processes which extend through the extravascular spaces of the bone marrow into the venous sinuses. Here the cytoplasm buds off to produce mature platelets which circulate with a lifespan of 9–12 days.[37] The differentiation of megakaryocytes appears to be controlled by several factors including IL-3, GMCSF, IL-6 and 'thrombopoietin'.[38–42] The identity of thrombopoietin has not been established, but may represent more than one entity, including Il-6 and GMCSF.[39,41,42]

Cell recruitment to tissues

The recruitment of cells from blood to tissue is without doubt a crucial event in the inflammatory response since the proliferation of cell populations associated with inflammatory reactions cannot be explained only by local replication; mature neutrophils, for instance, do not have the capacity to divide. Microscopic evidence, furthermore, has demonstrated the process of inflammatory cell migration through vascular endothelium and connective tissues. This recruitment represents a response to factors released at the site of inflammation which both affect adhesion molecules on the endothelium and migrating cells and provide a signal which attracts the inflammatory cell towards the area of inflammation. There has been intense investigation into molecules that can induce leucocyte migration. Although *in vivo* techniques, such as 'skin windows', have been used to observe cell migration in response to induced inflammatory reactions, *in vitro* methods are more useful for identifying the factors that induce migration of specific cell types. The observations on chemotaxis, described below, are based largely on these *in vitro* methods.

Two principal methods have been used. The first is the direct observation of cell migration under agarose gel slabs[43] in which adjacent wells are cut to contain cells and potential chemoattractants; these diffuse through the agar and induce cell migration beneath the agar layer. The second method is based on the Boyden chamber,[40] which is composed of a container divided into two compartments by a porous membrane through which the cells migrate in response to a chemoattractant, placed in the lower chamber. The process of migration, if demonstrated to be in response to a concentration gradient of chemo-attractant is called chemotaxis. This is distinguished from the process called chemokinesis, which refers to a response which merely activates non-directional movement or random migration. Nevertheless, even chemokinesis represents the stimulation of cell migration and should not be ignored as a potential mechanism of cell recruitment.

Cell adhesion

The first event in the recruitment of inflammatory cells to tissue sites is adhesion to vascular endothelium. This is followed by diapedesis, where the cell moves through the endothelium and basement membrane and continues to migrate through connective tissue to the site of infection or inflammation. These processes rely on adhesion molecules on the surface of the inflammatory cells which interact with appropriate ligands on endothelium, epithelium and connective tissue molecules.

Integrins

The major adhesion molecules on granulocytes, monocytes and platelets that bind to receptors on endothelium and connective tissue proteins are the integrins.[45,46] This is a family of transmembrane glycoproteins, found on leucocytes, with heterodimeric structure consisting of α and β subunits. Each subfamily of integrin has a common β subunit, but individual members of the subfamilies have different α subunits. Thus the LEUCAM subfamily share the β_2 subunit (CD18) and the different α subunits (CD11a-c) distinguish the LEUCAM molecules, known as CD18/CD11a (LFA-1), CD18/CD11b (MAC-1, CR3 or Mol) and CD18/CD11c (p150/95). Another family of integrins comprise the ‘very late antigens’ (VLA). These have a common β_1 subunit. The α subunits distinguish recognised receptors for the connective tissue components fibronectin (VLA-3 and VLA-4), laminin (VLA-1, VLA-3 and VLA-6) and collagen (VLA-1, VLA-2, VLA-3). A third family of integrins, with β_2 subunits, include the receptor for vitronectin and a platelet receptor, gpIIb/IIIa.[47] Although platelets are not motile cells, this and other adhesion molecules are important for platelet aggregation and adhesion. The ligands for all integrins except CD18/CD11a include the amino acid sequence arg-gly-asp (RGD peptide), which is found on a variety of proteins including C3bi and fibrinogen;[48–50] CD18/CD11b also binds bacterial lipopolysaccharides.[50] The conformation of the RGD appears to confer some selectivity regarding the integrin to which it binds.[47]

Intercellular adhesion molecules (ICAM)

The ligands for CD18/CD11a are the ICAMs. The first member of this family of transmembrane proteins was ICAM-1 (CD54),[51] which is expressed most strongly on vascular endothelium but also on leucocytes,[52] demonstrating it has an important role in leucocyte-endothelial and leucocyte-leucocyte interactions. Two other members of the ICAM family have been identified; ICAM-2, which also binds CD18/CD11a,[53] and VCAM-1 (vascular cell adhesion molecule) which can be induced on endothelial cells and binds the integrin VLA-4.[54] Neither of these molecules has the RGD peptide in its sequence.

Selectins

Another family of cell adhesion molecules are the selectins. These molecules, of which three have been identified, have N-terminal lectin and epidermal growth factor-like domains but no RGD sequences.[55] The molecule designated ELAM-1 can be induced on endothelial cells but is not found on leucocytes. No ligand has been identified for this molecule, but it has been shown to cause neutrophil adhesion and migration.[55,56] A second selectin, GMP-140 (granule membrane protein), is a component of platelet and endothelial cells and induces rapid neutrophil adhesion to activated endothelium.[57] A third selectin, expressed in lymphoid tissues, designated Mel-14 in mice, is also known as the lymphocyte homing receptor.[58]

Modulation of cell adhesion

The wide distribution of cell adhesion molecules and their ligands (or complementary receptors) raises the question of how cell recruitment is initiated and how the process can be selective for certain inflammatory cell types. In addition, since adhesion is followed by continued cell motility, the adhesive interaction must be reversible.

The quantitative distribution of families of adhesion molecules such as integrins on blood leucocytes may not be uniform and specific cells express requirements for different endothelial receptors. For example, all granulocytes and monocytes express LEUCAM integrins and the CD18-ICAM interaction has been shown to be important for the adhesion to endothelium of monocytes,[59] neutrophils[60] basophils[61] and eosinophils.[62] Nevertheless, in leucocyte adhesion deficiency syndrome, an inherited deficiency of the CD18 molecule, eosinophils remain capable of migrating to inflamed tissues.[63] This suggests that eosinophils are less dependent upon the CD18/ICAM-1 mechanism than other non-lymphocytic leucocytes and indicates the role for a variety of adhesion molecules in different cells.

The functional and quantitative expression of several adhesion molecules are modulated by activating factors. Although ICAM-1 is present at 'basal' levels on tissues such as endothelium, its expression is increased in inflamed tissues[52] and a number of cytokines can increase the expression of this molecule thus regulating the rate and possibly specificity of cell adhesion. This process is to some extent tissue specific; interferon-γ (IFN-γ) strongly enhances ICAM-1 expression on epidermal keratinocytes, but has only a weak effect on endothelium. In contrast, ICAM-1 expression is increased strongly on endothelium by interleukin-1 (IL-1), bacterial lipopolysaccharide and tumour necrosis factor α (TNF-α), which has little effect on keratinocytes.[52,64,65] The different effects of cytokines on endothelial ICAM-1 expression are also evident in the time-course of responses,[66] maximum effects taking about 24 hours with rapid recovery to basal levels after withdrawal of the cytokine. The selectin ELAM-1 is only detected on endothelial cells that have been activated[55] but, in contrast to ICAM-1, induction by cytokines is rapid, reaching a maximum effect at four hours with a slow recovery. The expression of ICAM-2 might not be regulated by cytokines.[51] The GMP-140 protein has been shown to be induced on endothelium by phorbol ester and also histamine,[57] suggesting potential regulation by activated mast cells.

The functions of integrins can also be regulated, but in a way that differs fundamentally from ICAM-1 or ELAM. Thus agonists causing platelet activation have been shown to result in ligand binding by gpIIb/IIIa[67] and exposure of neutrophils to a variety of activating factors results in increased ligand binding by CD18/CD11b and CD18/CD11a.[68–70] This modulation of ligand binding, which is reversed rapidly, appears to be effected through increased affinity for ligand, without increased expression of receptor numbers.[68,70,71] A change in affinity of neutrophil associated and purified CD18/CD11b, for C3bi, has been demonstrated in response to a lipid (integrin modulating factor; IMF-1), produced transiently by activated neutrophils.[72] The change in affinity appears to be due to a conformational change within the adhesion molecule.[72] This observation may set a precedent for further studies of the autocrine and paracrine modulation of adhesion molecules. Furthermore, the principle of receptor modulation, including changes in receptor affinity state, has implications regarding other inflammatory cell receptors for activating factors.

The nature of the cell population induced to adhere to an inflammatory endothelial site therefore appears to be controlled by a complex modulation of receptors on endothelial and blood inflammatory cells. This involves not only the identities and affinities of the adhesion molecules expressed, but also the time-course within which they are available. This reversible expression is important in breaking the cell attachment and allowing the cell to detach or commence diapedesis. Another determinant in the inflammatory cell response is the nature of the chemotactic factors released at the tissue site.

Chemotactic factors

Inflammatory cells are responsive to chemotactic factors from many sources and these often have the ability to activate other cell functions. In infections, bacteria release potent factors, of which the most extensively studied are the N-formylated peptides, for which monocytes and granulocytes have surface receptors. The peptides with the highest affinities for these receptors have an N-terminal methionine or norleucine residue and two or three more hydrophobic amino acids. Thus the chemotactic factor that is often used to study chemotaxis *in vitro* is N-formyl-methionyl-leucyl-phenylalanine (fmlp).

The host tissues themselves are the source of many chemotactic factors. The activation of complement results in the release of C3a, which is chemotactic.[73] Another chemotactic peptide derived from complement activation is C5a, which induces migration in neutrophils,[74] basophils,[75] eosinophils[22] and monocytes.[76] Further humoral factors known to induce chemotaxis are antigen-antibody complexes, which attract neutrophils,[77] and thrombin which is chemotactic for monocytes.[78] Inflammatory cells themselves release a wide range of chemotactic factors, some of which, like leukotriene B4 (LTB4), are derived from several cell types and can also induce chemotaxis in most leucocytes.[76,22,79] Some appear to be more selective in their chemotactic potential. Thus interleukin-8 (IL-8) is particularly chemotactic for neutrophils;[80] IL-5,[81] platelet-activating factor[82] and eosinophil chemotactic factor of anaphylaxis (ECF-A)[22] for eosinophils; IL-3 for mast cells[83] and transforming growth factor β (TGF-β)[84] for monocytes. This is not a comprehensive list, nor can these chemotactic factors be regarded as totally specific in the cells which they influence; TGF-β, for instance, is chemotactic for T lymphocytes[85] and also neutrophils, but only within a narrow range of concentrations.[86] Nevertheless, the potency of each factor appears to be relatively discriminatory and this may contribute to the pattern of cell recruitment.

In addition to producing chemotactic factors directly, inflammatory cells can, as a consequence of tissue damage, induce the release of chemotactic activity in the form of extracellular matrix proteins or peptides derived from these proteins. Monocytes and neutrophils have been shown to respond to fibronectin,[87] collagen,[88,89] laminin,[90] and elastin.[91]

The identification of chemotactic factors summarised above is largely the result of *in vitro* studies with isolated materials. The situation *in vivo* will, of course, be represented by a complex mixture of factors existing together. The effects of multiple factors are as yet unknown and will be dictated not only by the qualitative composition of chemotactic molecules, but also their effective concentrations. Leucocytes are exquisitely sensitive to the concentrations of chemotactic and activating factors. For instance, it has been calculated that a neutrophil can respond to a concentration gradient of fmlp that changes by as little as 2% of the cell's length.[92] Despite this sensitivity to chemo-attractant concentrations, the cell's response is apparent over several orders of magnitude, with a characteristic dose-response curve (Figure 3.5) demonstrating maximum chemotaxis at the optimal concentration of chemo-attractant, but decreasing response at lower or higher concentrations. It is possible that this phenomenon represents a mechanism that induces cell movement towards the chemotactic signal but prevents further migration once the cell encounters the tissue site from which the signal emanates and at which the concentration of chemo-attractant is highest. Furthermore, the cells 'adapt' with time

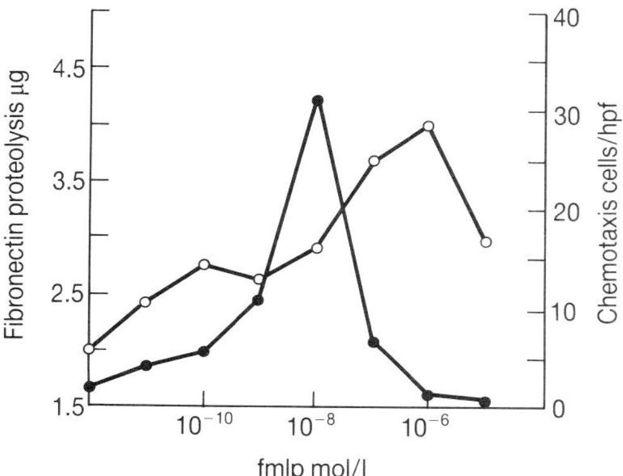

Fig. 3.5 The response of neutrophils to fmlp. Dark squares show the chemotactic response in a modified Boyden chamber system. Light squares show their ability to digest extracellular fibronectin.

to a constant concentration of chemo-attractant and cease responding until the concentration changes, or perhaps respond to another chemo-attractant. Interestingly, the concentration inducing maximum chemotactic response is often different from that which causes activation of other cell functions. In the case of fmlp, this represents concentrations differing by two orders of magnitude; the optimal concentration for chemotaxis is 10^{-8}mol/l whereas that for superoxide production and induction of extracellular proteinase activity is 10^{-6}mol/l (see Figure 3.5). Thus the activation of antimicrobial and potentially tissue damaging functions will be delayed until the cell has moved to the appropriate site.

The ability of a cell to orientate itself and move within a concentration gradient is dependent upon the polarisation of the cell when it adheres or moves in response to an appropriate signal. This involves the polarisation of receptors, which appear to be expressed on the adherent or leading aspect of the cell; this phenomenon has been observed with respect to neutrophil receptors for immunoglobulin Fc, formyl peptides, TNF-α and C3b[93–95] (this receptor is CD18/CD11a). This 'redistribution' of receptors can also involve an alteration in the receptor affinity for ligand and may be associated with changes in the cells' responses to ligand binding.[95] This undoubtedly will result from changes in intracellular signalling pathways but the mechanism remains unknown at present. It is possible that 'new' populations of receptors are distributed at the cell surface or, alternatively, it might prove to be another example of modulation of receptor affinity status.[72]

Potential mechanisms of tissue damage

The products of inflammatory cells can influence pathological tissue changes in two fundamental ways: either through direct damage to host cells and connective tissue proteins, or by activating these mechanisms in other cells. The molecular mechanisms responsible can also, for convenience, be classified as those produced *de novo* upon cell activation, and the release or activity of preformed, stored materials, particularly granule contents such as proteolytic enzymes.

The respiratory burst

Oxygen metabolites, or reactive oxygen intermediates, are produced by activated monocytes and granulocytes by the membrane-bound NADPH-oxidase system that utilises glucose and oxygen. As a result of an electron transfer chain, a variety of highly reactive products is released, which are toxic to micro-organisms. The importance of this mechanism in bacterial killing is illustrated by the syndrome chronic granulomatous disease in which affected individuals, unable to elicit the respiratory burst, are susceptible to infections.[26,96] The enzyme NADPH-oxidase, thought to be a flavoprotein, catalyses the reduction of oxygen by one electron to form superoxide radical (0_2-).[97] Two molecules of 0_2- can interact spontaneously (dismutation) to form molecular oxygen and hydrogen peroxide, but this reaction is also catalysed by a metallo-enzyme, superoxide dismutase. In the presence of halide ions, of which chloride is likely to be the most important physiologically, peroxidases (the peroxidase of eosinophils and myeloperoxidases of neutrophils, monocytes and other cells are not identical molecules[98,99]) catalyse the reduction of peroxidase to hypochlorous acid, a precursor of chloramines, and free chloride, which are powerful antimicrobial agents. Myeloperoxidase can also catalyse the reduction of peroxide to water. A further theoretical product is the generation of extremely reactive hydroxyl radical from superoxide or peroxide in the presence of free iron (the Haber-Weiss reaction). Since most iron is protein-bound, the significance of this potential product is not clear. Most of the products of the oxidative burst are extremely short-lived. Superoxide anion is rapidly dismuted and the enzymes catalase and myeloperoxidase would dispose of peroxide rapidly.

Platelets may have an important role in protecting tissues such as endothelium from damage due to inflammatory cell oxidants. They contain large quantities of catalase,[100] superoxide dismutases[101] and components of the glutathione redox system.[102] Functionally, platelets have been shown to have very effective reducing powers *in vitro*[101] and to protect against oxidant mediated tissue changes *in vivo*.[103] Since platelet adhesion is enhanced by oxidants *in vitro*,[100,104] they may be 'recruited' more effectively to sites of potential oxidant damage. Because of the highly reactive nature of these oxidants (hence their effective antimicrobial role) they will interact rapidly with available substrates. Methionine, for instance, is abundant as the free amino acid and as a component of proteins and is oxidised by peroxide. In this way, reactive products would be effectively chelated. Paradoxically, however, this might lead to the potential oxidative inactivation of host proteins. Oxidative inactivation of the serine proteinase α 1-proteinase inhibitor (α 1-antitrypsin), by the formation of methionine sulphoxide at the protein's reactive site, has been proposed as a mechanism that leads to connective tissue destruction by neutrophil serine proteinases such as elastase.[105] The potential of the products of the oxidative burst to cause pathological tissue damage is, like other cell products, determined by their expression and survival outside the cell. Superoxides are produced in and adjacent to the plasma membrane, typically within the phagocytic vacuole. Nevertheless, the reaction can be induced with a number of agents in non-phagocytosing inflammatory cells. This can be elicited with phorbol esters and fmlp.[106]

Cytokines can induce the phenomenon of 'priming'; they may not themselves be effective at activating the oxidative burst, but prime the cells to a reaction on subsequent exposure to or if co-incubated with other agents.[107] Neutrophil adherence, mediated through integrins, appears to be a prerequisite for superoxide production in response to activating agents including GMCSF, GCSF and TNF.[108–109] The induction of superoxide release by inflammatory cells is therefore, like other functions, controlled by complex combinations of signals and cell interactions; the production of superoxide anion by neutrophils in response to immune complexes is, for example, enhanced by the presence of platelets, an effect attributed to the release of nucleotides.[110] This may seem paradoxical in view of the potential *protective* role of platelets outlined above. A further twist is that platelet activating factor (PAF), which is produced by granulocytes and macrophages, can also prime cells including neutrophils and eosinophils.[111,112] This illustrates the complex nature of cell interactions and suggests caution in the interpretation of results obtained from *in vitro* experiments that are inevitably reductionist in nature.

Although superoxides have been shown, at very high concentrations, to degrade fibronectin,[113] experiments with neutrophils suggest that superoxides contribute relatively little directly to connective tissue damage, which appears to be the result of proteolytic enzymes.[114,115] They might, however, potentiate the effects of proteinases through the oxidative inactivation of proteinase inhibitors[105,116] and activate proteinases.[117] Superoxides, nevertheless, have been implicated in the pathogenesis of diseases through their ability to be cytotoxic[118] and this may occur at the interface of activated leucocytes and potential target cells such as endothelium. This might be due to their direct effects on target cells, or through synergy with other cytotoxic molecules, such as defensins.[119]

Proteinases and other cytotoxic proteins

Proteolytic enzymes are by definition capable, within the limits of their specificities and other determining factors such as cofactors and pH, to elicit damage to connective tissue proteins. They also have the potential to damage cellular tissue by attacking surface proteins. This might lead to cell death or cell detachment through proteolysis of adhesion molecules or proteins to which the cells are attached. Other proteins, without proteinase activity, also have direct cytotoxic properties through a variety of actions. Enzymes capable of hydrolysing carbohydrates and lipases may contribute to tissue damage by degrading non-protein substrates.

Cytotoxic proteins

The eosinophil contains, within its specific granules, several cationic proteins with cytotoxic potential. These basic proteins appear not to be a component of other inflammatory cells. The major basic protein (MBP) is the major constituent of the specific granule core.[120] It has a molecular weight of 14000 and is rich in arginine residues.[121] The protein is toxic to parasites including helminths, protozoa[22] and bacteria.[122] It is also toxic to mammalian cells[123] and can influence other cells, for instance by activating histamine release from mast cells and basophils.[124] Small amounts of MBP have been detected in basophils;[22] it is not known whether this is the result of low levels of synthesis or uptake of the protein. Three other proteins with cytotoxic potential are located in the matrix component of the specific granules.[120] Eosinophil cationic protein (ECP), molecular weight 21000, is antihelminthic,[125] antibacterial[122] and cytotoxic to mammalian cells including neurones.[126] Another neurotoxic protein[126] is eosinophil derived neurotoxin (EDN), molecular weight 18500, which has a homologous structure to ECP.[127] The mechanism by which these proteins damage parasites and host cells is not clear, but is probably related to their basic properties and, in the case of ECP, results in the formation of lytic pores in target cell membranes.[128] The presence of MBP in the extracellular fluids of patients with eosinophilia[121] demonstrates that this protein and the other granule proteins might be released from eosinophils as a result of cell activation and degranulation. Several factors that activate eosinophils and cause degranulation have been described, including opsonisation with IgG or IgA,[129] TNF,[22] GMCSF and IL-3.[130] Two non-proteinase basic proteins, azurocidin or CAP 37, and CAP 57[131,132] with antimicrobial and potential cytotoxic activity have also been identified in the azurophil granules of neutrophils.

Neutrophil azurophil granules also contain a family of four antimicrobial peptides named defensins. These are cyclic[133] single-chain peptides, molecular weight about 4000, which are rich in arginine residues and each has six cysteine residues with three intrachain disulphide bonds. Three of the defensins (called HNP 1–3) are identical in structure in all but the final N-terminal amino acid. Two, HNP-1 and HNP-3, are 29 residues long whereas HNP-2 has 29 amino acids.[134] The fourth defensin, HNP-4, which is less abundant than HNP 1–3, also shares less structural homology.[135] The human defensins show a large degree of structural homology with defensins of the rabbit, rat and guinea pig,[136] and even with antimicrobial peptides of insects suggesting an ancient lineage for these peptides.[137] Defensins are toxic to bacteria, fungi and enveloped viruses[136] which they kill by the production of ion channels in the target membranes.[138] They can also kill human cells including endothelial cells[139] but in contrast to microbial killing, the toxicity to mammalian cells appears to be effected in two stages. The first, reversible and rapid (five minutes), is associated with the formation of pores which are permeable to small molecules. In the continued presence of defensins, the cells become permeable to larger molecules and are lysed after one to six hours.[140] This second 'lytic' phase is sensitive to inhibitors of protein synthesis and, although the mechanism of lysis is not determined, it is suggested that the defensin molecules might enter the target cell.

The cyclic structure of defensins is reminiscent of the doughnut-shaped protein complex formed during the lytic sequence of complement activation; this tempts one to speculate that the defensin molecule might be inserted into the membrane of the target molecule, forming a cylindrical pore. The cytotoxic potential of defensins has so far only been demonstrated with purified material. Defensins have not yet been located outside the neutrophil. Nevertheless, other azurophil granule components have been detected in extracellular fluids such as pus and defensins would presumably also be present and may therefore come into contact with other cells. Neutrophils cannot be easily persuaded, with activating stimuli, to shed their azurophil granules.[115] Indeed, after stimulation of neutrophils with the potent activating phorbol esters, or during phagocytosis, only 3–8% of the cells' defensins were released.[141] The pericellular environment around adherent neutrophils is thought to be the site where azurophil granule contents, such as proteinases, are most likely to be active.[115,142] This may be for two reasons: firstly, exclusion of inhibitors from the pericellular zone and secondly, because the molar concentrations of azurophil contents may be relatively high. The serum protein α_2-macroglobulin binds defensins[143] and because of its large size (molecular weight 75 KDa) would be excluded effectively from the pericellular space. Nevertheless, the long time required for purified defensins to elicit cell lysis suggests that a neutrophil would not remain adherent to a target cell long enough for defensins to be effective. A metabolising neutrophil might, however, produce superoxides and these can work synergistically with defensins in producing cell lysis,[119] suggesting a potential role for these molecules in host tissue damage.

Proteinases

Proteolytic enzymes are present in monocytes, mast cells, neutrophils and platelets, each cell containing a distinctive complement. With the exception of monocytes and macrophages, the proteinases are stored in cytoplasmic granules; monocytes and macrophages, although having stored proteinases, can also synthesise and secrete proteolytic enzymes that are not stored within the cell. Furthermore, these cells produce distinctive ranges of proteinases which are classified into four groups: serine proteinases, metalloproteinases, cysteine (thiol) proteinases and aspartic proteinases.

The serine proteinases comprise a large group, some of which appear to be members of a supergene family including non-proteinase proteins. Rat mast cell proteinases, which are similar to human mast cell chymase,[144] human neutrophil elastase, cathepsin G, proteinase 3 (also called APG7 or P29), azurocidin (or CAP37, not a proteinase) and lymphocyte proteinase, and the mouse lymphocyte granzymes, all share considerable homology in the N-terminal region (Table 3.1).[131,132,143–149] Mast cell tryptase is not a member of this group.[144] The proteins are translated as proproteins which, in the case of the enzymes, are not active until cleavage of the propeptide, which occurs rapidly after translation.[150] The considerable homology around the proprotein region suggests that these proteins are processed by similar proteinases in all the cells and species expressing these sequences; this enzyme(s) has not been identified. These serine proteinases all have neutral pH optima and are therefore effectively inactive within the storage granules; pHs compatible with enzyme activity will occur in the phagolysosome or outside the cell.

In the case of human mast cells, chymase and tryptase are stored in the same secretory granules although, as described previously, chymase is absent from mast cells at some tissue sites. Tryptase has been detected in blood[151] and other body fluids in association with histamine,[152] suggesting that degranulation of mast cells involves the release of this enzyme and possibly also chymase. These enzymes have been shown to digest a number of protein substrates. Chymase cleaves

Table 3.1 The published amino acid sequences of the pro-dipeptides and 18 N-terminus residues of the 'mature' processed protein, of some serine proteinases and granule proteins from mouse, rat and human granulocytes and lymphocytes. The amino acids in italics denote major homologies between proteins from different species and cells. Note that there are also other major intraspecies homologies. The published references from which the sequences were obtained are cited in the text.

Protein	Pro-dipeptide	Protein N-terminus
Human		
Neutrophil elastase	S E	I V G G R RAR P H A W P F M V S L
Cathepsin G	G E	I I G G R E SR P H S R P Y M A Y L
Proteinase 3 (APG7 or P29)	A E	I V G G H E AQ P H S R P Y M A S L
Azurocidin (CAP37)		I V G G R KAR P H Q F P F L A S I
Lymphocyte proteinase	G E	I I G G H E A KP H S R P Y M AY L
Rat		
Mast cell proteinase I		I I G G V E S R P H S R P Y M A H L
Mast cell proteinase II	E E	I I G G V E S I P H S R P Y M A H L
Mouse		
Granzymes BGH	G E	I I G G H E V K P H S R P Y M A L L
Granzyme C	E E	I I G G M E I S P H S R P Y M A Y Y
Granzyme D	E E	I I G G H V V K P H S R P Y M A F V
Granzyme E	E E	I I G G H V V K P H S R P Y M A F V
Granzyme F	E E	I I G G H E V K P H S R P Y M A R V

substance P, angiotensin I (to produce angiotensin II) and extracellular matrix proteins. It can also cooperate with histamine in producing a wheal and flare reaction.[144] Tryptase can activate the extracellular 'matrix' metalloproteinases, prostromelysin and procollagenase, secreted by macrophages as inactive precursors, and fibrinogen as well as several other proteins, and also behaves as a fibroblast growth factor.[153] Since tryptase and chymase are inactivated by proteinase inhibitors, including $\alpha_1$antitrypsin, $\alpha_1$antichymotrypsin and $\alpha_2$macroglobulin, it may be that their activity is restricted to pericellular environments. Nevertheless, their potential to be secreted in large amounts from the cell and their wide-ranging activities suggest they contribute to inflammatory and pathological processes.

In contrast to mast cells, neutrophils do not readily degranulate their azurophil granules, in which three major serine proteinases are found with myeloperoxidase. These are neutrophil elastase, cathepsin G and proteinase 3. Elastase derives its name from the ability to attack elastin, which is relatively resistant to proteinases. It can also hydrolyse other connective tissue components including laminin,[154] collagen[155] and proteoglycan.[156] For this reason, and the abundance of neutrophils, elastase has been implicated in the pathogenesis of a number of diseases, particularly those, such as pulmonary emphysema, where damage to elastin as well as other connective tissue proteins is thought to be an important feature.[157] Cathepsin G is a chymotrypsin-like enzyme. The natural protein substrates for this enzyme have not been studied in detail although it can work synergistically with elastase in elastin degradation.[158] Cathepsin G, like other proteinases, also has properties *in vitro* that seem to have little to do with a proteolytic role; cathepsin G can behave as an agonist for platelet activation.[159] Proteinase 3 is also able to degrade elastin but its pH optimum for this activity is pH 6.5 whereas that of elastase is at pHs between seven and nine[160].

The neutrophil secondary granules contain, in addition to lactoferrin, lysozyme, a vitamin B-binding protein, fmlp receptors and a procollagenase of the metalloproteinase class that is stored in an inactive form that can be activated by oxidation hypochlorous acid.[161] Another metalloproteinase, gelatinase, which can degrade denatured type I collagen, is present in the neutrophil and this also might be activated by oxidants.[162] There is some debate as to whether this proteinase is stored in the specific granules[163] or a distinct population, tertiary granules.[164]

Macrophages synthesise and secrete at least four metalloproteinases, produced by other cells including fibroblasts, belonging to a supergene family, the 'matrix metalloproteinases'.

Stromelysin,[165,166] can digest fibronectin, laminin, proteoglycans and collagens type IV and IX. Two macrophage gelatinases, or type IV collagenases,[167,168,169] of 72 KDa and 92 KDa, can degrade collagens type IV, V and X as well as denatured collagen (gelatin). The fourth matrix metalloproteinase produced by macrophages is 'interstitial' collagenase[169] that can degrade collagens type I, II, III and X. These enzymes are not stored within the cell and are produced as pro-enzymes which must be activated. The potential for secretion, and therefore synthesis, of these enzymes is greater in macrophages than in monocytes.[169] Whether human macrophages can produce a metallo-elastase has been the subject of controversy. Murine macrophages are known to produce a metallo-elastase[170] but attempts to identify such an enzyme from human monocytes or macrophages were, with one exception[171] unsuccessful,[172,173] or detected enzyme activity[174] that could be attributed[175] to the presence of neutrophil elastase and cathepsin G in these cells.[176] This might be due to uptake by macrophages, or a residue of 'neutrophil' proteinases synthesised during development in the bone marrow.[177] Metallo-elastase activity has now been demonstrated convincingly by alveolar macrophages cultured on insoluble elastin substrate, the activity being most apparent after 24 hours in culture[178] and appears to be due to the activity of the 92 KDa and 72 KDa collagenases.[179] Macrophages also contain the lysosomal cysteine proteinases, including cathepsin B[180,181] and cathepsin L.[182] Cathepsin B can degrade a number of substrates including the connective tissue proteins collagen and proteoglycan[183,184] and cathepsin L is elastolytic[185] although these enzymes function at acidic pH and tend to be denatured at pHs above neutral.[186] Macrophages also produce neutral serine proteinases, such as plasminogen activator[187] and the acidic aspartic proteinase cathepsin D.[188] Macrophages therefore contain, synthesise and secrete proteinases capable of degrading a wide spectrum of potential substrates in a wide range of environmental conditions.

Platelets also contain proteolytic enzymes[189] including a serine elastase distinct from neutrophil elastase.[190] Little is known about the structure or biological significance of this enzyme.

Extracellular activity of leucocyte proteinases

As outlined above, degranulation following the activation of mast cells is associated with the release of proteinases,[121] which might reflect an extracellular role for these enzymes in killing of parasites. In contrast, activation of neutrophils with phorbol esters, phagocytosis or cytokines such as TNF-α, interleukin-1α (IL-1) and GMCSF activates these cells without a significant release of azurophil contents.[115,141,191–194] This phenomenon probably reflects the essentially intracellular functions of neutrophil azurophil proteins and enzymes; that is, the killing and decomposition of phagocytosed micro-organisms. Clearly, in view of the huge numbers of neutrophils often recruited to inflammatory foci, it would be potentially catastrophic if large quantities of cytotoxic proteins were released into the extracellular environment. Nevertheless, living neutrophils can digest extracellular proteins, although this activity appears to be limited to the pericellular area of adherent cells in contact with the protein substrate.[142] This proteolysis can occur even if proteinase inhibitors are present in the culture medium, suggesting that these are excluded from the pericellular space.[116,142,195] The proteolytic activity can be increased with the addition of activating factors including fmlp, bacterial lipopolysaccharide, TNF-α, IL-1 and IFN-γ,[115,196,197] but, as for superoxide production,[106,108,109] only if the cells are adherent. Since 'basal' levels of superoxide production can be elicited by non-adherent neutrophils, this suggests that activation of some functions of neutrophils is dependent on cell adherence and might be regulated by the altered expression of cytokine receptors,[95] perhaps mediated through 'coupling' to the status of adhesion molecules. A degree of limited extracellular proteolysis by neutrophils is probably a normal consequence of cell adhesion and migration and has even been proposed as a requirement for the penetration of these cells through connective tissues.[198] Why this mechanism might sometimes lead to pathological consequences is the subject of continuing study.

Macrophages also contain lysosomal enzymes which are presumably involved in the digestion of ingested material. Nevertheless, they also secrete newly synthesised proteinases that may be important for functions including killing of micro-organisms and the remodelling of connective tissue. Their ability to digest extracellular protein has been attributed to several proteinases, including plasminogen activator,[187] the metallocollagenases[178,179] and cathepsin L;[182] although cathepsin L functions only at acidic pH, it has been shown that the pH beneath macrophages can be acidic.[199] The reasons why different investigators have implicated different proteinases in this process is not clear. The conditions of cell culture might influence the secretion of particular enzymes; hence it was only after prolonged culture on elastin that the metallo-elastase activity of macrophages was evident.[178] This suggests the possibility that the substrates available to macrophages might determine which enzymes are expressed. Furthermore, macrophages synthesise and secrete proteinase inhibitors including the serine proteinase inhibitors,[34] cysteine proteinase inhibitors (cystatins[200]) and the tissue inhibitors of metalloproteinases,[201] of which two (TIMP-1 and TIMP-2) have been identified.[202] The extracellular activity of proteinases released by these cells will be determined by the inhibitors present in the extracellular environment, which will be excluded to some degree from the pericellular space,[203] and those actively secreted by the macrophages themselves. Nevertheless, the ability to express such a wide range of proteinases demonstrates a versatile potential to degrade connective tissue proteins and damage host cells.

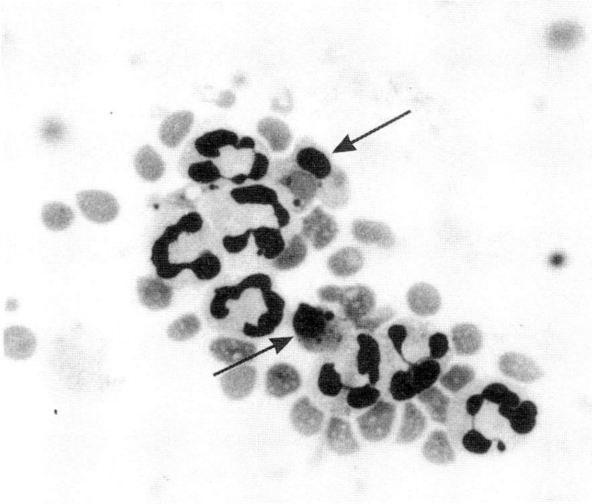

(a)

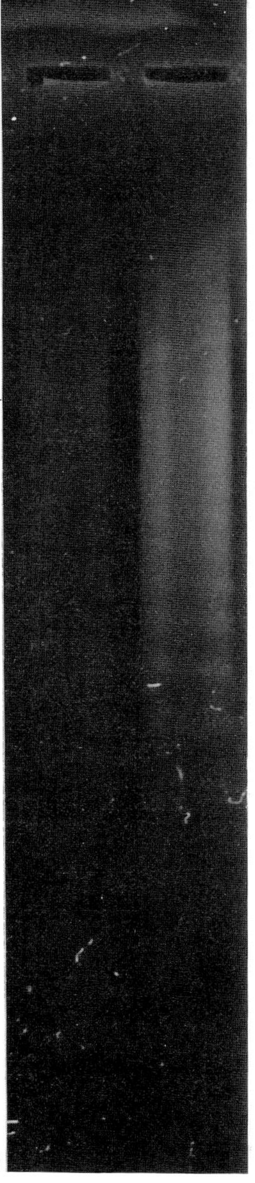

(b)

Fig. 3.6 (a) Neutrophils maintained in culture for 24 hours. Most of the cells shown demonstrate the typical polymorphonuclear morphology of neutrophils but two cells (arrowed) have the typical appearance associated with apoptosis. (b) Agarose gel electrophoresis of DNA preparations stained with ethydium bromide. DNA is separated by size, smaller fragments moving faster towards the bottom of the gel. Track 1 shows DNA from newly isolated blood neutrophils. Track 2 shows DNA fragmentation in apoptotic neutrophils aged in culture.

Cell death

The fate of inflammatory cells after recruitment to tissues is not yet well understood. It is thought unlikely that they re-enter the circulation but, were they to disintegrate within the tissues, their contents including cytotoxic proteins and proteinases would be released extracellularly and cause extensive lysis of cells and proteins. Nevertheless, despite massive accumulations of granulocytes, inflammatory and infective processes normally resolve with no pathological consequences.[204] Experiments with neutrophils now suggest that these cells are removed intact and disposed of by macrophages as a consequence of apoptosis. Apoptosis is a form of 'programmed cell death' which can be identified by characteristic morphological and biochemical changes in the cell. The morphological changes include nuclear condensation with the formation of membrane bound, chromatin containing bodies, cell rounding, loss of microvilli, dilation of endoplasmic reticulum and fusion of cytoplasmic vesicles with the cell membrane. In addition, apoptosis is associated with fragmentation of DNA (by specific endonucleases) which can be detected by gel electrophoresis.[205,206] The specific cleavage of the chromosomal DNA effectively shuts down cell functions, and the cell contents are safely packaged as 'apoptotic bodies'. Changes in the cell surface properties appear to enable these apoptotic cells to be recognised by others, including tissue macrophages. Neutrophils isolated from the blood and maintained in culture demonstrate apoptotic changes after about 24 hours (Figure 3.6). It has been demonstrated that these apoptotic cells are engulfed, intact, by macrophages,[207,208] probably through a recognition mechanism involving vitronectin receptors,[209] without activation of other macrophage functions. This process has also been observed *in vivo*.[210] Eosinophils have also been observed to undergo apoptosis *in vitro* and were recognised and ingested by macrophages. The apoptotic process was delayed by IL-5, GMCSF and IL-3.[211,212] Apoptosis of neutrophils and leukaemic myeloid cells has been shown to be accelerated by inhibitors of protein and RNA synthesis.[213,214] The fate of macrophages themselves is not known, but they might also succumb eventually to apoptosis and be removed by cannibalistic macrophages or other cells.

Apoptosis therefore represents a mechanism whereby neutrophils at inflammatory sites can be disposed of without the release of their contents, which are presumably safely digested within the macrophage. The rate of cell death appears to be capable of regulation and the process might prove to be as important as activation of cells in determining the outcome of inflammation.

References

1. Hubscher SG, Clements D, Elias E, McMaster P. Biopsy findings in cases of rejection of liver allografts. *J Clin Pathol* 1985; **38,** 1366–1373.
2. Wright DGD. Pathology of rejection. In: *Liver Transplantation*, Calne RY (ed). London: Grune and Stratton, 1983.
3. Snover DC, Sibley RK, Freese DK *et al.* Orthotopic liver transplantation: a pathological study of 63 serial liver biopsies from 17 patients with special reference to diagnostic features and natural history of rejection. *Hepatology* 1984; **4,** 1212–1222.
4. Demetris AJ, Lasky S, van Thiel DH, Starzl TE, Dekker A. Pathology of hepatic transplantation: a review of 62 adult allograft recipients immunosuppressed with cyclosporin/steroid regimen. *Am J Path* 1985; **118,** 151–161.
5. Foster PF, Sankary HN, Hart M, Ashmann M, Williams JW. Blood and graft eosinophilia as precursors of rejection in human liver transplantation. *Transplantation* 1989; **47,** 72–74.
6. Foster P, Sankary HN, Williams JW, Bhattacharyya A, Coleman J, Ashmann M. Morphometric inflammatory cell analysis of human liver allograft biopsies. *Transplantation* 1991; **51,** 873–876.
7. Adams DH, Burnett D, Stockley RA, Elias E. Patterns of leukocyte chemotaxis to bile after liver transplantation. *Gastroenterology* 1989; **97,** 433–438.
8. Adams DH, Wang LF, Burnett D, Stockley RA, Neuberger JM. Neutrophil activation – an important cause of tissue damage during liver allograft rejection? *Transplantation* 1990; **50,** 86–91.
9. Foster PF, Bhattacharyya A, Sankary HN, Coleman J, Ashmann M, Williams JW. Eosinophil cationic protein's role in human hepatic allograft rejection. *Hepatology* 1991; **13,** 1117–1125.
10. Blaies DM, William JF. A simplified method for staining mast cells with astra blue. *Stain Tech* 1981; **56,** 91–94.
11. Schwartz LB. Monoclonal antibodies against human mast cell tryptase demonstrate shared antigenic sites on subsets of tryptase and selective localisation of the enzyme to mast cells. *J Immunol* 1985; **134,** 526–531.
12. Irani AA, Schechter NM, Craig SS, De Blois G, Schwartz LB. Two types of human mast cells that have distinct neutral protease compositions. *Proc Nat Acad Sci USA* 1986; **83,** 4464–4468.
13. Schwartz LB, Huff TF. Mast cells. In: *The Lung: Scientific Foundations*, Crystal RG, West JB (eds). New York: Raven Press Ltd, 1991.
14. Plaut M, Pierce JH, Watson CJ, Hanley-Hyde J, Nordan RP, Paul WE. Mast cell lines produce lymphokines in response to cross-linkage of

$F_{c\epsilon}RI$ or to calcium ionophores. *Nature* 1989; **339,** 64–67.

15. Davies RJ, Devalia JL. Epithelial cells. *Brit Med Bull* 1992; **48,** 85–96.
16. Ihle JN, Keller JR, Oroszlan S *et al.* Biological properties of homogeneous interleukin 3. I. Demonstration of WEHI-3 growth factor activity, mast cell growth factor activity, p cell stimulating factor activity, colony stimulating factor activity, and histamine-producing cell-stimulating factor activity. *J Immunol* 1983; **131,** 282–287.
17. Bainton DF, Ullyot JL, Farquhar MG. The development of neutrophilic polymorphonuclear leucocytes in human bone marrow: origin and content of azurophil and specific granules. *J Exp Med* 1971; **134,** 907–934.
18. MacGlashan DW, Lichtenstein LM. Basophils. In: *The Lung: Scientific Foundations*, Crystal RG, West JB (eds). New York: Raven Press Ltd, 1991.
19. Denburg JA, Messner H, Lim B, Jamal N, Telizyn S, Bienenstock J. Clonal origin of human basophil/mast cells from circulating multipotent hemopoietic progenitors. *Exp Hematol* 1985; **13,** 185–188.
20. Butterworth AE. Cell-mediated damage to helminths. *Adv Parasitol* 1988; **23,** 143–235.
21. Weller PF. The immunobiology of eosinophils. *N Engl J Med* 1991; **324,** 1110–1118.
22. Slifman NR, Adolphson CR, Gleich GJ. Eosinophils: biochemical and cellular aspects. In: *Allergy: Principles and Practice*, Middleton E, Reed CE, Ellis EF, Adkinson NF, Yunginger JW (eds). St Louis: CV Mosby, 1988.
23. Spry CJF. *Eosinophils: A Guide to the Scientific and Medical Literature*. Oxford: Oxford University Press, 1988.
24. Sonoda Y, Arai N, Ogawa M. Humoral regulation of eosinophilopoiesis in vitro: analysis of the targets of interleukin-3, granulocyte/macrophage colony-stimulating factor (GM-CSF), and interleukin-5. *Leukemia* 1989; **3,** 14–18.
25. Clutterbuck EJ, Hirst EM, Sanderson CJ. Human interleukin-5 (IL-5) regulates the production of eosinophils in human bone marrow cultures: comparison and interaction with IL-1, IL-3, IL-6 and GMCSF. *Blood* 1989; **73,** 1504–1512.
26. Lehrer RI, Ganz T, Selsted ME, Babior BM, Curnutte JT. Neutrophils and host defense. *Ann Intern Med* 1988; **109,** 127–142.
27. Sullivan R. Haemopoietic colony stimulating factors: biological functions and clinical potentials. *Am J Respir Cell Molec Biol* 1990; **3,** 283–284.
28. Athens JW, Raab SO, Haab OP *et al.* Leukokinetic studies. III. The distribution of granulocytes in the blood of normal subjects. *J Clin Invest* 1961; **40,** 159–164.
29. Athens JW, Haab OP, Raab SO *et al.* Leukokinetic studies. XI. Blood granulocyte kinetics in polycythemia vera, infection and myelofibrosis. *J Clin Invest* 1965; **44,** 778–788.
30. Dougherty GJ, McBride WH. Monocyte differentiation *in vitro*. In: *Human Monocytes*, Zembala M, Asherson GL (eds). San Diego: Academic Press Ltd, 1989.
31. Stanley ER. The macrophage colony-stimulating factor, CSF-1. *Methods in Enzymology* 1985; **116,** 564–587.
32. Bitterman PB, Salzman LE, Adelberg S, Ferrans VJ, Crystal RG. Alveolar macrophage replication: one mechanism for the expansion of the mononuclear phagocyte population in the chronically inflamed lung. *J Clin Invest* 1984; **74,** 460–469.
33. Lasser A. The mononuclear phagocyte system: a review. *Hum Pathol* 1983; **14,** 108–126.
34. Nathan CF. Secretory products of macrophages. *J Clin Invest* 1987; **79,** 319–326.
35. Sibille Y, Reynolds HY. Macrophages and polymorphonuclear neutrophils in lung defense and injury. *Am Rev Respir Dis* 1990; **141,** 471–501.
36. Wintrobe MM, Lee GR, Boggs DR *et al.* Platelets and megakaryocytes. In: *Clinical Hematology* Philadelphia: Lea and Febiger, 1981.
37. Hawker LA, Finch CA. Thrombokinetics in man. *J Clin Invest* 1969; **48,** 963–974.
38. Williams N. Stimulators of megakaryocyte development and platelet production. *Prog Growth Factor Res* 1990; **2,** 81–95.
39. Dessypris EN, Chuncharunee S, Frierson KE. Thrombopoiesis-stimulating factor: its effects on megakaryocyte colony formation in vitro and its relation to granulocyte-macrophage colony-stimulating factor. *Exp Hematol* 1990; **18,** 754–757.
40. Vannucchi AM, Grossi A, Rafanelli D, Ferrini PR. *In vivo* stimulation of megakaryocytopoiesis by recombinant murine granulocyte-macrophage colony-stimulating factor. *Blood* 1990; **76,** 1473–1480.
41. Nagasawa T, Orita T, Matsushita J *et al.* Thrombopoietic activity of human interleukin-6. *FEBS Lett* 1990; **260,** 176–178.
42. McDonald TP, Cottrell MB, Swearingen CJ, Clift RE. Comparative effects of thrombopoietin and interleukin-6 on murine megakaryocytopoiesis and platelet production. *Blood* 1991; **77,** 735–740.
43. Nelson RD, Herron MJ. Agarose method for human neutrophil chemotaxis. In: *Immunochemical Techniques*, Part L: *Chemotaxis and Inflammation. Methods in Enzymology*,

Vol. 162, DiSabato G (ed). San Diego: Academic Press, 1988.
44. Falk W, Goodwin RH, Leonard EJ. A 48-well microchemotaxis assembly for rapid and accurate measurement of leukocyte migration. *J Immunol Methods* 1980; **33,** 239–247.
45. Albeda SM, Buck CA. Integrins and other cell adhesion molecules. *Faseb J* 1990; **4,** 2868–2880.
46. Springer TA. Adhesion receptors of the immune system. *Nature* 1990; **346,** 425–434.
47. Ruoslahti E, Pierschbacker MD. New perspectives in cell adhesion: RGD and integrins. *Science* 1987; **238,** 491–497.
48. Diamond MS, Staunton DE, de Fougerolles AR *et al.* ICAM-1 (CD54): a counter-receptor for Mac-1 (CD11b/CD18). *J Cell Biol* 1990; **111,** 3129–3139.
49. Wright SD, Weitz JI, Huang AJ, Levin SM, Silverstein SC, Loike JD. Complement receptor type three (CD11b/CD18) of polymorphonuclear leukocytes recognises fibrinogen. *Proc Nat Acad Sci USA* 1988; **85,** 7734–7738.
50. Wright SD, Levin SM, Jong MTC, Chad Z, Kabbash LG. CR3 (CD11b/CD18) expresses one binding site for Arg-Gly-Asp-containing peptides and a second site for bacterial lipopolysaccharide. *J Exp Med* 1989; **169,** 175–183.
51. Makgoba MW, Saunders ME, Gunther Luce GE *et al.* ICAM-1 a ligand for LFA-1 dependent adhesion of B, T and myeloid cells. *Nature* 1988; **331,** 86–88.
52. Dustin M, Rothlein R, Bhhan AK, Dinarello CA, Springer TA. Induction by IL-1 and IFNγ: tissue distribution, biochemistry and function of a natural adherence molecule (ICAM-1). *J Immunol* 1986; **137,** 245–254.
53. Staunton DE, Dustin ML, Springer TA. Functional cloning of ICAM-2, a cell adhesion ligand for LFA-1 homologous to ICAM-1. *Nature* 1989; **339,** 61–63.
54. Lobb RR. VCAM-1 on activated endothelium interacts with the leukocyte integrin VLA-4 at a site distinct from the VLA-4/fibronectin binding site. *Cell* 1990; **60,** 577–584.
55. Bevilacqua MP, Stengelin S, Gimbrone MA, Seed B. ELAM-1: an inducible receptor for neutrophils related to complement regulatory proteins and lectins. *Science* 1988; **243,** 1160–1164.
56. Luscinskas FW, Brock AF, Arnout MA, Gimbrone MA. ELAM-1 dependent and leucocyte [CD11/CD18] dependent mechanisms contribute to PMN leucocyte adhesion to cytokine-activated human vascular endothelium. *J Immunol* 1989; **142,** 2257–2263.
57. Geng J-G, Bevilacqua MP, Moore KL *et al.* Rapid neutrophil adhesion to activated endothelium mediated by GMP-140. *Nature* 1990; **343,** 757–760.
58. Bowen BR, Nguyen T, Lasky LA. Characterization of a human homologue of the murine peripheral lymph node homing receptor. *J Cell Biol* 1989; **109,** 421–427.
59. Te Velde AA, Keizer GD, Figdor CG. Differential function of LFA-1 family molecules (CS11 and CD18) in adhesion of human monocytes to melanoma and endothelial cells. *Immunology* 1987; **61,** 261–267.
60. Smith CW, Rothlein R, Hughes BJ *et al.* Recognition of an endothelial determinant for CD18-dependent human neutrophil adherence and transendothelial migration. *J Clin Invest* 1988; **82,** 1746–1756.
61. Bochner BS, Peachell PT, Brown KE, Schleimer RP. Adherence of human basophils to cultured human umbilical vein endothelial cells. *J Clin Invest* 1988; **81,** 1355–1364.
62. Wegner CD, Gundel RH, Reilly P, Haynes N, Gordon Letts L, Rothlein R. ICAM-1 in the pathogenesis of asthma. *Science* 1990; **247,** 416–418.
63. Anderson DC, Schmalsteig FC, Finegold MJ *et al.* The severe and moderate phenotypes of heritable Mac-1, LFA-1 deficiency: their quantitative definition and relation to leukocyte dysfunction and clinical features. *J Infect Dis* 1985; **152,** 668–689.
64. Montefort S, Holgate ST. Adhesion molecules and their role in inflammation. *Respir Med* 1991; **85,** 91–99.
65. Dustin ML, Singer KH, Tuck DT, Springer TA. Adhesion of T lymphocytes to epidermal keratinocytes is regulated by IFNγ and is mediated by ICAM-1. *J Exp Med* 1988; **167,** 1323–1340.
66. Pober JS, Gimbrone MA, Lopierre LA *et al.* Overlapping patterns of activation of human endothelial cells by IL-1, TNF and IFNγ. *J Immunol* 1986; **137,** 1893–1896.
67. Coller BS. Activation affects access to the platelet receptor for adhesive glycoproteins. *J Cell Biol* 1986; **103,** 451–456.
68. Wright SD, Meyer BC. Phorbol esters cause sequential activation and deactivation of complement receptors on polymorphonuclear leukocytes. *J Immunol* 1986; **136,** 1759–1764.
69. Lo SK, van Seventer G, Levin SM, Wright SD. Two leukocyte receptors (CD11a/CD18 and CD11b/CD18) mediate transient adhesion to endothelium by binding to different ligands. *J Immunol* 1989; **143,** 3325–3329.
70. Lo SK, Detmers PA, Levin SM, Wright SD. Transient adhesion of neutrophils to endothelium. *J Exp Med* 1989; **169,** 1779–1793.
71. Vedder NB, Harlan JM. Increased surface expression of CD11b/CD18 (Mac-1) is not required for stimulated neutrophil adherence to cultured endothelium. *J Clin Invest* 1988; **81,** 676–682.

72. Hermanowski-Vosatka A, Van Strijp JAG, Swiggard WJ, Wright SD. Integrin modulating factor-1: a lipid that alters the function of leukocyte integrins. *Cell* 1992; **68,** 341–352.
73. Bokisch VA, Muller-Eberhard HJ, Cochrane CG. Isolation of a fragment (C3a) of the third component of human complement containing anaphylotoxin and chemotactic activity and description of an anaphylotoxin inactivator in human serum. *J Exp Med* 1969; **129,** 1109–1130.
74. Toews GB, Vial WC. The role of C5 in polymorphonuclear leukocyte recruitment in response to *Streptococcus pneumoniae*. *Am Rev Respir Dis* 1984; **129,** 82–86.
75. Lett-Brown MA, Boetcher DA, Leonard EJ. Chemotactic responses of normal human basophils to C5a and to lymphocyte-derived chemotactic factor. *J Immunol* 1976; **117,** 246–252.
76. Verghese MW, Snyderman R. Chemotaxis and chemotactic factors. In: *Human Monocytes*, Zembala M, Asherson GL, (eds). San Diego: Academic Press Ltd, 1989.
77. Boyden S. The chemotactic effect of mixtures of antibody and antigen on polymorphonuclear leukocytes. *J Exp Med* 1962; **115,** 453–466.
78. Bar-Shavit R, Kahn AJ, Wilner GD, Fenton JW. Monocyte chemotaxis: stimulation by specific exosite region in thrombin. *Science* 1983; **220,** 728–731.
79. Martin TR, Raugi G, Merritt TL, Henderson WR. Relative contribution of leukotriene B4 to the neutrophil chemotactic activity produced by the resident human alveolar macrophage. *J Clin Invest* 1987; **80,** 1114–1124.
80. Baggiolini M, Walz A, Kunkel SL. Neutrophil activating peptide-1/interleukin-8, a novel cytokine that activates neutrophils. *J Clin Invest* 1989; **84,** 1045–1049.
81. Wang JM, Rambaldi A, Biondi A, Chen ZG, Sanderson CJ, Mantovani A. Recombinant human interleukin-5 is a selective eosinophil chemoattractant. *Eur J Immunol* 1989; **19,** 701–705.
82. Wardlaw AJ, Moqbel R, Cromwell O, Kay AB. Platelet activating factor. A potent chemotactic and chemokinetic factor for human eosinophils. *J Clin Invest* 1986; **78,** 1701–1706.
83. Matsuura N, Zetter BR. Stimulation of mast cell chemotaxis by interleukin-3. *J Exp Med* 1989; **138** 1421–1426.
84. Wahl SM, Hunt DA, Wakefield LM *et al.*, Transforming growth factor type β induces monocyte chemotaxis and growth factor production. *Proc Nat Acad Sci USA* 1987; **84,** 5788–5792.
85. Adams DH, Hathaway M, Shaw J, Burnett D, Elias E, Strain AJ. Transforming growth factor-β induces human T lymphocyte migration *in vitro*. *J Immunol* 1991; **147,** 609–612.
86. Fava RA, Olsen NJ, Postlethwaite AE *et al.* Transforming growth factor β1 (TGF-β1) induced recruitment to synovial tissues: implications for TGF-β-driven synovial inflammation and hyperplasia. *J Exp Med* 1991; **173,** 1121–1132.
87. Clark RAF, Wilkner NE, Doherty DE, Norris DA, Howell SE. Cryptic 120-kDa fibroblastic cell-binding fragment. *J Cell Biol* 1988; **263,** 2115–2123.
88. Laskin DL, Kimura T, Sakakibara S, Riley JD, Berg RA. Chemotactic activity of collagen-like polypeptides for human peripheral blood neutrophils. *J Leuk Biol* 1986; **39,** 255–266.
89. Postlethwaite AE, Kang AH. Collagen and collagen-peptide induced chemotaxis of human blood monocytes. *J Exp Med* 1976; **143,** 1299–1307.
90. Bryant G, Rao CN, Brentani M *et al.* A role for the laminin receptor in leukocyte chemotaxis *J Leuk Biol* 1987; **41,** 220–227.
91. Senior RM, Hinek A, Griffin GL, Pipoly DJ, Crouch EC, Mecham RP. Neutrophils show chemotaxis to type IV collagen and its 7S domain and contain a 67 kD type IV collagen-binding protein with pectin properties. *Am J Respir Cell Mol Biol* 1989; **1,** 479–487.
92. Zigmond SH. Chemotactic response of neutrophils. *Am J Respir Cell Molec Biol* 1989; **1** 451–453.
93. Sullivan SJ, Daukas G, Zigmond SH. Asymmetric distribution of the chemotactic peptide receptor on polymorphonuclear leukocytes. *J Cell Biol* 1984; **99,** 1461–1467.
94. Shield JM, Haston WS. Behaviour of neutrophil leucocytes in uniform concentrations of chemotactic factors: contraction waves, cell polarity and persistence. *J Cell Sci* 1985; **74,** 75–93.
95. Chamba A, Stockley RA, Burnett D. Effects of neutrophil adherence on the characteristics of receptors for tumor necrosis factor-α. *FEBS Lett* 1991; **282,** 373–376.
96. Curnette JT, Whitten DM, Babior BM. Defective superoxide production by granulocytes from patients with chronic granulomatous disease. *N Engl J Med* 1974; **290,** 593–597.
97. Babior BM. The respiratory burst of phagocytes. *J Clin Invest* 1984; **73,** 599–601.
98. Bolscher BGJM, Plat H, Wever R. Some properties of human eosinophil peroxidase; a comparison with other peroxidases. *Biochim Biophys Acta* 1984; **784,** 177–186.
99. Ten RM, Pease LR, McKean DJ, Bell MP, Gleich GJ. Molecular cloning of the human eosinophil peroxidase. Evidence for the existence of a peroxidase multigene family. *J Exp Med* 1989; **169,** 1757–1769.
100. Del Principe D, Menichelli A, de Matteis W, di

Corpo D, Giuilio S, Finazzi-Agro A. Hydrogen peroxide has a role in the aggregation of human platelets. *FEBS Lett* 1985; **185,** 142–146.
101. Handin RI, Karabin R, Boxer GJ. Enhancement of platelet function by superoxide anion. *J Clin Invest* 1977; **59,** 959–965.
102. Bryant RW, Simon TC, Bailey JM. Role of glutathione perxidase and hexose monophosphate shunt in the platelet hypoxogenase pathway. *J Biol Chem* 1982; **257,** 14937–14943.
103. Heffner JE, Cook JA, Halushka PV. Human platelets modulate edema formation in isolated rabbit lungs. *J Clin Invest* 1989; **84,** 757–764.
104. Salvemini D, de Nucci G, Sneddon JM, Vane JR. Superoxide anions enhance platelet adhesion and aggregation. *Br J Pharmacol* 1989; **97,** 1145–1150.
105. Johnson D, Travis J. The oxidative inactivation of human α-l-proteins inhibitor: further evidence for methionine at the reactive center. *J Biol Chem* 1979; **254,** 4022–4026.
106. Nathan C. Neutrophil activation on biological surfaces. Massive secretion of hydrogen peroxide in response to products of macrophages and lymphocytes. *J Clin Invest* 1987; **80,** 1550–1560.
107. Kownatzki E, Kapp A, Uhrich S. Modulation of human neutrophilic functions by recombinant human tumor necrosis factor and recombinant human lymphotoxin. Promotion of adherence, inhibition of chemotactic migration and superoxide anion release from adherent cells. *Clin Exp Immunol* 1988; **74,** 143–148.
108. Nathan CF. Respiratory burst in adherent human neutrophils: triggering by colony-stimulating factors CSF-GM and CSF-G. *Blood* 1989; **73,** 301–306.
109. Nathan C, Srimal S, Farber C *et al.* Cytokine-induced respiratory burst of human neutrophils: dependence on extracellular matrix proteins and CD11/CD18 integrins. *J Cell Biol* 1989; **109,** 1341–1349.
110. Ward PA, Cunningham TW, McCulloch KK, Phan SH, Powell J, Johnson KJ. Platelet enhancement of O_2-responses in stimulated human neutrophils. Identification of platelet factor as adenine nucleotide. *Lab Invest* 1988; **58,** 37–47.
111. Gay JC, Beckman JK, Zabog KA, Lukens JN. Modulation of neutrophil oxidative responses to soluble stimuli by PAF. *Blood* 1986; **67,** 931–936.
112. Zoratti EM, Sedgwick JB, Bates ME, Vrtis RF, Geiger K, Busse WW. Platelet-activating factor primes human eosinophil generation of superoxide. *Am J Respir Cell Mol Biol* 1992; **6,** 100–106.
113. Vissers MC, Winterbourne CC. Oxidative damage to fibronectin. I. The effects of the neutrophil myeloperoxidase system and HOCL. *Arch Biochem Biophys* 1991; **285,** 53–59.
114. Rice WG, Weiss SJ. Regulation of proteolysis at the neutrophil-substrate interface by secretory leukoprotease inhibitor. *Science* 1991; **249,** 178–181.
115. Chamba A, Afford SC, Stockley RA, Burnett D. Extracellular proteolysis of fibronectin by neutrophils: characterization and the effects of recombinant cytokines. *Am J Respir Cell Mol Biol* 1991; **4,** 330–337.
116. Weiss SJ, Regiani S. Neutrophils degrade subendothelial matrices in the presence of alpha-1-proteinase inhibitor. Cooperative use of lysosomal proteinases and oxygen metabolites. *J Clin Invest* 1984; **73,** 1297–1303.
117. Shah SV, Baricos WH, Basci A. Degradation of human glomerular basement by stimulated neutrophils. Activation of a metalloproteinase(s) by reactive oxygen metabolites. *J Clin Invest* 1987; **79,** 25–31.
118. Cross CE, Halliwell B, Borish ET *et al.* Oxygen radicals and human disease. *Ann Intern Med* 1987; **107,** 526–545.
119. Lichtenstein A, Ganz T, Selsted M, Lehrer R. Synergistic cytolysis mediated by hydrogen peroxide combined with peptide defensins. *Cell Immunol* 1988; **114,** 104–110.
120. Peters MS, Rodriguez M, Gleich GJ. Localization of human eosinophil major basic protein, eosinophil cationic protein and eosinophil-derived neurotoxin by immunoelectron microscopy. *Lab Invest* 1986; **54,** 656–662.
121. Barker RL, Loegering DA, Arakawa KC, Pease LA, Gleich GJ. Cloning and sequence analysis of the human gene encoding eosinophil major basic protein. *Gene* 1990; **86,** 285–289.
122. Lehrer RI, Szklarek D, Barton A, Ganz T, Hamann KJ, Gleich GJ. Antibacterial properties of eosinophil major basic protein and eosinophil cationic protein. *J Immunol* 1989; **142,** 4428–4434.
123. Gleich GJ, Frigas E, Loegering DA, Wassom DL, Steinmuller D. Cytotoxic properties of the eosinophil major basic protein. *J Immunol* 1979; **123,** 2925–2927.
124. O'Donnell MC, Ackerman SJ, Gleich GJ, Thomas LL. Activation of basophil and mast cell histamine release by eosinophil granule major basic protein. *J Exp Med* 1983; **157,** 1981–1991.
125. Ackerman SJ, Gleich GJ, Loegering DA, Richardson BA, Butterworth AE. Comparative toxicity of purified human eosinophil granule cationic proteins for schistosomula of *Schistosoma mansoni. Am J Trop Med Hyg* 1985; **34,** 735–745.
126. Durack DT, Sumi SM, Klebanoff SJ. Neurotoxicity of human eosinophils. *Proc Nat Acad Sci USA* 1979; **76,** 1443–1447.
127. Hamann KJ, Barker RL, Loegering DA, Pease

LR, Gleich GJ. Nucleotide sequence of human eosinophil-derived neurotoxin cDNA: identity of deduced amino acid sequence with certain human non-secretory ribonucleases. *Gene* 1989; **83,** 161–167.

128. Young JDE, Peterson CGB, Venge P, Cohn ZA. Mechanism of membrane damage mediated by human eosinophil cationic protein. *Nature* 1986; **321,** 613–616.
129. Abu-Ghazaleh R, Fujisawa T, Mestecky J, Kyle RA, Gleich GJ. IgA-induced eosinophil degranulation. *J Immunol* 1989; **142,** 2393–2400.
130. Fujisawa T, Abu-Ghazaleh R, Kita H, Sanderson CJ, Gleich GJ. Regulatory effect of cytokines on eosinophil degranulation. *J Immunol* 1990; **144,** 642–646.
131. Pohl J, Pereira HA, Martin NM, Spitznaegel JK. Amino acid sequence of CAP 37, a human neutrophil granule-derived antibacterial and monocyte-specific chemotactic glycoprotein structurally similar to neutrophil elastase. *FEBS Lett* 1990; **272,** 200–204.
132. Pereira HA, Spitznaegel JK, Winton EF *et al.* The ontogeny of a 57-kD cationic antimicrobial protein of human polymorphonuclear leukocytes: localization to a novel granule population. *Blood* 1990; **76,** 825–834.
133. Selsted ME, Harwig SS. Determination of the disulphide array in the human defensin HNP-2. *J Biol Chem* 1989; **264,** 4003–4007.
134. Selsted ME, Harwig SSL, Granz T, Schilling JW, Lehrer RI. Primary structure of three human neutrophil defensins. *J Clin Invest* 1985; **76,** 1436–1439.
135. Wilde GC, Griffith JE, Marra MN, Snable JL, Scott RW. Purification and characterization of human neutrophil peptide 4, a new member of the defensin family. *J Biol Chem* 1989; **264,** 11200–11203.
136. Ganz T, Selsted ME, Lehrer RI. Defensins. *Eur J Haematol* 1990; **44,** 1–8.
137. Lambert J, Keppi E, Dimarcq JL *et al.* Insect immunity: isolation from the blood of the dipteran *Phormia terranovae* of two insect antibacterial peptides with sequence homology to rabbit lung macrophage bactericidal peptides. *Proc Nat Acad Sci USA* 1989; **86,** 262–266.
138. Lehrer RI, Barton A, Daher KA, Harwig SS, Ganz T. Interaction of human defensins with *Escherichia coli*: mechanism of bactricidal activity. *J Clin Invest* 1989; **84,** 553–561.
139. Okrent DG, Lichtenstein AK, Ganz T. Direct cytotoxicity of polymorphonuclear leukocyte granule proteins to human lung-derived cells and endothelial cells. *Am Rev Respir Dis* 1990; **141,** 179–185.
140. Lichtenstein A. Mechanism of mammalian cell lysis mediated by peptide defensins. Evidence for an initial alteration of the plasma membrane. *J Clin Invest* 1991; **88,** 93–100.
141. Ganz T. Extracellular release of antimicrobial defensins by polymorphonuclear leukocytes. *Infect Immunity* 1987; **55,** 568–571.
142. Campbell EJ, Campbell MA. Pericellular proteolysis by neutrophils in the presence of proteinase inhibitors: effects of substrate opsonization. *J Cell Biol* 1988; **106,** 667–676.
143. Panyutich A, Ganz T. Activated α2-macroglobulin is a principal defensin-binding protein. *Am J Respir Cell Mol Biol* 1991; **5,** 101–106.
144. Caughey GH. The structure and airway biology of mast cell proteinases. *Am J Respir Cell Mol Biol* 1991; **4,** 387–394.
145. Wilde CG, Snable JL, Griffith JE, Scott RW. Characterization of two azurophil granule proteases with active-site homology to neutrophil elastase. *J Biol Chem* 1990; **265,** 2038–2041.
146. Campanelli D, Detmers PA, Nathan CF, Gabay JE. Azurocidin and a homologous serine protease from neutrophils. Differential antimicrobial and proteolytic properties. *J Clin Invest* 1990; **85,** 904–915.
147. Jenne DE, Tschopp J, Ludemann J, Utecht B, Gross WL. Wegener's autoantigen decoded. *Nature* 1990; **346,** 520.
148. Salvesen G, Farley D, Shuman J, Przybyla A, Reilly C, Travis J. Molecular cloning of human cathepsin G: structural similarity to mast cell and cytotoxic T lymphocyte proteinases. *Biochemistry* 1987; **26,** 2289–2293.
149. Jenne D, Rey C, Haeflinger JA, Qiao BY, Groscurth P, Tschopp J. Identification and sequencing of cDNA clones encoding the granule-associated serine protease granzymes D, E, and F of cytolytic T lymphocytes. *Proc Nat Acad Sci USA* 1988; **85,** 4814–4818.
150. Salvesen G, Enghild JJ. An unusual specificity in the activation of neutrophil serine proteinase zymogens. *Biochemistry* 1990; **29,** 5304–5308.
151. Schwartz LB, Metcalfe DD, Miller JS, Earl H, Sullivan T. Tryptase levels as an indicator of mast cell activation in systemic anaphylaxis and mastocytosis. *N Engl J Med* 1987; **316,** 1622–1626.
152. Wenzel SE, Fowler AA, Schwartz LB. Activation of pulmonary mast cells by bronchoalveolar allergen challenge. *In vivo* release of histamine and tryptase in atopic subjects with and without asthma. *Am Rev Respir Dis* 1988; **137,** 1002–1008.
153. Ruoss SJ, Hartmann T, Caughey GH. Mast cell tryptase is a mitogen for cultured fibroblasts. *J Clin Invest* 1991; **88,** 493–499
154. Heck LW, Blackburn WD, Irwin MH, Abrahamson DR. Degradation of basement membrane laminin by human neutrophil elastase and

cathepsin G. *Am J Pathol* 1990; **136,** 1267–1274.

155. Pipoly DJ, Crouch EC. Degradation of native type IV procollagen by human neutrophil elastase. Implications for leukocyte-mediated degradation of basement membrane. *Biochemistry* 1987; **26,** 5748–5754.
156. McGowan SE. Mechanisms of extracellular matrix proteoglycan degradation by human neutrophils. *Am J Respir Cell Mol Biol* 1990; **2,** 271–279.
157. Weiss SJ. Tissue destruction by neutrophils. *N Engl J Med* 1989; **320,** 365–376.
158. Boudier C, Holle C, Bieth JG. Stimulation of the elastolytic activity of leucocyte elastase by leucocyte cathepsin G. *J Biol Chem* 1981; **256,** 10256–10258.
159. Selak MA, Chignard M, Smith JB. Cathepsin G is a strong platelet agonist released by neutrophils. *Biochem J* 1988; **251,** 293–299.
160. Kao RC, Wehner NG, Skubitz KM, Gray BH, Hoidal JR. Proteinase 3. A distinct human polymorphonuclear leukocyte proteinase that produces emphysema in hamsters. *J Clin Invest* 1988; **82,** 1963–1973.
161. Weiss SJ, Peppin G, Ortiz X, Ragsdale C, Test ST. Oxidative autoactivation of latent collagenase by human neutrophils. *Science* 1985; **227,** 747–749.
162. Peppin GJ, Weiss SJ. Activation of the endogenous metalloproteinase, gelatinase, by triggered human neutrophils. *Proc Nat Acad Sci USA* 1986; **83,** 4322–4326.
163. Hibbs MS, Bainton DF. Human neutrophil gelatinase is a component of specific granules. *J Clin Invest* 1989; **84,** 1395–1402.
164. Dewald B, Bretz U, Baggiolini M. Release of gelatinase from a novel secretory compartment of human neutrophils. *J Clin Invest* 1982; **70,** 518–525.
165. Wilhelm SM, Collier IE, Kronberger A *et al.* Human skin fibroblast stromelysin: structure, glycosylation, substrate specificity and differential expression in normal and tumorigenic cells. *Proc Nat Acad Sci USA* 1987; **84,** 6725–6729.
166. Wilhem SE, Murphy G, Angel P *et al.* Comparison of human stromelysin and collagenase by cloning and sequence analysis. *Biochem J* 1986; **240,** 913–916.
167. Wilhelm SM, Collier IE, Marmer BL, Eisen AZ, Grant GA, Goldberg GI. SV40-transformed human lung fibroblasts secrete a 92-kDa type IV collagenase which is identical to that secreted by normal human macrophages. *J Biol Chem* 1989; **264,** 17213–17221.
168. Hibbs MS, Hoidal JR, Kang AH. Expression of a metalloproteinase that degrades native type V collagen and denatured collagens by cultured human alveolar macrophages. *J Clin Invest* 1987; **80,** 1644–1650.
169. Welgus HG, Campbell EJ, Cury JD *et al.* Neutral metalloproteinases produced by human mononuclear phagocytes. Enzyme profile, regulation, and expression during cellular development. *J Clin Invest* 1990; **86,** 1496–1502.
170. Banda MJ, Werb Z. Mouse macrophage elastase. Purification and characterization as a metalloproteinase. *Biochem J* 1981; **193,** 589–605.
171. Sandhaus RA, McCarthy KM, Musson RA, Henson PM. Elastolytic proteinases of the human macrophage. *Chest* 1983; **83** (suppl), 60–62.
172. Green MR, Lin JS, Berman LB *et al.* Elastolytic activity of alveolar macrophages in normal dogs and human subjects. *J Lab Clin Med* 1979; **94,** 549–562.
173. Hinman LM, Stevens CA, Matthay RA, Gee JBL. Elastase and lysosomal activities in human alveolar macrophages. Effects of cigarette smoking. *Am Rev Respir Dis* 1980; **121,** 263–271.
174. De Cremoux H, Hornebeck W, Jourand MC, Bignon J, Robert L. Partial characterization of an elastase-like enzyme secreted by human and monkey alveolar macrophages. *J Pathol* 1978; **125,** 171–177.
175. Burnett D, Afford SC, Campbell EJ, Rios-Mollineda RA, Buttle DJ, Stockley RA. Evidence for lipid-associated serine proteases and metalloproteases in human bronchoalveolar lavage fluid. *Clin Sci* 1988; **75,** 601–607.
176. Kargi HA, Campbell EJ, Kuhn C. Elastase and cathepsin G of human monocytes: heterogeneity and subcellular localization to peroxidase-positive granules. *J Histochem Cytochem* 1990; **38,** 1179–1186.
177. Senior RM, Connolly NL, Campbell EJ, Welgus HG, Burnett D. Human mononuclear phagocytes produce different proteinases at different stages of differentiation: observations with TPA-differentiated U-937 cells. In: *Pulmonary Emphysema and Proteolysis: 1986*, Taylor JC, Mittman C (eds). London: Academic Press Ltd, 1987.
178. Senior RM, Connolly NL, Cury JD, Welgus HG, Campbell EJ. Elastin degradation by human alveolar macrophages. A prominent role of metalloproteinase activity. *Am Rev Respir Dis* 1989; **139,** 1251–1256.
179. Senior RM, Griffin GLL, Fliszar CJ, Shapiro SD, Goldberg GI, Welgus HG. Human 92- and 72-kilodalton type IV collagenases are elastases. *J Biol Chem* 1991; **266,** 7870–7875.
180. Morland B. Cathepsin B activity in human blood monocytes during differentiation *in vitro*. *Scand J Immunol* 1985; **22,** 9–16.
181. Howie AJ, Burnett D, Crocker J. The distri-

bution of cathepsin B in human tissues. *J Pathol* 1985; **145,** 307–314.

182. Reilly JJ, Mason RW, Chen P *et al.* Synthesis and processing of cathepsin L, an elastase, by human alveolar macrophages. *Biochem J* 1989; **257,** 493–498.
183. Burleigh MC, Barrett AJ, Lazarus GS. Cathepsin B1. A lysosomal enzyme that degrades native collagen. *Biochem J* 1974; **137,** 387–389.
184. Roughley PJ. The degradation of cartilage proteoglycans by tissue proteinases. *Biochem J* 1977; **167,** 639–646.
185. Mason RW, Johnson DA, Barrett AJ, Chapman HA. Elastinolytic activity of human cathepsin L. *Biochem J* 1986; **233,** 925–927.
186. Barrett AJ. Cathepsin B, cathepsin H and cathepsin L. *Methods Enzymol* 1981; **80,** 535–561.
187. Chapman HA, Reilly JJ, Kobzik L. Role of plasminogen activator in degradation of extracellular matrix protein by live human alveolar macrophages. *Am Rev Respir Dis* 1988; **137,** 412–419.
188. Lesser M, Chang JC, Galicki NI, Edelman J, Cardozo C. Cathepsin B and D activity in alveolar macrophages from rats with pulmonary granulomatous inflammation or acute lung injury. *Agents Actions* 1989; **28,** 264–271.
189. Leoncini G, Balestrero F, Maresca M. Lysosomal enzymes in human blood platelets. *Cell Biochem Funct* 1985; **3,** 121–126.
190. James HL, Wachtfogel YT, James PL, Zimmerman M, Colman RW, Cohen AB. A unique elastase in human blood platelets. *J Clin Invest* 1985; **76,** 2330–2337.
191. Ozaki Y, Ohashi T, Kume S. Potentiation of neutrophil function by recombinant DNA-produced interleukin 1a. *J Leuk Biol* 1987; **42,** 621–627.
192. Kapp A, Zeck-Kapp G, Danner M, Luger TA. Human granulocyte-macrophage colony stimulating factor: an effective direct activator of human polymorphonuclear neutrophilic granulocytes. *J Invest Dermatol* 1988; **91,** 49–55.
193. Ozaki Y, Ohashi T, Niwa Y, Kume S. Effect of recombinant DNA-produced tumor necrosis factor on various parameters of neutrophil function. *Inflammation* 1988; **2,** 297–309.
194. Yonemaru M, Stephens KE, Ishizaka A *et al.* Effects of tumor necrosis factor on PMN chemotaxis, chemoluminescence, and elastase activity. *J Lab Clin Med* 1989; **114,** 674–681.
195. Schalkwijk J, van den Berg WB, van de Putte LBA, Joosten LAB. Elastase secreted by activated polymorphonuclear leucocytes causes chondrocyte damage and matrix degradation in intact articular cartilage: escape from inactivation by alpha-1-proteinase inhibitor. *Br J Exp Pathol* 1986; **68,** 81–88.
196. Burnett D, Chamba A, Hill SL, Stockley RA. Neutrophils from subjects with chronic obstructive lung disease show enhanced chemotaxis and extracellular proteolysis. *Lancet* 1987; **2,** 1043–1046.
197. Burnett D, Chamba A, Hill SL, Stockley RA. Effects of plasma, tumour necrosis factor, endotoxin and dexamethasone on extracellular proteolysis by neutrophils from healthy subjects and patients with emphysema. *Clin Sci* 1989; **77,** 35–41.
198. Sandhaus RA. Elastase may play a central role in neutrophil migration through connective tissue. In: *Pulmonary Emphysema and Proteolysis: 1986*, Taylor JC, Mittman C (eds). London: Academic Press Ltd, 1987.
199. Silver IA, Murrills RJ, Etherington DJ. Microelectrode studies on the acid environment beneath adherent macrophages and osteoclasts. *Exp Cell Res* 1988; **175,** 266–276.
200. Barrett AJ, Rawlings ND, Davies ME, Machleidt W, Salvesen G, Turk V. Cysteine proteinase inhibitors of the cystatin superfamily. In: *Research Monographs in Cell and Tissue Physiology. Vol. 12: Proteinase Inhibitors*, Barrett AJ, Salvesen G (eds). Amsterdam: Elsevier, 1986.
201. Albin RJ, Senior RM, Welgus HG, Connolly NL, Campbell EJ. Human alveolar macrophages secrete an inhibitor of metalloproteinase elastase *in vitro*. *Am Rev Respir Dis* 1987; **135,** 1281–1285.
202. Stetler-Stevenson WG, Krutzsch HC, Liotta LA. Tissue inhibitor of metalloproteinase (TIMP-2). A new member of the metalloproteinase inhibitor family. *J Biol Chem* 1989; **264,** 17374–17378.
203. Wright SD, Silverstein SC. Phagocytosing macrophages exclude proteins from the zones of contact with opsonised targets. *Nature* 1984; **309,** 359–361.
204. Haslett C, Henson PM. Resolution of inflammation. In: *The Molecular and Cellular Biology of Wound Repair*, Clark RAF, Henson PM (eds). New York: Plenum Publishing, 1988.
205. Wyllie AH, Kerr JFR, Currie AR. Cell death: the significance of apoptosis. *Int Rev Cytol* 1980; **68,** 251–306.
206. Alison MR, Sarraf CE. Apoptosis: a gene-directed programme of cell death. *J Roy Coll Physicians Lond* 1992; **26,** 25–35.
207. Newman SL, Henson JE, Henson PM. Phagocytosis of senescent neutrophils by human monocyte-derived macrophages and rabbit inflammatory macrophages. *J Exp Med* 1982; **156,** 430–442.
208. Savill JS, Wyllie AH, Henson JE, Walport MJ, Henson PM, Haslett C. Macrophage phagocytosis of aging neutrophils in inflammation. Programmed cell death in the neutrophil leads to its

recognition by macrophages. *J Clin Invest* 1989; **83,** 865–875.

209. Savill JS, Dransfield I, Hogg N, Haslett C. Vitronectin receptor-mediated phagocytosis of cells undergoing apoptosis. *Nature* 1990; **343,** 170–173.

210. Grigg JM, Savill JS, Sarraf C, Haslett C, Silverman M. Neutrophil apoptosis and clearance from neonatal lungs. *Lancet* 1991; **338,** 720–722.

211. Stern M, Meagher L, Savill J, Haslett C. Eosinophils undergo apoptosis and are recognised and ingested as whole cells by macrophages. *Am Rev Respir Dis* 1991; **143** (suppl), A331 (abstract).

212. Tai PC, Sun L, Spry CJ. Effects of IL-5, granulocyte/macrophage colony-stimulating factor (GM-CSF) and IL-3 on the survival of human blood eosinophils *in vitro*. *Clin Exp Immunol* 1991; **85,** 312–316.

213. Whyte MKB, Meagher LCM, Haslett C. Modulation of programmed cell death (apoptosis) in the neutrophil. *Am Rev Respir Dis* 1991; **143** (suppl), A330 (abstract).

214. Martin SJ, Lennon SV, Bonham AM, Cotter TG. Induction of apoptosis (programmed cell death) in human leukemic HL-60 cells by inhibition of RNA or protein synthesis. *J Immunol* 1990; **145,** 1859–1867.

4

Inflammatory cytokines

C Dinarello

Introduction

The polypeptide cytokines interleukin-1 (IL-1) and tumour necrosis factor (TNF) affect nearly every tissue and organ system, induce the expression of a variety of genes and synthesis of several proteins which, in turn, induce acute and chronic inflammatory changes. IL-1 and TNF are often implicated as key mediators of the biological responses to lipopolysaccharide (LPS), infection and inflammatory stimulants. Most studies on the biology of IL-1 and TNF have been carried out by injecting either cytokine into animals but human subjects have also been injected with recombinant IL-1 or TNF and the results confirm that the injection of either cytokine can mimic a disease state, particularly acute infection or inflammation. However, in either situation, the biological responses of humans or experimental animals to LPS can also result in the synthesis of other cytokines, which could mediate the host response to infection and inflammation. A good example of this is the cytokine IL-8, which causes neutrophil infiltration and activation. Is there a role for IL-8 and other related cytokines in the host response to infection which is independent of IL-1 and TNF? How much of the response to infection or injury is, in fact, due to either IL-1 or TNF? Although various agents for reducing the synthesis and/or for antagonising the effects of IL-1 and TNF have been proposed, the recent cloning of a naturally occurring IL-1 receptor antagonist (IL-1ra) and the finding of a naturally occurring soluble receptor for TNF have allowed examination of the extent of the biological responses to disease that are altered by specific blockade of IL-1 or TNF. The ability of the IL-1ra to block IL-1 key receptors in animals without agonist activities has reduced the severity of diseases in which LPS plays a prominent role, such as *E. coli* shock, lethal bacterial sepsis, inflammatory bowel disease, and the cellular infiltration following LPS. Similarly, blocking TNF with anti-TNF antibodies or soluble TNF receptors has reduced susceptibility to infection in mice and baboons. These results demonstrate that both IL-1 and TNF play essential roles in mediating responses to infection and inflammation.

Interleukin-1

Interleukin-1 (IL-1) is the term for two polypeptides (IL-1α and IL-1β) that possess a wide spectrum of inflammatory, metabolic, physiological, haematopoietic, and immunological properties. Although both forms of IL-1 are distinct gene products, they recognise the same cell surface receptors and share biological activities. With the exception of skin keratinocytes, some epithelial cells and certain cells in the central nervous system, significant amounts of mRNA coding for IL-1 are not observed in health in most other cells. However, there is a dramatic increase in IL-1 production by a variety of cells in response to infection, microbial toxins, inflammatory agents, products of activated lymphocytes, complement, and clotting components. In some diseases, notably myeloid leukemia, the IL-1β gene appears to be spontaneously expressed.

IL-1 was originally described in the 1940s as a heat-labile protein found in acute granulocytic exudate fluid, which, when injected into animals or humans, produced fever. At that time, it was called endogenous pyrogen.[1] When injected into animals, endogenous pyrogen caused decreases in plasma iron and zinc levels, produced neutrophilia, induced the appearance of a colony stimulating activity, and triggered the synthesis of hepatic amyloid A protein. Several substances originally described for their biological activities have been indentified as IL-1. 'Lymphocyte activating factors', described by Gery, Waksman and Bach, were macrophage products which augmented thymocyte proliferation to mitogens. It was subsequently demonstrated that homogeneous, purified endogenous pyrogen also augmented T cell responses to mitogens[2] and hence 'lymphocyte activating factor' appeared to be a property of the endogenous pyrogen molecule (reviewed in ref 3.) Leucocytic endogenous mediator[4,5] mononuclear cell factor,[6] catabolin,[7] osteoclast activating factor,[8] haemopoietin-1,[9] lymphocyte proliferation promoting factor of neutrophils,[10] melanoma growth inhibition factor,[11] and tumour inhibitory factor-2[12] have all been shown to be IL-1.

Considerable interest has focused on IL-1 as a mediator of the systemic 'acute phase' responses. A single injection of 10–100 ng/kg of either IL-1 form into experimental animals results in fever, neutrophilia, increased circulating levels of colony stimulating factors, IL-6, hypozincaemia, hypoferraemia, increased hepatic acute phase proteins synthesis, decreased albumin, anorexia, sleep, ACTH release and other manifestations of the response. At higher doses (5 μg/kg), IL-1 induces hypotension and leucopenia. Recent phase I clinical trials of intravenously administered IL-1 (10 ng–1 μg/kg) have confirmed the systemic effects of IL-1 reported in animals, particularly fever and hypotension.[13,14]

Genomic organisation of IL-1

Two IL-1 cDNAs were cloned in 1984; IL-1β was cloned from human blood monocytes[15] and IL-1α from the mouse macrophage line P388D.[16] These two forms correspond to the two forms of endogenous pyrogen that were described by their distinct iso-electric points;[17] IL-1β has a pI of 7.2 and IL-1α a pI of 5.3. Subsequent to the description of these two cDNAs, IL-1α or β have been cloned for the human, cow, pig, rabbit, rat and mouse. The entire genomic sequences for each IL-1 form have also been reported; the human IL-1β gene is 7.8 kb[18] and the human IL-1α is 10.5 kb.[19] Each gene contains seven exons coding for the processed IL-1 mRNA. The 3′ end contains a 7 nucleotide repetitive motif shared by other LPS-inducible cytokines;[20] these sequences may cause mRNA instability which is 'stabilised' by LPS. The genes for IL-1β and IL-1α are located on chromosome 2.[21]

Protein structure of IL-1

Within the various animal species of mature IL-1β, the sequence of amino acids is conserved in the range of 75–78% whereas the α sequence is conserved 60–70%. Comparison between the β and α forms of IL-1 within each species, however, reveals that the amino acid homology is only 25%. Although both IL-1β and α have glycosylation sites, glycosylation by expression in yeast has not increased specific activity over that of the non-glycosylated form.[22]

Since IL-1β and IL-1α trigger the same receptors, some regions of each form may contain minimal structural requirements for receptor activation. Four approaches have been employed to investigate this, using (1) biological activity of synthetic subpeptides; (2) antibodies to synthetic subpeptides; (3) site-specific mutagenesis, and (4) X-ray crystallographic analysis. In each experimental approach, T cells and fibroblasts which express the p80 or IL-1 receptor type I (IL-1RtI) have been used to assess biological activity or receptor binding. Although IL-1 subpeptides have some biological activity, their specific activities are low. The carboxyl terminal of the mature IL-1β appears to retain some biological activity.[23] A subpeptide of IL-1β from 208–240 (amino acid number refers to pro-IL-1) possesses sleep and pyrogenic properties but lacks T cell activation[24] whereas subpeptide 237–269 antagonises mature IL-1 effects on T cells.[25] A nonapeptide consisting of residues 163–171 activates T cells, stimulates glycosaminoglycan synthesis, is an adjuvant and recruits anti-tumour reactivity *in vivo*, but lacks pro-inflammatory and pyrogenic properties.[26,27] A pentapeptide (165–169) is highly exposed and is more potent than the nonapeptide.[27] A 21 amino acid subpeptide of human IL-1β (165–186) exhibits fibroblast activity.[28]

Data from site-directed mutagenesis suggest that the two cysteine residues in mature IL-1β are required for full activity,[29] whereas the exposed lysines are not.[30] In general, the various muteins generated by specific amino acid substitutions have not changed the overall structure of IL-1 determined by circular dichroism or proton magnetic resonance. The effects of site-specific mutagenesis on IL-1 activity and receptor binding have been reviewed.[31] The histidine at position 146 or the single tryptophan in IL-1β is required for biological and receptor-binding activity.[32] N-terminal mutations have also yielded muteins of IL-1β with altered biological and receptor-binding activity[33,34,35,36] suggesting that N-terminal amino acids, particularly the arginine at 120, play an important role in either stabilising the tertiary structure or by direct interaction with receptor-binding domains. A single point substitution in the human IL-1β of arginine 127 to glycine results in a 100-fold loss in biological activity on T cells without diminishing receptor-ligand binding.[37]

Attempts to separate the immunostimulatory from pro-inflammatory properties have yielded several IL-1 muteins. Substitution of arginine to glycine at position 120 of IL-1β results in a mutein which is devoid of any pyrogenic property but retains the ability to stimulate ACTH release.[38] Changing the aspartic acid at position 151 to tyrosine in the mature IL-1α results in loss of PGE_2 induction and fibroblast growth but retention of T cell responses.[39] This mutein also antagonises IL-1α and β induction of PGE_2 and functions like a receptor antagonist.

Mature human IL-1β has been crystallised and its tertiary structure analysed at a resolution of 2 and 3 A.[31,40] The three-dimensional analysis reveals 12 β strands held together by hydrogen bonds. Well-conserved amino acids are on the surface of the molecule. Two amino acids (glutamic acid at 212 and proline at 234) have >35% of their side chains accessible to solvent.[31] The glutamic acid could be critical for biological effects since selective destruction of glutamic acid residues results in dramatic loss of biological activity.[41] The nonapeptide (163–171) corresponds to a loop between β strands 4 and 5. The overall folding of the 12 β strands is similar to that found in the soybean trypsin inhibitor but there is no biological activity of the molecule.[42]

Control of transcription

The amount of IL-1β mRNA found in stimulated human peripheral blood mononuclear cells (PBMC) is usually 25- to 50-fold greater than the α form.[43] The two forms of IL-1 appear to be under separate transcriptional control.[44,45] A critical aspect of understanding IL-1 gene expression in a variety of cells is the exquisite sensitivity to LPS. This is particularly the case with human blood monocytes, which synthesise IL-1 when stimulated by 10–20 pg/ml of LPS; routine tissue culture media often contain this and greater amounts of LPS. In order to evaluate IL-1 transcription and translation, water and tissue culture media should be subjected to ultrafiltration by hydrophobic membranes to remove exogenous IL-1-inducing substances.[46] Using these conditions, there is no evidence of IL-1β or α gene expression in circulating PBMC of healthy subjects by northern hybridisation, *in situ* hybridisation or polymerase chain reaction. However, adherence of PBMC to glass or polystyrene triggers IL-1β gene expression, but, in the strict absence of LPS, gene expression occurs without translation into IL-1 protein.[47] Circulating human blood in plastic tubing at 200 ml/minute for four hours at 37°C under strict LPS-free conditions does not trigger transcription.[48] Numerous reports of 'spontaneous' IL-1 production in various disease states such as AIDS or in the laboratory by infection of mononuclear cells with the HIV are likely to be artifactual because of the LPS contamination.[49,50,51]

Using LPS and other microbial products, transcription of IL-1β mRNA is rapid; in macrophage cell lines, endothelial, smooth muscle, and blood mononuclear cells, LPS-stimulated IL-1β mRNA transcription is observed within 15 minutes.[47,52,53,54,55] Following stimulation by LPS, peak accumulation of IL-1β mRNA occurs at 3–4 hours, is sustained for 6–8 hours and then decreases rapidly. Studies suggest that there is synthesis of a transcriptional repressor as well as increases in the half-life of the mRNA.[54,55] On the other hand, using IL-1 as a stimulus of its own gene expression, steady state levels are slower to rise and are sustained for 30 hours.[56]

Translational control

Transcription and translation of IL-1 are distinct and dissociated processes. Transcription without translation can be observed following adherence of blood monocytes to surfaces, or exposure to recombinant C5a, β-glucan polymers, or calcium ionophore;[45,47,48,57] in each case, steady state mRNA levels for IL-1β are comparable to those using 1 ng/ml of LPS but unlike LPS, there is no translation of the IL-1 mRNA into protein. The half-life of mRNA is unchanged using these stimuli, suggesting that accelerated destruction of mRNA is not the explanation for the failure of translation.[57] Cells containing untranslated IL-1 mRNA are 'primed' and small amounts of other stimuli (LPS or IL-1 itself) rapidly trigger translation and usually result in more IL-1 synthesis than non-primed cells. Another stimulus, heat-killed *Staphyloccocus epidermidis*, delivers a primarily translational signal.[47]

Processing of pro-IL-1

The first translation product of IL-1 is the pro-IL-1 31-KDa precursor. Without a clear signal peptide, a considerable amount of the pro-IL-1 that is synthesised remains cell associated.[58,59,60] The localisation of cell associated IL-1 is almost entirely cytoplasmic, rather than in the endoplasmic reticulum, Golgi, or plasma membrane fraction.[61,62] There is evidence that cytosolic IL-1 can be localised to non-clathrin coated vesicles,[61] microtubules,[63] or lysosomes.[64] Pro-IL-1α but not IL-1β is phosphorylated at serine 90[65,66] and presumably phosphorylated pro-IL-1α would be more resistant to proteolytic cleavage or transport to the extracellular space, although there is no direct evidence to support this explanation. The half-life of cell associated IL-1α is 15 hours whereas that of IL-1β is 2.5 hours.[67]

The amount of IL-1 that is 'secreted' depends upon the cell type and the conditions of stimulation. The monocyte/macrophage appears to be efficient in its secretion of IL-1β compared to endothelial, smooth muscle cells and fibroblasts. As much as 70% of the IL-1β is secreted by PBMC in 24 hours whereas IL-1α remains cell associated during the first 20 hours. Increasing the content of plasma proteases in the culture medium does not change the secretion of IL-1α.[59] Unlike stimulation by LPS, IL-1β induction by IL-1α or IL-2 remains cell associated.[68,69]

It is still unclear how IL-1 is transported from the cytosol to the extracellular compartment and how it is cleaved to its mature peptides. Secretion of the 31 KDa IL-1 precursor and processing to its mature peptide appear to be linked events, although studies suggest that pro-IL-1β is secreted intact and then later cleaved by various enzymes present in inflammatory tissue.[58,67,70] Mature IL-1β has an N-terminus at the alanine position 117[71] but other naturally occurring N-termini have been reported.[72] Pro-IL-1β and a 22 KDa partially cleaved peptide are found in the supernates of monocytes,[58,73] demonstrating that the pro-IL-1β is secreted prior to generation of the mature peptide. Some stimuli selectively increase secretion and processing, as originally proposed by Igal Gery, such as phagocytic stimuli and calcium ionophores.[74] Murine pro-IL-1α can be mannosylated[75] and both human pro-IL-1α and IL-1β can be myristylated.[76] These metabolic alterations to the IL-1 precursors are likely to facilitate the localisation of IL-1 to subcellular compartments such as the lysosomes[64] or transport to the plasma membrane.

Elastase, plasmin, cathepsin G, collagenase and serine proteases as well as the surface enkephalinase have been implicated in the cleavage of pro-IL-1β into its 17.5 KDa mature carboxyl fragment.[58,74,77,78,79] A monocyte specific protease has been described that specifically cleaves IL-1β at the alanine position.[80] This protease is not found in fibroblasts but rather in monocytes and monocyte cell lines. Blockade of specific pro-IL-1 processing enzymes has been proposed as a possible strategy for preventing the effects of IL-1 in disease. Zidovudine decreases the amount of IL-1β secreted by human monocytes without affecting the total synthesis of IL-1.[81] However, there appears to be more than a single protease which cleaves the precursor into active IL-1 peptides.[70]

A calcium activated neutral protease (calpain, EC 3.4.22.17) has been described which processes IL-1α.[82] Inhibitors of serine proteases prevent the appearance of mature and smaller molecular weight IL-1 peptides.[58] The 17.5 KDa IL-1 mature peptide, as well as other subfragments detected by bio-assay following gel filtration,[83] are routinely found in human plasma, urine, and peritoneal, pleural and joint fluids. These fragments are probably cleaved via trypsin sensitive sites. Human IL-1β contains several cleavage sites for serine proteases. In preparations of recombinant IL-1, we have identified a 5488-Da C-terminal peptide, generated at the lysine-lysine-lysine site of human IL-1β, which could represent the active C-terminal fragment.[25]

Membrane IL-1

IL-1 activity has been described after fixation of macrophages and called 'membrane bound' IL-1.[84] 'Membrane bound' IL-1 is active on lymphocyte and several non-lymphocytic cells. The 'membrane' IL-1 appears to be almost exclusively IL-1α in that histochemical and neutralising antibodies to IL-1α rather than IL-1β have been effective. In addition to macrophages, membrane IL-1 has been detected on endothelial and dendritic cells and fibroblasts. A biochemical mechanism for pro-IL-1α anchoring to the cell membrane has been proposed via lectin-like binding since D-mannose dissociates the activity and the immunoprecipitable IL-1.[75] Alternatively, IL-1α may be bound to its surface receptor as has been shown for TNF.[85] Recent controversy has focussed on whether membrane IL-1 is a functioning integral membrane protein or whether the bio-activity of membrane IL-1 is due to leakage of IL-1 from inadequately fixed cells. Studies by Mizel and others have shown that 1% paraformaldehyde fixation for 15 minutes at room temperature results in IL-1 leakage.[77,86] Other investigators have shown that following this standard fixation method, IL-1 (β and α) is secreted, although in decreasing amounts, for up to 96 hours. However, macrophages tested for biological activity 144 hours after fixation continue to retain T cell stimulating activity which is specifically neutralised by anti-IL-1α,[87] suggesting that membrane IL-1 is still present. It is unclear how membrane IL-1 is oriented on the surface of the cell so that its structural components are available for binding to IL-1 receptors.

IL-1 receptors

The initial studies on the binding of radio-labelled IL-1 were carried out using a variety of cells in which there appeared to be a single class of intermediate affinity receptor (KDa ranging from 200 pM to 1 nM) and relatively few receptors (200/cell). Although the IL-1 receptor(s) was specific in that it did not recognise other cytokines, the binding did not distinguish between IL-1α or IL-1β. Either IL-1α or IL-1β competed for binding of each other on T and fibroblast cell lines. In general, the binding correlated with the capacity of the cells to respond to IL-1, although this was not always the case. Subsequently, cell lines were found which expressed unusually high numbers of receptors (5–20,000);[88,89] however, in general, non-transformed cells taken from fresh tissues or circulating blood leucocytes express few receptors (100–200 per cell) and this low number of IL-1R expressed on responding cells represents one of the fundamental aspects of the biology of IL-1.

Cross-linking of radio-labelled IL-1 revealed that there were several proteins which specifically bound IL-1 at 30, 68, 80, 105 and 220 KDa. Of these, two molecular weight IL-1 binding proteins were prominent. On T cells and fibroblasts, an 80 KDa IL-1 receptor was consistently observed whereas B cell lines possessed a 68 KDa IL-1 binding protein. These two binding proteins have now been shown to be separate gene products;[90,91] they are recognised as the two major IL-1 receptor molecules. The p80 IL-1R is called the IL-1RtI and the p68 is the IL-1RtII. The other molecular weight IL-1 binding proteins (putative receptors)[89,92] may be related to either the p80 or p68 receptor or represent other IL-1 receptors or associated binding proteins as is the case with IL-2R. The 105 KDa IL-1 binding protein may represent a heavily glycosylated IL-1R and the 220 KDa, observed by many investigators, may be a dimer of the IL-1RtI with IL-1 as cross-linking ligand, similar to the case for the TNF, fibroblast growth factor and the platelet derived growth factor receptors.

Compared to other cytokines such as the interferons and colony stimulating factors, there is little species specificity of IL-1's biological effects on using a variety of mammals and even reptiles and fish. However, there is evidence that species specificity can play a role in some biological responses. Human IL-1β triggers ACTH release from rats whereas human IL-1α does not.[93] However, when rat IL-1s are expressed and tested in the rat homologous system, rat IL-1α is ten times more potent than human IL-1α.[94] Biological responses involving cells which express primarily the type II receptor appear to be more species restricted than cells bearing the type I receptor.

The IL-1 receptor type I (IL-1RtI)

The IL-1RtI has been cloned from mouse and human cells.[95] It is found on T cells, fibroblasts, keratinocytes, endothelial cells, synovial lining cells, chrondrocytes, and hepatocytes. Although a p80 IL-1R has been reported on purified human blood monocytes and has the characteristic ability to internalise IL-1,[96] other studies suggest that murine macrophages do not express the type I receptor.[91] The type I receptor belongs to the immunoglobulin superfamily. There is an extracellular segment which contains the three domains homologous to immunoglobulins. The extracellular segment has several sites for glycosylation; there is a single transmembrane portion of approximately 21 amino acids and a cytosolic region. This cytosolic region has no homology with any known protein kinase but the serine/threonine residues are phosphorylated soon after IL-1 binds to the extracellular domains.[97] The possibility exists that the higher molecular weight IL-1 binding proteins represent glycosylated variants of the IL-1RtI.[98] Some T cells respond to subpicomolar concentrations of IL-1 without possessing demonstrable IL-1 binding.[99] One explanation is that low receptor occupancy is sufficient to trigger intracellular events. This is supported by the observation that less than 5% receptor occupancy triggers phosphorylation of the remaining IL-1RtI.[97] On the other hand, synovial sarcoma cell line with high affinity type I receptors does not manifest a biological response to IL-1,[100] suggesting either tumour-related mutations in the IL-1RtI or a dysfunction in signal transduction.

The extracellular segment of the type I receptor has been expressed in HeLa cells as a separate molecule and binds IL-1 with the same affinity as the complete receptor on cell surface membranes. Using this soluble receptor, one IL-1α molecule binds to one truncated receptor.[101] Transfection of cells with different deletion mutants of the receptor reveals that the outer two domains are involved with ligand binding. Using antibodies to various synthetic peptides which represent 4 hydrophilic amino acid segments distributed throughout the extracellular domains, only antibodies to a 17 amino acid segment in the outermost Ig domain blocks the binding of IL-1.[102] Glycosylation also contributes to IL-1 binding to the type I receptor and different patterns and types of sugar linkages differ on cells.[98]

Using various T and fibroblast cell lines of human or murine cell origin, there is still no consensus whether the IL-1R on these cells express a single binding affinity[103] or two classes of binding affinity.[88] Some reports clearly indicate two classes of receptor binding but this finding is inconsistent. The multiple glycosylation sites on the IL-1RtI may have a role in receptor expression, affinities and specificies. Lectins block the binding of IL-1 on T cells; however, cells of separate lineage are affected by different lectins with different sugar specificies.[98] The evidence suggests that N- and O-glycosylation patterns on cells differ and this may affect the binding of IL-1α or β.

After binding, IL-1 is internalised but internalisation of IL-1 bound to truncated mutants of the type I extracellular domains can occur without a full signal transduction taking place. Internalised IL-1 bound to the type I receptor is not degraded[103] and is found in the nuclear compartment after several hours.[104,105] Although this translocation implies a nuclear site for IL-1 biological activity, biological responses such as rapid changes in arachidonic acid metabolism take place within a few minutes and are distinct from the growth and gene expression properties of IL-1.

IL-1RtII

The initial observation of the IL-1RtII was on Epstein-Barr virus (EBV) transformed B cells.[106] It was then shown that the IL-1R on various B cell lines, including the Raji human B cell lymphoma line, has a distinctly different molecular weight (68 KDa) and differed in many respects to the IL-1R on T cells and fibroblasts.[107,108,109] The type II receptor is also a member of the immunoglobulin superfamily with three Ig-like domains in the extracellular segment; there is 28% amino acid homology between the extracellular portions of the type I and II receptors[110] and a highly homologous transmembrane segment. One major difference between the type I and II receptor is the truncated cytoplasmic portion of the type II receptor which accounts for the lower molecular weight of the type II receptor and may explain the differences in signal transduction reported for IL-1 on B cells.

At present, the IL-1RtII is found on B cell lineages, neutrophils and bone marrow cells. Besides being a different gene product, the type II receptor differs from the type I receptor in binding affinities, on and off rates, regulation of its surface expression and the type of signal transduced. For example, at 37°C, 60–70% of the IL-1RtI is internalised within five minutes by an azide sensitive mechanism and remains inside the cell for 12 hours, whereas IL-1 bound to the type II receptor remains in the surface for as long as 60 minutes and is poorly internalised.[107] IL-1 bound to the IL-1RtI is internalised and only a small amount is degraded[111] whereas that bound to the type II receptor is found in extracellular fluid in a degraded form. These results suggest that there are different vesicles and acidification mechanisms for the two receptors.

The half-life of the type II receptor on B cells is shorter (two hours) than that for the type I receptor on T cells (5–12 hours).[108] B cells exhibit a heterogeneous population of IL-1R and some lines express both p80 and p68 receptors.[112] Some EBV B cell lines bind IL-1α with greater affinity than IL-1β.[112] The Raji cell IL-1RtII has more binding sites for IL-1β than α (2000 vs. 400).[109] The type II receptor on Raji cells transduces a signal which results in IL-2R, c-Ha-ras, and c-myc gene expression[108] but the type II receptor on neutrophils[113] 'primes' cells for other neutrophil agonists. IL-1 binding to neutrophils results in increased arachidonic acid metabolism with 60 minutes of exposure.[114,115] This rapid effect on neutrophil arachidonic acid metabolism may be the 'priming' effect of IL-1 on neutrophils. The activity of IL-1 on neutrophils is not due to changes in cytosolic calcium.[116]

Tumour necrosis factor

TNF was initially identified in the circulation of animals following the injection of endotoxin. It was also discovered in the supernates from stimulated macrophage cell lines, where its property as an inhibitor of lipoprotein lipase led to its being named 'cachectin', because it produced a wasting syndrome when chronically administered to mice. The amino acid sequences of TNF[117] are identical to cachectin.[118] TNF, a product of stimulated monocytes and macrophages, is also produced by lymphocytes, endothelial cells and keratinocytes. A structurally related polypeptide, initially isolated from activated T cells, is lymphotoxin. Lymphotoxin and TNF produce similar biological changes in a variety of cells.

Structure of TNF

Both mature TNF (often called TNFα) and lymphotoxin (often called TNFβ) have the same molecular weight of 17 KDa, and similar to IL-1, have a precursor form that can remain intracellularly.[119] However, this precursor form of 26 KDa is readily processed and TNF is secreted from cells of macrophagic origin[120] and when induced *in vivo*,[121] rapidly appears in the circulation. The amino sequence of TNFα and lymphotoxin are closely related[117] and both molecules are recognised by the same cell membrane receptor. The isolation and expression of genomic DNA for TNF has been reported.[122] TNFα trimerises into a stable form and it is the trimer rather than the monomer (17 KDa) that is biologically active.[123] An important note of caution, however: antigenic recognition assays for detecting TNF recognise the monomeric form whereas only the biological form is active. Therefore, it is possible to measure large amounts of TNF in body fluids without biological activity. Like IL-1β and IL-1α, TNF and lymphotoxin are sufficiently structurally distinct molecules that antibodies produced to each cytokine do not cross-react with the other cytokine.

TNF receptors

Just as TNFα and TNFβ represent two distinct but related gene products, there are two structurally related receptors for TNF which recognise both forms of TNF. These were initially recognised as TNF 'inhibitors' and, as with the IL-1 'inhibitor', the TNF 'inhibitor' was originally found in the urine.[85] After careful affinity purification, the TNF urinary inhibitors were shown to be the soluble (extracellular) forms of the two receptors for TNF.[124] The entire cDNA for each TNF receptor has been reported.[125,126] The type I TNF receptor is 75 KDa and the type II is 55 KDa. They are also known as TNF binding protein I and TNF binding protein II when referring to their respective extracellular forms (also called soluble TNF receptors).

There is no evidence that IL-1 receptors act cooperatively, as do the two (α and β) IL-2 receptors. However, the two TNF receptors appear to trigger their cytotoxicity signal by a simple cross-linking or receptor aggregation. This mechanism of action of TN was elegantly demonstrated in experiments where antibodies to either of the TNF cell surface receptors cross-linked with anti-F(ab')2 were sufficient to deliver a signal to the cells which mimicked the action of *bona fide* TNF.[127]

Biological activities of TNF in humans

Although originally studied for its ability to kill tumour cells *in vitro* as well as when injected in tumour bearing mice, the widespread biological effects of TNF on mesenchymal and other cells have been the focus of studies related to its inflammatory properties, particularly in mediating synovial cell activity and cartilage and bone degradation. Moreover, recombinant human TNF has been injected into human subjects and many of its systemic effects, such as fever, leucopenia, and hypotension, which were studied in animals, have been observed in humans.[128] When humans are injected intravenously with LPS, the leucopenia which develops rapidly correlates directly with the circulating level of TNF.[121] When TNF (1 μg/kg) is injected as a bolus intravenously into healthy human subjects, there is an immediate fall in circulating neutrophils followed by a leucocytosis. Lymphopenia remains for a more prolonged time.[129] The levels of lactoferrin are elevated in the circulation during the time of neutropenia, suggesting neutrophil activation[129] and there is a 40-fold increase in circulating IL-6 levels. Fever and headache accompany the response. At this dose of TNF, there is no significant fall in systemic blood pressure.[130] There is also evidence that following TNF injection, there is activation of several clotting parameters, including an increase in plasminogen activator inhibitor levels.[130]

Other biological activities of TNF

TNF has been shown to activate T cells[131] and induce the expression of IL-2 receptors. B cells are also stimulated by TNF. The molar concentration of TNF required to stimulate immunocompetent cells is one or two orders of magnitude greater than IL-1.[131] Since TNF induces the synthesis and release of immunostimulatory polypeptides such as IL-1 and IL-6 from monocytes, fibroblasts and endothelial cells, it is possible that these cytokines augment the action of TNF on lymphocytes. Some investigators have attempted to separate a direct action of TNF on lymphocytes from that secondary to the induction of IL-1 or IL-6. It also appears that, unlike IL-1, the immunostimulatory effects of TNF are species specific.

Nearly every non-immunological biological property of IL-1 has also been observed with TNF. These include fever,[132] the induction of PGE_2 and collagenase synthesis in a variety of tissues,[133] bone and cartilage resorption inhibition of lipoprotein lipase,[118] increases in hepatic acute phase proteins and complement components, and a decrease in albumin synthesis.[134] Slow wave sleep and appetite suppression are also observed following the injection of TNF.[135] Both molecules induce fibroblast proliferation and collagen synthesis. The cytotoxic activity of TNF differs from that of IL-1. IL-1 is inactive on a variety of tumour targets for which TNF is a potent cytotoxin whereas IL-1 exhibits cytotoxic effects on melanoma cells which are unaffected by TNF. Another difference between IL-1 and TNF is that IL-1 can function as a cofactor for stem cell activation (haemopoietin-1 activity),[9] whereas TNF suppresses bone marrow colony formation.[136] Both IL-1 and TNF induce the synthesis of colony stimulating factors.[137,138]

In experimental animals, TNF produces hypotension, leucopenia and local tissue necrosis. On a weight basis in rabbits, TNF is more potent than IL-1 in producing shock.[139] However, in humans, IL-1β or IL-1α, when given intravenously,[14] appear to be more potent than TNF in producing hypotension.[130] Administration of anti-TNF antibodies to baboons[140] or rabbits prevents the shock induced by endotoxin.[141] The shocklike responses to TNF probably reflect effects on the vascular endothelium. TNF stimulates PGI_2, PGE_2, and platelet activating factor production by cultured endothelium. In addition, like IL-1, TNF stimulates procoagulant activity, leukocyte adherence, and plasminogen activator inhibitor on these cells. TNF also induces a capillary leak syndrome.

Despite the similarities, receptors for TNF and IL-1 are distinct and specific. Furthermore, IL-1 down-regulates its own receptor[142] as well as that of TNF.[143] The most likely explanation is that TNF and IL-1 stimulate similar intracellular messages by different pathways and alter the same cascade of intracellular metabolites. Of note is the fact that TNF stimulates human neutrophil oxidative metabolism, whereas IL-1 does not.

The biological effects of IL-1 relevant to disease

Biological effects of IL-1 in humans

IL-1α and IL-1β have been administered to humans in phase I trials. Systemic administration of intravenous IL-1 from 10–100 ng/kg has produced fever, sleepiness, anorexia, generalised myalgias, arthralgias, headache, some gastrointestinal disturbances; at higher doses, hypotension has been observed.[13,14] The subcutaneous route is associated with fewer side effects. Laboratory data show that IL-1 can increase both circulating neutrophils and platelets.[13] In general, the early experiences in humans are consistent with previous observations in the rabbit and other animals. In the following section, the multiple biological activities of IL-1 are based on animal and *in vitro* studies.

Expression of various genes in cells exposed to IL-1

IL-1 induces a wide variety of genes, some by inducing new transcripts such as serum amyloid A (SAA)[144] or IL-1 itself[68] whereas others represent stabilisation and prolongation of mRNA half-life, for example GM-CSF.[145,146,147] IL-1 also suppresses the expression of other genes, for example albumin, cytochrome P450 and aromatase, by reducing new transcription. IL-1 reduces the surface expression of its own type I receptor by accelerated mRNA degradation.[142] In TSH stimulated thyrocytes, IL-1 inhibits gene expression for thyroglobulin and thyroid peroxidase. In isolated rat adrenal glomerulosa cells stimulated with angiotensin II, aldosterone biosynthesis is reduced by fM concentrations of IL-1, probably by reduced mRNA transcripts. In human marrow stromal cells, IL-1 selectively increases the c-abl proto-oncogene 6 kb but not the 5 kb transcript. The JE and KC genes which are platelet derived growth factor inducible genes are also induced by fM levels of IL-1. In general, IL-1 stimulates new transcripts for several proto-oncogenes.[148]

The mechanism of IL-1 induced genes may involve the activation of nuclear factors. Two such factors have been shown to be IL-1 inducible: NF ϰ-B[149] and AP-1.[150] An IL-1 responsive element was described in the IL-2 promoter gene which shares homology with phorbol ester inducible sequences and is recognised by the nuclear factor AP-1. The signal transduction mechanism for nuclear factors may be different in cells of different origins. Table 4.1 summarises the effect of IL-1 on gene expression. It should be pointed out that the expression of some lymphokine genes by IL-1 requires the presence of another stimulant, particularly lectins or agents which raise cytosolic calcium.

Table 4.1 IL-1 and TNF induced gene expression or gene suppression[1]

Increased gene expression	Suppression of gene expression
IL-1, IL-2, IL-3, IL-4,	Albumin
IL-5, IL-6, IL-7, IL-8	Cytochrome P450
TNFα, TNFβ, INFβ-1	Lipoprotein lipase
GM-CSF, G-CSF, M-CSF	Aromatase
IL-2R (Tac antigen)	Aldosterone
Metallothionein; Ceruloplasmin	Thyroglobulin
Complement; C2; Factor B	Thyroid peroxidase
Manganese superoxide dismutase	Prepro-insulin
Cyclooxygenase, phospholipase A2	
Platelet derived growth factor (AA)	
Adhesion molecules	
Oncogenes (c-fos; c-myc; c-jun)	
G-protein α-i-2-subunit	
Interferon regulatory factor	
Tissue and urinary plasminogen activator	
Plasminogen activator inhibitor	
Preproendothelin-1	
Corticotropin releasing factor and pro-opiomelanocortin	
Amyloid A and amyloid beta proteins	
Collagenases and stromelysin	

[1]IL-1 and TNF do not affect the expression of the list of genes in all cells

Central nervous system

In contrast to molecules of similar size, IL-1 does not cross the blood–brain barrier and enter the substance of the central nervous system. In cats given large doses of LPS, third cerebroventricular levels of biologically active IL-1 are not detected.[151] However, the rapid (five minutes) induction of fever, sleep and the release of a variety of neuropeptides suggest that IL-1 readily affects structures in the central nervous system. It is likely that IL-1 acts on the special endothelial cells of the periventricular organs where the blood–brain barrier is interrupted; furthermore, arachidonic acid metabolites are released from these cells. IL-1Rs are found distributed throughout the brain but glial and possibly neuronal cells synthesise IL-1. This endogenously produced IL-1 may be acting as a co-factor in synaptic transmission.

Hepatocytes

IL-1 induces two- or three-fold increases in normal hepatic proteins but the synthesis of pathological proteins can increase 100-fold to 1000-fold. One such protein, serum amyloid A (SAA) protein, contributes to the development of secondary amyloidosis. IL-1 also induces hepatocytes to synthesise fibrinogen, complement components, factor B, metallothionen, and various clotting factors. In isolated hepatocytes, IL-1 decreases the transcription of RNA coding for albumin, transferrin, lipoprotein lipase and cytochromes. IL-1 stimulates fatty acid synthesis by increasing hepatic citrate levels.[152] Some of IL-1's effects on hepatocytes may be via the intermediate production of IL-6.

Catabolic effects of IL-1

Although early studies suggested that IL-1 played a role in the negative nitrogen balance often associated with chronic disease by inducing muscle proteolysis, subsequent studies have not confirmed this.[153] However, IL-1 probably contributes to the development of negative nitrogen balance because it induces reduced food intake in experimental animals, although tachyphylaxis develops to the anorectic property of IL-1.[154] IL-1 also induces hypoglycaemia and this effect may be due to the ability of IL-1 to increase the synthesis of glucose transporters and thus increase intracellular glucose levels.[155] IL-1-induced anorexia is thought be due to a direct effect on the liver which subsequently affects the hypothalamic appetite centre.[156] This concept is supported by a study in which systemically administered antibodies to the IL-1RtI block the weight loss associated with inflammation.[157]

Vascular effects of IL-1

The systemic effects of high dose (>1μg/kg) IL-1 following an intravenous injection into animals include hypotension, increased systemic vascular resistance, depressed myocardial function, lactic acidosis, leucopenia, thrombocytopenia, vascular leak, pulmonary congestion, and tissue neutrophilic infiltration with necrosis. The hypotensive effects of intravenously administered IL-1 in humans have been observed at doses below 1 μg/kg and hypotension is the major clinical response limiting the maximal dose tolerated to 300 ng/kg.[14] The hypotensive effect of IL-1 may be via various mechanisms. The hypotension following IL-1 injection into rabbits is blocked by cyclo-oxygenase inhibitors.[139] Arterial perfusion with IL-1 increases prostanoid synthesis which lowers the pain threshold to bradykinin.[158] A single large dose of IL-1 (>500 μg/kg) is not nearly as lethal as the same or lower doses divided into two separate injections.[159,160] TNF potentiates these effects of IL-1 whereas pre-treatment with cyclo-oxygenase inhibitors blocks the response to the combination of TNF and IL-1.[139] IL-1 inhibits vascular smooth muscle contraction[161] independent of prostaglandin synthesis. The inhibition of smooth muscle contraction by IL-1 appears to be due to an L-arginine dependent increase in nitric oxide production leading to increased guanylate cyclase activity.[162]

Cultured endothelial cells exposed to IL-1 increase the expression of adhesion molecules which enhances the adherence of leucocytes to endothelial surfaces. These IL-1 treated endothelial cells also increase procoagulant activity, tissue factor, PGE_2, PGI_2, PAF, plasminogen activator inhibitor production,[163,164] enhancement of thrombin induced von Willebrand's factor, and the synthesis of other cytokines including IL-1 itself.[52] IL-1 increases smooth muscle cell synthesis of itself,[165] other cytokines and platelet derived growth factor[166] and serves as an autocrine growth factor for smooth muscle cells.[167] These effects of IL-1 are thought to play a role in the development of atherosclerosis and neovascularisation. On the other hand, the pro-inflammatory effect of IL-1 on endothelial cells plays a role in vasculitis[168] and inhibition of cell growth perhaps by down-regulation of receptors for fibroblast growth factor.[169]

Endocrine effects of IL-1

IL-1 effects on insulin production are reviewed above. Low doses of IL-1 increase spermatogenesis whereas high doses are suppressive. IL-1 inhibits human chorionic gonadotropin induced testosterone synthesis. Other IL-1 effects have been reported on granulosa cell function.[170] IL-1 inhibits the function of thyrocytes,[171] and stimulates PGE formation; in addition, thyrocytes appear to synthesise an IL-1-like molecule. Although adrenal tissue shows evidence of IL-1 staining, perfusion of adrenal tissue with IL-1 increases steroid synthesis induced by ACTH.

Within ten minutes of an intravenous injection of IL-1, several neuropeptides are released into the systemic circulation; increased corticotropin releasing factor, ACTH, vasopressin and somatostatin are induced by IL-1 whereas IL-1 inhibits thyroid releasing hormone induced prolactin release. The effect of IL-1 on ACTH release is via a cyclo-oxygenase metabolite pathway and IL-1 acts synergistically with IL-6 in the induction of ACTH (R. Neta, personal communication). It has been proposed that IL-1 induced corticosteroids (via direct and indirect ACTH action) represent a biological negative feedback loop since corticosteroids inhibit cytokine gene expression. The IL-1 induced corticosteroids have some protective effect since adrenalectomised mice are markedly sensitive to the lethal effects of IL-1 induction.[159]

Haematopoietic effects of IL-1

There are various levels at which IL-1 affects haematopoiesis.[172,173] IL-1 induces the production of GM-CSF, G-CSF, M-CSF, IL-3 and other cytokines; it acts synergistically with CSFs and other cytokines on haematopoiesis, regulates the cell cycle of the haematopoietic progenitor cell, and protects early progenitor cells from cytotoxic agents. Protection of the early progenitor cell may be due to cell cycle changes.[174] IL-1 enhances CSF synthesis from a variety of cells, particularly bone marrow stromal cells,[137,138,175] and increased production can be through new mRNA transcription or, as in the case of GM-CSF, through stabilisation of mRNA.[147,172] IL-1 acts synergistically with IL-3, IL-6, G-CSF and GM-CSF in the induction of specific lineage and multilineage colonies.[9,176] IL-1 also increases the survival of progenitor cells *in vitro*. IL-1 by itself has no effect on stem cell proliferation or differentiation but requires colony stimulating factors such as IL-3 and GM-CSF. Stem cell factor by itself also has no effect but synergises with CSFs;[177] it is possible that IL-1's activity on stem cells is due to induction of stem cell factor.

The necessary co-factor for colony formation after bone marrow treatment with cytotoxic drugs was originally described as 'haemopoietin-1' (H-1); during molecular cloning, H-1 was identified as IL-1α. There are no differences between the two forms of IL-1 for H-1 activity. *In vivo*, the H-1 activity of IL-1 acts on the early progenitor stem cell's responsiveness to CSF as well as inducing the CSF. A single injection of IL-1 stimulates circulating CSF in normal mice, protects stem cells, and accelerates the return of granulocytes following cytotoxic drugs or irradiation.[178,179,180,181]

Following a single injection of IL-1 (<1 μg/kg) into animals there are increased circulating granulocytes[182] and precursor forms[183] which seem to be a direct effect of IL-1 and not mediated by IL-6. The peak elevation in circulating neutrophils in animals has been four hours and similar kinetics have been reported in humans given IL-1.[13,14] Higher doses of IL-1 result in granulocytopenia due to adherence of circulating granulocytes to endothelium. In patients receiving IL-1 (68 ng/kg), receptors (type II) for IL-1 on circulating neutrophils were initially reduced but after 6–8 hours, there was up to a six-fold increase in IL-1 binding sites.[184] Similar findings were obtained by adding IL-1 directly to neutrophils *in vitro*.

Recent studies in humans suggest that IL-1 directly stimulates platelet production.[13] Although this effect may be due to a synergy between IL-1 and IL-3, no changes in plasma IL-3 levels were observed during IL-1 treatment. The effect of IL-1 on platelet counts was observed at relatively low IL-1 doses of 1 or 10 ng/kg. After five daily intravenous injections of IL-1 into patients with cancer, there were no significant increases in peripheral platelet counts but on the sixth day and for the next five days, there was a rapid increase from approximately 250,000 to 350,000 which reached peak elevations on day ten and then slowly decreased to baseline counts on day 28. There was no statistically significant difference between 1 and 10 ng/kg doses of IL-1β. These data support the concept that IL-1 is acting on an early and primitive stem cell and are supported by animal studies.[185] In cynomolgus primates, IL-1 is more effective in releasing haematopoietic stem cells into the peripheral circulation than IL-3 and GM-CSF.[186]

The continued use of IL-1 *in vivo* is associated with the induction of TNF which exerts a suppressive effect on haematopoiesis.[187] In rabbits and human PBMC, IL-1 induces TNF gene expression and circulating TNF.[188] IL-1 can also be directly suppressive on erythropoiesis but this suppression can be overcome with erythropoietin.[189]

IL-1-induced non-specific resistance to infection and injury

Early studies on non-specific resistance to infection employed bacterial products which induce IL-1. IL-1 was tested in such models and was shown to afford protection and could replace bacterial products in the induction of this resistance. IL-1 is most effective when administered 24 hours prior to the challenge. Pretreatment with IL-1 has been used in a variety of models: infection in normal and granulocytopenic mice, LPS in mice with severe liver failure, hyperoxia in rats, immune colitis in rabbits, anaphylaxis in guinea pigs, lethal radiation in mice, and malaria. The most consistent finding is the lack of effect if the IL-1 is delayed beyond the onset of the pathological process leading to death or inflammation.

Although in models of infection in granulocytopenic mice there is the possibility of IL-1 accelerating bone marrow recovery, this is not the mechanism of protection and neither is protection related to a cyclo-oxygenase product.[190] However, protection against colitis and hyperoxia are mediated, in part, by IL-1 stimulated prostaglandins.[191,192] Explanations for how a single, low dose of IL-1 can be so effective in affording protection include IL-1's ability to down-regulate the TNF and IL-1 receptors,[142,193] induce oxygen scavenger molecules, or induce corticosteroids. Table 4.2 summarises the biological effects of IL-1.

Table 4.2 Biological effects of IL-1

Immunological properties
T-cell activation:synergism with IL-6 for IL-2 synthesis
Increased IL-2R expression
B-cell activation via induction of IL-6; synergy with IL-4
Natural killer activity: synergism with IL-2 and IFN
Lymphokine gene expression

Pro-inflammatory properties
Fever, sleep, anorexia, neuropeptide release
Gene expression for complement; suppression of P450 synthesis
Endothelial cell activation
Neutrophilia
Increased adhesion molecule expression
Neutrophil priming, eosinophil degranulation
Hypotension, myocardial suppression, shock, death
Neutrophil tissue infiltration (via IL-8)
Beta islet cell cytotoxicity
Amino acid turnover; hyperlipidaemia
Cyclo-oxygenase and lipoxygenase gene expression
Synthesis of collagenases and collagens; osteoblast activation

Protective effects
Malaria
Bacterial infections
Lethal radiation
Early stem cell
Hyperoxia
Inflammatory bowel disease
Histamine release

Comparison of IL-1, TNF and IL-6

IL-1 and TNF

The biological properties of TNF are remarkably similar to those of IL-1, particularly the non-immunological effects of IL-1 (see Table 4.3). Some lymphocyte activating properties of IL-1 or IL-6 are shared with TNF, but these require considerably higher concentrations of TNF than of IL-1 or IL-6. Both IL-1 and TNF induce fever by direct stimulation of hypothalamic PGE_2 synthesis.[132] Levels of circulating TNF rise rapidly in human subjects injected with LPS.[121,194] IL-1 and TNF both increase CSF *in vitro* and *in vivo*. On a weight basis in rabbits, TNF is more potent than IL-1 in producing shock.[139] Administration of anti-TNF antibodies to rabbits or baboons prevents the shock induced by LPS but IL-1 levels are suppressed by anti-TNF therapy, suggesting

Table 4.3 Comparison of IL-1, TNF and IL-6

Biological property	IL-1	TNF	IL-6
Endogenous pyrogen fever	+	+	+
Slow wave sleep	+	+	−
Hepatic acute phase proteins	+	+	+
T cell activation	+	+	+
B cell activation	+	+	+
B cell Ig synthesis	−	−	+
Fibroblast proliferation	+	+	−
Sten cell activation (haemopoietin-1)	+	−	+
Non-specific resistance to infection	+	+	+
Radioprotection	+	+	−
Cyclo-oxygenase, PLA_2 gene expression	+	+	−
Synovial cell activation	+	+	−
Endothelial cell activation	+	+	−
Shock syndrome	+	+	−
Induction of IL-1, TNF and IL-8	+	+	−
Induction of IL-6	+	+	−

that IL-1 is under the control of TNF in some models.[195]

Synergism between IL-1 and TNF

When the two cytokines are used together in experimental studies, the net effect often exceeds the additive effect of each cytokine. Potentiation or frank synergism between these two molecules has been demonstrated in studies on fibroblast production of PGE_2, the cytotoxic effect on certain tumour cells, and when administered to tumour bearing mice. IL-1 acts synergistically with TNF to protect rats exposed to lethal hyperoxia or radiation. IL-1 cytotoxic effects on the insulin producing beta cells of the islets of Langerhans are dramatically augmented by TNF. Rats receiving intravenous infusions of IL-1 or TNF manifest metabolic changes reflected in plasma amino acid levels but, when given together, negative nitrogen balance and muscle proteolysis can be demonstrated. Although high doses (10–20 μg/kg) of TNF produce a shocklike state with tissue damage, IL-1 and TNF act synergistically to produce haemodynamic shock and pulmonary haemorrhage at doses of only 1 μg/kg when given together.[139] The synergism between these two cytokines seems to be due to second message molecules rather than up-regulation of cell receptors; in fact, IL-1 reduces TNF receptors.[143,196]

IL-1 and IL-6

In some models, the production of IL-6 appears to be under the control of IL-1; for example, mice subjected to an inflammatory event induced by intramuscular turpentine fail to produce IL-6 when pretreated with anti-IL-1 receptor antibodies.[157] In baboons injected with *E. coli*, anti-TNF antibodies prevent the appearance of IL-6 in the circulation.[195] Like IL-1 and TNF, IL-6 is an endogenous pyrogen and an inducer of acute phase responses. Since IL-1 and TNF induce IL-6, levels of IL-6 often correlate with the amount of fever and disease in patients. Many studies demonstrate that IL-6 levels are elevated in patients with a variety of infectious diseases. The best correlation of the severity of an infectious disease with any cytokine is clearly with the levels of IL-6, not IL-1 or TNF. However, it is important to note that unlike IL-1 and TNF, there is no evidence, except for one paper,[197] that IL-6 is a lethal cytokine. IL-6 does not cause shock in mice or primates regardless of the amount given, either alone or with TNF. IL-6 does not induce endothelial cell adhesion molecules and it does not stimulate the genes for cyclo-oxygenase, phospholipase A_2 or nitric oxide synthase. Finally, unlike soluble receptors for TNF and IL-1 which bind and *reduce* their respective biological activities, soluble p80 receptors for IL-6 *enhance* the activity of this cytokine.[198,199]

IL-6 suppresses LPS- and TNF-induced IL-1 production.[120] In general, IL-6 appears to be an anti-inflammatory peptide. Of considerable importance is the observation that IL-6 acts as haemopoietin-1 on bone marrow cultures.[9] The spectrum of acute phase proteins induced by IL-6 includes many antiproteases with anti-inflammatory properties.

IL-1 antagonism

It appears that nature developed several mechanisms for blocking the activity of IL-1. Naturally occurring substances which *specifically* inhibit IL-1 have been detected in the serum of human volunteers injected with bacterial LPS,[200] urine of febrile patients,[201] plasma following haemodialysis,[202] supernatants of human monocytes adhering to IgG coated surfaces[203] and urine of patients with monocytic leukaemia.[204] An IL-1 specific inhibitory molecule of 52–66 KDa secreted from a human myelomonocytic cell line,[205] and the mouse macrophage cell line P388D,[206] have also been reported. Another inhibitory material isolated from the urine of pregnant women has been identified as uromodulin, a glycosylated form of the Tamm-Horsfall protein. The carbohydrate portion of uromodulin binds IL-1 as well as TNF and other cytokines and is thus non-specific. IL-1 inhibitory activities have also been reported from virus infected monocytes, blood neutrophils, UV-exposed keratinocytes, Epstein-Barr infected B cell lines, and from normal submandibular glands.

The IL-1 receptor antagonist (IL-1ra) was originally called the 'IL-1 inhibitor';[203,204,207,208] it was a 23–25 KDa protein purified from the urine of patients with monocytic leukaemia.[204,208,209] Natural IL-1 inhibitor blocked the ability of IL-1 to stimulate synovial cell PGE_2 production, thymocyte proliferation, and decreased insulin release from isolated pancreatic islets.[204,208,210,211] It appears that the IL-1-specific inhibitory activity found in the serum during endotoxaemia[200] is probably the IL-1ra[212] but the IL-1-specific inhibitor for the M20 myelomonocytic cell line[205] does not share identity with the IL-1ra.[213] In each case, the IL-1 inhibitory activity was shown to prevent IL-1 but not IL-2 or mitogen induced T cell proliferation. The 'IL-1 inhibitor' blocked the binding of IL-1 to receptors on T cells and fibroblasts but did not affect the binding of TNF or IL-2 to their receptors.[208,211] The IL-1 inhibitor also did not bind to IL-1 itself.

Using the IL-1 inhibitor purified from adherent monocytes,[203,214] N-terminal sequence was obtained and the molecule was cloned.[215] The cDNA sequence codes for a polypeptide of approximately 17 KDa; the 25 KDa molecular weight is due to glycosylation. The amino acid sequence deduced from the cDNA revealed a 26% amino acid homology to IL-1β and a 19% homology to IL-1α. Conserved amino acids as defined by Dayoff[216] revealed a 41% homology of the IL-1ra to IL-1β and 30% to IL-1α. The IL-1ra was also cloned from U937 cells and reported as the interleukin-1 receptor antagonist protein (IRAP).[217]

Similar to the purified naturally occurring IL-1 urinary inhibitor,[208] the recombinant IL-1 inhibitor competes with the binding of IL-1 to its cell surface receptors. Because of its sequence homology and mode of action, the IL-1 inhibitor was re-named the IL-1 receptor antagonist. Recombinant human IL-1ra expressed by *E. coli* is not glycosylated but blocks binding of IL-1 as well as the glycosylated natural form. Antibodies produced to the recombinant human IL-1ra recognise the purified urinary IL-1 inhibitor of Seckinger and Dayer, establishing that the IL-1 inhibitor and IL-1ra are the same molecule.[218]

The IL-1ra blocks IL-1 activity *in vitro* and *in vivo*. *In vitro*, the IL-1ra competes with IL-1 for occupancy of the IL-1RtI on T cells and fibroblasts with nearly the same affinity as that for *bone fide* IL-1 but without demonstrable agonist activity.[214] To date, attempts to show agonist activity of IL-1ra on a variety of cells *in vitro* have failed. Humans have been injected with large amounts of IL-1ra and symptoms or signs of agonist properties have not been observed. In a phase I trial of the IL-1ra, blood levels were in excess of 20 μg/ml and there were no indications of altered homoeostatic parameters.[219]

When IL-1ra occupies the type I receptor, there is no evidence of internalisation nor of protein kinase activity. Early reports showed that in murine pre-B cell lines which express only the p68 IL-1R (IL-1RtII), there was no blockade of IL-1 binding by the IL-1ra.[214,217,220] However, the human IL-1ra blocks the binding of IL-1 to human cells bearing the IL-1RtII such as neutrophils and B cells[221,222] as well as human peripheral myelomonocytic leukaemia cells.[223] In addition, IL-1ra blocks the binding of IL-1β to human blood monocytes, a type II receptor bearing cell.[224] Using murine T cells (IL-1RtI), the human IL-1ra blocks the binding of IL-1 at nearly equimolar concentration; however, a 10–50-fold molar excess of the IL-1ra is required to block the binding of human IL-1 to human type II receptor bearing cells.[221]

It is not surprising that recombinant IL-1ra will block the activity of IL-1 in various animal models of disease. Rabbits[225] or baboons[226] injected with IL-1 develop hypotension which is reversed by prior administration of the IL-1ra. However, a larger question remains: during acute or chronic disease several cytokines are produced but what is the effect of specific blockade of IL-1? The results of several studies have now been published and demonstrate that IL-1 receptor blockade significantly reduces the severity of several inflammatory diseases (reviewed in[227]).

Effect of IL-1ra on septic shock

The administration of the IL-1ra prevents death in rabbits exposed to LPS.[225] The intravenous injection of *E. coli* suspensions to rabbits produces several parameters of the septic shock syndrome, namely hypotension, decreased systemic vascular resistance, leucopenia, thrombocytopenia and tissue damage. When rabbits were pretreated with the IL-1ra, only a transient and mild hypotensive episode was observed whereas severe and sustained hypotension with a 50% mortality was observed in control rabbits.[228] There were also reduced numbers of tissue infiltrating neutrophils. The circulating levels of TNF and IL-1β were unchanged. IL-1ra also blocks the shock syndrome induced by Staphylococci,[229] a model where IL-1 levels correlate with the degree of hypotension.[230] The interpretation of these results suggests that TNF may be responsible for the initial fall in blood pressure but that IL-1 is playing an essential role in the progression of the shock state. The human IL-1ra also prevents lethal *Klebsiella pneu-*

moniae sepsis in newborn rats[221] and *E. coli* induced hypotension in baboons.[226]

In mice, administration of IL-1ra will prevent LPS induced elevation of circulating colony stimulating factors and the early part of LPS induced tolerance.[231] In addition, IL-1ra prevents LPS induced hypoglycaemia[231] and death due to high doses of LPS.[232] Intratracheal injection of LPS to mice results in a pulmonary infiltrative neutrophilic response which is blocked by prior systemic injection of IL-1ra.[233] Table 4.4 illustrates those disease processes where IL-1ra has reduced the severity of disease in the model.

Table 4.4 Reduction in severity by human IL-1ra in animal models of various diseases

Death in rabbits from endotoxin (LPS)[225,228]
Death in mice from endotoxin (LPS)[23]
Death in newborn rats from *Klebsiella pneumoniae*[251]
Haemodynamic shock and tissue damage in rabbits from *E. coli*[228]
Haemodynamic shock in rabbits from *Staphylococcus epidermidis*[229]
Haemodynamic shock and death in baboons from *E. coli*[226]
Cerebral malaria in mice[252]
Streptococcal wall induced arthritis in rats[253]
Collagen induced arthritis in mice[254]
Inflammatory bowel disease in rabbits[236]
Onset of spontaneous diabetes in BB rats[255]
Hypoglycaemia and CSF production in mice following endotoxin[256]
Poliferation and CSF production of acute myeloblastic leukaemia cells[223]
Poliferation of chronic myelogenous leukaemia cells[257]
Neutrophil accumulation in inflammatory peritonitis[258]
Sciatic nerve regeneration in mice[259]
Graft *versus* host disease in mice[260]
Experimental enterocolitis in rats[261]
Indomethacin induced intestinal ulceration in rats[261]
LPS induced pulmonary inflammation in rats[233]

The IL-1ra in immune complex induced colitis

A role for IL-1 has been proposed in the pathogenesis of inflammatory bowel disease. Three studies support this conclusion: (1) rabbit colonic tissue releases large amounts of PGE_2 and LTB_4 for several hours following a brief period of perfusion with IL-1;[234] (2) there is a reduction in the severity of colonic inflammation in rabbits pretreated with a single low dose of IL-1 24 hours before the induction of colitis;[235] and (3) the degree of inflammation, oedema and necrosis in colonic tissue correlates with the tissue levels of IL-1 in these tissues.[236] Although IL-1 levels and tissue injury correlate, these data do not necessarily support an essential role for IL-1 in the pathogenesis of colitis in this model, as other inflammatory cytokines may also be involved. However, when rabbits were pretreated with the IL-1ra, a marked decrease in tissue inflammatory cell infiltration, oedema and necrosis was observed.[236] In addition, decreased PGE_2 was measured in the rectal lumen despite the fact that IL-1 tissue levels were unchanged.[237] Together, these data demonstrate that blockade of IL-1 prevents the onset and development of the inflammatory lesion in this model of immune complex induced colitis. Although the events leading up to the production of IL-1 in this model of colitis are still unclear, LPS from the colonic lumen may be playing a role.

Other effects of the IL-1ra

The recombinant IL-1ra blocks IL-1 augmentation of thymocyte proliferation to mitogens, IL-1 induced synovial cell PGE_2 synthesis, and collagenase synthesis from chondrocytes.[238] In order to inhibit 50% of these IL-1 induced responses *in vitro*, 100-fold excess IL-1ra is required.[238] The IL-1ra also blocks the production of IL-1 induced IL-1, TNF and IL-6 from human PBMC as well as from purified monocytes.[224] However, 50% inhibition is observed at equimolar ratio whereas at 10-fold molar excess of IL-1ra to IL-1, a complete inhibition is observed.[224] In a rabbit model of meningeal inflammation, the IL-1ra blocks cerebrospinal pleocytosis induced by cerebroventricular IL-1[239] and this requires 5000-fold excess IL-1ra to block 90% of the IL-1 induced pleocytosis. A similar study has shown that intracerebroventricular injection of 100 μg of the IL-1ra (10,000-fold excess) blocks non-rapid eye movement sleep and fever induced by 10 ng of IL-1β given by the same route.[240] Systemic injection of 100-fold molar excess of the IL-1ra blocks 95% of the fever due to the intravenous injection of IL-1 in rabbits. Administration of the IL-1ra to rats with adjuvant arthritis has reduced the severity of the joint lesions.

Balance of IL-1 and IL-1ra production

IL-1ra is synthesised in septic animals and humans with a variety of infectious or inflammatory diseases. The balance between the amount and secretion of IL-1 and its receptor antagonist may be critical in some diseases. IL-1 and IL-1ra gene expression and protein synthesis are differently regulated.[203,241] For example, IL-1β is transcribed and synthesised in cells before IL-1ra. The dysregulation in production of the agonist and antagonist in human disease has recently been studied by Rambaldi and Cozzolino who examined spontaneous gene expression for IL-1β and IL-1ra in fresh cells from patients with acute myelogenous leukaemia.[223] Cells from each of 11 patients studied spontaneously expressed the gene for IL-1β whereas the leukaemic cells from only one of 11 patients expressed IL-1ra following stimulation.

Large amounts of circulating IL-1ra have been found during experimental endotoxaemia in humans[212] in sepsis,[242] or in systemic juvenile rheumatoid arthritis.[243] In several studies on circulating IL-1β during infection in humans, levels rarely exceed 500 pg/ml.[194,244] During experimental endotoxaemia in humans, levels of IL-1β reach a maximal concentration of 150–200 pg/ml after 3–4 hours, and then fall rapidly; in these same individuals, the peak levels of IL-1ra occur after four hours, exceed the concentration of IL-1β by 100-fold and are sustained for 12 hours.[212] During *E. coli* sepsis in baboons, peak IL-1ra levels occur 8–10 hours later.[242] Thus, production of a small amount of IL-1 but a large amount of the IL-1ra appears to be a natural response in some clinical situations. Endogenously produced IL-1ra probably contributes to limiting the severity of disease, but may be inadequate in overwhelming infection or acute inflammation. Providing exogenous IL-1ra in some of these latter situations may have beneficial effects as observed in animal models.

IL-1ra, with a classical signal peptide, is readily secreted into the extracellular compartment whereas in the same cell culture, only 50% of IL-1β and less than 10% of IL-1α is secreted. An intracellular form of IL-1ra without a signal peptide has been described in keratinocytes[245] and it is speculated that intracellular IL-1ra in these cells acts to counter the biological activity of IL-1α which remains in the cytosolic compartment. However, this is not the case in human monocytes stimulated with endotoxin where nearly all of their IL-1α is intracellular but less than 10% of IL-1ra remains in these cells. Nevertheless, the concept that intracellular IL-1α is biologically active has received recent experimental support[246] and the balance of IL-1 to IL-1ra should be considered for both intracellular and extracellular compartments.

Soluble IL-1R proteins

The extracellular domain of the IL-1RtI has been expressed and shown to bind both forms of IL-1. Unlike soluble TNF, IL-6 and INFγ receptors which occur naturally,[85,199] soluble IL-1R have yet to be found naturally. When the recombinant soluble IL-1RtI was given to mice undergoing heart transplantation, survival of the heterotopic allografts was increased. Lymph nodes directly injected with allogeneic cells have reduced hyperplasia with the use of the soluble IL-1RtI.[247] However, it is unclear from these experiments how many of the effects of the soluble type I receptor are due to decreased inflammation rather than decreased immunoresponsiveness. There are no data suggesting that the type I IL-1R is naturally shed; however, conditioned media from the IL-1RtII bearing Raji cells contain the soluble form (35–45 KDa) of the IL-1RtII.[248]

TNF antagonism

The effects of monoclonal antibodies to TNF have been discussed above. However, antibody therapies in humans have their limitations and hence attention has been focused on the use of soluble receptors for TNF which have the distinct advantage of being natural products and unlikely to induce an antibody response. Soluble TNFRs, which represent the extracellular domains of the two TNFRs (TNFRtI and TNFRtII), were initially discovered in the urine of healthy humans,[85,124,127] suggesting that they are constantly being produced. The soluble TNFRs are proteolytic cleavage products, not separate products of alternate mRNA splicing as is the case with other receptors such as the IL-4 receptor. Circulating levels of soluble TNFRtI in the serum or plasma of healthy humans are in the 1–2 ng/ml range[249] and are elevated in patients during infection and with metastatic disease. Like IL-1ra, the host response to infection includes a brisk production of antagonistic molecules.

The effects of blocking TNF using the soluble forms of the TNFRtI are the same as those due to antibodies. A reduction in *E. coli* induced shock in baboons (L. Moldawer, personal communication) and death in mice from LPS[250] have been observed when animals are treated with soluble TNFR. Clinically, the amounts of soluble TNFR required to block these events are high but the use of chimeric molecules where the soluble TNFR is linked covalently to the Fc portion of Ig results in prolonged circulating half-life and greater effectiveness than the native form.

Unlike antibodies to the IL-1RtI which block IL-1 responses, antibodies to the TNF receptor are not blocking but rather induce a TNF response.[127] The mechanism of action of TNF appears to be cross-linking of two receptors and the cross-linked receptors are responsible for triggering signal transduction. Thus, there are four possible modes of antagonism to IL-1 (IL-1ra, anti-IL-1, anti-IL-1R and soluble IL-1R) whereas for TNF antagonism, there is at present only anti-TNF and soluble TNFR. Regardless of the approach taken, the data consistently show that blocking either IL-1 or TNF (using any of the available antagonistic molecules) reduces the severity of, and sometimes abolishes, the consequences of infectious and inflammatory disease processes. What does this mean in terms of the role of either IL-1 or TNF? The current interpretation is that *both* IL-1 and TNF orchestrate the deleterious effects of infection and injury and that blocking the activity of either one of these cytokines prevents the full consequences of the disease. This interpretation is consistent with the known synergistic effects of IL-1 and TNF.

Acknowledgements
These studies are supported by NIH Grant AI 15614. The author thanks Drs K Aiura, BD Clark, JA Gelfand, EV Granowitz, T Ikejima, J Mancilla, LC Miller, D Poutsiaka, R Porat, E Vannier, G Wakabayashi, Sheldon M Wolff and K Ye.

References

1. Atkins E. Pathogenesis of fever. *Physiol Rev* 1960; **40,** 580–646.
2. Rosenwasser LM, Dinarello CA, Rosenthal AS. Adherent cell function in murine T-lymphocyte antigen recognition. IV. Enhancement of murine T-cell antigen recognition by human leukocytic pyrogen. *J Exp Med* 1979; **150,** 709–714.
3. Dinarello CA, Cannon JG, Wolff SM. New concepts on the pathogenesis of fever. *Rev Infect Dis* 1988; **10,** 168–189.
4. Kampschmidt RF. Leukocytic endogenous mediator/endogenous pyrogen. In: *The Physiologic and Metabolic Responses of the Host*, Powanda MC, Canonico PG (eds). Amsterdam: Elsevier/North Holland, 1981.
5. Merriman CR, Pulliam LA, Kampschmidt RF. Comparison of leukocytic pyrogen and leukocytic endogenous mediator. *Proc Soc Exp Biol Med* 1977; **154,** 224–227.
6. Krane SM, Conca W, Stephenson ML, Amento EP, Goldring MB. Mechanisms of matrix degradation in rheumatoid arthritis. *Ann N Y Acad Sci* 1990; **580,** 340–354.
7. Saklatvala J, Sarsfield SJ, Townsend Y. Pig interleukin 1: purification of two immunologically different leukocyte proteins that cause cartilage resorption, lymphocyte activation, and fever. *J Exp Med* 1985; **162,** 1208–1222.
8. Dewhirst FE, Stashenko PP, Mole JE, Tsurumachi T. Purification and partial sequence of human osteoclast-activating factor: identity with interleukin 1 beta. *J Immunol* 1985; **135,** 2562–2568.
9. Moore MA, Warren DJ. Synergy of interleukin 1 and granulocyte colony-stimulating factor: *in vivo* stimulation of stem-cell recovery and hematopoietic regeneration following 5-fluorouracil treatment of mice. *Proc Nat Acad Sci USA* 1987; **84,** 7134–7138.
10. Mori S, Goto F, Goto K *et al.* Cloning and sequence analysis of a cDNA for lymphocyte proliferation potentiating factor of rabbit neutrophils: identification as rabbit interleukin-1β. *Biochem Biophys Res Comm* 1988; **150,** 1237–1243.
11. Nishida T, Nishino N, Takano M *et al.* cDNA cloning of IL-1 alpha and IL-1 beta from mRNA of U937 cell line. *Biochem Biophys Res Comm* 1987; **143,** 345–352.
12. Fryling C, Dombalagian M, Burgess W, Hollander N, Schreiber BB, Heimovich J. Purification and characterization of tumor inhibitory factor-2: its identity to interleukin-1. *Cancer Res* 1989; **49,** 3333–3337.
13. Tewari A, Buhles WC Jr, Starnes HF Jr. Preliminary report: effects of interleukin-1 on platelet counts. *Lancet* 1990; **336,** 712–714.
14. Smith J, Urba W, Steis R *et al.* Interleukin-1 alpha: Results of a phase I toxicity and immunomodulatory trial. *Am Soc Clin Oncol* 1990; **9,** 717.
15. Auron PE, Webb AC, Rosenwasser LJ *et al.*

Nucleotide sequence of human monocyte interleukin 1 precursor cDNA. *Proc Nat Acad Sci USA* 1984; **81,** 7907–7911.
16. Lomedico PT, Gubler R, Hellmann CP *et al.* Cloning and expression of murine interleukin-1 cDNA in *Escherichia coli. Nature* 1984; **312,** 458–462.
17. Dinarello CA, Goldin NP, Wolff SM. Demonstration and characterization of two distinct human leukocytic pyrogens. *J Exp Med* 1974; **139,** 1369–1381.
18. Clark BD, Collins KL, Gandy MS, Webb AC, Auron PE. Genomic sequence for human prointerleukin 1 beta: possible evolution from a reverse transcribed prointerleukin 1 alpha gene. *Nucleic Acids Res* 1986; **14,** 7897–7914.
19. Furutani Y, Notake M, Fukui T *et al.* Complete nucleotide sequence of the gene for human interleukin 1 alpha. *Nucleic Acids Res* 1986; **14,** 3167–3179.
20. Caput D, Beutler B, Hartog K, Thayer R, Brown-Shimer S, Cerami A. Identification of a common nucleotide sequence in the 3′-untranslated region of mRNA molecules specifying inflammatory mediators. *Proc Nat Acad Sci USA* 1986; **83,** 1670–1674.
21. Webb AC, Collins KL, Auron PE *et al.* Interleukin-1 gene (IL1) assigned to long arm of human chromosome 2. *Lymphokine Res* 1986; **5,** 77–85.
22. Casagli MC, Borri MG, Bigio M *et al.* Different conformation of purified human recombinant interleukin 1 beta from *Escherichia coli* and *Saccharomyces cerevisiae* is related to different level of biological activity. *Biochem Biophys Res Comm* 1989; **162,** 357–363.
23. Rosenwasser LJ, Webb AC, Clark BD *et al.* Expression of biologically active human interleukin 1 subpeptides by transfected simian COS cells. *Proc Nat Acad Sci USA* 1986; **83,** 5243–5246.
24. Obalj F, Opp M, Cady AB *et al.* Interleukin 1α and an interleukin 1β fragment are somnogenic. *Am J Physiol*; **259,** R437–R446.
25. Palaszynski EW. Synthetic C-terminal peptide of IL-1 functions as a binding domain as well as an antagonist for the IL-1 receptor. *Biochem Biophy Res Comm* 1987; **147,** 204–211.
26. Antoni G, Presentini R, Perni F *et al.* Interleukin 1 and its synthetic peptides as adjuvants for poorly immunogenic vaccines. *Adv Exp Med Biol* 1989; **251,** 153–160.
27. Boraschi D, Antoni G, Perni F *et al.* Defining the structural requirements of a biologically active domain of human IL-1β. 1990; **1,** 21–26.
28. Herzbeck H, Blum B, Ronspeck W *et al.* Functional and molecular characterization of a monoclonal antibody against the 165–186 peptide of human IL-1 beta. *Scand J Immunol* 1989; **30,** 549–562.
29. Kamogashira T, Masui Y, Ohmoto Y *et al.* Site-specific mutagenesis of the human interleukin-1 beta gene: structure-function analysis of the cysteine residues. *Biochem Biophys Res Comm* 1988; **150,** 1106–1114.
30. Yem AW, Zurcher-Neely HA, Richard KA, Staite ND, Heinrikson RL, Deibel MR Jr. Biotinylation of reactive amino groups in native recombinant human interleukin-1 beta. *J Biol Chem* 1989; **264,** 17691–17697.
31. Preistle JP, Schar HP, Grutter MG. Crystallographic refinement of interleukin 1 beta at 2.0 A resolution. *Proc Nat Acad Sci USA* 1989; **86,** 9667–9671.
32. Gronenborn AM, Wingfield PT, McDonald HR, Schmeissner U, Clore GM. Site directed mutants of human interleukin-1 alpha: a 1H-NMR and receptor binding study. *FEBS Lett* 1988; **231,** 135–138.
33. Daumy GO, Merenda JM, McColl AS *et al.* Isolation and characterization of biologically active murine interleukin-1 alpha derived from expression of a synthetic gene in *Escherichia coli. Biochim Biophys Acta* 1989; **998,** 32–42.
34. Richard KA, Yem AW, Deibel MR Jr, Staite ND. Isolation and bioactivities of three IL-1 beta N-terminal variants. *Agents Actions* 1989; **27,** 268–270.
35. Huang JJ, Newton RC, Horuk R *et al.* Muteins of human interleukin-1 that show enhanced bioactivities. *FEBS Lett* 1987; **223,** 294–298.
36. Lillquist JS, Simon PL, Summers M, Jonak Z, Young PR. Structure-activity studies of human IL1 beta with mature and truncated proteins expressed in *Escherichia coli. J Immunol* 1988; **141,** 1975–1981.
37. Gehrke L, Jobling SA, Paik LS, McDonald B, Rosenwasser LJ, Auron PE. A point mutation uncouples human interleukin-1 beta biological activity and receptor binding. *J Biol Chem* 1990; **265,** 5922–5925.
38. Naito Y, Fukata J, Masui Y *et al.* Interleukin-1 beta analogues with markedly reduced pyrogenic activity can stimulate secretion of adrenocorticotropic hormone in rats. *Biochem Biophys Res Comm* 1990; **167,** 103–109.
39. Yamayoshi M, Ohue M, Kawashima H *et al.* A human IL-1α derivative which lacks prostaglandin E_2 inducing activity and inhibits the activity of IL-1 through receptor competition. *Lymph Res* 1990; **9,** 405–413.
40. Priestle JP, Schar HP, Grutter MG. Crystal structure of the cytokine interleukin-1 beta. *EMBO J* 1988; *7,* 339–343.
41. Dinarello CA, Bendtzen K, Wolff SM. Studies

on the active site of human leukocytic pyrogen. *Inflammation* 1982; **6,** 63–78.

42. Richard KA, Speziale SC, Staite ND *et al.* Soybean trypsin inhibitor (SBTI) shares some structural homology with interleukin-1 (IL-1) and was tested for IL-1 bioactivity. *Agents Actions* 1989; **27,** 265–267.
43. Demczuk S, Baumberger C, Mach B, Dayer JM. Expression of human IL 1 alpha and beta messenger RNAs and IL 1 activity in human peripheral blood mononuclear cells. *J Mol Cell Immunol* 1987; **6,** 255–265.
44. Turner M, Chantry D, Barrett K, Feldmann M. Regulation of expression of human IL-1 alpha and IL-1 beta genes. *J Immunol* 1989; **143,** 3556–3561.
45. Yamoto K, el-Hajjaoui Z, Koeffler HP. Regulation of levels of IL-1 mRNA in human fibroblasts. *J Cell Physiol* 1989; **139,** 610–616.
46. Schindler R, Dinarello CA. Ultrafiltration to remove endotoxins and other cytokine-inducing materials from tissue culture media and parenteral fluids. *Bio Techniques* 1990; **8,** 408–413.
47. Schindler R, Clark BD, Dinarello CA. Dissociation between interleukin-1β mRNA and protein synthesis in human peripheral blood mononuclear cells. *J Biol Chem* 1990; **265,** 10232–10237.
48. Schindler R, Lonnemann G, Shaldon S, Koch KM, Dinarello CA. Transcription, not synthesis, of interleukin-1 and tumor necrosis factor by complement. *Kidney Int* 1990; **37,** 85–93.
49. Molina J-M, Scadden DT, Amirault C *et al.* Human immunodeficiency virus does not induce interleukin-1, interleukin-6, or tumor necrosis factor in mononuclear cells. *J Virology* 1990; **64,** 2901–2906.
50. Molina JM, Scadden DT, Byrn R, Dinarello CA, Groopman JE. Production of tumor necrosis factor alpha and interleukin 1 beta by monocytic cells infected with human immunodeficiency virus. *J Clin Invest* 1989; **84,** 733–737.
51. Molina J-M, Schindler R, Ferriani R *et al.* Production of cytokines by peripheral blood monocytes/macrophages infected with human immunodeficiency virus type 1 (HIV-1). *J Inf Dis* 1990; **161,** 888–893.
52. Libby P, Ordovas JM, Birinyi LK, Auger KR, Dinarello CA. Inducible interleukin-1 gene expression in human vascular smooth muscle cells. *J Clin Invest* 1986; **78,** 1432–1438.
53. Libby P, Ordovas JM, Auger KR, Robbins AH, Birinyi LK, Dinarello CA. Endotoxin and tumor necrosis factor induce interleukin-1 gene expression in adult human vascular endothelial cells. *Am J Pathol* 1986; **124,** 179–185.
54. Fenton MJ, Clark BD, Collins KL, Webb AC, Rich A, Auron PE. Transcriptional regulation of the human prointerleukin 1 beta gene. *J Immunol* 1987; **138,** 3972–3979.
55. Fenton MJ, Vermeulen MW, Clark BD, Webb AC, Auron PE. Human pro-IL-1 beta gene expression in monocytic cells is regulated by two distinct pathways. *J Immunol* 1988; **140,** 2267–2273.
56. Schindler R, Ghezzi P, Dinarello CA. IL-1 induces IL-1. IV. IFN-γ suppresses IL-1 but not lipopolysaccharide-induced transcription of IL-1. *J Immunol* 1990; **144,** 2216–2222.
57. Schindler R, Gelfand JA, Dinarello CA. Recombinant C5a stimulates transcription rather than translation of IL-1 and TNF; cytokine synthesis induced by LPS, IL-1 or PMA. *Blood* 1990; **76,** 1631–1638.
58. Auron PE, Warner SJ, Webb AC *et al.* Studies on the molecular nature of human interleukin 1. *J Immunol* 1987; **138,** 1447–1456.
59. Lonnemann G, Endres S, van der Meer JW, Cannon JG, Koch KM, Dinarello CA. Differences in the synthesis and kinetics of release of interleukin 1 alpha, interleukin 1 beta and tumor necrosis factor from human mononuclear cells. *Eur J Immunol* 1989; **19,** 1531–1536.
60. Endres S, Cannon JG, Ghorbani R *et al. In vitro* production of IL-1beta, IL-1alpha, TNF, and IL-2 in healthy subjects: distribution, effect of cyclooxygenase inhibition and evidence of independent gene regulation. *Eur J Immunol* 1989; **19,** 2327–2333.
61. Rubartelli A, Cozzolino F, Talio M, Sitia R. A novel secretory pathway for interleukin-1 beta, a protein lacking a signal sequence. *EMBO J* 1990; **9,** 1503–1510.
62. Singer II, Scott S, Hall GL, Limjuco G, Chin J, Schmidt JA. Interleukin 1 beta is localised in the cytoplasmic ground substance but is largely absent from the Golgi apparatus and plasma membranes of stimulated human monocytes. *J Exp Med* 1988; **167,** 389–407.
63. Baldari CT, Telford JL. The intracellular precursor of IL1 beta is associated with microtubules in activated U937 cells. *J Immunol* 1989; **142,** 785–791.
64. Bakouche O, Brown DC, Lachman LB. Subcellular localization of human monocyte interleukin 1: evidence for an inactive precursor molecule and a possible mechanism for IL 1 release. *J Immunol* 1987; **138,** 4249–4255.
65. Beuscher HU, Nickells MW, Colten HR. The precursor of interleukin-1 alpha is phosphorylated at residue serine 90. *J Biol Chem* 1988; **263,** 4023–4028.
66. Kobayashi Y, Appella E, Yamada M, Copeland TD, Oppenheim JJ, Matsushima K. Phosphorylation of intracellular precursors of human IL-1. *J Immunol* 1988; **140,** 2279–2287.

67. Hazuda DJ, Lee JC, Young PR. The kinetics of interleukin 1 secretion from activated monocytes. Differences between interleukin 1 alpha and interleukin 1 beta. *J Biol Chem* 1988; **263,** 8473–8479.
68. Dinarello CA, Ikejima T, Warner SJ *et al.* Interleukin 1 induces interleukin 1. I. Induction of circulating interleukin 1 in rabbits *in vivo* and in human mononuclear cells *in vitro*. *J Immunol* 1987; **139,** 1902–1910.
69. Numerof RP, Kotick AN, Dinarello CA, Mier JW. Pro-interleukin-1β production by a subpopulation of human T cells, but not NK cells, in response to interleukin-2. *Cell Immunol* 1990; **130,** 118–128.
70. Hazuda DJ, Strickler J, Kueppers F, Simon PL, Young PR. Processing of precursor interleukin-1 beta and inflammatory disease. *J Biol Chem* 1990; **265,** 6318–6322.
71. Van Damme J, De Ley M, Opdenakker G, Billiau A, De Somer P. Homogeneous interferon-inducing 22K factor is related to endogenous pyrogen and interleukin-1. *Nature* 1985; **314,** 266–268.
72. Knudsen PJ, Dinarello CA, Strom TB. Purification and characterization of a unique human interleukin 1 from the tumor cell line U937. *J Immunol* 1986; **136,** 3311–3316.
73. Beuscher HU, Guenther C, Roellinghoff M. IL-1 beta is secreted by activated murine macrophages as biologically inactive precursor. *J Immunol* 1990; **144,** 2179–2183.
74. Suttles J, Giri JG, Mizel SB. IL-1 secretion by macrophages. Enhancement of IL-1 secretion and processing by calcium ionophores. *J Immunol* 1990; **144,** 175–182.
75. Brody DT, Durum SK. Membrane IL-1: IL-1α precursor binds to the plasma membrane via a lectin-like interaction. *J Immunol* 1989; **143,** 1183.
76. Bursten SL, Locksley RM, Ryan JL, Lovett DH. Acylation of monocyte and glomerular mesangial cell proteins. *J Clin Invest* 1988; **82,** 1479–1486.
77. Suttles J, Carruth LM, Mizel SB. Detection of IL-1α and IL-1β in the supernatants of paraformaldehyde-treated human monocytes. Evidence against a membrane form of IL-1. *J Immunol* 1990; **144,** 170–174.
78. Pierart ME, Najdovski T, Appelboom TE, Deschodt-Lanckman MM. Effect of human endopeptidase 24.11 ('enkephalinase') on IL-1-induced thymocyte proliferation activity. *J Immunol* 1988; **140,** 3808–3811.
79. Black RA, Kronheim SR, Cantrell M *et al.* Generation of biologically active interleukin-1 beta by proteolytic cleavage of the inactive precursor. *J Biol Chem* 1988; **263,** 9437–9442.
80. Kostura MJ, Tocci MJ, Limjuco G *et al.* Identification of a monocyte specific pre-interleukin 1 beta convertase activity. *Proc Nat Acad Sci USA* 1989; **86,** 5227–5231.
81. Weiss L, Haeffner-Cavaillon N, Gilquin J, Kazatchkine MD. Zidovudine inhibits functional extracellular monocytic interleukin-1. *AIDS* 1990; **4,** 255–257.
82. Kobayashi Y, Yamamoto K, Saido T, Kawasaki H, Oppenheim JJ, Matsushima K. Identification of calcium-activated neutral protease as a processing enzyme of human interleukin 1 alpha. *Proc Nat Acad Sci USA* 1990; **87,** 5548–5552.
83. Cannon JG, Dinarello CA. Increased plasma interleukin-1 activity in women after ovulation. *Science* 1985; **227,** 1247–1249.
84. Kurt-Jones EA, Beller DI, Mizel SB, Unanue ER. Identification of a membrane-associated interleukin-1 in macrophages. *Proc Nat Acad Sci USA* 1985; **82,** 1204.
85. Engelmann H, Aderka D, Rubinstein M, Rotman D, Wallach D. A tumor necrosis factor-binding protein purified to homogeneity from human urine protects cells from tumor necrosis factor toxicity. *J Biol Chem* 1989; **264,** 11974–11980.
86. Minnich-Carruth LL, Suttles J, Mizel SB. Evidence against the existence of a membrane form of murine IL-1α. *J Immunol* 1989; **142,** 526.
87. Bailly S, Ferrua B, Fay M, Gougerot-Pocidalo M-A. Paraformaldehyde fixation of LPS-stimulated human monocytes: technical parameters permitting the study of membrane IL-1 activity. *Eur Cytokine Net* 1990; **1,** 47–51.
88. Lowenthal JW, MacDonald HR. Binding and internalization of interleukin-1 by T-cells. Direct evidence from high and low affinity classes of interleukin-1 receptors. *J Exp Med* 1986; **164,** 1060–1072.
89. Savage N, Puren AJ, Orencole SF, Ikejima T, Clark BD, Dinarello CA. Studies on IL-1 receptors on D10S T-helper cells: demonstration of two molecularly and antigenically distinct IL-1 binding proteins. *Cytokine* 1989; **1,** 23–25.
90. Bomsztyk K, Sims JE, Stanton TH *et al.* Evidence for different interleukin 1 receptors in murine B- and T-cell lines. *Proc Nat Acad Sci USA* 1989; **86,** 8034–8038.
91. Chizzonite R, Truitt T, Kilian PL *et al.* Two high-affinity interleukin 1 receptors represent separate gene products. *Proc Nat Acad Sci USA* 1989; **86,** 8029–8033.
92. Kroggel R, Martin M, Pingoud V, Dayer J-M, Resch K. Two-chain structure of the interleukin-1 receptor. *FEBS Lett* 1988; **229,** 59–62.
93. Uehara A, Gottscall PE, Dahl RR, Arimura A. Stimulation of ACTH release by human interleu-

kin-1b but not interleukin-1a, in conscious, freely moving rats. *Biochem Biophys Res Comm* 1987; **146,** 1286–1290.

94. Naito Y, Fukata J, Tominaga T *et al.* Adrenocorticotropin hormone releasing activities of interleukins in a homologous *in vivo* system. *Biochem Biophy Res Comm* 1989; **164,** 1262–1267.
95. Sims JE, March CJ, Cosman D *et al.* cDNA expression cloning of the IL-1 receptor, a member of the immunoglobulin superfamily. *Science* 1988; **241,** 585–589.
96. Uhl J, Newton RC, Giri JG, Sandlin G, Horuk R. Identification of IL-1 receptors on human monocytes. *J Immunol* 1989; **142,** 1576–1581.
97. Gallis B, Prickett KS, Jackson J *et al.* IL-1 induces rapid phosphorylation of the IL-1 receptor. *J Immunol* 1989; **143,** 3235–3240.
98. Mancilla J, Ikejima I, Clark BD, Orencole SF, Sirko S, Dinarello CA. Lectin binding suggests different glycosylation patterns of IL-1 receptors on different cells. *Cytokine* 1989; **1,** 95.
99. Rosoff PM, Savage N, Dinarello CA. Interleukin-1 stimulates diacylglycerol production in T lymphocytes by a novel mechanism. *Cell* 1988; **54,** 73–81.
100. End D, Garrabrant T. Characterization of a high affinity interleukin-1 (IL-1) specific binding site in a human synovial sarcoma (Hs431) cell line. *Lymph Res* 1990; **9,** 167–171.
101. Dower SK, Wignall JM, Schooley K *et al.* Retention of ligand binding activity by the extracellular domain of the IL-1 receptor. *J Immunol* 1989; **142,** 4314–4320.
102. Clark BD, Ikejima T, Mancilla J *et al.* An antibody to a 17 amino acid synthetic peptide of the 80 kDa IL-1R blocks both binding and biological activity. *Cytokine* 1989; **90** (abs).
103. Qwarnstrom EE, Page RC, Gillis S, Dower SK. Binding, internalization, and intracellular localization of interleukin-1 beta in human diploid fibroblasts. *J Biol Chem* 1988; **263,** 8261–8269.
104. Curtis BM, Widmer MB, deRoos P, Qwarnstrom EE. IL-1 and its receptor are translocated to the nucleus. *J Immunol* 1990; **144,** 1295–1303.
105. Mizel SB, Kilian PL, Lewis JC, Paganelli KA, Chizzonite RA. The interleukin 1 receptor. Dynamics of interleukin 1 binding and internalization in T cells and fibroblasts. *J Immunol* 1987; **138,** 2906–2912.
106. Matsushima K, Akahoshi T, Yamada M, Furutani Y, Oppenheim JJ. Properties of a specific interleukin-1 receptor on human Epstein-Barr virus-transformed B lymphocytes: identity of the receptor for IL-1a and IL-1b. *J Immunol* 1986; **136,** 4496–4500.
107. Horuk R, Huang JJ, Covington M, Newton RC. A biochemical and kinetic analysis of the interleukin-1 receptor. Evidence for differences in molecular properties of IL-1 receptors. *J Biol Chem* 1987; **262,** 16275–16278.
108. Horuk R, McCubrey JA. The interleukin-1 receptor in Raji human B cell lymphoma cells. *Biochem J* 1989; **260,** 657–663.
109. Scapigliati G, Ghiara P, Bartalini A, Taglibue A, Boraschi D. Differential binding of IL-1α and IL-1β to receptors on B and T cells. *FEBS Lett* 1989; **243,** 394–398.
110. Dower SK, McMahan C, Flack J *et al.* Molecular characterization of two types of interleukin-1 receptor coding peptides on murine and human cells. *J Leuk Biol* 1990; **1** (suppl), 103.
111. Matsushima K, Yodoi J, Tagaya Y, Oppenheim JJ. Down-regulation of interleukin-1 receptor expression by IL-1 and fate of internalised 125-I-labeled IL-1b in a human large granular lymphocyte cell line. *J Immunol* 1986; **137,** 3183–3188.
112. Benjamin D, Wormsley S, Dower SK. Heterogeneity in interleukin (IL)-1 receptors expressed on human B cell lines. Differences in the molecular properties of IL-1 alpha and IL-1 beta binding sites. *J Biol Chem* 1990; **265,** 9943–9951.
113. Parker KP, Benjamin WR, Kaffka KL, Kilian PL. Presence of IL-1 receptors on human and murine neutrophils. Relevance to IL-1-mediated effects in inflammation. *J Immunol* 1989; **142,** 537–542.
114. Conti P, Cifone MG, Alesse E, Reale M, Fieschi C, Dinarello CA. *In vitro* enhanced thromboxane B2 release by polymorphonuclear leukocytes and macrophages after treatment with human recombinant interleukin 1. *Prostaglandins* 1986; **32,** 111–115.
115. Borish L, Rosenbaum R, McDonald B, Rosenwasser LJ. Recombinant interleukin-1 beta interacts with high-affinity receptors to activate neutrophil leukotriene B4 synthesis. *Inflammation* 1990; **14,** 151–162.
116. Georgilis K, Schaefer C, Dinarello CA, Klempner MS. Human recombinant interleukin 1 beta has no effect on intracellular calcium or on functional responses of human neutrophils. *J Immunol* 1987; **138,** 3403–3407.
117. Nedwin GE, Naylor SL, Sakaguchi AY *et al.* Human lymphotoxin and tumor necrosis factor genes: structure, homology and chromosomal localization. *Nucleic Acids Res* 1985; **13,** 6361–6373.
118. Beutler B, Cerami A. Cachectin: more than a tumor necrosis factor. *N Engl J Med* 1987; **316,** 379–385.
119. Kriegler M, Perez C, DeFay K, Albert I, Lu SD. A novel form of TNF/cachectin is a cell surface cytotoxic transmembrane protein: ramifications

for the complex physiology of TNF. *Cell* 1988; **53,** 45–53.

120. Schindler R, Mancilla J, Endres S, Ghorbani R, Clark SC, Dinarello CA. Correlations and interactions in the production of interleukin-6 (IL-6), IL-1, and tumor necrosis factor (TNF) in human blood mononuclear cells: IL-6 suppresses IL-1 and TNF. *Blood* 1990; **75,** 40–47.
121. Michie HR, Manogue KR, Spriggs DR *et al.* Detection of circulating tumor necrosis factor after endotoxin administration. *N Engl J Med* 1988; **318,** 1481–1486.
122. Korn JH, Mory Y, Ziberstein A, Holtmann H, Revel M, Wallach D. Cloning of genomic DNA for tumor necrosis factor and efficient expression in CHO cells. *Lymphokine Res* 1988; **7,** 349–358.
123. Jones EY, Stuart DI, Walker NPC. Structure of tumor necrosis factor. *Nature* 1989; **338,** 225–228.
124. Engelmann H, Novick D, Wallach D. Two tumor necrosis factor-binding proteins purified from human urine. Evidence for immunological cross-reactivity with cell surface tumor necrosis factor receptors. *J Biol Chem* 1990; **265,** 1531–1536.
125. Dembric Z, Loetscher H, Gubler U *et al.* Two human TNF receptors have similar extracellular but distinct intracellular domain sequences. *Cytokine* 1990; **2,** 231–237.
126. Nophar Y, Kemper O, Brakebusch C *et al.* Soluble forms of tumor necrosis factor receptors (TNF-Rs). The cDNA for the type I TNF-R, cloned using amino acid sequence data of its soluble form, encodes both the cell surface and a soluble form of the receptor. *EMBO J* 1990; **9,** 3269–3278.
127. Engelmann H, Holtmann H, Brakebusch C *et al.* Antibodies to a soluble form of a tumor necrosis factor (TNF) receptor have TNF-like activity. *J Biol Chem* 1990; **265,** 14497–14504.
128. Chapman PB, Lester TJ, Casper ES *et al.* Clinical pharmacology of recombinant human tumor necrosis factor in patients with advanced cancer. *J Clin Oncol* 1987; **5,** 1942–1951.
129. Van der Poll T, van Deventer SJH, Hack CE *et al.* Effects of leukocytes following injection of tumor necrosis factor into healthy humans. *Blood* 1991; **79,** 693–698.
130. Van der Poll T, Bueller HR, ten Cate H *et al.* Activation of coagulation after administration of tumor necrosis factor to normal subjects. *N Engl J Med* 1990; **322,** 1622–1627.
131. Ranges GE, Zlotnik A, Espevik T, Dinarello CA, Cerami A, Palladino MAJ. Tumor necrosis factor alpha/cachectin is a growth factor for thymocytes. Synergistic interactions with other cytokines. *J Exp Med* 1988; **167,** 1472–1478.
132. Dinarello CA, Cannon JG, Wolff SM *et al.* Tumor necrosis factor (cachectin) is an endogenous pyrogen and induces production of interleukin 1. *J Exp Med* 1986; **163,** 1433–1450.
133. Dayer JM, Beutler B, Cerami A. Cachectin/tumor necrosis factor stimulates collagenase and prostaglandin E_2 production by human synovial cells and dermal fibroblasts. *J Exp Med* 1985; **162,** 2163–2168.
134. Perlmutter DH, Dinarello CA, Punsal PI, Colten HR. Cachectin/tumor necrosis factor regulates hepatic acute phase gene expression. *J Clin Invest* 1986; **78,** 1349–1354.
135. Shoham S, Davenne D, Cady AB, Dinarello CA, Krueger JM. Recombinant tumor necrosis factor and interleukin 1 enhance slow-wave sleep. *Am J Physiol* 1987; **253,** R142–R149.
136. Zucali JR, Broxmeyer HE, Gross MA, Dinarello CA. Recombinant human tumor necrosis factors alpha and beta stimulate fibroblasts to produce hemopoietic growth factors *in vitro*. *J Immunol* 1988; **140,** 840–844.
137. Zucali JR, Dinarello CA, Oblon DJ, Gross MA, Anderson L, Weiner RS. Interleukin 1 stimulates fibroblasts to produce granulocyte-macrophage colony-stimulating activity and prostaglandin E_2. *J Clin Invest* 1986; **77,** 1857–1863.
138. Bagby GCJ, Dinarello CA, Wallace P, Wagner C, Hefeneider S, McCall E. Interleukin 1 stimulates granulocyte macrophage colony-stimulating activity release by vascular endothelial cells. *J Clin Invest* 1986; **78,** 1316–1323.
139. Okusawa S, Gelfand JA, Ikejima T, Connolly RJ, Dinarello CA. Interleukin 1 induces a shock-like state in rabbits. Synergism with tumor necrosis factor and the effect of cyclooxygenase inhibition. *J Clin Invest* 1988; **81,** 1162–1172.
140. Tracey K, Fong Y, Hesse DG *et al.* Anti-cachectin/TNF monoclonal antibodies prevent septic shock during lethal bacteremia. *Nature* 1987; **330,** 662–664.
141. Mathison JC, Wolfson E, Ulevitch RJ. Participation of tumor necrosis factor in the mediation of gram negative bacterial lipopolysaccharide-induced injury in rabbits. *J Clin Invest* 1988; **81,** 1925–1937.
142. Ye K, Clark BD, Dinarello CA. Interleukin-1β downregulates gene and surface expression of interleukin-1 receptor type I by destabilising its mRNA whereas interleukin-2 increases its expression. *Immunol* 1991; **75,** 427–434.
143. Holtmann H, Wallach D. Down regulation of the receptors for tumor necrosis factor by interleukin 1 and 4 beta-phorbol-12-myristate-13-acetate. *J Immunol* 1987; **139,** 1161–1167.
144. Ramadori G, Sipe JD, Dinarello CA, Mizel SB, Colten HR. Pretranslational modulation of acute phase hepatic protein synthesis by murine recom-

binant interleukin 1 (IL-1) and purified human IL-1. *J Exp Med* 1985; **162,** 930–942.

145. Ernst TJ, Ritchie AR, Demetri GD, Griffin JD. Regulation of granulocyte- and monocyte-colony stimulating factor mRNA levels in human blood monocytes is mediated primarily at a post-transcriptional level. *J Biol Chem* 1989; **264,** 5700–5703.

146. Demetri GD, Zenzie BW, Rheinwald JG, Griffin JD. Expression of colony-stimulating factor genes by normal human mesothelial cells and human malignant mesothelioma cell lines *in vitro*. *Blood* 1989; **74,** 940–946.

147. Griffin JD, Cannistra SA, Sullivan R, Demetri GD, Ernst TJ, Kanakura Y. The biology of GM-CSF: regulation of production and interaction with its receptor. *Int J Cell Cloning* 1990; **1,** 35–44.

148. Bottazzi B, Nobili N, Mantovani A. Expression of c-fos proto-oncogene in tumor-associated macrophages. *J Immunol* 1990; **144,** 4878–4882.

149. Shirakawa F, Mizel SB. *In vitro* activation and nuclear translocation of NF-kappa B catalyzed by cyclic AMP-derived protein kinase and protein kinase C. *Mol Cell Biol* 1989; **9,** 2424–2430.

150. Muegge K, Williams TM, Kant J *et al.* Interleukin-1 costimulatory activity on the interleukin-2 promoter via AP-1. *Science* 1989; **246,** 249–251.

151. Coceani F, Lees J, Dinarello CA. Occurrence of interleukin-1 in cerebrospinal fluid of the conscious cat. *Brain Res* 1988; **446,** 245–250.

152. Grunfeld C, Soued M, Adi S, Moser AH, Dinarello CA, Feingold KR. Evidence for two classes of cytokines that stimulate hepatic lipogenesis: relationships among tumor necrosis factor, interleukin-1 and interferon-alpha. *Endocrinology* 1990; **127,** 46–52.

153. Moldawer LL, Andersen C, Gelin J, Lundholm KG. Regulation of food intake and hepatic protein synthesis by recombinant derived cytokines. *Am J Physiol* 1988; **254,** G450–456.

154. Mrosovsky N, Molony LA, Conn CA, Kluger MJ. Anorexic effects of interleukin-1 in the rat. *Am J Physiol* 1989; **257,** R1315–1321.

155. Bird TA, Davies T, Baldwin SA, Saklatvala J. Interleukin-1 regulates the glucose transporter of fibroblasts. *J Biol Chem* 1990; **265,** 13578–13583.

156. Hellerstein MK, Meydani SN, Meydani M, Wu K, Dinarello CA. Interleukin-1-induced anorexia in the rat. Influence of prostaglandins. *J Clin Invest* 1989; **84,** 228–235.

157. Gershenwald JE, Fong YM, Fahey TJ *et al.* Interleukin 1 receptor blockade attenuates the host inflammatory response. *Proc Nat Acad Sci USA* 1990; **87,** 4966–4970.

158. Schweizer A, Feige U, Fontana A, Muller K, Dinarello CA. Interleukin-1 enhances pain reflexes. Mediation through increased prostaglandin E_2 levels. *Agents Actions* 1988; **25,** 246–251.

159. Bertini R, Bianchi M, Ghezzi P. Adrenalectomy sensitizes mice to the lethal effects of interleukin 1 and tumor necrosis factor. *J Exp Med* 1988; **167,** 1708–1712.

160. Butler LD, Layman NK, Cain RL *et al.* Interleukin-1 induced pathophysiology. *Clin Immunol Immunopathol* 1989; **53,** 400–421.

161. Beasley DS, Cohen RA, Levinsky NG. Interleukin-1 inhibits contraction of vascular smooth muscle. *J Clin Invest* 1989; **83,** 331–335.

162. Beasley D, Schwartz JH, Brenner BM. Interleukin 1 induces prolonged L-arginine-dependent cyclic guanosine monophosphate and nitrite production in rat vascular smooth muscle cells. *J Clin Invest* 1991; **87,** 602–608.

163. Dejana E, Breviario F, Erroi A *et al.* Modulation of endothelial cell functions by different molecular species of interleukin 1. *Blood* 1987; **69,** 695–699.

164. Rossi V, Breviario F, Ghezzi P, Dejana E, Mantovani A. Prostacyclin synthesis induced in vascular cells by interleukin-1. *Science* 1985; **229,** 174–176.

165. Warner SJC, Auger KR, Libby P. Human interleukin 1 induces interleukin 1 gene expression in human vascular smooth muscle cells. *J Exp Med* 1987; **165,** 1316–1331.

166. Raines EW, Dower SK, Ross R. Interleukin-1 mitogenic activity for fibroblasts and smooth muscle cells is due to PDGF-AA. *Science* 1989; **243,** 393–396.

167. Libby P, Warner SJ, Friedman GB. Interleukin 1: a mitogen for human vascular smooth muscle cells that induces the release of growth-inhibitory prostanoids. *J Clin Invest* 1988; **81,** 487–498.

168. Movat HZ, Burrowes CE, Cybulsky MI, Dinarello CA. Acute inflammation and a Shwartzman-like reaction induced by interleukin-1 and tumor necrosis factor. Synergistic action of the cytokines in the induction of inflammation and microvascular injury. *Am J Pathol* 1987; **129,** 463–476.

169. Cozzolino F, Torcia M, Aldinucci D *et al.* Interleukin-1 is an autocrine regulator of human endothelial cell growth. *Pro Nat Acad Sci USA* 1990; **87,** 6487–6490.

170. Gottschall PE, Katsuura G, Arimura A. Interleukin-1 b is more potent than interleukin-1 a in suppressing follicle stimulating hormone differentiation of ovarian granulosa cells. *Biochem Biophy Res Comm* 1989; **163,** 764–770.

171. Bendtzen K, Buschard K, Diamant M, Horn T, Svenson M. Possible role of IL-1, TNF, and IL-6 in insulin-dependent diabetes melitus and autoimmune thryoid disease. *Lymphokine Res* 1988; **8,** 335–340.

172. Bagby GC Jr. Interleukin-1 and hematopoiesis. *Blood Rev* 1989; **3,** 152–161.
173. Fibbe WE, Falkenburg JHF. Regulation of hematopoiesis by interleukin-1. *Biotherapy* 1990; **1,** 263–276.
174. Neta R, Sztein MB, Oppenheim JJ, Gillis S, Douches SD. The *in vivo* effects of interleukin-1. I Bone marrow cells are induced to cycle after administration of interleukin-1. *J Immunol* 1987; **139,** 1861–1866.
175. Zsebo KM, Yuschenkoff VN, Schiffer S *et al.* Vascular endothelial cells and granulopoiesis: interleukin-1 stimulates release of G-CSF and GM-CSF. *Blood* 1988; **71,** 99–103.
176. Bradley TR, Williams N, Kriegler AB, Fawcett J, Hodgson GS. *In vivo* effects of interleukin-1 alpha on regenerating mouse bone marrow myeloid colony forming cells after treatment with 5-fluorouracil. *Leukemia* 1989; **3,** 893–986.
177. McNiece I, Langely K, Zsebo K. Recombinant human stem cell factor synergises with CSF's and EPO to stimulate colony formation of myeloid and erythroid cells. *Blood* 1990; **76** (suppl), 154a.
178. Oppenheim JJ, Neta R, Tiberghien P, Gress R, Kenny JJ, Longo DL. Interleukin-1 enhances survival of lethally irradiated mice treated with allogeneic bone marrow cells. *Blood* 1989; **74,** 2257–2263.
179. Fibbe WE, van der Meer JWM, Falkenburg JHF, Hamilton MS, Kluin PM, Dinarello CA. A single low dose of human recombinant interleukin 1 accelerates the recovery of neutrophils in mice with cyclophosphamide-induced neutropenia. *Exp Hematol* 1989; **17,** 805–808.
180. Neta R, Oppenheim JJ, Douches SD. Interdependence of the radioprotective effects of human recombinant interleukin 1 alpha, tumor necrosis factor alpha, granulocyte colony-stimulating factor, and murine recombinant granulocyte-macrophage colony-stimulating factor. *J Immunol* 1988; **140,** 108–111.
181. Schwartz GN, MacVittie TJ, Vigneulle RM *et al.* Enhanced hematopoietic recovery in irradiated mice pretreated with interleukin-1 (IL-1). *Immunopharmacol Immunotoxicol* 1987; **9,** 371–389.
182. Ulich TR, del Castillo J, Keys M, Granger GA, Ni R-X. Kinetics and mechanisms of recombinant human interleukin 1 and tumor necrosis factor-α-induced changes in circulating numbers of neutrophils and lymphocytes. *J Immunol* 1987; **139,** 3406–3415.
183. Van Damme J, Opdenakker G, DeLey M, Heremans H, Billiau A. Pyrogenic and haematological effects of the interferon-inducing 22K factor (interleukin-1) from human leukocytes. *Clin Exp Immunol* 1986; **66,** 303–311.
184. Shieh J-H, Gordon MS, Peterson RHF, Jakubowski AA, Gabrilove JL, Moore MAS. Modulation of cytokine receptors and superoxide production in neutrophils treated with IL-1 *in vitro* and *in vivo*. *Blood* 1990; **76** (suppl), 165a.
185. Williams DE, Morrissey PJ. Alterations in megakaryocyte and platelet compartments following *in vivo* IL-1 beta administration to normal mice. *J Immunol* 1989; **142,** 4361–4365.
186. Gasparetto C, Smith C, Gillio A, Stoppa A, Muench M, Moore MAS. Enrichment of peripheral blood stem cells with cytokine treatment in a preclinical primate model. *Blood* 1990; **76** (suppl), 541a.
187. Gasparetto C, Laver J, Abboud M *et al.* Effect of interleukin-1 on hemopoietic progenitors: evidence of stimulatory and inhibitory activities in a primate model. *Blood* 1989; **74,** 547–550.
188. Ikejima T, Ikusawa S, Ghezzi P, van der Meer JWM, Dinarello CA. IL-1 induces TNF in human PBMC *in vitro* and a circulating TNF-like activity in rabbits. *J Inf Dis* 1990; **162,** 215–221.
189. Johnson CS, Keckler DJ, Topper MI, Braunschweiger PG, Furmanski P. *In vivo* hemopoietic effects of recombinant interleukin-1 alpha in mice: stimulation of granulocytic, monocytic, megakaryocytic, and early erythroid progenitors, suppression of late stage erythropoiesis, and reversal of erythroid suppression with erythropoietin. *Blood* 1989; **73,** 678–683.
190. van der Meer JWM, Barza M, Wolff SM, Dinarello CA. A low dose of recombinant interleukin 1 protects granulocytopenic mice from lethal gram-negative infection. *Proc Nat Acad Sci USA* 1988; **85,** 1620–1623.
191. White CW, Ghezzi P. Protection against pulmonary oxygen toxicity by interleukin-1 and tumor necrosis factor: role of antioxidant enzymes and effect of cyclooxygenase inhibitors. *Biother* 1989; **1,** 361–367.
192. Vannier E, Lefort J, Bachelet M, Lelouch-Tubiana A, Terlain B, Vargastig BB. Lipopolysaccharide from *E. coli* modulates anaphylatic bronchoconstriction of actively sensitised guinea pigs. *Am Rev Resp Dis* 1989; **139,** A355.
193. Wallach D, Holtmann H, Engelmann H, Nophar Y. Sensitization and desensitization to lethal effects of tumor necrosis factor and IL-1. *J Immunol* 1988; **140,** 2994–2999.
194. Cannon JG, Tompkins RG, Gelfand JA *et al.* Circulating interleukin-1 and tumor necrosis factor in septic shock and experimental endotoxin fever. *J Inf Dis* 1990; **161,** 79–84.
195. Fong Y, Tracey KJ, Moldawer LL *et al.* Antibodies to cachectin/tumor necrosis factor reduce interleukin 1β and interleukin 6 appearance during lethal bacteremia. *J Exp Med* 1989; **170,** 1627–1633.
196. Wallach D, Holtmann H, Aderka D *et al.* Mechanisms which take part in regulation of the re-

sponse to tumor necrosis factor. *Lymphokine Res* 1989; **8,** 359–363.

197. Starnes HF, Pearce MK, Twari A, Yim JM, Zou J-C, Abrams JS. Anti-monoclonal antibodies protect against lethal *Escherichia coli* infection and lethal tumor necrosis factor-α challenge in mice. *J Immunol* 1990; **145,** 4185–4191.
198. Novick D, Engelmann H, Wallach D, Leitner O, Revel M, Rubinstein M. Purification of soluble cytokine receptors from normal human urine by ligand-affinity and immunoaffinity chromatography. *J Chromatogr* 1990; **510,** 331–337.
199. Novick D, Engelmann H, Wallach D, Rubinstein M. Soluble cytokine receptors are present in normal human urine. *J Exp Med* 1989; **170,** 1409–1414.
200. Dinarello CA, Rosenwasser LJ, Wolff SM. Demonstration of a circulating suppressor factor of thymocyte proliferation during endotoxin fever in humans. *J Immunol* 1981; **127,** 2517–2519.
201. Liao Z, Grimshaw RS, Rosenstreich DL. Identification of a specific interleukin-1 inhibitor in the urine of febrile patients. *J Exp Med* 1984; **159,** 125–136.
202. Shaldon S, Koch KM, Bingel M, Granolleras C, Deschodt G, Dinarello CA. Modulation of plasma interleukin-1 and its circulating protein inhibitor (CPI) by hemodialysis and hemofiltration. *Kidney Int* 1987; **31,** 245(abstract).
203. Arend WP, Joslin FG, Thompson RC, Hannum CH. An IL-1 inhibitor from human monocytes. Production and characterization of biologic properties. *J Immunol* 1989; **143,** 1851–1858.
204. Seckinger P, Dayer JM. Interleukin-1 inhibitors. *Ann Inst Pasteur/Immunol* 1987; **138,** 461–516.
205. Barak V, Treves AJ, Yanai P *et al.* Interleukin-1 inhibitory activity secreted by a human myelomonocytic cell line (M20). *Eur J Immunol* 1986; **16,** 1449–1452.
206. Isono N, Kumagai K. Production of interleukin-1 inhibitors by the murine macrophage cell line P388D which produces interleukin-1. *Microbial Immunol* 1989; **33,** 43–57.
207. Arend WP, Joslin FG, Massoni RJ. Effects of immune complexes on production by human monocytes of interleukin 1 or an interleukin 1 inhibitor. *J Immunol* 1985; **134,** 3868–3875.
208. Seckinger P, Lowenthal JW, Williamson K, Dayer JM, MacDonald HR. A urine inhibitor of interleukin-1 activity that blocks ligand binding. *J Immunol* 1987; **139,** 1546–1549.
209. Mazzei GJ, Seckinger PL, Dayer JM, Shaw AR. Purification and characterization of a 26-kDa competitive inhibitor of interleukin 1. *Eur J Immunol* 1990; **20,** 683–689.
210. Dayer-Metroz MD, Wollheim CB, Seckinger P, Dayer JM. A natural interleukin 1 (IL-1) inhibitor counteracts the inhibitory effect of IL-1 on insulin production in cultured rat pancreatic islets. *J Autoimmun* 1989; **2,** 163–171.
211. Balavoine JF, de Rochemonteix B, Williamson K, Seckinger P, Cruchaud A, Dayer JM. Prostaglandin E_2 and collagenase production by fibroblasts and synovial cells is regulated by urine-derived human interleukin 1 and inhibitor(s). *J Clin Invest* 1986; **78,** 1120–1124.
212. Granowitz EV, Santos A, Poutsiaka DD *et al.* Circulating interleukin-1 receptor antagonist levels during experimental endotoxemia in humans. *Lancet* 1991; **338,** 1423–1424.
213. Barak V, Peritt D, Flechner I *et al.* The IL-1 specific inhibitor from the M20 myelomonocytic cell line is distinct from the IL-1 receptor antagonist. *Lymphokine Cytokine Res* 1991; **10,** 437–442.
214. Hannum CH, Wilcox CJ, Arend WP *et al.* Interleukin-1 receptor antagonist activity of a human interleukin-1 inhibitor. *Nature* 1990; **343,** 336–340.
215. Eisenberg SP, Evans RJ, Arend WP *et al.* Primary structure and functional expression from complementary DNA of a human interleukin-1 receptor antagonist. *Nature* 1990; **343,** 341–346.
216. Dayoff MO, Barker WC, Hunt LT. Establishing homologies in protein sequences. *Meth Enzymol* 1983; **91,** 524–545.
217. Carter DB, Deibel MRJ, Dunn CJ *et al.* Purification, cloning, expression and biological characterization of an interleukin-1 receptor antagonist protein. *Nature* 1990; **344,** 633–638.
218. Seckinger P, Klein-Nulend J, Alander C, Thompson RC, Dayer JM, Raisz LG. Natural and recombinant human IL-1 receptor antagonists block the effects of IL-1 on bone resorption and prostaglandin production. *J Immunol* 1990; **145,** 4181–4184.
219. Granowitz EV, Porat R, Gelfand JA, *et al.* Effects of intravenous interleukin-1 receptor antagonist in healthy human subjects. *Cytokine* 1991; **3,** 501(abs).
220. Young P, Kumar V, Lillquist J *et al.* A site-specific mutant of IL-1 beta with reduced activity but wild type binding. *Lymphokine Res* 1990; **9,** 599.
221. Granowitz EV, Mancilla J, Clark BD, Dinarello CA. The IL-1 receptor antagonist inhibits IL-1 binding to the type II IL-1 receptor. *J Biol Chem* 1991; **266,** 14147–14150.
222. McCall E, Tracey DE. IL-1 receptor antagonist recognises the type II R on human neutrophils. *FASEB J* 1991; **5,** in press.
223. Rambaldi A, Torcia M, Bettoni S *et al.* Modulation of cell proliferation and cytokine production in acute myeloblastic leukemia by interleukin-1 receptor antagonist and lack of its

expression by leukemic cells. *Blood* 1990; **76,** 114a.
224. Granowitz EV, Clark BD, Vannier E, Callahan MV, Dinarello CA. Interleukin-1 receptor antagonist inhibits interleukin-1 induced cytokine synthesis by human monocytes. *Clin Res* 1991; **39,** 462A.
225. Ohlsson K, Bjork P, Bergenfeldt M, Hageman R, Thompson RC. Interleukin-1 receptor antagonist reduces mortality from endotoxin shock. *Nature* 1990; **348,** 550–552.
226. Fischer E, Marano MA, Zee KJ *et al.* IL-1 receptor blockade improves survival and hemodynamic performance in *E Coli* septic shock but fails to alter host responses to sublethal endotoxemia, *J Clin Invest*; **89:** 1551–1557.
227. Dinarello CA, Thompson RC. Blocking IL-1: effects of IL-1 receptor antagonist *in vitro* and *in vivo*. *Immunol Today* 1991; **12,** 407–410.
228. Wakabayashi G, Gelfand JA, Burke JF, Thompson RC, Dinarello CA. A specific receptor antagonist for interleukin-1 prevents *Escherichia coli*- induced shock. *FASEB J* 1991; **5,** 338–343.
229. Aiura K, Gelfand JA, Wakabayashi G *et al.* Interleukin-1 receptor antagonist blocks Staphylococcal induced shock in rabbits. *Cytokine* 1991; **3,** 498(abs).
230. Wakabayashi G, Gelfand JA, Jung WK, Connolly RJ, Burke JF, Dinarello CA. *Staphylococcus epidermidis* induces complement activation, tumor necrosis factor and interleukin-1, a shock-like state and tissue injury in rabbits without endotoxemia. *J Clin Invest* 1991; **87,** 1925–1935.
231. Henricson BE, Neta R, Vogel SN. An interleukin-1 receptor antagonist blocks lipopolysaccharide-induced colony stimulating factor production and early endotoxin tolerance. *Infect Immun* 1991; **59,** 1188–1192.
232. Alexander HR, Doherty GM, Buresh CM, Venzon DJ, Norton JA. A recombinant human receptor antagonist to interleukin-1 improves survival after lethal endotoxemia in mice. *J Exp Med* 1991; **173,** 1029–1032.
233. Ulich TR, Yin SM, Guo KZ, Del CJ, Eisenberg SP, Thompson RC. The intratracheal administration of endotoxin and cytokines. III. The interleukin-1 (IL-1) receptor antagonist inhibits endotoxin- and IL-1-induced acute inflammation. *Am J Pathol* 1991; **138,** 521–524.
234. Cominelli F, Nast CC, Dinarello CA, Gentilini P, Zipser RD. Regulation of eicosanoid production in rabbit colon by interleukin-1. *Gastroenterology* 1989; **97,** 1400–1405.
235. Cominelly F, Nast CC, Llerena R, Dinarello CA, Zipser RD. Interleukin-1 suppresses inflammation in rabbit colitis: mediation by endogenous prostaglandins. *J Clin Invest* 1990; **85,** 582–586.
236. Cominelli F, Nast CC, Clark BD *et al.* Interleukin-1 gene expression, synthesis and effect of specific IL-1 receptor blockade in rabbit immune complex colitis. *J Clin Invest* 1990; **86,** 972–980.
237. Cominelli F, Llerena R, Clark BD, Nast CC, Thompson RC, Dinarello CA. *In vivo* anti-inflammatory properties of recombinant interleukin-1 receptor antagonist (IL-1ra). *Lymph Res* 1992; in press.
238. Arend WP, Welgus HG, Thompson RC, Eisenberg SP. Biological properties of recombinant human monocyte-derived interleukin-1 receptor antagonist. *J Clin Invest* 1990; **85,** 1694–1697.
239. Ramilo O, Saez-Llorens X, Mertsola J *et al.* Tumor necrosis factor α/cachectin and interleukin-1β initiate meningeal inflammation. *J Exp Med* 1990; **172,** 497–507.
240. Opp MR, Krueger JM. Interleukin 1-receptor antagonist blocks interleukin 1-induced sleep and fever. *Am J Physiol* 1991; **260,** R453–R457.
241. Poutsiaka D, Clark BD, Vannier E, Dinarello CA. Production of interleukin-1 receptor antagonist and interleukin-1β by peripheral blood mononuclear cells is differentially regulated. *Blood* 1991; **78,** 1275–1281.
242. Fischer E, Poutsiaka DD, Van Zee KJ, Rack CS *et al.* Levels of interleukin-1 receptor antagonist cerculates in experimental inflammation and in human disease. *Blood*. In Press.
243. Prieur AM, Kaufmann MT, Griscelli C, Dayer JM. Specific interleukin-1 inhibitor in serum and urine of children with systemic juvenile chronic arthritis. *Lancet* 1987; **2,** 1240–1242.
244. Cannon JG, Gelfand JA, Tompkins RG, Hegarty MT, Burke JF, Dinarello CA. Plasma IL-1β and TNFα levels in humans following cutaneous injury. In: *The Physiological and Pathological Effects of Cytokines*, Dinarello CA, Kluger MJ, Powanda MC, Oppenheim JJ (eds). New York: Wiley-Liss, 1990.
245. Haskill S, Martin M, VanLe L *et al.* cDNA cloning of a novel form of the interleukin-1 receptor antagonist associated with epithelium. *Pro Nat Acad Sci USA* 1991; **88,** 3681–3685.
246. Maier JAM, Voulalas P, Roeder D, Masiag T. Extension of the life span of human endothelial cells by an interleukin-1a antisense oligomer. *Science* 1990; **249,** 1570–1574.
247. Fanslow WC, Sims JE, Sassenfeld H *et al.* Regulation of alloreactivity *in vivo* by a soluble form of the interleukin-1 receptor. *Science* 1990; **248,** 739–742.
248. Giri J, Newton RC, Horuk R. Identification of soluble interleukin-1 binding protein in cell-free

supernatants. *J Biol Chem* 1990; **265,** 17416–17419.

249. Liabakk NB, Sundan A, Waage A *et al.* Development of immunoassays for the detection of soluble tumour necrosis factor receptors. *J Immunol Methods* 1991; **141,** 237–243.

250. Lesslauer W, Tabuchi H, Gentz M *et al.* Recombinant soluble TNF receptor proteins inhibit LPS-induced lethality in mice. *Cytokine* 1991; **3,** 497(abstract).

251. Mancilla J, Garcia P, Dinarello CA. IL 1 receptor antagonist can either protect or enhance the lethality of *Klebsiella pneumoniae* sepsis in newborn rats. *Cytokine* 1991; **3,** 502 (abs).

252. van der Meer JWM. IL-1ra blocks effects of cerebral malaria. *Cytokine* 1991; **3,** 497 (abs).

253. Schwab JH, Anderle SK, Brown RR, Dalldorf FG, Thompson RC. Pro- and anti-inflammatory roles of IL-1 in recurrence of bacterial cell wall-induced arthritis in rats. *Inf Immun* 1991; **59,** 4436–4442.

254. Wooley PH, Whalen JD, Chapman DL *et al.* The effect of an interleukin-1 receptor antagonist protein on type II collagen and antigen-induced arthritis in mice. *Arthritis and Rheumat* 1990; **33,** S20(abstract).

255. Dayer-Metroz MD, Duhamel D, Rufer N *et al.* IL-1ra delays the spontaneous autoimmune diabetes in the BB rat. *Eur J Clin Invest* 1991; **22,** A50 (abstract).

256. Henricson BE, Neta R, Vogel SN. An interleukin-1 receptor antagonist blocks lipopolysaccharide-induced colony-stimulating factor production and early endotoxin tolerance. *Infect Immun* 1991; **59,** 1188–1191.

257. Estrov Z, Kurzrock R, Wetzler M *et al.* Suppression of CML colony growth by IL-1 receptor antagonist and soluble IL-1 receptors: a novel application for inhibitors of IL-1 activity. *Blood* 1991; **78,** 1476–1484.

258. McIntyre KW, Stepan GJ, Kolinsky DK *et al.* Interleukin-1 receptor antagonist blocks acute inflammatory responses to IL-1 and other agents *in vivo*. *J Exp Med* 1991; **173,** 931–939.

259. Guenard V, Dinarello CA, Weston PJ, Aebischer P. Peripheral nerve regeneration is impeded by interleukin-1 receptor antagonist released from a polymeric guidance channel. *J Neurosci Res* 1991; **29,** 396–400.

260. McCarthy PL, Abhyankar S, Neben S *et al.* Inhibition of interleukin-1 by interleukin-1 receptor antagonist prevents graft versus host disease. *Blood* 1991; **78:** 1915–1918.

261. Sartor RB, Holt LC, Bender DE, Murphy ME, McCall RD, Thompson RC. Prevention and treatment of experimental enterocolitis with a recombinant interleukin-1 receptor antagonist. *Gastroenterology* 1991; **100,** A613(abstract).

5

T cell cytokines

M Salmon and A Akbar

Introduction

Trying to understand cytokines can be a depressing business. The development of this field is an elegant example of what could be called circular progress in science. The first stirrings came in the late 1960s, when it became clear that soluble factors derived from antigen stimulated cell cultures could have effects on other aspects of immunity. The term lymphokine was coined by Dumonde *et al.* in 1969[1] to embrace all such factors. In the 1970s lymphokine research was a slightly disreputable thing to be involved in. A large number of biological functions were described in rather obscure assay systems, many of which seemed to illustrate historical links with alchemy more than anything particularly relevant to immunophysiology. Little sense was made of all this until some of the factors were cloned in the late 1970s and early 1980s. Lymphokines became respectable. The numerical classification of interleukins was conceived at this time, when it became clear that many different assays were actually measuring the same molecules.[2] It seemed within our grasp to understand intercellular signalling within the immune system. Coupled to an increasingly precise picture of the direct molecular interactions of cell–cell contact, immunoregulation could be sewn up. All that was needed was to clone the full set of cytokines, and see what they do . . . Life of course didn't stay simple for very long.

Not only could individual cytokines do a lot of different things (pleitropy) but it became clear very quickly that many different cytokines could do the same thing (redundancy). There was an exquisitely painful little twist: cytokines interact with each other. Indeed, it seems that almost any process within the immune system is regulated by a complex interaction of cytokines; part of a dynamic network maintaining a precise equilibrium. The actions of even two molecules together can rarely be predicted from those of the molecules separately. As there are now at least 20 well documented cytokines, and a number of neural peptides can have cytokine-like effects, the potential complexity of the regulatory language written by these molecules is enormous.

The term cytokine is now used to refer to all such soluble regulatory molecules produced in or influencing the immune system. This is probably more accurate than 'lymphokine', and better than the slightly pedantic fad of referring to lymphokines and monokines (derived from monocyte/macrophages), since many of these molecules are produced by several different cell types.

Cytokines produced by T cells

What actually is it that characterises a cytokine? This may seem rather a silly question, but failure to address it has been the cause of a lot of confusion and apparent contradictions in the field. To illustrate this we should consider the ways in which cytokines are measured. Detection of mRNA sequences coding for a particular molecule is extremely specific and can be performed using either mRNA extracted from populations of cells and blotted onto filters,[3] or by in-situ hybridisation.[4] This approach can be useful to show that a cytokine is actually being produced at a specific site, rather than imported from elsewhere. However, it depends heavily on the assumption that the mRNA will necessarily be translated into protein, which is not invariably the case. The translated protein itself can be measured either by immunocytochemistry or ELISA assays. This seems definitive, but it doesn't necessarily follow that the protein was produced where it was detected, and these assays give no information about the biological function of that protein. Many cytokine inhibitors and cleaved inactive cytokines have been described which are still immunoreactive. Bio-assays tend to circumvent this problem, but of course specificity is extraordinarily difficult to guarantee. For example, a few years ago the T cell growth factor assay was considered a specific measure of IL-2, but it is now clear that IL-4, IL-7, IL-9 and IL-12 all enhance this activity, or even replace it, while TGFβ suppresses it.[5] Monoclonal antibodies are often used in various ways to improve specificity, but it's very difficult to predict the effects of unknown cytokines, or particular combinations. This dichotomy between measuring the molecule or its function has created a lot of controversy and a fair amount of acrimonious debate over the last ten years. There isn't really an answer; most people now tend to measure whatever is most pertinent to the question asked, or more pragmatically, whatever they can.

In this section some of the basic biochemistry and observed functions of the major cytokines known to be produced by T cells will be described (Table 5.1). The distinction is a trifle arbitrary. Many of the cytokines characteristically thought of as T cell derived, like IL-2 and IFNγ, are also produced by other cells. On the other hand molecules like IL-6 and TNFα, which are more characteristic of stromal cells or macrophages, are also produced by T cells and play a significant part in their biology.

The functions described for individual cytokines should not be seen as definitive, or necessarily even characteristic of these molecules. As will be discussed later, cytokines interact, and the resulting effects are often very difficult to predict.

Interleukin-2 (IL-2)

Interleukin-2 is an essential autocrine growth factor for the activation and function of most, if not all, T cells.[6] However, IL-2 also promotes the growth and differentiation of B lymphocytes and NK cells, as well as macrophage activation. The induction of so-called lymphokine activated killer (LAK) cells, principally by IL-2, has received a great deal of attention. The precursors appear to

Table 5.1 Major characteristics of the T cell derived cytokines

Lymphokine	Length (amino acids)	Principal actions
Interleukin-2	133	T cell growth factor. Also activates NK cells, regulates B cell function
Interleukin-3	134–140	Growth factor for bone marrow stem cells, also activation of mast cells and basophils
Interleukin-4	120	B cell growth and differentiation factor
Interleukin-5	115	Eosinophil differentiating factor. In mice, IL-5 is also an important B cell differentiating factor
Interleukin-6	189	B cell growth and differentiation, T cell co-stimulation. Induction of acute phase response
Interleukin-8	72	Neutrophil chemotaxis and activation
Interleukin-9	126	Helper T cell growth factor
Interleukin-10	160	Inhibits IL-2 and IFN-γ production
Interferon-γ	146	Macrophage activation, Class II MHC regulation, B cell differentiation. Promotes NK cell function
Tumor necrosis factor α & β	α157 β171	T cell growth factor, macrophage activation. Endothelial cell activation, and fever induction
Transforming growth factor β	112 (β1)	Macrophage activation. Lymphocyte inhibition. Regulates B cell function

be NK cells,[7] so this is really a parallel description of the potentiating action of IL-2 on this population. In terms of inflammation and general immunity, IL-2 induced NK cells are probably most important for producing high levels of IFNγ.[8]

The high affinity IL-2 receptor is a heterodimer (two dissimilar chains).[9] The p55 α chain (Tac antigen) is expressed in gross excess, has a very low affinity for IL-2, and has no signalling capacity. The β chain (p75) has an affinity intermediate to the chain and the high affinity receptor. NK cells constitutively express the β chain, which is used as a functional receptor in the absence of the α chain. Both components are up-regulated on activation of T cells; the high affinity receptor is actually stabilised by bound IL-2.[10] The receptor is believed to associate with other peptides in the membrane associated with signalling.[9]

Interleukin-3 (IL-3)

Interleukin-3 is a growth factor for bone marrow stem cells and B cell precursors,[11] but it is difficult to see this as a major physiological role since IL-3 seems to be exclusively produced by CD4+ peripheral T cells. However, IL-3 has agonistic effects on mast cells and basophils,[12] and also enhances class II MHC expression and IL-1 production by macrophages. The IL-3 receptor is a 140 KDa glycoprotein with cytoplasmic signalling capacity.

Interleukin-4 (IL-4)

Originally called B cell stimulating factor-1 (BSF-1), IL-4 plays a major role in promoting growth and differentiation of B cells, particularly in regulating isotype switching.[13] IL-4 promotes IgG1 formation and is essential for IgE production; simultaneously reducing expression of IgG2a and b as well as IgG3.[13] IL-4 also up-regulates class II MHC expression on B cells along with CD23, which appears itself to have wide regulatory activity. IL-4 is also a T cell growth factor. In some mouse clones it appears to be *the* autocrine growth factor.[14] This lymphokine acts directly on a very wide range of cells including macrophages, mast cells, reticulocytes and B cell precursors. This rather contradictory molecule seems to antagonise the effects of IFNγ in many systems, and also the colony stimulating functions of IL-3 and GM-CSF.[15] IL-4 can directly activate macrophages, leading to increased MHC class II expression. However, in dynamic systems, particularly where T cells are also present, IL-4 may have precisely opposite net effects, since it also down-regulates IL-1, TNF, IL-2 receptor and IFNγ production.

The IL-4 receptor is closely related to the β chain of the IL-2 receptor, and also to the IL-6 receptor.[16] The intracellular domain is critically important for signal transduction, but we don't yet know how because its sequence does not have typical signalling motifs.

Interleukin-5 (IL-5)

This lymphokine was first described as a mouse B cell growth factor (BCGF II)[17] as it seemed to parallel the effects of IL-4 in some respects. However its B cell specific actions are rather circumscribed, largely promoting previously differentiated activity. In humans, it does not even seem to do that, indeed no B cell specific actions of IL-5 have been described outside the mouse. IL-5 is a major factor for the differentiation and maturation of eosinophils in both species.[18]

Interleukin-6 (IL-6)

IL-6 has five alternative names including: IFNβ2, B cell stimulation factor 2 (number 1 was IL-4), B cell differentiation factor, hybridoma growth factor and hepatocyte stimulating factor. This is certainly an impressive range of activities, but of course in combination with other molecules, the effects of IL-6 are actually much more complex (reviewed in [19]). In general, IL-6 is predominantly produced by macrophages, though primed T cells after activation can be a major source. However low levels of IL-6 are produced by virgin T cells; this is the only cytokine other than IL-2 reported from such cells. Many of the systemic actions of IL-6 are shared with IL-1 and TNF, and indeed several of the apparent functions of these molecules are mediated through local induction of IL-6. T cell derived IL-6 probably plays little role in the systemic response, unless produced directly in the liver by infiltrating cells. The 80 KDa IL-6 receptor, like the IL-4 receptor which is in the same rather small family, has no apparent signalling sequence, but it associates in the cell membrane with a 130 KDa protein which may transduce signals. The IL-6 receptor is very widely distributed on many cell types.

Interleukin-8 (IL-8)

A chemotactic molecule belonging to the Rantes group of cytokines, IL-8 is a small protein (8.4 KDa). Closely regulated by a range of other cytokines, it acts principally as a neutrophil attractant, though at low concentrations it seems preferentially to recruit primed lymphocytes.[20] The mouse equivalent of IL-8 (MIP-2) affects bone marrow stem cells, synergising with other cytokines to regulate myeloid progenitors.

Interleukin-9 (IL-9)

IL-9 is a growth factor which specifically promotes the proliferation of CD4+ helper T cells, but not CD8+ cytotoxic T cells. It may be involved in the non-specific amplification of immune responses. Little is known of the interactions of IL-9 with other cytokines.[21]

Interleukin-10 (IL-10)

Originally described as cytokine synthesis inhibitory factor (CSIF), IL-10 was identified in certain mouse T cell clones characterised as Th2 (see below).[22] The mRNA at least has since been found in very low amounts in stimulated peripheral T cells from both mouse and man.[23] IL-10 inhibits the production of IL-2 and IFNγ particularly, but also other cytokines.[22] It is likely to be involved in down-regulation of inflammatory immune processes, and perhaps indirectly controlling complex events like antibody isotype switching. IL-10 inhibits macrophage function, but in complete contrast it enhances B cell activation and differentiation. This is perhaps not surprising considering its inhibitory action on IFNγ production.

Interferon γ (IFNγ)

Interferon γ occurs in two glycosylated forms of 20 and 25 KDa. It has powerful agonistic effects on macrophage activation, NK cell cytotoxicity and lymphokine production.[24] In many systems IFNγ appears to counteract the effects of IL-4. Class II MHC expression is markedly up-regulated on many cells by IFNγ, but the IL-4 mediated up-regulation of class II on B cells is actually inhibited. Antibody isotypes are regulated by IFNγ, again antagonising the effects of IL-4.[13] IFNγ enhances IL-2 receptor expression on T cells, but inhibits production of IL-4 and IL-5, which may reflect a differential effect on cells in different stages of development.

The ability of IFNγ to induce high level class II MHC expression on somatic cells not usually connected with the immune system has been proposed by many as a mechanism of autoimmunity.[25] This is a difficult proposition, because expression of class II in the absence of appropriate second signals seems to lead to anergy rather than activation. Indeed, this may be a major mechanism of self tolerance.

The receptor for IFNγ is a single chain molecule with extensive intracellular targets for phosphorylation.[26] Predictably the receptor is very widely distributed on many different cell types, but there is evidence that IFNγ can operate without receptor mediated binding.

Tumour necrosis factor (TNF α and β)

There are two quite different forms of TNF, which have very little sequence similarity (about 30%) but they bind to the same receptor and appear to be functionally indistinguishable. They are also adjacent to each other on chromosome 6.[27] TNFα is produced by many cell types, particularly macrophages and also primed T cells. TNFβ or lymphotoxin, however, appears to be a purely T cell product. TNFβ is the larger of the two, 25 compared with 17 KDa. TNF induces profoundly aggressive macrophage activation in bacteraemia; indeed, there is evidence that much of the damage in conditions such as meningitis is caused by this molecule. It can act as an autocrine growth factor for T cells in some situations, but can inhibit haematopoiesis. Since both forms of TNF bind to the same 55 KDa receptor,[28] which is very widely distributed, it is not surprising that their actions are largely synonymous. Recent evidence, however, suggests that, like IFNγ, TNF may be able to bind directly to cell membranes, punching holes to act as ion channels in a manner analogous to the multimeric forms of perforin and the terminal attack complex of complement (C5-C9).[29] This is probably important in the cytotoxic actions of the molecules. It seems likely that T cell derived TNFα or β largely mediates effects on the local immune response, where synergy with IFNγ in particular seems markedly to enhance the effects of the latter cytokine.

Transforming growth factor β (TGFβ)

The transforming growth factors β are a group of about half a dozen distinct molecules which play a significant role in many aspects of immunoregulation, particularly during inflammation.[5] TGFβ is chemotactic for macrophages and activates them. In contrast most of its effects on lymphocytes are profoundly suppressive. TGFβ inhibits T cell and NK cell function, and B cell antibody production, though it actually enhances the production of IgA, synergising with IL-2 and, in the mouse, IL-5.[30] This is interesting, because TGFβ actually inhibits the production of both of these cytokines.

Cytokine interactions: synergy and antagonism

Regulation of B cell isotype expression

Cytokine interactions can affect immunity in two general ways: they may act together on the same cells to regulate complex events, or complementary cytokines may promote the synergistic interaction of different cells. The growth and differentiation of B lymphocytes provides an excellent model of cytokine interactions, since the system can be isolated effectively, and very clear endpoint effects can be measured.[13,31,32]

A number of T cell derived factors influence the various stages of B cell differentiation. IL-4 appears to act at all stages of the process, though not necessarily in the same way: IL-4 promotes the expression of IgM by pre-B cells, but actively inhibits earlier stages of B cell growth. IL-2, IFNγ and IL-6 all regulate late stages of mature B cell activation and plasma cell differentiation.

Immunoglobulin isotypes control the effects of specific antibody antigen interactions, for example complement fixation, or which cell types interact with specific antibodies or immune complexes. The isotype refers to the constant region of the heavy chain. The rearranged variable region (antigen binding site) of a particular immunoglobulin can be associated with each of the different constant regions in turn, by progressive gene splicing (Figure 5.1). The actual mechanism of re-arrangement is poorly understood, though at least one of the recombinase enzymes involved has been cloned. T cell cytokines play a major role in regulating isotype switching. Isolated B cells stimulated with bacterial lipopolysaccharide (LPS) show a complex pattern of lymphokine interactions (Table 5.2). IL-4 and IFNγ are completely mutually antagonistic in this system. IL-4 favours induction of IgG1 and is essential for IgE production, suppressing induction of other isotypes.[13] IFNγ favours IgG2a, suppressing IgG1 and IgE. The relative levels of these two cytokines dictate expression of the isotypes in a quite complex manner. Other cytokines appear to act synergistically in this system; IL-2, TGFβ and IL-5 (the latter only in mice) appear to be particularly important in regulating IgA production.[31] IL-6 can act on precommited IgA+ B cells to selectively promote IgA production.

Antibodies to IL-6 have a profoundly suppressive effect on immunoglobulin production by poke-weed mitogen (PWM) stimulated B cells, but this system, unlike LPS, is heavily T cell dependent. The effects of IL-6 may not be exclusively on the B cells.

The effect of microenvironments

The effects of specific cytokines in regulating a process such as isotype switching can be studied precisely, because the system can be isolated, and the effects of individual molecules and combinations calculated by direct experiment. However systems are not isolated *in vivo*. In the isotype switching example discussed above, IL-4 and IFNγ appear to play a critical and mutually antagonistic role, but it is equally clear that in a dynamic system any factor capable of regulating the production of these cytokines will itself indirectly regulate isotype switching.[32] It is the availability of cytokines within the microenvironment of a particular immune event and the regulation of their production which must be the key to understanding the network. How big is a lymphokine determined microenvironment? This is very difficult; IL-1, IL-6 and TNFα frequently operate systemically and may therefore play a role in modulating environments throughout the whole organism,[33] while IL-4 has been shown capable of directional secretion by T cells.[34] In other words the lymphokine can be secreted from one side of

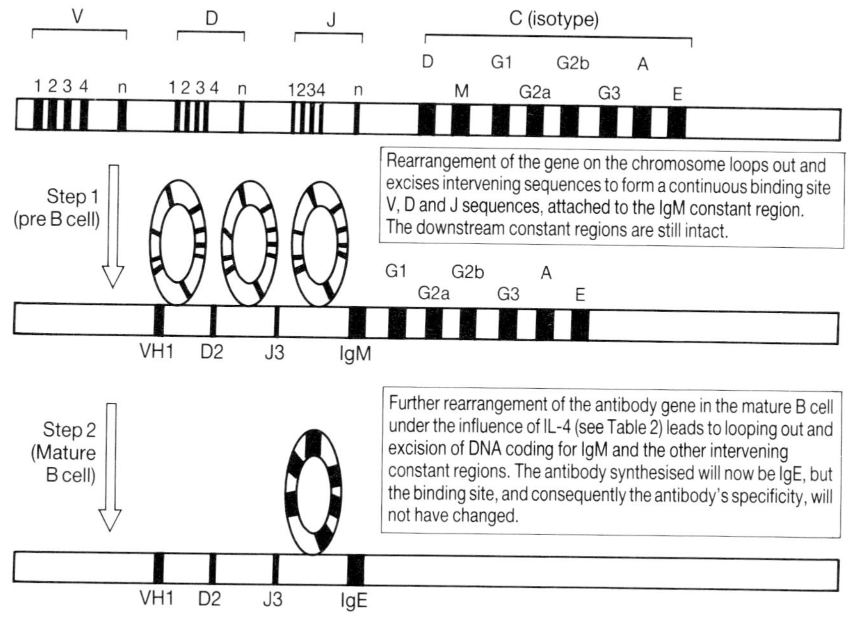

Fig. 5.1 Immunoglobulin heavy chain gene re-arrangement. The variable, diversity and joining sequences are re-arranged in pre-B cells to construct a functional antibody idiotype (antigen binding site). The heavy chain constant regions can subsequently be re-arranged in mature B cells, under the influence of cytokines, to attach different isotypes to the same idiotype.

Table 5.2 Cytokine mediated regulation of immunoglobulin isotype switching in LPS stimulated B cells

	IgM	IgG1	IgG2a	IgG2b	IgG3	IgA	IgE
LPS alone	++++	++		+	++		
IL-4	++*	++++	*	*	*		++++
IFN-γ	+++	+*	++++	+	+		*
IL-2	++++	++	+	+	++	+	
IL-5#	++++	++		+	++	+	@
TGFβ	++*	+*		+	+*	+	
IL-2+TGFβ	+++*	+*		+	++	++++	
IL-5+TGFβ	+++*	+*		+	+*	++	

* Actively suppresses the isotype
@ Enhances IL-4 induced IgE production
# Only functional in mice. May not induce class switching, but promotes previously differentiated production

the cell in the precise direction of the eliciting signal. This could mean the specific microenvironment is as small as the area of contact between two cells.

Regulation of T cell lymphokine production

Fine control of immune reactions appears to be achieved by precise combinations of cytokines. For this to be possible, T cells must have the capacity to separate the production of different lymphokines, either in time or in space. Essentially the question is this: how do T lymphocytes manage to deliver the right combination of lymphokines to the right place at the right time? A number of possible models have been proposed which fall broadly into three catagories:

1. Fixed heterogeneity;
2. Transient heterogeneity;
3. Coordinated regulation.

Working out the constraints applied to and by the production of cytokines will play an essential role in limiting the potential diversity of cytokine interactions within the network; in other words, make it a little easier to understand. Recognition of this has made the area topical but rather contentious, so each of the three main hypotheses will be discussed in more detail.

Fixed heterogeneity

In 1986 Mosmann *et al*. described a panel of T cell clones which fell into two distinct categories.[35,36] T helper 1 (Th1) clones synthesised IL-2, IFNγ and other cytokines which predominantly act on the cellular arm of the immune response, while Th2 clones produced IL-4 and IL-5 which principally regulate B cell immunity. Other cytokines seemed to be intermediate; IL-3, GM-CSF and TNFβ were produced equally by both sets of clones.

Subsequently it became apparent that many murine T cell clones fall into a third category, which has been termed Th0.[37] These cells make pretty well everything with very little selectivity. The Th1/Th2 segregation has become the most widely accepted model for lymphokine segregation, but there are certain difficulties with this interpretation. Firstly it has proved very difficult to produce either Th1 or Th2 clones of human T cells. The majority of reports have consistently failed to show such a pattern of lymphokine segregation[3,38] and in most of those which have purported to do so the segregation is only partial.[39] Both in mouse and in man, freshly isolated cells or those in culture for only a few weeks appear to fall into the Th0 category. Probably the best evidence for a physiological role for the Th1/Th2, model comes from allergy, and parasitic disease models such as Leishmania. In both systems, 'Th2-like' IL-4 producing cells have been isolated. A sceptic might point out that this is a bit of a self-fulfilling prophecy. Constitutively high levels of IgE are produced in both allergy and parasite infections. Since IL-4 is an absolute requirement for IgE synthesis, it is perhaps hardly surprising that comparatively high numbers of IL-4 secreting cells can be isolated from such conditions.

If Th1 and Th2 clones with fixed heterogeneity of lymphokine production are not an artifact of long term *in vitro* cultures, how do they arise? Virgin T cells on first challenge with antigen just make IL-2 (see below). These cells may then develop into pluripotential Th0 cells. The final differentiation event into a Th1 or Th2 state would take many cell cycles, and depend on a particular set of environmental signals. Alternatively, the virgin T cells many themselves be precommitted, requiring a number of cycles before they can effectively suppress the 'forbidden' genes (Figure 5.2).[40] Neither model is entirely satisfactory.

Transient segregation

Virgin T cells are very good at making IL-2 if stimulated but they make little else. In contrast, stimulated primed T cells produce rather less IL-2 on a unit basis, but they also make all of the other

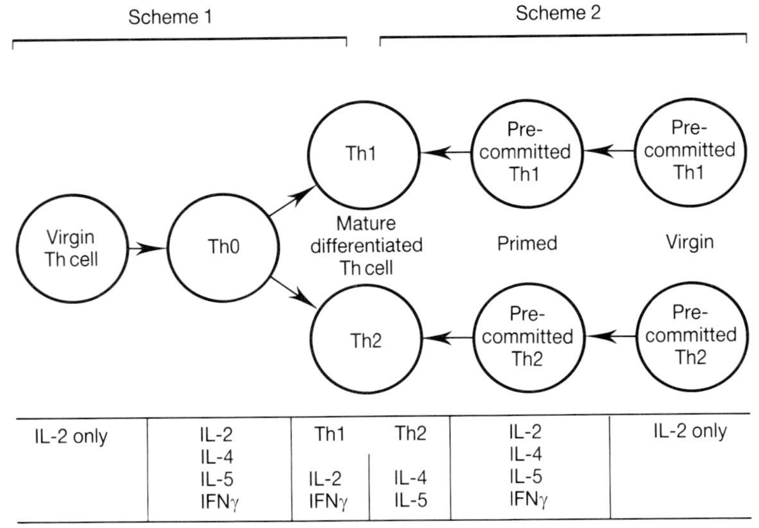

Fig. 5.2 Fixed heterogeneity of T cell cytokine production. Two possible schemes are illustrated for the generation of Th1 and Th2 cells. In the first, cells are pluripotential until the final stages of differentiation. In the second, T cells are precommitted but require many cycles to suppress specific cytokine genes.

T cell derived cytokines.[3] Since it is known that virgin T cells become primed after stimulation[3,41] this is a simple model of transient segregation of lymphokine synthesis; in other words non-permanent states in which T cells produce a restricted range of cytokines. Our own recent work suggests that primed T cells may also show such a transient segregation.[42]

The differentiation state of human T cells can be identified by their expression of different isoforms of the leucocyte common antigen CD45. Virgin T cells express CD45RA and high levels of CD45RB (B bright); primed T cells express CD45RO and also highly variable levels of CD45RB.[43] Actually the expression of CD45RO and RB is inversely proportional in primed T cells which form a continuous spectrum.[42] We have found that the B bright primed cells differentiate through a series of cycles into cells expressing very low levels of CD45RB (B dull cells). The key point is this: B bright cells make IL-2 and IFNγ very effectively, while B dull cells make IL-4, no IL-2, and very little IFNγ.[42] This provides a model for lymphokine segregation, in which different combinations of cytokine may be produced as a continuous spectrum by cells in various states of differentiation (Figure 5.3) There is no particularly good reason to assume that this process only goes one way. In rats, the CD45 isoform identified by an antibody called OX-22 seems very similar to CD45RB in humans. Bell and colleagues have shown that *in vivo*, cells which have differentiated to the OX-22 dull state can revert to an OX-22 bright phenotype, with the characteristic changes in function which that implies.[44] This seems to resolve one of the problems of the Th1/Th2 subset model: if the differentiation through Th0 (pluripotential) into Th1 or Th2 has occurred *in vivo* over the lifetime of an individual, and the cells have irreversibly differentiated, then why can't we isolate resting Th1 or Th2 cells?

Coordinated regulations

The cellular regulation of lymphokine gene expression operates principally at the level of transcription.[45] Regulatory elements 5′ (upstream) of the genes for IL-2, IL-4 and IFNγ show regions of close homology suggesting a degree of coordinated regulation by DNA binding proteins. There are three regions (each roughly 30 base pairs) of about 70% homology between the regulatory sequences of IL-2 and IL-4 genes, while two regions of complete homology exist between the IL-4 and IFNγ 5′ sequences.[46] Similar but quite distinct homologies are found between IL-2 and IFNγ.[47] Transcriptional regulation of IL-2 and to a lesser extent IFNγ has been mapped using deletion constructs, and by DNAse-1 footprinting.[45] Sites known to bind transcriptionally active factors such as NFκB have been identified. These observations suggest that a limited number of nuclear DNA binding proteins may interact with both unique and shared binding sites in a fairly complex manner, to regulate the expression of each of these lymphokines in the same cells in a coordinated fashion. Evidence from other systems suggests that quantitative regulation of transcription involves complex interactions of a number of DNA binding proteins acting together.[48]

At one level, this pattern of transcriptional regulation tells us something of the process necessary for the expression of any gene. However pat-

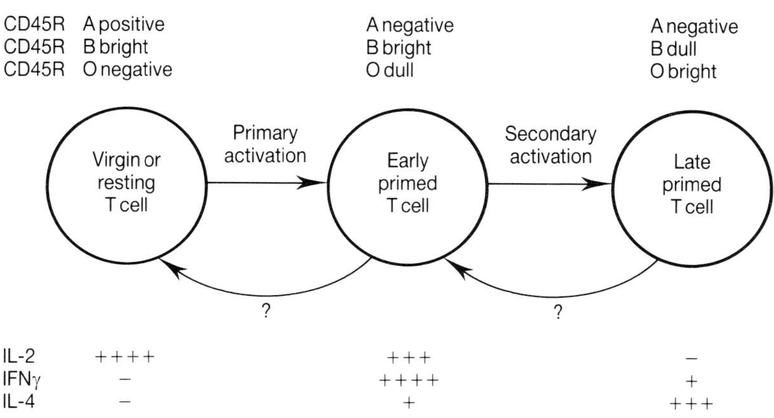

Fig. 5.3 Transient heterogeneity of cytokine production. Activated virgin T cells make IL-2 but little else. After a few cycles, they acquire the ability to produce IFN-γ. After further differentiation, they gradually lose the ability to produce both IL-2 and IFN-γ but begin to produce high levels of IL-4. Several lines of evidence suggest that this process is reversible.

terns which have emerged suggest that there is no particularly good reason why T cells should have to specialise at all. A pattern of closely co-ordinated regulation could mean that T cells produce lymphokines directly related to signals received from their environment, on an unrestricted basis.

It seems likely that aspects of all three of these models of lymphokine segregation play a part in regulating the immune system. If we can define the constraints applied to and by their coordinated production, then we may have the essential key to understanding the interactive network of cytokine function.

Cellular synergy in the response to allo-antigens

The immune response to transplanted tissue is often so intense that it leads to graft rejection even in the presence of potent immunosuppression. Why is it so powerful? Conventional recall antigens selectively activate primed CD45RO+ T cells. The precursor frequency for an antigen like tetanus toxoid is usually between 1 in 5000 and 1 in 50,000 in a primed individual. Allo-antigens are capable of stimulating about 10% of the T cell population *in vitro*, and they activate both CD45RO+ and CD45RA+ cells equally.[49] This activation of CD45RA+ cells has also been observed in rejecting renal allografts, and may profoundly increase the potency of the response.[50] As discussed above, CD45RA+ cells produce high levels of IL-2. This is super-optimal since adding further IL-2 has no effect on their function. However they produce no IL-4 and little IL-6; addition of either or both of these cytokines markedly increases both proliferation and cytokine production. In contrast, CD45RO+ primed cells produce a net excess of IL-4 and IL-6 but a deficit of IL-2 when stimulated with allo-antigen.[51,52] This suggests that the cells may synergise during activation, and indeed they do proliferate much more effectively if cultured in combination than either population cultured separately[52] (Figure 5.4). Why should such a synergy have evolved? It seems rather strange that any advantage could be gained from primed T cells synergising with virgin cells, because the precursor frequency for a recall antigen within the virgin population should be vanishingly small.

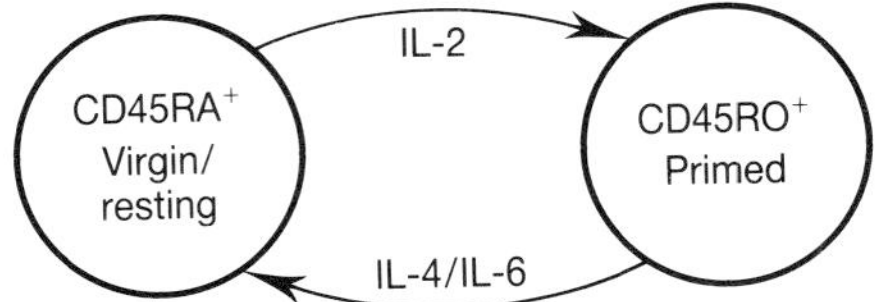

Fig. 5.4 Synergy between helper T cell subpopulations. During the response to allo-antigens, and possibly during the amplification of conventional antigen specific reactions, CD45RA+ and CD45RO+ helper T cells synergise with each other by responding to cytokines produced by the complementary subtype.

There are two possible explanations: firstly CD45RA+ T cells may not all be virgin; several lines of evidence suggest that a proportion of them may be resting memory cells. Perhaps synergy provides a mechanism for recall of such cells from the resting state, bypassing the stringent activation requirements of CD45RA+ cells. A second possibility is that synergy may be part of the non-specific amplification of immune responses. If fresh peripheral T cells are stimulated *in vitro* with a recall antigen, about 40% will be activated after six days. This is 500 to 5000 times more than would be expected from the precursor frequency. Immune responses are certainly specific in their induction, but markedly less so in their effects. For clearing a pathogen this has obvious value. For tissue transplantation, synergy makes the allo-reactive immune response very difficult to control.[53]

Summary

The cytokine network is not a system in itself; it is a means of communication within and between systems, at its broadest encompassing the whole organism. Cytokines can act synergistically, but also with incredibly fine specificity. IL-4, for example, can be secreted in the precise direction of the inducing stimulus.[34] The most characteristic features of cytokines in general are their ability to interact, and their propensity to exert quite distinct effects on different cells.

Non-linear mathematical models will eventually help us to understand this network, but it will not be an easy task. At the moment research is focusing on the relationship between the regulation of cytokine production, microenvironments and specific models of cytokine action. The critical association of IL-4 with the induction of IgE antibodies, for example, has provided a great deal of impetus to the study of allergic and parasitic disease models, where all three areas can be investigated.[54]

The last 20 years have seen the solution of a number of apparently insurmountable problems in immunology. Perhaps the best example is our understanding of immune recognition structures (Figure 5.2). No theory or model available at the time was able to predict the pattern of gene rearrangement which Tonegawa and others so elegantly showed. Perhaps we just need a new paradigm.

References

1. Dumonde DC, Wolstencroft RA, Panayi GS, Matthew M, Morley J, Howson WT. 'Lymphokines'. Non-antibody mediators of cellular immunity generated by lymphocyte activation. *Nature* 1969; **224,** 38–41.
2. Aarden A, Brunner TK, Cerottini JC, Dayer JM *et al.* Revised nomenclature for antigen non-specific T cell proliferation and helper factors. *J Immunol* 1979; **123,** 2928–2929.
3. Salmon M, Kitas GD, Bacon PA. Production of lymphokine mRNA by CD45R+ and CD45R helper T cells from human peripheral blood, and by human CD4+ T cell clones. *J Immunol* 1989; **143,** 907–912.
4. Pardue ML. In situ hybridisation. In: *Nucleic Acid Hybridisation: A Practical Approach*, Hames BD, Higgins SJ (eds). Oxford: IRL Press, 1985.
5. Wahl SM, McCartney-Francis N, Mergenhagen SE. Inflammatory and immunomodulatory roles of TGFβ. *Immunol Today* 1989; **10,** 258–262.
6. Watson J. Continuous proliferation of murine antigen specific helper T lymphocytes in culture. *J Exp Med* 1979; **150,** 1510–1519.
7. Philips JH, Lanier LL. Dissection of the lymphokine activated killer phenomenon. *J Exp Med* 1986; **164,** 814–819.
8. Djeu JY. Production of interferon by natural killer cells. *Clin Immunol Allergy* 1983; **3,** 561–568.
9. Hatakeyama M, Kono T, Kobayashi N *et al.* Interaction of the IL-2 receptor with the src-family kinase p56:^{lck} identification of novel intermolecular association. *Science* 1991; **252,** 1523–1528.
10. Smith KA. Interleukin-2: inception, impact and implications. *Science* 1988; **240,** 1169–1176.
11. Ihle JN, Keller J, Oroszlan, Henderson ZE *et al.* Biologic properties of homologous interleukin-3. Demonstration of WEHI-3 growth factor activity, P-cell stimulating factor activity, colony stimulating factor activity and histamine producing cell stimulating factor activity. *J Immunol* 1983; **131,** 282–289.
12. Schrader J, Lewis SJ, Clarke-Lewis I, Culvenor JG. The persisting (P) cell: histamine content, regulation by a T cell-derived factor, origin from a bone marrow precursor, and relationship to mast cells *Proc Nat Acad Sci USA* 1981; **78,** 323–327.
13. Coffman RL, Savelkoul HE, Lebman DA. Cytokine regulation of immunoglobulin isotype switching and expression. *Semin Immunol* 1989; **1,** 55–76.
14. Hu-Li J, Shevach EM, Mizuguchi J, Ohara J, Mosmann T, Paul WE. B cell stimulatory factor-1 (interleukin 4) is a potent co-stimulant for normal resting T lymphocytes. *J Exp Med* 1987; **165,** 157–172.
15. Paul WE, Ohara J. B-cell stimulatory factor-1/interleukin-4. *Ann Rev Immunol* 1987; **5,** 429–459.
16. Cambier J. Transmembrane signalling in T lymphocyte dependant B lymphocyte activation. *Semin Immunol* 1989; **1,** 43–69.
17. Yokota T, Arai N, de Vries J *et al.* Molecular biology of interleukin 4 and interleukin 5 genes, and biology of their products that stimulate B cells, T cells and hemopoietic cells. *Immunol Rev* 1988; **102,** 137–163.
18. Sanderson CJ, Campbell HD, Young IG. Molecular and cellular biology of eosinophil differentiating factor (interleukin-5) and its effects on human and mouse B cells. *Immunol Rev* 1988; **102,** 29–50.
19. Van Snick J. Interleukin-6: an overview. *Ann Rev Immunol* 1990; **8,** 253–278.
20. Matsushima K, Morishita K, Yoshimura T *et al.* Molecular cloning of a human monocyte derived neutrophil chemotactic factor MDNCF and the induction of MDNCF mRNA by interleukin-1 and tumor necrosis factor. *J Exp Med* 1988; **167,** 1883–1894.
21. Yang Y-C, Ricciardi S, Ciarletta A, Calvetti J, Kelleher K, Clarke SC. Expression cloning of a cDNA encoding a novel hemopoietic growth factor: human homologue of murine T cell growth factor p40. *Blood* 1989; **74,** 1880–1884.
22. Fiorentino DF, Bond MW, Mosmann TR. Two types of mouse T helper cell IV. Th2 clones secrete a factor that inhibits cytokine production by Th1 cells. *J Exp Med* 1989; **170,** 2081–2095.
23. Moore KW, Viera P, Fiorentino DF, Trounstine ML, Khan TA, Mosmann TR. Homology of cytokine synthesis inhibitory factor (IL-10) to the Epstein-Barr virus gene BCRFI. *Science* 1990; **248,** 1230–1234.
24. Hamblin AS. *Lymphokines*. In Focus Series, Male D (ed). Oxford: Oxford University Press, 1988.

25. Bottazzo GF, Pujol Borrell R, Hanafusa T, Feldmann M. Role of aberrant HLA-DR expression and antigen presentation in induction of endocrine autoimmunity. *Lancet* 1983; **ii,** 1115–1119.
26. Friedman R, Stark GR. Alpha-interferon-induced transcription of HLA and metallothionein genes containing homologous upstream sequences. *Nature* 1985; **314,** 637–639.
27. Spies T, Morton CC, Nedospasor SA, Fiers W, Pious D, Strominger JL. Genes for the tumor necrosis factors alpha and beta are linked to the human major histocompatibility complex. *Proc Nat Acad Sci USA* 1986; **83,** 8699–8702.
28. Loetscher H. Molecular cloning and expression of the human 55 KD tumor necrosis factor receptor. *Cell* 1990; **61,** 351–357.
29. Kagan BL, Baldwin RL, Munoz D, Wisnieski BJ. Formation of ion permeable channels by tumor necrosis factor α. *Science* 1992; **255,** 1427–1430.
30. Coffman RL, Lebman DA, Schrader B. Transforming growth factor β specifically enhances IgA production by lipopolysaccharide-stimulated murine B lymphocytes. *J Exp Med* 1989; **170,** 1039–1045.
31. Esser C, Radbruch A. Immunoglobulin class switching: molecular and cellular analysis. *Ann Rev Immunol* 1990; **8,** 717–735.
32. Finkelman FD, Holmes J, Katoma IM *et al.* Lymphokine control of *in vivo* immunoglobulin isotype selection. *Ann Rev Immunol* 1990; **8,** 303–336.
33. Emery P, Salmon M. Systemic mediators of inflammation. *Br J Hosp Med* 1991; **45,** 164–168.
34. Poo WJ, Conrad L, Janeway CA. Receptor-directed focusing of lymphokine release by helper T cells. *Nature* 1988; **332,** 378–380.
35. Mosmann T, Cherwinski H, Bond MW, Giedlin MA, Coffman RL. Two types of murine helper T cell clone. I. Definition according to profiles of lymphokine activities and secreted proteins. *J Immunol* 1986; **136,** 2348–2355.
36. Kurt-Jones EA, Hamberg S, O'Hara J, Paul WE, Abbas AK. Heterogeneity of helper/inducer T lymphocytes 1. Lymphokine production and lymphokine responsiveness. *J Exp Med* 1986; **166,** 1774–1787.
37. Firestein GS, Roeder WD, Laxer JA *et al.* A new murine CD4+ T cell subset with an unrestricted cytokine profile. *J Immunol* 1989; **143,** 518–524.
38. Palliard X, De Waal Malefijt R, Yssel H *et al.* Simultaneous production of IL-2, IL-4 and IFNγ by activated human CD4+ and CD8+ T cell clones. *J Immunol* 1988; **141,** 849–855.
39. Plant M. Antigen-specific lymphokine secretory patterns in atopic disease. *J Immunol* 1990; **144,** 4497–4500.
40. Male D, Champion B, Cooke A, Owen M. Cytokines. In: *Advanced Immunology*, London: Gower, 1990.
41. Akbar A, Terry L, Timms A, Beverley PCL, Janossy G. Loss of CD45R and gain of UCHL-1 reactivity is a feature of primed T cells. *J Immunol* 1988; **140,** 2171–2178.
42. Salmon M, Pilling D, Borthwick N *et al.* Unpublished data, 1992.
43. Mason D, Powrie F. Memory CD4+ T cells in man form two distinct subpopulations defined by their expression of isoforms of the leucocyte common antigen, CD45. *Immunology* 1991; **70,** 427–433.
44. Bell EB, Sparshott SM. Interconversion of CD45R subsets of CD4 T cells *in vivo*. *Nature* 1990; **348,** 163–166.
45. Taniguchi T. Regulation of cytokine gene expression. *Ann Rev Immunol* 1988; **6,** 439–464.
46. Arai N, Nomura D, Villaret D, *et al.* Complete nucleotide sequence of the chromosomal gene for human IL-4 and its expression. *J Immunol* 1989; **142,** 274–282.
47. Fujita T, Shibuya H, Ohashi T, Yamanishi K, Taniguchi T. Regulation of human interleukin-2 gene: functional DNA sequences in the 5′ flanking region for the gene expression in activated T lymphocytes. *Cell* 1986; **46,** 401–407.
48. Maniatis T, Goodbourne S, Fischer JA. Regulation of inducible and tissue specific gene expression. *Science* 1987; **236,** 1237–1245.
49. Merkenschlager M, Terry L, Edwards R, Beverley PC. Limiting dilution analysis of proliferative responses in human lymphocyte populations defined by the monoclonal antibody UCHL1: implications for differential CD45 expression in T cell memory formation. *Eur J Immunol* 1988; **18,** 1653–1661.
50. Akbar AN, Amlot PL, Timms A, Lombardi G, Lechler R, Janossy G. The development of primed/memory CD8+ lymphocytes *in vitro* and in rejecting kidneys after transplantation. *Clin Exp Immunol* 1990; **81,** 225–231.
51. Salmon M, Kitas GD, Gaston JSH, Bacon PA. Interleukin-2 production and response by helper T cell subsets in man. *Immunol* 1988; **65,** 81–85.
52. Akbar AN, Salmon M, Ivory K, Taki S, Pilling D, Janossy G. Human CD4+ CD45RO+ and CD4+ CD45RA+ T cells synergise in response to alloantigens. *Eur J Immunol* 1991; **21,** 2517–2522.
53. Akbar AN, Salmon M, Janossy G. The synergy between naive and memory T cells during activation. *Immunol Today* 1991; **12,** 184–188.
54. Scott P, Pearce E, Cheever AW, Coffman RL, Sher A. Role of cytokines and CD4+ T cell subsets in the regulation of parasite immunity and disease. *Immunol Rev* 1989; **112,** 161–183.

6

Synthesis and actions of eicosanoids

CJ Hawkey and N Hudson

Introduction

Two families of membrane phospholipid derived autacoids (*autos* = self, *akos* = remedy) have been identified: the eicosanoids[1–7] (*eicosi* = 20 in Greek), and modified membrane phospholipids such as platelet activating factor (PAF).[8,9] Eicosanoids can be formed from three different 20-carbon polyunsaturated fatty acids, dihomo-gammalinoleic acid (DGLA – derived from linoleic acid) which contains three double bonds, arachidonic acid (which is most prevalent and contains four double bonds) and eicosapentaenoic acid (present principally in oily fish) which contains five double bonds. These fatty acids can be transformed by two main enzyme pathways: the microsomal cyclo-oxygenase enzyme which yields prostaglandins and thromboxane, and lipoxygenase enzymes which yields leukotrienes and other hydroperoxy fatty acid derivatives (Figure 6.1).

Cyclo-oxygenase products

Each of the three precursor fatty acids gives rise to a largely analogous series of cyclo-oxygenase and lipoxygenase products. The cyclo-oxygenase enzyme is attached to intracellular membranes and is found in microsomes after subcellular fractionation. Two double bonds are lost during synthesis of cyclo-oxygenase products so that DGLA gives rise to a series of prostaglandins and thromboxane containing one double bond (PGE_1, etc.), arachidonic acid to a series of prostaglandins containing two double bonds (PGE_2, etc.), and eicosapentaenoic acid to a series of prostaglandins containing three double bonds (PGE_3, etc.[1–4]). Prostaglandins A_2 to I_2 have been identified as products of arachidonic acid (Figure 6.2) and analogous one series prostaglandins from DGLA and three series prostaglandins from EPA have, with a few exceptions, been identified.

Prostaglandins A to C are biologically unimportant derivatives of E prostaglandins which arise during extraction procedures. Prostaglandins G_2 and H_2 are the immediate unstable products of the cyclo-oxygenase enzyme which are normally metabolised by second enzymatic steps to prostaglandins D_2, E_2 $F_2\alpha$ and I_2 (prostacyclin), or thromboxane A_2.[10]

Of these product, thromboxane A_2 and prostacyclin are very unstable, breaking down non-metabolically to thromboxane B_2 and 6-keto PGF 1α.[4,5] Prostaglandins are also metabolised locally, in the blood, liver and lungs, initially by 15-keto dehydrogenase and 13-reducatase enzymes. Subsequent complex metabolic steps involve β and omega oxidation of side chains. Major urinary metabolities of PGE_2, PGI_2 and TXB_2 have been identified.

Lipoxygenase products

Lipoxygenases are a family of enzymes which, in contrast to the co-enzyme, are located in the cytosol and which oxidise unsaturated fatty acids to lipid hydroperoxides *without* loss of double bonds.[6,7] Calcium plays an important role in activating lipoxygenase enzymes and is believed to act by stimulating translocation of the enzyme from the cytosol to the cell membrane.[11] The immediate products of arachidonic acid metabolism via the lipoxygenase pathways are hydroperoxyeicosatetraenoic acid (HPETES). Lipoxygenases acting at the five, 12 and 15 position are the main metabolites recognised. 5-lipoxygenase products

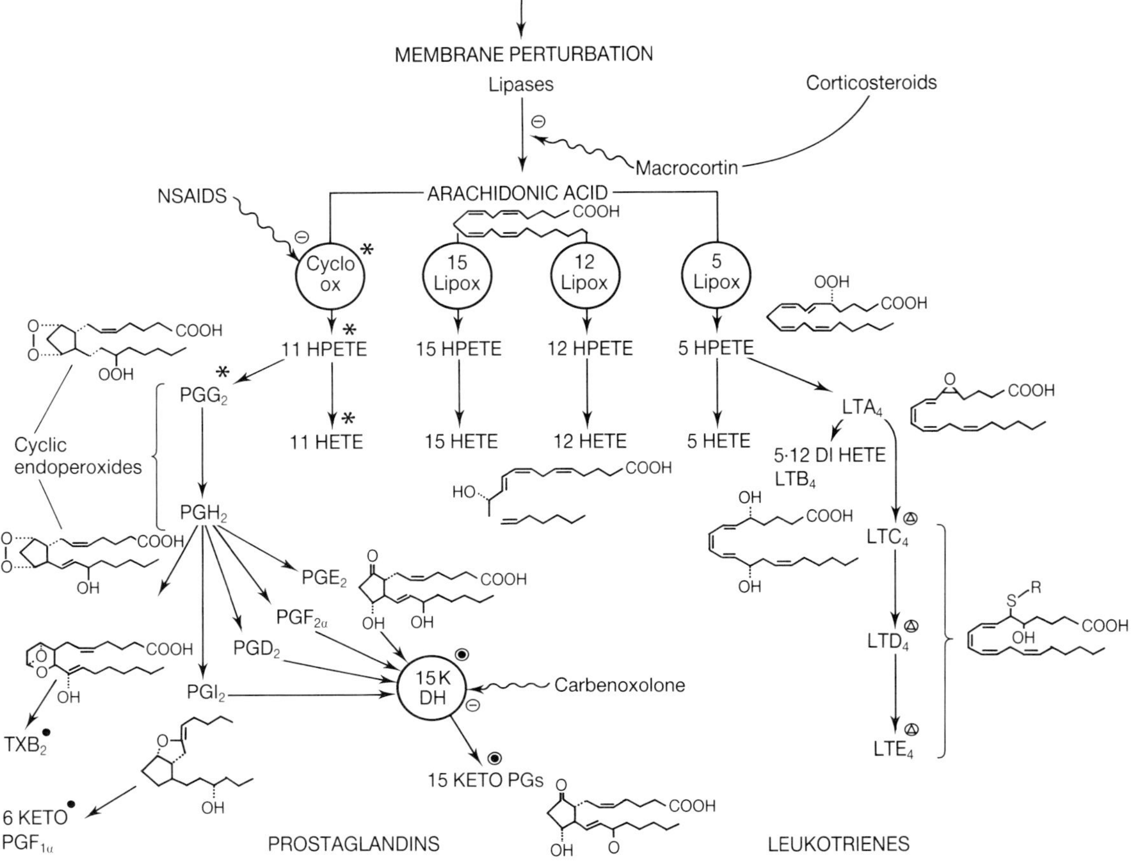

Fig. 6.1 Products of arachidonic acid metabolism[21] (reproduced by kind permission of *Gastroenterology*).

are best characterised biologically. As with prostaglandins, the most predominant family is that derived from arachidonic acid. However its members have four double bonds (LTB_4, etc.), since none is lost during synthesis.

The immediate product of arachidonic acid metabolites via the 5-lipoxygenase pathway is 5 HPETE, an unstable product which can then be converted into a stable 5 HETE or leukotriene A_4. This pivotal compound is subsequently transformed either by a hydrolase to leukotriene B_4, or conjugated with glutathione to form leukotriene C_4 (a much bigger molecule). Subsequent metabolic transformation (cleavage of glutamic acid and of glycine respectively) gives rise to LTD_4 and LTE_4. These peptide leukotrienes are now recognised to constitute the biological activity originally described as slow reacting substance of anaphylaxis.[12]

The capacity to produce eicosanoids is distributed widely throughout the body. However, many cells are specialised to favour production of one or a small number of eicosanoids. The most obvious example is the platelet which produces large quantities of thromboxane, together with some prostaglandin D_2 and 12 HETE; by contrast, endothelial cells produce large quantities of PGI_2. Moreover, within individual tissues some cells are more prominent sources of eicosanoids than others.

Control of synthesis

Release of substrate from membrane phospholipids is a major controlling mechanism for synthesis of both cyclo-oxygenase and lipoxygenase products although lipoxygenase pathways also re-

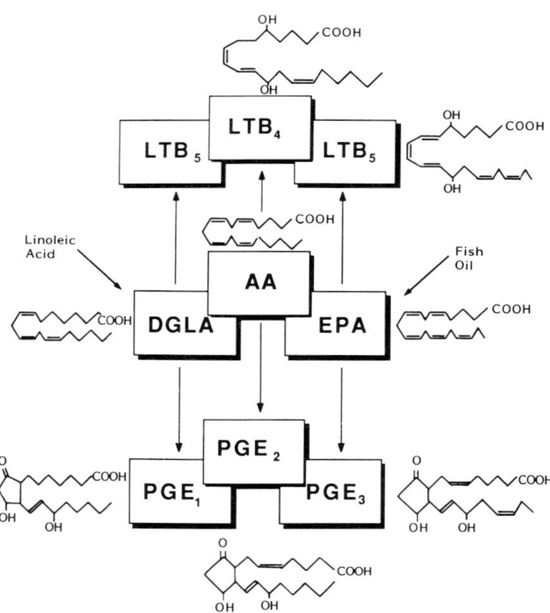

Fig. 6.2 Different familes of eicosanoids from different fatty acid precursors, illustrated for PGE_2 and LTB_4.

quire calcium for its activity. Substrate release largely occurs under the action of phospholipase A_2 or phospholipase C. These phospholipases can be activated in a number of ways by such stimuli as membrane perturbation (calcium influx), direct phospholipase A_2 activation, thrombin (cleavage of a peptide normally inhibitory to phospholipase A_2, cytokines and growth factors, bradykinin and the calcium ionophore. Many of the stimuli which stimulate synthesis of eicosanoids also cause release of PAF.

Many cells can elaborate lipocortins (also known as annexins[13]). These are endogenous inhibitors of phospholipase A_2. Synthesis of lipocortins is stimulated by corticosteroids and this is believed to be the main way in which corticosteroids inhibit the synthesis of eicosanoids.

Inhibitors of synthesis

Non-steroidal, anti-inflammatory drugs (NSAIDs) are well recognised as inhibitors of prostaglandin synthesis.[14] They act more directly than corticosteroids, binding to and inhibiting the activity of the cyclo-oxygenase enzyme with reduction of all products arising from a given cell. Substrate diversion with consequential enhanced lipoxygenase products is conceivable though little demonstrated. Cyclo-oxygenase inhibitors at high concentration may inhibit lipoxygenase pathways. Specific lipoxygenase inhibitors have also been developed, either binding directly to the enzyme or inhibiting translocation to the cell membrane.[11,15] Other drugs inhibit leukotriene synthesis by scavenging oxygen radicals.[16]

The spectrum of eicosanoid products can be profoundly influenced by modification of the membrane unsaturated fatty acid content achieved through dietary manipulation.[17] As well as changing the predominant family of products synthesised, modification of enzyme activity by differential feedback inhibition by different products also occurs.

Action of cyclo-oxygenase products

Receptors

The actions of prostaglandins and thromboxane are believed to be mediated largely through receptors[18,19] which display preferences for individual prostaglandins and are coupled through G proteins to two main second messenger systems.[19–21] Well recognised is stimulation of the adenyl cyclase enzyme with enhanced accumulation of cyclic AMP. In addition, cyclo-oxygenase products can also stimulate phospholipase C with formation of inositol triphosphate and diacyl glycerol, leading to increases in cytosolic calcium. These actions also lead to increased availability of substrate, and for further eicosanoid synthesis represent one of several positive feedback mechanisms. The interactions with PAF and cytokines (see section on interactions with other compounds) are other mechanisms.

As well as actions mediated via their products, there is good evidence that unsaturated fatty acids such as arachidonic acid can also have a role in direct second messenger signalling. For example, arachidonic acid activates protein kianse C directly.[22]

Actions

Eicosanoids influence the tone of smooth muscle from many sources.

Bronchial smooth muscle

E and I prostaglandins generally relax whilst D and F prostaglandins cause contraction of bronchial smooth muscle, as do thromboxane A_2, LTC_4 and D_4.[1,12]

Uterus

The effect of prostaglandins on uterine smooth muscle is complex and depends upon dose and reproductive status. Both E and F prostaglandins stimulate contraction of the pregnant uterus and can cause abortion.[1,23,24]

Gastro-intestinal smooth muscle

F prostaglandins contract both circular and longitudinal smooth muscle whilst E prostaglandins relax circular and contract longitudinal smooth muscle. These actions give rise to diarrhoea, cramps and reduced transit time.[25]

Vascular

D, E and I prostaglandins are generally vasodilator (although PGD_2 constricts pulmonary vessels and other blood vessels at high concentration).[1,26,27] F prostaglandins, TXA_2 and leukotrienes C_4 and D_4 are generally vasoconstrictor. PGI_2 and PGE_2 cause hypotension whilst thromboxane, LTC_4 and D_4 do so indirectly by inducing cardiac depression.[6,12,28,29] LTC_4 and D_4 can also lower blood pressure by constricting the microvasculature to cause plasma exudation.[6,12,29]

Platelets

Thromboxane A_2 induces platelet aggregation and release.[5,10] These can be inhibited by PGI_2, at physiological concentrations, leading to the medically important concept of a balance between platelet thromboxane and vascular prostacyclin as a possible determinant of susceptibility to vascular disease.[1,4]

Immune and inflammatory responses

The vasodilator effects of prostaglandins contribute to the vascular component of inflammatory responses including wheal and flare responses and plasma exudation. Leukotriene B_4 is a highly potent chemotactic agent for neutrophils, eosinophils and monocytes, promoting aggregation and degranulation, endothelial adherence and migration into sites of inflammation.[30] Since leukocytes are its main source, leukotriene B_4 may be particularly important in the secondary amplification of inflammatory reactions.

Immune responses

There is an increasing recognition that prostaglandins affect immune responses mediated by lymphocytes and macrophages. Following early observations[31–37] that E prostaglandins derived from macrophages and other sources could suppress immune responsiveness in lymphocytes and neutrophils[31–39] and that opposite effects could be obtained with indomethacin, it has become clear that there is a close interaction between prostaglandins and cytokines, best shown for interleukin 1. Prostaglandins have been shown both to mediate many of the effects of[35] and also to suppress synthesis of interleukin.[34] NSAID treatment may thus stimulate cytokine release[36,37] as well as suppressing some of their actions.[38] The full clinical significance of these changes is not fully elucidated.

Secretory responses

E and I prostaglandins inhibit gastric acid secretion (unusually by causing a fall in cyclic AMP) and also stimulate bicarbonate secretion by surface epithelial cells (with increases in cyclic AMP).[25,40] Mucus secretion (but probably not synthesis) is stimulated by prostaglandins. E and F prostaglandins also stimulate chloride secretion throughout the intestine, often resulting in diarrhoea.

Gastric cytoprotection

Low concentrations of prostaglandins can protect the gastric mucosa against a wide variety of damaging insults.[41] It is contentious whether this is due to an intrinsic 'cytoprotective' action or to an aggregate of potentially beneficial actions such as enhanced mucosal blood flow, bicarbonate secretion and mucus secretion.

Neural tissue

E and I prostaglandins and LTB_4 sensitise afferent nerve endings to a wide variety of stimuli, enhancing perception of pain.[32] In the hypothalamus, prostaglandins can induce fever and may mediate some of the actions of pyrogens.[1,24,32]

Renal effects of prostaglandins

As well as influencing renal blood flow substantially, prostaglandins have direct effects on renal tubules. E prostaglandins inhibit chloride and water reabsorption and (with PGI_2 and PGD_2) stimulate renin secretion.[1,28]

Endocrine and metabolic effects

E prostaglandins stimulate release of a large number of hormones, perhaps indicating a role in the normal control of hormone release. E prostaglandins are recognised to inhibit lipolysis in fat.[1]

Interactions with other compounds

Eicosanoids interact with other compounds in a complex and sometimes pivotal way, resulting in both positive and negative feedback. Positive feedback may result because of mutual amplification of release or activity of other compounds with pro-inflammatory actions. For example, eicosanoids and PAF interact in this way. PAF is released in inflammatory situations[42] and can stimulate further eicosanoid synthesis.[43,44] Equally it is clear that arachidonic acid and/or its metabolites are necessary for synthesis of PAF to occur.[42] Similarly, many of the actions of cytokines and growth factors such as interleukin 1 are dependent upon stimulation of prostaglandin synthesis and can be inhibited by cyclo-oxygenase inhibitors.[38] Conversely, prostaglandins modulate the production of cytokines and growth factors. For example, the production of cytokines in response to endotoxaemia is exaggerated in animals pretreated with NSAIDs.[45,46]

Primary abnormalities of eicosanoid metabolism

No primary abnormalities of eicosanoid metabolism have been clearly identified. Most changes (such as increased synthesis during inflammation) are secondary to accumulation and activation of inflammatory cells. Barter's syndrome is the only abnormality identified which might involve a primary alteration in eicosanoid production.[1,47] Barter's syndrome is characterised by a potassium losing state with decreased sensitivity to angiotensin. The latter, along with the accompanying hyperreninaemia and hyperaldosteronism, is reversed by indomethacin although the potassium loss is not.

Actions of eicosanoids illustrated by consequences of treatment

Prostaglandins

Prostaglandins and prostaglandin analogues are available as abortifacients, for the assistance of labour, for ulcer healing and prevention, and for preservation of arterial patency in severe peripheral vascular disease.[48] The most prominent consequences of prostaglandin administration are diarrhoea, abdominal cramps, uterine cramps and a high incidence of abortion in pregnant patients.[25,49]

Non-steroidal, anti-inflammatory drugs

The consequences of NSAID administration illustrate the importance of eicosanoids in blood flow, platelet function, uterine contraction and pain perception. These drugs are used principally in the symptomatic management of patients with arthritis and other painful conditions including dysmenorrhoea, biliary and renal colic, and disseminated malignancy. Indomethacin is sometimes used, rarely, to achieve closure of patent ductus arteriosis in neonates.[1] Aspirin at doses which selectively affect platelets is used in vascular disease. Full dose NSAIDs can have profound effects on blood flow to the brain (particularly indomethacin, with dizziness, confusion and headache as common side effects[50],) kidneys (with exacerbation of renal impairment, such as in liver disease[1]). Reduction in mucosal blood flow is one of several mechanisms by which these drugs lead to gastric ulceration.[25,51] By inhibiting thromboxane, the bleeding time is prolonged.[1] Prolongation of pregnancy by non-steroidal, anti-inflammatory drugs illustrates the importance of endogenous prostaglandins in onset of labour.[1] The response of dysmenorrheic women to NSAIDs illustrates the importance of prostaglandins in the symptomatology of this condition.

Thromboxane synthesis inhibitors and receptor antagonists

Compounds which selectively inhibit thromboxane synthesis to antagonise thromboxane receptors are under evaluation.[52–54] Like low dose aspirin, they inhibit platelet aggregation of prolonged bleeding time. They may have value in vascular disease, and illustrate the pivotal role of thromboxane in platelet behaviour.

5-lipoxygenase inhibitors

These are under evaluation for the treatment of inflammatory bowel disease, asthma and psoriasis.[11,15,16]

Leukotriene antagonists

Because of the exquisite sensitivity of bronchial smooth muscle to LTC_4 and LTD_4 (slow reacting substance of anaphylaxis) receptor antagonists are under evaluation, particularly in the management of asthma.[55,56] Individual adverse events have been associated with different lipoxygenase inhibitors and leukotriene receptor antagonists, but a pattern of adverse events which can be used to identify which of their actions are important in normal physiology analogous to that seen with NSAIDs for cyclo-oxygenase products has yet to emerge. Thus, whilst leukotriene antagonists illustrate the importance of these compounds in bronchoconstriction, they have not yet clarified what other actions of leukotrienes are important at physiological concentrations.

References

1. Moncada S, Vane JR. Pharmacology and endogenous roles of prostaglandin endoperoxides, thromboxane A_2 and prostacyclin. *Pharmacol Rev* 1979; **30,** 293–331.
2. Needleman P, Turk J, Jaksschik BA, Morrison AR, Lefkowith JB. Arachidonic acid metabolism. *Ann Rev Biochem* 1986; **55,** 69–102.
3. Campbell WB. Lipid-derived autacoids: eicosanoids and platelet activating factor. In: *The Pharmacological Basis of Therapeutics*, Goodman Gilman A, Goodmans, Gilman A (eds)., 1990.
4. Moncada S, Gryglewski R, Bunting S, Vane JR. An enzyme isolated from arteries transforms prostaglandin endoperoxides to an unstable substance that inhibits platelet aggregation. *Nature* 1976; **263,** 663–665.
5. Hamberg M, Svensson J, Samuelsson B. Thromboxane: a new group of biologically active compounds derived from prostaglandin endoperoxides. *Proc Nat Acad Sci USA* 1975; **72,** 2994–2998.
6. Samuelsson B, Dahlen SE, Lindgren JA, Rouzer CA, Serhan CN. Leukotrienes and lipoxins: structures, biosynthesis and biological effects. *Science* 1987; **237,** 1085–1272.
7. Yamamoto S. Mammalian lipoxygenases: molecular and catalytic properties. *Prostaglandins, Leukotrienes, Essent Fatty Acids* 1989; **35,** 219–229.
8. Snyder F. Biochemistry of platelet-activating factor: a unique class of biologically active phospholipids. *Proc Soc Exp Biol Med* 1989; **190,** 125–135.
9. Evans RD, Lund P, Williamson DH. Platelet-activating factor and its metabolic effects. *Prostaglandins, Leukotrienes, Essent Fatty Acids* 1991; **44,** 1–10.
10. Hamberg M, Svensson J, Wakabayashi T, Samuelsson B. Isolation and structure of two prostaglandin endoperoxides that cause platelet aggregation. *Proc Nat Acad Sci USA* 1974; **71,** 345–349.
11. Miller DK, Gillard JW, Vickers PJ, Sadowski S, Leveille C, Mancini JA. Identification and isolation of a membrane protein necessary for leukotriene production. *Nature* 1990; **343,** 278–281.
12. Piper PJ. Formation and actions of leukotrienes. *Physiol Rev* 1984; **64,** 744–761.
13. Flower RJ, Blackwell JG. Anti-inflammatory steroids induce biosynthesis of a phospholipase A2 inhibitor which prevents prostaglandin generation. *Nature* 1979; **278,** 456–459.
14. Vane JR. Inhibition of prostaglandin synthesis as a mechanism of action for aspirin like drugs. *Nature (New Biol)* 1971; **231,** 232–235.
15. Griswold DE, Marshall PJ, Webb EF *et al.* SK&F 86002: a structurally novel anti-inflammatory agent that inhibits lipoxygenase- and cyclooxygenase-mediated metabolism of arachidonic acid. *Biochem Pharmacol* 1987; **36,** 3463–3470.
16. Hawthorne AB, Boughton-Smith NK, Whittle BJH, Hawkey CJ. Colorectal leukotriene B_4 synthesis *in vitro* in inflammatory bowel disease: inhibition by the selective 5-lipoxygenase inhibitor BWA4C. *Gut* (in press).
17. Hawthorne AB, Filipowicz BL, Edwards TJ, Hawkey CJ. High dose eicosapentaenoic acid

ethyl ester: effects on lipids and neutrophil leukotriene production in normal volunteers. *Br J Clin Pharm* 1990; **30,** 187–194.
18. Kennedy I, Coleman RA, Humphrey PPA, Levy GP, Lumley P. Studies on the characterisation of prostanoid receptors: a proposed classification. *Prostaglandins* 1982; **24,** 667–689.
19. Halushka PV, Mais DE, Mayeux PR, Morinelli TA. Thromboxane, prostaglandin and leukotriene receptors. *Ann Rev Pharmacol Toxicol* 1989; **29,** 213–219.
20. Piomelli D, Volterra A, Dale N *et al.* Lipoxygenase metabolites of arachidonic acid as second messengers for presynaptic inhibition of Aplysia sensory cells. *Nature* 1987; **238,** 38–43.
21. Burch RM, Axelrod J. Dissociation of bradykinin-induced prostaglandin formation from phosphatidylinositol turnover in Swiss 3T3 fibroblasts: evidence for G protein regulation of phospholipase A2. *Proc Nat Acad Sci USA* 1987; **84,** 6374–6378.
22. Wood JN. Essential fatty acids and their metabolites in signal transduction. *Biochem Soc Trans* 1990; **18,** 785–786.
23. Goldberg VJ, Ramwell PW. Role of prostaglandins in reproduction. *Physiol Rev* 1975; **55,** 325–351.
24. Behrman HR. Prostaglandins in hypothalamo-pituitary and ovarian function. *Ann Rev Physiol* 1979; **41,** 685–700.
25. Hawkey CJ, Rampton DS. Prostaglandins and the gastrointestinal mucosa: are they important in its function, disease or treatment? *Gastroenterology* 1985; **89,** 1162–88.
26. Firth BJ, Winniford MD, Campbell WB, Hills LD. Hemodynamic effects of intravenous prostacyclin in stable angina pectoris. *Am J Cardio* 1983; **52,** 439–443.
27. Ishii N, Watanabe H, Irisawa C *et al.* Intracavernous injection of prostaglandin E1 for the treatment of erectile impotence. *J Urol* 1989; **141,** 323–325.
28. Lee JB. Cardiovascular renal effects of prostaglandins. *Arch Intern Med* 1974; **133,** 56–76.
29. Feuerstein G. Leukotrienes and the cardiovascular system. *Prostaglandins* 1984; **27,** 781–802.
30. Bray MA, Ford-Hutchinson AW, Smith MJH. Leukotriene B4: an inflammatory mediator *in vivo*. *Prostaglandins* 1981; **22,** 213–222.
31. Goodwin JS, Webb DR. Regulation of the immune response by prostaglandins. *Clin Immunol Immunopathol* 1980; **15,** 106–122.
32. Davies P, Bailey PJ, Goldenberg MM. The role of arachidonic acid oxygenation products in pain and inflammation. *Ann Rev Immunol* 1984; **2,** 335–357.
33. Boraschi D, Censini S, Bartalina M, Tagliabue A. Regulation of arachidonic acid metabolism in macrophages by immune and non-immune interferons. *J Immunol* 1985; **135,** 502–505.
34. Gilman SC, Chang J, Zeigler PR, Uhl J, Mochan J. Interleukin-1 activates phospholipase A2 in human synovial cells. *Arthritis Rheum* 1988; **31,** 126–130.
35. Monick M, Glazier J, Hunninghake GW. Human alveolar macrophages suppress Interleukin-1 (IL-1) activity via the secretion of prostaglandin E_2. *Am Rev Respir Dis* 1987; **135,** 72–77.
36. Oben JA, Wallace GR, Chain BM, Foreman JC. The stimulation of IL2 production by anti-rheumatic drugs. *Immunol* 1989; **67,** 328–332.
37. Petrini B, Wolk G, Wasserman J *et al.* Indomethacin modulation of monocyte cytokine release following pelvic irradiation for cancer. *Eur J Cancer* 1991; **27**(5), 591–594.
38. Dinarello CA. Interleukin-1 and interleukin-1 antagonism. *Blood* 1991; **77,** 1627–1652.
39. Weissman G, Smolen JE, Korchak HM. Release of inflammatory mediators from stimulated neutrophils. *N Eng J Med* 1980; **303,** 27–34.
40. Isselbacher KJ. The role of arachidonic acid metabolites in gastrointestinal homeostasis. Biochemical, histological and clinical gastrointestinal effects. *Drugs* 1987; **33** (suppl 1), 38–46.
41. Robert A, Nezamis JE, Lancaster C, Hanchar A. Cytoprotection by prostaglandins in rats. Prevention of gastric necrosis produced by alcohol, HCl, NaOH, hypertonic NaCl, and thermal injury. *Gastroenterology* 1979; **77,** 433–43.
42. Peplow PV, Mikhailidis DP. Platelet activating factor (PAF) and its relation to prostaglandins, leukotrienes and other aspects of arachidonic metabolism. *Prostaglandins, Leukotrienes Essent Fatty Acids* 1990; **41,** 71–82.
43. Kawaguchi H, Yasuda H. Effect of platelet activating factor on arachidonic acid metabolism in renal epithelial cells. *Biochim Biophys Acta* 1986; **875,** 525–534.
44. Lin AH, Morton DR, Gorman RR. Acetyl glyceryl ether phosphorycholine stimulates leukotriene B4 synthesis in human polymorphonuclear leukocytes. *J Clin Invest* 1982; **70,** 1058–1065.
45. Martiche PJ, Dunner RL, Ceska M, Suffredini AF. Detection of interleukin-8 and tumour necrosis factor in normal humans after intravenous endotoxin: the effect of anti inflammatory agents. *J Exp Med* 1991; **173,** 1021–1024.
46. Spinas GA, Blocsh D, Keller W, Zimmerli W, Cammisuli S. Pretreatment with ibuprofin augments circulating tumour necrosis factor-alpha, interleukin-6, and elastase during acute endotoeaxmia. *J Inf Dis* 1991; **163,** 89–95.
47. Ferris TF. Prostaglandins, potassium and Barter's syndrome. *J Lab Clin Med* 1978; **92,** 663–668.
48. Belch JJF, McArdle B, Pollock JG *et al.* Epopros-

tenol (prostacyclin) and severe arterial disease. A double-blind trial. *Lancet* 1983; **1,** 315–317.
49. Monk JP, Clissold SP. Misoprostol: a preliminary review of its pharmacodynamic and pharmacokinetic properties, and therapeutic efficacy in the treatment of peptic ulcer disease. *Drugs* 1987; **33,** 1–30.
50. Seideman P, von Arbin M. Cerebral blood flow and indomethacin drug levels in subjects with and without central nervous side effects. *Br J Clin Pharmacol* 1991; **31,** 429–432.
51. Hawkey CJ. Non-steroidal, anti-inflammatory drugs and ulcers: facts and figures multiply, but do they add up? *Br Med J* 1990; **300,** 278–284.
52. Patrignani P, Filabozzi P, Catella F, Pugliese F, Patrono C. Differential effects of dazoxiben, a selective thromboxane-synthase inhibitor, on platelet and renal prostaglandin-endoperoxide metabolism. *J Pharmacol Exp Ther* 1984; **228,** 472–477.
53. Le Breton GC, Venton DL, Enke SE, Halushka PV. 13-Azaprostanoic acid: a specific antagonist of the human blood platelet thromboxane/endoperoxide receptor. *Proc Nat Acad Sci USA* 1979; **76,** 4097–4101.
54. Hall RA, Gillard J, Guindon Y, Letts G, Champion E, Etnser D *et al.* Pharmacology of L-655,240 3 ([1-(4-chlorobenzyl)-5-fluoro-3-methyl-indol-2-yl],2,-2-dimethylpropanoic acid): a potent, selective thromboxane/prostaglandin endoperoxide antagonist. *Eur J Pharmacol* 1987; **135,** 193–201.
55. Jones TR, Zambini R, Biley M, Champion E, Charette L, Ford-Hutchison AW *et al.* Pharmacology of L-660,711 (MK-571): a novel potent and selective leukotriene D4 receptor antagonist. *Can J Physiol Pharmacol* 1989; **67,** 17–28.
56. Snyder DW, Fleisch JH. Leukotriene receptor antagonists as potential therapeutic agents. *Ann Rev Pharmacol Toxicol* 1989; **29,** 123–143.

7

Leucocyte adhesion in inflammation

R Rothlein and LA Scharschmidt

Introduction

Over the last ten years there has been an explosion in our understanding of the central role that leucocyte adhesion plays in the proper functioning of a host defence response. Our understanding has expanded across multiple academic and clinical disciplines including immunology, cell biology, physiology, molecular biology and biochemistry and is just now extending into clinical studies.

The role of leucocyte adhesion and the molecules involved in this process have been found to be critical for all aspects of specific and non-specific immunological reactions. These include leucocyte trafficking, antigen specific lymphocyte reactivity and various effector functions of leucocytes such as cell mediated cytolysis and phagocytosis of opsonised targets. In general, the molecules involved in leucocyte adhesion can be divided into several different gene superfamilies that mediate different functions. The integrin gene superfamily of adhesion molecules facilitate most leucocyte attachment to and migration through endothelium and extracellular matrices. This family of adhesion molecules also mediates effector functions of leucocytes such as cell mediated cytolysis, in which effector cells and target cells must adhere prior to lysis, as well as homotypic and heterotypic adhesions required for antigen presentation and subsequent clonal expansion.[1–3] Intercellular adhesion molecule 1 (ICAM-1), ICAM-2, ICAM-3 and VCAM-1 (also called INCAM-1) as well as CD2 and LFA-3 are adhesion molecules that are members of the immunoglobulin gene superfamily. The ICAMs and VCAM mediate the same functions in part as some of the integrins since they are ligands for members of the integrin superfamily.[4–6] CD2 and LFA-3 together form a receptor/ligand pair that play a role in T cell adhesion and activation.[7]

Another family of adhesion molecules, the selectins, functionally are more limited than the leucocyte integrins and are thought to mediate the initial attachment of neutrophils and some lymphocytes to endothelium in inflammatory lesions, as well as direct the natural traffic of lymphocytes to peripheral lymphoid tissue.[8–9] To date, three selectins have been identified. These selectin molecules differ from one another by their cellular distribution, their time of appearance after stimulation and the specific ligand(s) which they recognise and bind. They are similar in that they all consist of an amino C-type lectin domain, a single EGF-like domain and a variable number (depending on the selectin) of short consensus repeats with homology to those found in complement binding proteins (reviewed in[8,10]).

L-selectin is expressed on most leucocytes and plays a role in neutrophil homing to inflammatory lesions and lymphocyte homing to peripheral lymph nodes. L-selectin is shed from neutrophil surfaces at the same time that MAC-1 is up-regulated, leading to the idea that L-selectin acts as a brake to slow neutrophils down at a site of inflammation. Once slowed, CD18/ICAMs interactions take over to allow the cell to migrate from circulation to the inflammatory lesion. To facilitate migration, however, L-selectin is shed from the neutrophil surface, thus minimising the adhesive forces holding the cell in the lumen of the vessel.[11,12] Antibodies to L-selectin inhibit neutrophil/endothelial cell interactions both *in vitro* and *in vivo*.[13,14]

E-selectin is expressed only on activated endothelial cells and is induced with inflammatory cytokines such as interferon gamma and IL-1.[15] *In vitro*, E-selectin has been shown to mediate, in

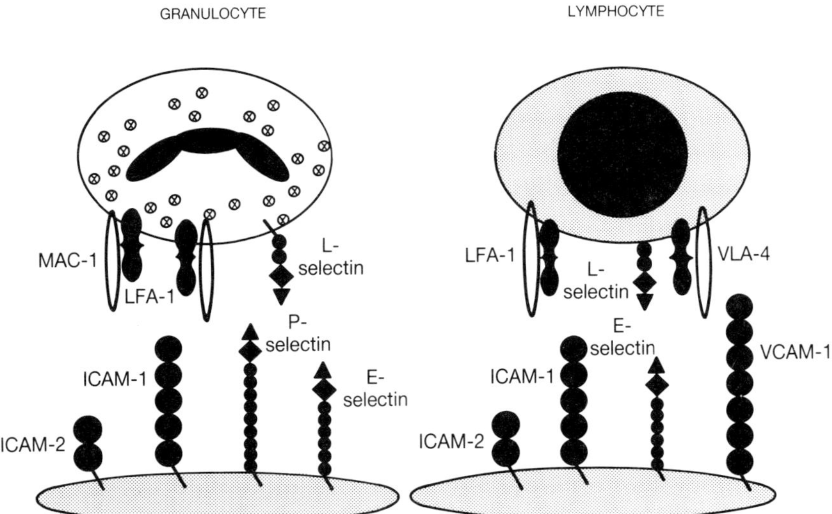

Fig. 7.1 Adhesion molecules involved in lymphocyte and neutrophil attachment to activated endothelium.

part, neutrophil and a subset of lymphocyte adhesion to endothelium.[16,17] *In vivo*, antibodies to E-selectin inhibit neutrophil trafficking to lungs in both non-human primates and in rats.[18,19]

P-selectin is expressed on platelets and endothelium. Like E-selectin, P-selectin is inducible. However, unlike E-selectin, P-selectin exists in intracellular pools and its expression is induced within minutes on endothelium exposed to mediators such as thrombin or histamine. P-selectin is also thought to mediate neutrophil/endothelial cell interactions as well as platelet endothelial cell interaction.[20] All the selectins are thought to bind to specific carbohydrates through their lectin-like domain. In the case of E-selectin this has been shown to be the case.[21,22]

Another adhesion molecule, CD44, has also been shown to function in the inflammatory response but does not fall into any of the above mentioned gene superfamilies.[23]

While it is obvious that there is an ever-expanding number of leucocyte adhesion molecules being identified on both the leucocyte and the target cells to which they adhere, in this chapter we will concentrate on perhaps the most fully characterised receptor/ligand combination. The receptors are members of the CD11, CD18 family of adhesion molecules (LFA-1, MAC-1, p150, 95) and the ligand is CD54 (intercellular adhesion molecule-1; ICAM-1).

Leucocyte adhesion – CD18 family

By way of background, it is clear that leucocyte/leucocyte and leucocyte/target cell adhesion is a necessary event for the host defence system to function normally in inflammation. Leucocytes must attach to endothelial cells lining blood vessels prior to migrating from the circulation to inflamed lesion.[24,25] Specific immunological processes involving lymphocytes such as antibody production or the generation and elaboration of antigen specific T cells necessitate lymphocytes first adhering to antigen presenting cells.[26] Finally, for leucocytes to perform effector functions such as lysis of target cells, they must first attach to these cells so that high concentrations of lytic mediators secreted by the leucocyte can be attained locally at the leucocyte/target cell junction.[27]

Through two lines of evidence obtained during the last ten years, the CD18 family of molecules on leucocytes has been implicated as being partially responsible for mediating leucocyte adhesion to cellular substrates. The CD18 family or LFA-1 family of adhesion molecules consists of CD11a, CD18 (LFA-1); CD11b, CD18 (MAC-1) and CD11c, CD18 (p150, 95) (reviewed in[1,3,28]). These molecules, which are distributed in various combinations on all leucocytes, are all heterodimers with distinct alpha subunits that associate with a common beta subunit. Structurally, the leucocyte adhesion molecules are members of the integrin superfamily and specifically they belong to the beta 2 subgroup. Although the leucocyte adhesion molecules mediate adhesion processes, they are unlike most other integrins in that they appear to recognise ligands that, for the most part, do not contain RGD sequences and their activity is dependent on Mg^{++} rather than Ca^{++}.[29–31]

Primary evidence to show the function of these molecules and, in fact, the importance of leucocyte adhesion in the generation and maintenance of inflammation has been elucidated in many experimental systems in which monoclonal antibodies to these molecules, used as antagonists, were found to inhibit multiple events associated with inflammation.

In vitro, monoclonal antibodies to CD18 or CD11a inhibit lymphocyte mediated lytic events such as cytotoxic T cell activity and natural killer cell activity[32–34] and lymphocyte trafficking processes such as attachment of lymphocytes to vascular endothelium and epidermal cells.[35,36] Furthermore these monoclonal antibodies inhibited *in vitro* models of general and/or specific immunological responsiveness such as antibody formation, mitogen and antigen induced T cell proliferation, and the mixed lymphocyte response (MLR).[37–40] All of these processes have in common the requirement for cell/cell interaction. The mechanism by which these antibodies to the adhesion molecules inhibit the above processes is thought to be mediated by their ability to antagonise the interaction of the appropriate CD18 family member with its ligand(s) rather than cellular elimination since these antibodies have not been shown to be cytotoxic themselves either in the presence of complement or in the presence of cells capable of mediating antibody dependent cellular cytotoxicity (ADCC).[34]

Monoclonal antibodies to CD18 and to CD11 also inhibit granulocyte function such as attachment to endothelium,[41] homotypic aggregation,[42] binding to iC3b coated particles[42,43] and ADCC.[34] These observations suggest that the CD18 family of adhesion molecules plays a role in processes involved in acute inflammation as well as those involved in specific immunological processes.

The second line of evidence that suggested an important role of the CD18 family came from the identification of a group of individuals who, due to genetic defects, were unable to express the normal number of leucocyte adhesion molecules on their cell surfaces.[44–46] These patients were classified into a severely deficient group (expressing between 0–1% of the normal number of adhesion molecules on the leucocyte surface) and a moderately deficient group (expressing between 2–10% of the normal number of adhesion molecules on the leucocyte surface).[47] Both groups of individuals presented with delayed umbilical cord separation, frequent skin infections with little leucocyte infiltrate and no pus formation. The severely deficient patients, in addition to the above, also had depressed T cell responses presumably because of defective antigen presenting capacity due to the inability of the T cell to attach to the antigen presenting cell. *In vitro*, lymphocytes from these individuals behaved as normal lymphocytes in the presence of anti-LFA-1 monoclonal antibodies. They had defective proliferative and effector responses in assays requiring cell/cell interactions.[48]

A ligand of LFA-1 is ICAM-1 which was functionally identified by screening antibodies from hybridomas generated from spleen cells of mice immunised against LFA-1 deficient lymphocytes for their ability to inhibit an LFA-1 dependent homotypic adhesion assay.[31,49] One antibody was identified and it was subsequently shown that the antigen that was affinity purified using this antibody, when inserted into planar membranes or immobilised on plastic, was able to mediate lymphocyte adhesion.[50,51] This adhesion was inhibitable by monoclonal antibodies directed against either ICAM-1 or LFA-1. Structurally, ICAM-1 is a member of the immunoglobulin supergene family with five Ig-like domains, a single membrane spanning region and a short cytoplasmic tail.[52,53] Further characterisation of ICAM-1 revealed that it was induced *in vitro* on multiple cell types including haematopoietic cells, endothelial cells and fibroblasts with IL-1a, IL-1b, TNFα, TNFβ and/or IFNγ depending on the cell type.[36,54–56] Functionally, anti-ICAM-1 monoclonal antibodies inhibited *in vitro* assays such as MLRs,[40] antigen induced proliferation,[38] cytotoxic T cell activity,[57,58] and granulocyte and lymphocyte attachment to endothelium.[41,59,60] Furthermore, when ICAM-1 was transfected into L cells expressing low amounts of HLA-DR molecules, enhanced class II restricted proliferation was attained when compared to L cells expressing the HLA-DR alone[61] and ICAM-1 defective mutants were unable properly to present antigen to mouse T cells.[62] These data suggested that, like the CD18 family of adhesion molecules, ICAM-1 expression on endothelial cells and other cell types was critical for the normal function of the host defence system.

Equally as suggestive is the expression of ICAM-1 at sites of inflammation. There is a low constitutive expression of ICAM-1 on venule endothelial cells; however, its expression is markedly increased at inflammatory sites.[54] Furthermore, there is an increased ICAM-1 expression on multiple cell types including keratinocytes in inflammatory skin lesions,[63,64] transplanted liver bile duct and perivenular hepatocytes during rejection[65] or, in cases of primary biliary cirrhosis,[18] endothelium in the brain surrounding multiple sclerosis plaques and experimental allergic encephalitis lesions in man and rodent respectively,[56,66–71] transplanted kidney glomeruli and tubules during rejection,[72] as well as lung epithelial cells following antigen provocation.[73] Increased ICAM-1 is also found on melanoma cells following metastasis.[74,75]

Anti-ICAM-1

The *in vivo* activity of anti-ICAM-1 monoclonal antibody has been assessed in several animal models of inflammation. Anti-ICAM-1 monoclonal antibody has been shown to inhibit neutrophil influx into rabbit lungs following systemic activation with phorbol esters.[76] Furthermore, anti-ICAM-1 monoclonal antibody mitigated eosinophil influx and airway hyper-responsiveness in a non-human primate model of antigen induced airway hyper-responsiveness.[73] Finally, it was recently reported that anti-ICAM-1, when given as the sole form of immunosuppressive therapy daily from two days prior to nine days post-transplant, increased the time to rejection of allogeneic kidneys in non-human primate recipients. The average time of allograft survival more than doubled from an average of less than ten days in the untreated animals to greater than 22 days in the treated animals.[72] Similar results were found in a non-human primate heterotopic heart transplant model using the same dosing regimen as above.[77] Anti-ICAM-1 monoclonal antibody also reversed acute allograft rejection episodes in the kidney transplant model described above. In this case monkeys were transplanted with cyclosporin A (CyA) being used as the immunosuppressive therapeutic agent. CyA doses were then tapered until subtherapeutic levels were achieved as detected by the onset of rejection monitored as a rise in serum creatinine. At this point, anti-ICAM-1 was administered daily for ten days while the subtherapeutic dose of CyA was maintained. Results of these experiments reveal that anti-ICAM-1 reversed the rise in serum creatinine in all animals tested as well as markedly prolonging the kidney allograft survival time.[72]

A rabbit model of spinal cord ischaemia/reperfusion was also shown to be sensitive to anti-adhesion monotional antibodies. Antibodies to either CD18 or ICAM-1 allowed the rabbit to be subjected to longer ischaemic times without any apparent deleterious effects.[78,79] In a model of haemorrhagic shock in non-human primates, anti-CD18 reduced the fluid requirements necessary to maintain cardiac output to a level of normal monkeys not subjected to shock while anti-ICAM-1 was not effective in this model.[80] More recently it was reported that anti-ICAM-1 antibodies were effective in inhibiting a Schwartzman type reaction in rabbits. In this model, a stimulus such as LPS was administered subcutaneously to rabbits on day 0 and subsequent injection of a neutrophil activating agent such as zymosan was administered 24 hours later along with technetium labelled red blood cells. Haemorrhage was measured four hours after that by monitoring the amount of radioactivity that had accumulated at the site of the LPS injection. The results from these experiments suggest that anti-ICAM-1 or anti-CD18 antibody given prior to the initial subcutaneous priming or the systemic challenge markedly reduced the amount of haemorrhage in these animals compared to saline or irrelevant antibody controls.[81] Finally, it was recently reported that a mouse anti-rat ICAM-1 was able to inhibit the development of a rat model of antigen induced arthritis by blocking the priming of antigen reactive cells.[82]

While all of these experiments show that anti-ICAM-1 and anti-CD18 inhibit inflammatory responses both *in vitro* and *in vivo* by blocking leucocyte adhesion, it is not clear which stage of the inflammatory process is most dependent on the CD18/ICAM-1 interactions. There is stong evidence to suggest that inhibition of CD18/ICAM-1 interactions results in fewer cells entering the inflammatory lesions in MAb treated animals as typified by the reduction of eosinophils found in the multiple antigen challenged primate lung previously mentioned.[73] However, since the primate was exposed to antigen in the presence of the inhibitory MAb, this reduction in infiltrating cells may be a result of a suppressed immunological response to the antigen which in turn reduced the amount of eosinophil chemoattractant generated, thus manifesting in a reduced cellular infiltrate, or it may simply be due to the inability of CD18 molecules on eosinophils to interact with their ligands on endothelium, thus inhibiting their ability to migrate to the inflamed lung. Furthermore, in the prophylactic model of kidney transplantation where the anti-ICAM-1 was given as the sole immunosuppressive agent, histological examination of the kidney clearly showed a reduction in the number of inflammatory cells found in the kidney prior to rejection. This suggests that anti-ICAM-1 inhibited the trafficking of lymphocytes through the endothelium to the transplanted organ tissue.[72,83] However, again this could be explained by the inhibition of antigen presentation at the time of transplant which would then mitigate the inflammatory response which then reduced the signal for cellular infiltration. That CD18/ICAM-1 plays a role in antigen presentation was elegantly shown when cells were transformed with both CD4 alone or CD4 and ICAM-1 and in some instances reactive T cells responded much more efficiently to the co-transfected cells than the CD4 expressing cells alone.[61] That the inhibition of CD18/ICAM-1 interactions blocks more than just leucocyte trafficking became convincingly apparent in the therapeutic protocol of non-human primate kidney transplantation where anti-ICAM-1 MAb reversed an acute rejection episode. Biopsies from the kidney revealed a moderate cell infiltrate in the face of a reversal of a rising serum creatinine level, suggesting that no damage was being mediated by alloreactive lymphocytes.[72] Thus, in this case, the mechanism of inhibition is thought to be mediated through inhibition of effector T cell/target cell conjugation.

One final point must also be made. Until recently we thought of the CD18 family of adhesion molecules as being somewhat passive in that they simply acted by facilitating leucocyte adhesion. Now data suggest that the interaction of CD18 molecules with ligands acts as a co-stimulatory signal for leucocytes. Immobilised anti-LFA-1 in conjunction with anti-CD3 causes a greater calcium influx in lymphocytes than anti-CD3 alone.[84] This concept was further developed when it was shown that lymphocytes were more responsive when plated on a bed of ICAM-1 than when plated on a control protein.[85,86] Thus it is possible that even if lymphocytes bind to appropriate cellular substrates in the presence of appropriate anti-adhesion MAb, the lack of the co-stimulatory signal then renders them impotent.

Conclusion

The inhibition of CD18/ICAM-1 interactions inhibits leucocyte trafficking, antigen presentation and leucocyte mediated cytolysis. It is unclear which of these three inhibitory processes is most responsible for the dramatic reduction in the inflammatory responses described to date and summarised in this chapter. It will probably be a combination of all three. Regardless, it is clear that antagonists of these interactions offer an exciting new target to prevent inflammatory responses associated with transplantation, autoimmunity and acute inflammation.

References

1. Martz E. LFA-1 and other accessory molecules functioning in adhesions of T and B lymphocytes. *Human Immunol* 1987; **18,** 3–37.
2. Kishimoto TK, Larson RS, Corbi AL, Dustin ML, Staunton DE, Springer TA. The leukocyte integrins. *Adv Immunol* 1989; **46,** 149–182.
3. Springer TA. Adhesion receptors of the immune system. *Nature* 1990; **346,** 425–434.
4. Dustin ML, Staunton DE, Springer TA. Supergene families meet in the immune system. *Immunol Today* 1988; **9,** 213–215.
5. Rice GE, Munro JM, Bevilacqua MP. Inducible cell adhesion molecule 110 (INCAM-110) is an endothelial receptor for lymphocytes: a CD11/CD18-independent adhesion mechanism. *J Exp Med* 1990; **171,** 1369–1374.
6. Carlos TM, Schwartz BR, Kovach NL *et al.* Vascular cell adhesion molecule-1 mediates lymphocyte adherence to cytokine-activated cultured human endothelial cells. *Blood* 1990; **76,** 965–970.
7. Springer TA. Cell adhesion: a birth certificate for CD2. *Nature* 1991; **353,** 704–705.
8. Springer TA, Lasky LA. Cell adhesion: sticky sugars for selectins. *Nature* 1991; **349,** 196–197.
9. Von Andrian UH, Chambers JD, McEvoy LM, Bargatze RF, Arfors KE, Butcher EC. Two-step model of leukocyte-endothelial cell interaction in inflammation: distinct roles for LECAM-1 and the leukocyte β_2 integrins *in vivo*. *Proc Nat Acad Sci USA* 1991; **88,** 7538–7542.
10. Butcher EC. Leukocyte-endothelial cell recog-

nition: three (or more) steps to specificity and diversity. *Cell* 1991; **67,** 1033–1036.

11. Kishimoto TK, Jutila MA, Berg EL, Butcher EC. Neutrophil MAC-1 and MEL-14 adhesion proteins inversely regulated by chemotactic factors. *Science* 1989; **245,** 1238–1241.
12. Kishimoto TK. A dynamic model for neutrophil localisation to inflammatory sites. *J NIH Res* 1991; **3,** 75–77.
13. Abbassi O, Lane CL, Krater S, *et al.* Canine neutrophil margination mediated by lectin adhesion molecule-1 *in vitro*. *J Immunol* 1991; **147,** 2107–2115.
14. Jutila MA, Rott L, Berg EL, Butcher EC. Function and regulation of the neutrophil MEL-14 antigen *in vivo*: comparison with LFA-1 and MAC-1. *J Immunol* 1989; **143,** 3318–3324.
15. Bevilacqua MP, Pober JS, Mendrick DL, Cotran RS, Gimbrone MA. Identification of an inducible endothelial-leukocyte adhesion molecule, E-LAM 1. *Proc Nat Acad Sci USA* 1987; **84,** 9238–9242.
16. Smith CW, Kishimoto TK, Abbassi O, *et al.* Chemotactic factors regulate lectin adhesion molecule-1 (LECAM-1) – dependent neutrophil adhesion to cytokine-stimulated endothelial cells *in vitro*. *J Clin Invest* 1991; **87,** 609–618.
17. Picker LJ, Kishimoto TK, Smith CW, Warnock RA, Butcher EC. ELAM-1 is an adhesion molecule for skin-homing T cells. *Nature* 1991; **349,** 796–799.
18. Adams DH, Hubscher SG, Shaw J, *et al.* Increased expression of intercellular adhesion molecule 1 on bile ducts in primary biliary cirrhosis and primary sclerosing cholangitis. *Hepatology* 1991; **14,** 426–431.
19. Mulligan MS, Varani J, Dame MK, *et al.* Role of endothelial-leukocyte adhesion molecule 1 (ELAM-1) in neutrophil-mediated lung injury in rats. *J Clin Invest* 1991; **88,** 1396–1406.
20. Larsen E, Celi A, Gilbert GE, *et al.* PADGEM protein: a receptor that mediates the interaction of activated platelets with neutrophils and monocytes. *Cell* 1989; **59,** 305–312.
21. Phillips ML, Nudelman E, Gaeta FCA *et al.* ELAM-1 mediates cell adhesion by recognition of a carbohydrate ligand, sialyl-Le^x. *Science* 1990; **250,** 1130–1132.
22. Polley MJ, Phillips ML, Wayner E, *et al.* CD62 and endothelial cell-leukocyte adhesion molecule 1 (ELAM-1) recognise the same carbohydrate ligand, sialyl-Lewis x. *Proc Nat Acad Sci USA* 1991; **88,** 6224–6228.
23. Shimizu Y, van Seventer GA, Siraganian R, Wahl L, Shaw. Dual role of the CD44 molecule in T cell adhesion and activation. *J Immunol* 1989; **143,** 2457–2463.
24. Perry MA, Granger DN. Role of CD11/CD18 in shear rate-dependent leukocyte-endothelial cell interactions in cat mesenteric venules. *J Clin Invest* 1991; **87,** 1798–1804.
25. Argenbright LW, Letts LG, Rothlein R. Monoclonal antibodies to the leukocyte membrane CD18 glycoprotein complex and to intercellular adhesion molecule-1 inhibit leukocyte-endothelial adhesion in rabbits. *J Leukocyte Biol* 1991; **49,** 253–257.
26. Lipsky PE, Rosenthal AS. Macrophage-lymphocyte interaction. II Antigen-mediated physical interactions between immune guinea pig lymph node lymphocytes and syngeneic macrophages. *J Exp Med* 1975; **141,** 138.
27. Bierer BE, Burakoff SJ. T cell adhesion molecules. *FASEB* 1988; **2,** 2584–2590.
28. Springer TA, Dustin ML, Kishimoto TK, Marlin SD. The lymphocyte function-associated LFA-1, CD2, and LFA-3 molecules: cell adhesion receptors of the immune system. *Ann Rev Immunol* 1987; **5,** 223–252.
29. Martz E. Immune lymphocyte to tumor cell adhesion: magnesium sufficient, calcium insufficient. *J Cell Biol* 1980; **84,** 584–598.
30. Martz E, Parker WL, Gately MK, Tsoukas CD. The role of calcium in the lethal hit of T lymphocyte-mediated cytolysis. *Adv Exp Biol Med* 1982; **146,** 121–143.
31. Rothlein R, Springer TA. The requirement for lymphocyte function-associated antigen 1 in homotypic leukocyte adhesion stimulated by phorbol ester. *J Exp Med* 1986; **163,** 1132–1149.
32. Krensky AM, Sanchez-Madrid F, Robbins E, Nagy J, Springer TA, Burakoff SJ. The functional significance, distribution, and structure of LFA-1, LFA-2, and LFA-3: cell surface antigens associated with CTL-target interactions. *J Immunol* 1983; **131,** 611–616.
33. Sanchez-Madrid F, Nagy J, Robbins E, Simon P, Springer TA. A human leukocyte differentiation antigen family with distinct alpha subunits and a common beta subunit: the lymphocyte function-associated antigen (LFA-1), the C3bi complement receptor (OKM1/Mac-1), and the p150,95 molecule. *J Exp Med* 1983; **158,** 1785–1803.
34. Kohl S, Springer TA, Schmalstieg FC, Loo LS, Anderson DC. Defective natural killer cytotoxicity and polymorphonuclear leukocyte antibody-dependent cellular cytotoxicity in patients with LFA-1/OKM-1 deficiency. *J Immunol* 1984; **133,** 2972–2978.
35. Haskard D, Cavender D, Beatty P, Springer T, Ziff M.T lymphocyte adhesion to endothelial cells: mechanisms demonstrated by anti-LFA-1 monoclonal antibodies. *J Immunol* 1986; **137,** 2901–2906.
36. Dustin ML, Singer KH, Tuck DT, Springer TA. Adhesion of T lymphoblasts to epidermal kera-

tinocytes is regulated by interferon gamma and is mediated by intercellular adhesion molecule-1 (ICAM-1). *J Exp Med* 1988; **167,** 1323–1340.

37. Davignon D, Martz E, Reynolds T, Kürzinger K, Springer TA. Monoclonal antibody to a novel lymphocyte function-associated antigen (LFA-1): mechanism of blocking of T lymphocyte-mediated killing and effects on other T and B lymphocyte functions. *J Immunol* 1981; **127,** 590–595.
38. Dougherty GJ, Murdoch S, Hogg N. The function of human intercellular adhesion molecule-1 (ICAM-1) in the generation of an immune response. *Eur J Immunol* 1988; **18,** 35–39.
39. Dougherty GJ, Hogg N. The role of monocyte lymphocyte function-associated antigen 1 (LFA-1) in accessory cell function. *Eur J Immunol* 1987; **17,** 943–947.
40. Boyd AW, Wawryk SO, Burns GF, Fecondo JV. Intercellular adhesion molecule 1 (ICAM-1) has a central role in cell-cell contact-mediated immune mechanisms. *Proc Nat Acad Sci USA* 1988; **85,** 3095–3099.
41. Smith CW, Rothlein R, Hughes BJ, Mariscalco MM, Schmalstieg FC, Anderson DC. Recognition of an endothelial determinant for CD18-dependent neutrophil adherence and transendothelial migration. *J Clin Invest* 1988; **82,** 1746–1756.
42. Anderson DC, Miller LJ, Schmalstieg FC, Rothlein R, Springer TA. Contributions of the Mac-1 glycoprotein family to adherence-dependent granulocyte functions: structure-function assessments employing subunit-specific monoclonal antibodies. *J Immunol* 1986; **137,** 15–27.
43. Beller DI, Springer TA, Schreiber RD. Anti-Mac-1 selectively inhibits the mouse and human type three complement receptor. *J Exp Med* 1982; **156,** 1000–1009.
44. Anderson DC, Springer TA. Leukocyte adhesion deficiency: an inherited defect in the Mac-1, LFA-1, and p150,95 glycoproteins. *Ann Rev Med* 1987; **38,** 175–194.
45. Todd RF, Freyer DR. The CD11/CD18 leukocyte glycoprotein deficiency. *Hem/Onc Clinics NA* 1988; **2,** 13–31.
46. Kishimoto TK, O'Connor K, Springer TA. Leukocyte adhesion deficiency: aberrant splicing of a conserved integrin sequence causes a moderate deficiency phenotype. *J Biol Chem* 1989; **264,** 3588–3595.
47. Anderson DC, Schmalstieg FC, Finegold MJ, *et al.* The severe and moderate phenotypes of heritable Mac-1, LFA-1 deficiency: their quantitative definition and relation to leukocyte dysfunction and clinical features. *J Inf Dis* 1985; **152,** 668–689.
48. Mentzer SJ, Bierer BE, Anderson DC, Springer TA, Burakoff SJ. Abnormal cytolytic activity of lymphocyte function-associated antigen-1-deficient human cytolytic T lymphocyte clones. *J Clin Invest* 1986; **78,** 1387–1391.
49. Rothlein R, Dustin ML, Marlin SD, Springer TA. A human intercellular adhesion molecule (ICAM-1) distinct from LFA-1. *J Immunol* 1986; **137,** 1270–1274.
50. Marlin SD, Springer TA. Purified intercellular adhesion molecule-1 (ICAM-1) is a ligand for lymphocyte function-associated antigen 1 (LFA-1). *Cell* 1987; **51,** 813–819.
51. Makgoba MW, Sanders ME, Luce GEG *et al.* ICAM-1: definition by multiple antibodies of a ligand for LFA-1 dependent adhesion of B, T and myeloid cell. *Nature* 1988; **331,** 86–88.
52. Staunton DE, Marlin SD, Stratowa C, Dustin ML, Springer TA. Primary structure of intercellular adhesion molecule 1 (ICAM-1) demonstrates interaction between members of the immunoglobulin and integrin supergene families. *Cell* 1988; **52,** 925–933.
53. Simmons D, Makgoba MW, Seed B. ICAM, an adhesion ligand of LFA-1, is homologous to the neural cell adhesion molecule NCAM. *Nature* 1988; **331,** 624–627.
54. Dustin ML, Rothlein R, Bhan AK, Dinarello CA, Springer TA. Induction by IL-1 and interferon, tissue distribution, biochemistry, and function of a natural adherence molecule (ICAM-1). *J Immunol* 1986; **137,** 245–254.
55. Pober JS, Gimbrone Jr MA, Lapierre LA *et al.* Overlapping patterns of activation of human endothelial cells by interleukin 1, tumor necrosis factor and immune interferon. *J Immunol* 1986; **137,** 1893–1896.
56. Frohman EM, Frohman TC, Dustin ML *et al.* Induction of ICAM-1 expression on human fetal astrocytes by interferon-gamma, tumor necrosis factor-alpha and interleukin-1: relevance to intracerebral antigen presentation. *J Neuroimmunol* 1989; **23,** 117–124.
57. Mentzer SJ, Rothlein R, Springer TA, Faller DV. Intercellular adhesion molecule-1 (ICAM-1) is involved in the cytolytic T lymphocyte interaction with human synovial cells. *J Cell Physiol* 1988; **137,** 173–178.
58. Makgoba MW, Sanders ME, Luce GEG *et al.* Intercellular adhesion molecule-1 (ICAM-1) monoclonal antibody inhibits cytotoxic T lymphocyte recognition. *Ann NY Acad Sci* 1989; **532,** 427–428.
59. Smith CW, Marlin SD, Rothlein R, Toman C, Anderson DC. Cooperative interactions of LFA-1 and Mac-1 with intercellular adhesion molecule-1 in facilitating adherence and transendothelial migration of human neutrophils *in vitro*. *J Clin Invest* 1989; **83,** 2008–2017.

60. Dustin ML, Springer TA. Lymphocyte function associated antigen-1 (LFA-1) interaction with intercellular adhesion molecule-1 (ICAM-1) is one of at least three mechanisms for lymphocyte adhesion to cultured endothelial cells. *J Cell Biol* 1988; **107,** 321–331.
61. Altmann DM, Hogg N, Trowsdale J, Wilkinson D. Cotransfection of ICAM-1 and HLA-DR reconstitutes human antigen-presenting cell function in mouse L cells. *Nature* 1989; **338,** 512–514.
62. Dang LH, Michalek MT, Takei F, Benaceraff B, Rock KL. Role of ICAM-1 in antigen presentation demonstrated by ICAM- 1 defective mutants. *J Immunol* 1990; **144,** 4082–4091.
63. Vejlsgaard GL, Ralfkiaer E, Avnstorp C, Czajkowski M, Marlin SD, Rothlein R. Kinetics and characterisation of intercellular adhesion molecule-1 (ICAM-1) expression on keratinocytes in various inflammatory skin lesions and malignant cutaneous lymphomas. *J Amer Acad Dermatol* 1989; **20,** 782–790.
64. Griffiths CEM, Nickoloff BJ. Keratinocyte intercellular adhesion molecule-1 (ICAM-1) expression precedes dermal T lymphocytic infiltration in allergic contact dermatitis (*Rhus dermatitis*). *Am J Pathol* 1989; **135,** 1045–1053.
65. Adams DH, Hubscher SG, Shaw J, Rothlein R, Neuberger JM. Intercellular adhesion molecule 1 on liver allografts during rejection. *Lancet* 1989; **2,** 1122–1125.
66. Sobel RA, Mitchell ME, Fondren G. Intercellular adhesion molecule-1 (ICAM-1) in cellular immune reactions in the human central nervous system. *Am J Pathol* 1990; **136,** 1309–1316.
67. Raine CS, Lee SC, Scheinberg LC, Duijvestijn AM, Cross AH. Adhesion molecules on endothelial cells in the central nervous system: an emerging area in the neuroimmunology of multiple sclerosis. *Clin Immunol Immunopathol* 1990; **57,** 173–187.
68. Cannella B, Cross AH, Raine CS. Upregulation and coexpression of adhesion molecules correlate with relapsing autoimmune demyelination in the central nervous system. *J Exp Med* 1990; **172,** 1521–1524.
69. Cannella B, Cross AH, Raine CS. Adhesion-related molecules in the central nervous system: upregulation correlates with inflammatory cell influx during relapsing experimental autoimmune encephalomyelitis. *Lab Invest* 1991; **65,** 23–31.
70. Raine CS. Multiple sclerosis: A pivotal role for the T cell in lesion development. *Neuropathol Appl Neurobiol* 1991; **17,** 265–274.
71. Wilcox CE, Ward AMV, Evans A, Baker D, Rothlein R, Turk JL. Endothelial cell expression of the intercellular adhesion molecule-1 (ICAM-1) in the central nervous system of guinea pigs during acute and chronic relapsing experimental allergic encephalomyelitis. *J Neuroimmunol* 1990; **30,** 43–51.
72. Cosimi AB, Conti D, Delmonico FL *et al*. *In vivo* effects of monoclonal antibody to ICAM-1 (CD54) in nonhuman primates with renal allografts. *J Immunol* 1990; **144,** 4604–4612.
73. Wegner CD, Gundel RH, Reilly P, Haynes N, Letts LG, Rothlein R. Intercellular adhesion molecule-1 (ICAM-1) in the pathogenesis of asthma. *Science* 1990; **247,** 456–459.
74. Matsui M, Temponi M, Ferrone S. Characterization of a monoclonal antibody-defined human melanoma-associated antigen susceptible to induction by immune interferon. *J Immunol* 1987; **139,** 2088–2095.
75. Natali P, Nicotra MR, Cavaliere R *et al*. Differential expression of intercellular adhesion molecule 1 in primary and metastatic melanoma lesions. *Cancer Res* 1990; **50,** 1271–1278.
76. Barton RW, Rothlein R, Ksiazek J, Kennedy C. The effect of anti-intercellular adhesion molecule-1 on phorbol-ester-induced rabbit lung inflammation. *J Immunol* 1989; **143,** 1278–1282.
77. Flavin T, Rothlein R, Faanes R, Ivens K, Starnes V. Monoclonal antibody against intercellular adhesion molecule (ICAM)-1 prolongs cardiac allograft survival in cynomolgus monkeys. *Transplant Proc* 1990; **23,** 533–534.
78. Clark WM, Madden KP, Rothlein R, Zivin JA. Reduction of central nervous system ischemic injury in rabbits using leukocyte adhesion antibody treatment. *Stroke* 1991; **22,** 877–883.
79. Clark WM, Madden KP, Rothlein R, Zivin JA. Reduction of central nervous system ischemic injury by monoclonal antibody to intercellular adhesion molecule. *J Neurosurg* 1991; **75,** 623–627.
80. Mileski WJ, Winn RJ, Vedder NB, Pohlman TH, Harlan JM, Rice CL. Inhibition of CD18-dependent neutrophil adherence reduces organ injury after hemorrhagic shock in primates. *Surgery* 1990; **108,** 206–212.
81. Argenbright LW, Barton RW. The Schwartzman response: a model of ICAM-1 dependent vasculitis. *Agents Actions* 1991; **34,** 208–210.
82. Iigo Y, Takashi T, Tamatani T *et al*. ICAM-1-dependent pathway is critically involved in the pathogenesis of adjuvant arthritis in rats. *J Immunol* 1991; **147,** 4167–4171.
83. Cosimi AB, Geoffrion C, Anderson T, Conti D, Rothlein R, Colvin RB. Immunosuppression of cynomolgus recipients of renal allografts by R6.5, a monoclonal antibody to intercellular adhesion molecule-1. In: *Leukocyte Adhesion Molecules*, Springer TA, Anderson DC, Rosenthal AS, Rothlein R (eds). New York: Springer-Verlag, 1989.
84. Wacholtz MC, Patel SS, Lipsky PE. Leukocyte function-associated antigen 1 is an activation mol-

ecule for human T cells. *J Exp Med* 1989; **170,** 431–448.

85. Van Seventer GA, Shimizu Y, Horgan KJ, Shaw S. The LFA-1 ligand ICAM-1 provides an important costimulatory signal for T cell receptor-mediated activation of resting T cells. *J Immunol* 1990; **144,** 4579–4586.

86. Van Seventer GA, Newman W, Shimizu Y *et al.* Analysis of T cell stimulation by superantigen plus major histocompatibility complex class II molecules or by CD3 monoclonal antibody: costimulation by purified adhesion ligands VCAM-1, ICAM-1, but not ELAM-1. *J Exp Med* 1991; **174,** 901–913.

SECTION II

Immune Mechanisms in Rejection

8

Antigen presentation and allo-immunity

R Gill, L Hao and K Lafferty

Introduction

Early observations of the allograft response indicated that there were particularly strong 'transplantation antigens' which could elicit a violent immune response to the grafted tissues. Tremendous gains have been made in our current understanding of the allograft response, especially the central role of major histocompatability complex (MHC) antigens as the prime molecules controlling this response. The molecular nature of antigen presentation, in particular, has seen great advances over the past decade. However, a lingering problem with our understanding of antigen presentation in the allograft response can be stated as a transplantation paradox composed of three propositions:

1. The process of allograft rejection involves the recognition of transplantation antigens carried on the grafted tissues;
2. The allograft response must be included among the most violent immune responses that occur *in vivo*;
3. Transplantation antigens in their molecular form are extremely weak immunogens.[1]

The paradox is that this violent immune reaction, dependent on antigen recognition, involves a response to antigens which are inherently weakly immunogenic.[1,2] A key proposition of this chapter is that presentation of allogeneic MHC antigens is required, but is not *sufficient* for the activation of the rejection response.

Antigen presentation and direct allorecognition

During the 1970s it became clear that T cell responses were not directed against nominal antigens per se but rather involved antigen recognition in association with MHC antigens. This phenomenon of MHC restriction pointed to the central role of MHC molecules in controlling the immune response.[3] The notion of antigen recognition with MHC has been refined by the working model of Bjorkman *et al.*[4] whereby peptide antigen fragments are physically associated with MHC class I molecules in a peptide binding groove in the external domain of the MHC molecules. This notion was extrapolated to encompass peptide interaction with class II MHC as well.[5]

The processing and presentation of peptide antigens appears to involve two primary pathways depending on the origin of the antigen: endogenous and exogenous. Endogenous antigens are derived from proteins degraded in the cytosol and transported into the endoplasmic reticulum where they preferentially associate with class I MHC antigens.[6] Studies utilising acid elution of affinity purified class I molecules revealed that class I MHC associated peptides were invariably 8–9 amino acids in length.[7–9] Studies by Townsend *et al.* indicated that peptide–MHC binding is necessary for the surface expression of class I MHC by stabilising the association of the class I heavy chain with β_2-microglobulin.[6]

The association of antigens with class II, unlike class I MHC, does not involve cytosolic molecules but rather involves the exogenous pathway of antigen presentation. MHC class II molecules derive their peptides from extracellular proteins captured by cellular phagocytosis and endocytosis. Such proteins are degraded in cellular acidic vesicles where peptide fragments associate with class II MHC molecules. In contrast to class I MHC antigen, neither initial class II heterodimer assembly nor intracellular transport appears to be dependent on tight peptide binding.[10] Further, acid elution of affinity purified class II molecules revealed that class II associated peptides were up to double the length of those peptides dissociated from class I MHC molecules.[11]

The allograft response actually represents atypical recognition/presentation of MHC molecules. Rather than presenting processed antigens to self T cells, polymorphic residues of MHC antigens are themselves the recognition determinants. Like self MHC restricted responses, allogeneic class I MHC molecules elicit primarily CD8 T cell responses while class II MHC molecules elicit CD4 T cell responses.[12] However, the recognition of polymorphic determinants of allogeneic MHC antigens does not explain the extraordinarily high precursor frequency of alloreactive cells, which is orders of magnitude greater than the frequency of cells reactive to exogenous antigens presented to self by MHC antigens. The role of processed peptide antigens associated with MHC described above may provide part of the answer to the high alloreactive precursor frequency.

An early model to explain the high frequency of alloreactive T cells was suggested by Matzinger and Bevan[13] who proposed that allorecognition, like self MHC restricted responses, involved the set of T cells which recognised common cellular antigens in association with allogeneic MHC. Thus, the allogeneic MHC was in effect 'reshuffling' the range of self antigens which could be recognised by T cells by presenting them on a novel restricting element(s). The high alloreactive precursor frequency was not merely a reflection of cells recognising allo-MHC per se, but rather a large repertoire of T cells seeing a variety of antigens in the context of the new MHC molecule to which the host was not tolerant. Current models of MHC–antigen interaction make this a particularly attractive hypothesis, especially considering that a peptide–MHC interaction may be *necessary* for class I MHC antigen expression.[6] Thus the co-recognition of the allogeneic MHC–peptide complex may be important for allogeneic recognition. The requirement for the MHC–peptide interaction (at least for class I MHC), plus recent studies indicating that self antigens are constitutively processed and presented by antigen presenting cells (APC),[11,14] provides a molecular basis for the original hypothesis of Matzinger and Bevan.

A different view of the high alloreactive precursor frequency relates to the positive selection of the T cell repertoire on self MHC molecules in the thymus.[15,16] According to this view, since the positive selection of T cells in the thymus requires a bias towards MHC, a relatively large frequency of T cells would react with high affinity to slight variations in the allogeneic MHC molecule. This model does not require the co-recognition of peptides with allogeneic MHC, unlike the Matzinger/Bevan model; the polymorphic MHC residues might themselves be the recognition structure. Even if peptide interaction with MHC is necessary for stable MHC conformation,[6] a *specific* peptide may not be required for the alloreactive T cell interaction. However, this model does not *exclude* the possibility of co-recognition of the allo-MHC-peptide complex. There is no *a priori* reason to assume that alloreactive T cells cannot display both types of allorecognition. Experimental evidence is consistent with the view that some T cell clones exhibit a fine specificity for polymorphic MHC residues without any apparent co-recognition requirement for a specific peptide,[17] while other alloreactive clones appear to require a putative species specific peptide interaction with the allogeneic MHC for recognition.[17,18] The proportion of alloreactive T cells which require co-recognition of MHC+peptide versus recognition of polymorphic MHC residues alone remains to be clarified.

Indirect presentation of allo-antigens

The discussion above refers to the *direct* presentation of allogeneic MHC antigens expressed on the cell surface. This form of recognition would allow for both class I (CD8) and class II (CD4) MHC restricted T cells to recognise the allo-antigens. However, *indirect* allo-antigen presentation can also occur whereby grafted antigens can be presented by host APC (Figure 8.1). In this case antigens which are shed from the cell surface or released by dead cells will be processed and presented like any exogenous

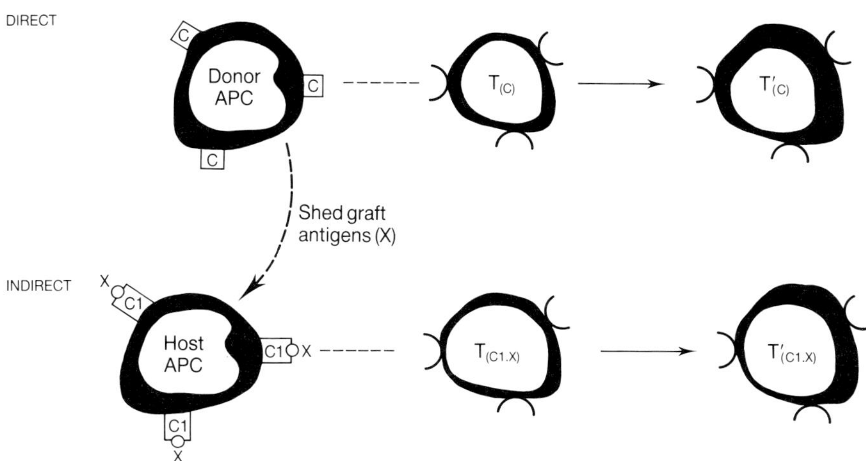

Fig. 8.1 Direct and indirect allo-antigen presentation. Allo-antigens can be recognised on the surface of donor cells as intact cell surface molecules ('c' referring to the donor MHC), the direct pathway of allo-presentation. Alternatively, antigens shed from the graft (generically termed 'x') can be processed by host APCs and presented in association with self-MHC (c2), the indirect pathway of allo-presentation. Note that T cells generated by the direct reaction will be graft specific, whereas T cells generated by the indirect pathway will not be graft specific but rather will be restricted by host MHC molecules.

antigen. Also, both MHC and non-MHC allo-antigens would be capable of being presented to host T cells in the context of self MHC. Importantly, T cells reactive to antigens presented by the indirect pathway would not be graft specific but would be restricted to self MHC antigens. Further, the processing of exogenous antigens by this indirect pathway would result primarily in presentation by class II MHC antigens and so would lead to the activation of CD4 T cells preferentially.

Despite advances in the understanding of the molecular nature of allorecognition, positive and negative selection of the T cell repertoire in the thymus, and the phenomenon of MHC restriction in T cell activation, we still do not have an explanation of why MHC molecules (as opposed to other cell surface molecules) serve such a major role in controlling the immune response. As mentioned above, when isolated from the cell surface, MHC antigens make quite weak immunogens.[1] We favour the view that MHC antigens are the control molecules of the immune response not simply because they present peptide antigens but because they also have a key *functional* role in the response as well (see below).

The two signal model for T cell activation

The association of degraded peptide antigens, derived from both intracellular and extracellular sources, with MHC molecules might lead to the assumption that this molecular complex is the basis of immunogenicity to responsive T cells (either antigen specific or alloreactive). However, as previously stated, a transplantation paradox is that the allograft response is a violent reaction to molecules which are weak immunogens when isolated from the cell surface.[1] Further, the immunogenicity of allogenic cells is a *viable* cell function; when APCs are metabolically inactivated, they lose their ability to stimulate alloresponses despite retaining recognisable MHC antigens.[19–21] MHC antigens, therefore, do not appear to be *intrinsically* immunogenic. The two signal model for T cell activation helps explain this problem.[22] This model was derived from the Bretcher/Cohn model for B cell activation, which proposed that two signals were required for activation.[23] Signal 1 was provided by engagement of the B cell receptor and signal 2 by engagement of a second epitope on the antigenic molecule by a second receptor of different specificity (below).

The two signal model for T cell activation was developed in Canberra at the same time that

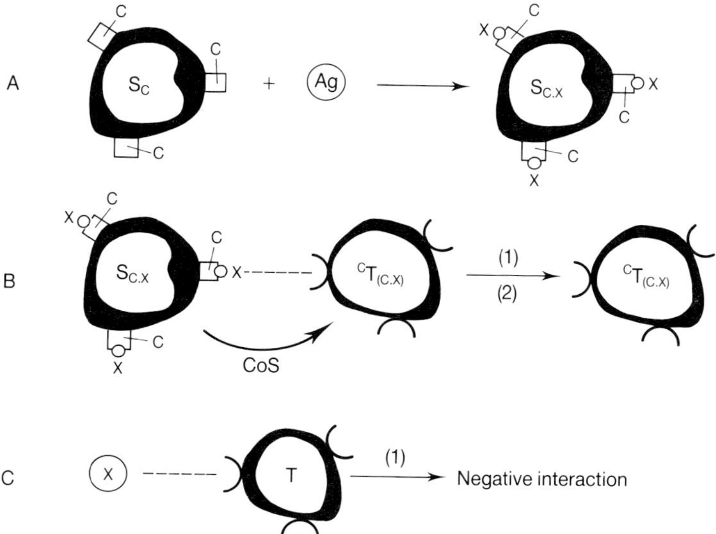

Fig. 8.2 The two signal model for T cell activation based on the function of a control molecule, c, which regulates release of the co-stimulator, the second signal in the process of T cell activation. *Reaction A*: Antigen (Ag) is taken up and processed by the stimulating cell, S_c, which carries a control molecule, c, on its surface. Processed antigen is converted to peptide structures, x, which are coupled to c and carried to the cell surface where the complex is presented as the complex c.x. *Reaction B*: Antigen presented as c.x on the stimulating cell is recognised by a T cell of specificty c.x (the left superscript denotes the T cell genotype, the right subscript in parentheses denotes the T cell specificity). This recognition provides signal (1) for the T cell. Engagement of c.x on the surface of the stimulating cell activates release of the co-stimulator, providing the second signal for T cell induction. *Reaction C*: The interaction with the epitope x alone provides signal (1) for the T cell and may result in a negative interaction.

Doherty and Zinkernagel, also working in Canberra, were unravelling the MHC restriction of T cell responses.[3] A question much discussed at that time concerned why T cells were so biased towards MHC antigen recognition. Was Lewis Thomas correct when he proposed that T cells were the surveillance system of the body, recognising and responding to variance of self such as nascent tumours? The immune surveillance concept did provide an explanation for the violence of the allograft response, and Doherty and Zinkernagel saw it as providing an attractive explanation for MHC restriction of immune responses; the responding T cells were thought to be responding to altered-self components.[3] Why MHC antigens were so important in terms of the definition of self was not explained. Moreover, the concept of immune surveillance could not deal with the central problem raised by the transplantation paradox: the failure of isolated MHC antigens to induce allograft immunity.[21]

These loose threads in the theoretical fabric could be drawn together with a two signal model for T cell activation.[22] This theory proposes that the antigen presenting cell (APC) plays an active role in the process of T cell activation by providing both the source of antigen (signal 1) and a source of co-stimulator (CoS) activity which provides the second signal for T cell induction (see Figure 8.2). Only cells capable of elaborating the CoS would be capable of activating the responding T cell. This means that MHC molecules would be presented in two distinct forms: APCs capable of CoS production (stimulating or S^+ phenotype) would be capable of activating primary T cells whereas allo-antigens on the surface of cells incapable of CoS production (non-stimulating or S^- phenotype) would present the same MHC antigens but would not stimulate responsive T cells due to the inability to elaborate the second signal.

If the production of a CoS by the active APC (the S^+ cell) was regulated by a control molecule on the surface of that cell, then engagement of this molecule would be required in order to signal CoS release from the APC.

Antigens or antigenic epitopes (generically termed 'x') which were recognised in association with this control molecule would be highly immunogenic, and the T cell responses would be biased towards recognition of the control molecule c, because engagement of molecule c would be a requirement for CoS production (see Figure 8.2). Recognition of epitope 'x' alone by the T cell would only provide signal 1 and would thus be a negative interaction. Alloreactivity was now explained as an 'abnormal' immune reaction in which allogeneic control molecules were recognised because of *genetic* rather than *antigenic* alterations (Figure 8.3). Moreover, strong allo-antigens were those molecules that could function as control molecules (MHC antigen); other allo-antigens (non-MHC antigen) would be weak immunogens. That is, there would be two classes of allo-antigen, major and minor histocompatibility antigens, based on the ability of these antigens to serve as control structures for release of the second signal.

Experimental analysis based on the *in vitro* mixed lymphocyte reaction demonstrated that the development of strong alloresponses required differences at the MHC locus of the interacting cells.[24] Thus, MHC antigens were behaving as the control molecules of the immune system, and for this reason were the restricting element for T cell responses to foreign antigen. We would propose that MHC plays such a dominant role in controlling immune responses not only due to its role as a presenting/recognition structure, but also due its *functional* role, critical for the release of the CoS.

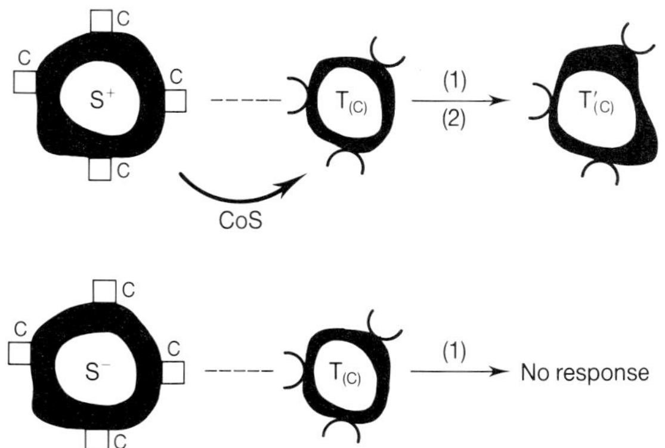

Fig. 8.3 Theory of alloreactivity. According to this model, the allogeneic control molecule (c) itself becomes part of the recognition structure for the responsive T cell. Allo-antigen presentation by an S+ cell will provide both a source of antigen (signal 1) and a source of co-stimulator (signal 2) required by T cell activation. Allo-antigen presented on the surface of an S- cell will not be directly immunogenic because these cells cannot provide a source of the second signal.

The two signal model provided a solution to the transplantation paradox; MHC antigens were only strong immunogens when they functioned as control molecules of the immune system; that is, when presented on the surface of metabolically active APCs. Tissue immunogenicity was a function of living cells because CoS production, an essential requirement for T cell activation, was a function of the *viable* cell. This model also explained why MHC antigens, the control molecules of the immune system, restricted T cell responses. This model implied that MHC antigens were not strong immunogens per se and that the barrier to transplantation was S^+ cells carried in the graft, suggesting that tissue immunogenicity might be reduced by removal of active APCs from a graft prior to transplantation (see below).

Alteration of tissue immunogenicity: the passenger leucocyte model

The notion that allo-antigen presentation between S^+ and S^- cells within the graft represent qualitatively different forms of antigen presentation led back to an early concept that graft immunogenicity can be reduced by appropriate tissue pretreatment.[25] If tissue immunogenicity is due to a small proportion of resident S^+ cells – the 'passenger leucocytes' – then removal or inactivation of these cells prior to grafting should facilitate allograft acceptance.[22] Tissue pretreatment has been strikingly successful for facilitating allograft acceptance of endocrine tissues. Work in the mid 1970s indicated that pretreatment of thyroid tissues in 95% O_2 culture would facilitate long term graft acceptance in non-immunosuppressed, allogeneic recipient mice.[26] This technique was later applied to the modification of pancreatic islet allograft immunogenicity.[27,28] Grafting experimentally induced diabetic mice with untreated islet allografts results in initial return to euglycaemia followed by a rapid return to hyperglycaemia due to graft rejection (see Figure 8.4). Following organ culture in 95% O_2 for seven days, islet allografts survive and function indefinitely in recipient mice. Application of 95% O_2 culture has also allowed successful islet allografting in rats[29,30] and even in outbred mice,[31] though short term immunosuppression with cyclosporin A was

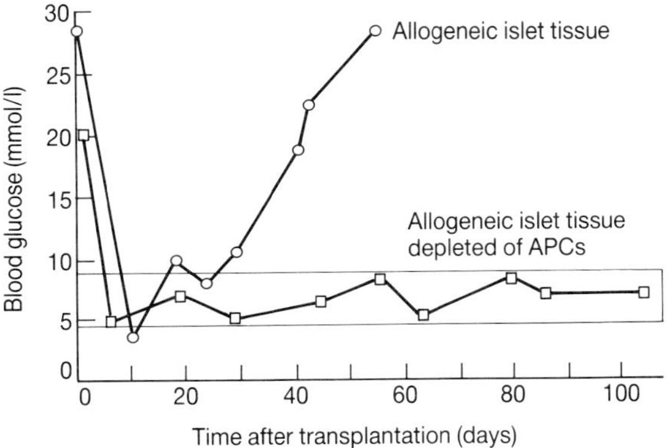

Fig. 8.4 Function of the cultured islet allograft. Untreated pancreatic islets (open circles) transplanted to allogeneic animals briefly return the blood sugar to the normal range but animals return to hyperglycaemia in two to three weeks due to rejection. Allogeneic tissue depleted of APCs (open squares) can be grafted to animals without any immunosuppression and continue to function for an indefinite period.

necessary for long term graft survival in this later study.

A variety of other tissue pretreatment techniques have also led to long term islet allograft acceptance, including graft pretreatment with ultraviolet (UV) irradiation,[32] low temperature culture,[33] anti-Ia or dendritic cell antibodies,[34–36] and low pH media.[37] Hegre and coworkers[38] have shown that perinatal rat islets isolated by *in vitro* cultivation are accepted in non-immunosuppressed, allogeneic recipients. Further, appropriate graft pretreatment techniques have led to prolonged graft acceptance of a variety of tissues including thyroid and parathyroid,[26,39,40] ovarian tissue,[41] and keratinocytes.[42]

This wide range of techniques with a variety of tissues and donor–recipient strain combinations indicate that allograft acceptance can be facilitated by appropriate pretreatment of the graft.

Antigenicity versus immunogenicity of MHC allo-antigens

A key question centres on the mechanism whereby pretreated tissues survive in immunocompetent, allogeneic recipients. Is the immunogenicity of cultured grafts altered due to the modulation of graft antigens, as proposed by Jacobs,[43] or by the elimination/inactivation of passenger leucocytes? This issue has become important due to the more recent finding that hyperbaric oxygen culture of thryoid tissue leads to reduced MHC antigen expression on the graft.[39,44] Studies by Hullet *et al.*,[39] show that thyroid grafts cultured in hyperbaric oxygen survive even in recipient mice primed against donor antigens. These results suggested that the regulation of graft antigen expression may play a role in subsequent graft survival. Although antigen modulation may occur during some forms of organ culture, a variety of evidence indicates that this modulation in not *necessary* for allograft acceptance. That is, loss of immunogenicity does not require a loss of antigenicity on the graft.

Batchelor's group studied the role of antigen expression in long term kidney allograft survival and found that kidney grafts would survive in immunologically enhanced, allogeneic recipient rats. When such long surviving kidney allografts were transplanted from the primary to a secondary recipient of the same haplotype, the kidney did not elicit allo-immunity in the untreated, secondary recipient.[45] Significantly, the failure of long surviving kidney grafts to activate a rejection response could not be attributed to a lack of either class I or class II antigen expression in the graft, leading these investigators to conclude that the effect resulted from a loss of donor derived passenger leucocytes in the graft while in the primary recipient. They later showed that immunisation with donor strain dendritic cells (a source of S^+ cells) in very low numbers would trigger rejection of the established kidney graft.[46] Clearly, the antigens of the grafted kidney could not elicit allo-immunity but could serve as a target of immune destruction once the animal was primed.

Islet allografts cultured in 95% O_2 are also vulnerable to rejection by active immunisation of the recipient.[47] Challenge of the recipient animal with donor-type S^+ cells during the immediate post-transplant period triggers acute rejection of the established islet graft. Active immunisation of the host also triggers the rejection of established cultured thyroid[48] and keratinocyte[42] allografts. These results illustrate the distinction between graft antigenicity and immunogenicity; the cultured graft cannot trigger allograft immunity but can serve as a target for immune destruction.

The issue of class II MHC immunogenicity was elegantly examined in transplantation studies by

Markmann *et al.*[49] by taking advantage of tissue specific class II MHC expression in transgenic mice. Donor animals were I-E$^-$ mice carrying a class II I-E transgene under control of the insulin promoter (ins-I-E), leading to tissue specific, ectopic expression of the I-E molecule on the surface of pancreatic islet β cells.[50] Importantly, such animals did not express the I-E transgene product on lymphoid cells. They then transplanted foetal pancreas from the ins-I-E mice into I-E$^-$, non-transgenic parental strain mice. Despite high expression of the transgene on the β cell surface, such foetal pancreas grafts did not trigger allo-immunity. However, immunising recipient mice with I-E$^+$ spleen cells (a source of I-E bearing S$^+$ cells) triggered prompt rejection of the ins-I-E graft, indicating that the transgenic foetal pancreas could serve as a target for immune destruction. What these experiments clearly demonstrated was that class II MHC antigen is not *inherently* immunogenic and therefore is not sufficient to trigger allograft immunity.

LaRosa[44] recently tested the role of donor antigen expression on the survival of cultured thyroid allografts. In these experiments, thyroid grafts were cultured in 95% O_2 to reduce tissue immunogenicity. These cultured thyroid grafts were then grafted directly or pretreated with IFNγ to induce high levels of class I MHC antigen expression on the graft. Whereas fresh (uncultured) thyroid grafts were uniformly rejected, the acceptance of cultured grafts was not altered with IFNγ treatment of the graft. That is, acceptance of the cultured graft was not due simply to the alteration of antigen expression. Our own recent work with cultured islet allografts produced a similar result (Table 8.1). In this case, islet allografts which were pretreated by 95% O_2 culture to reduce tissue immunogenicity[28] were also incubated in IFNγ, resulting in vast enhancement of donor MHC class I expression. Despite this induction of MHC antigen expression, the IFNγ treated grafts survived in untreated allogeneic recipients (Table 8.1).

Taken together, these varied studies indicate that neither class I nor class II MHC allo-antigen is the primary barrier to allografting.

The role of indirect antigen presentation in allo-immunity

The studies mentioned above suggest that tissue immunogenicity can be modified prior to grafting. This pretreatment would be expected to affect the direct pathway of allogeneic presentation by eliminating donor-derived APC (see Figure 8.1). However, graft antigens could still be released from grafted tissues, processed and presented by host APCs leading to the activation of host CD4 T cells (see Figure 8.1). As mentioned previously, this helper cell would not be graft specific but would be restricted to the host MHC. A key question centres on whether this putative helper cell can provide help for the activation of graft reactive T cells, resulting in graft rejection? *In vitro* experiments from a variety of systems have clearly shown that factors (especially IL-2) produced by T cells of one specificity (helper cells) can drive the activation of T cells with another specificity.[24,51–53] This type of bystander reaction forms the basis of the prevailing view of T–T collaboration.[24,51]

Table 8.1 Survival of cultured, IFNγ treated islet allografts

Group	Islet culture	IFNγ treated	n	Graft survival (days)
BALB/c → CBA				
1.	–	–	10	6, 7, 9, 11, 12, 14, 15, 25, 28, >100
2.	+	–	4	>39, >49, >49, >74
3.	+	+	4	>49, >49, >74, >74
C57B1/6 → BALB/c				
1.	–	–	10	9, 13, 14, 14, 15, 15, 16, 17, 18, 19, 24, >100, >100
2.	+	–	2	>30, >81
3.	+	+	2	>30, >81

Streptozotocin-induced diabetic mice were grafted with 400 allogeneic islets which were either untreated (immunogenic) or were pretreated for seven days in 95% O_2 culture[28] to reduce tissue immunogenicity (islet culture). Where indicated, cultured islets were incubated from days 5–7 of culture in 300 U/ml recombinant IFNγ. Such treatment resulted in profound enhancement of class I MHC expression throughout the graft. No detectable enhancement of class II MHC expression by this procedure was found.

Though bystander T cell help occurs readily *in vitro*, two lines of evidence challenge its role *in vivo* for the activation of graft specific immunity. First, the fact that pretreated tissues survive in a wide variety of systems (see above) would provide empirical evidence that help provided by the indirect pathway of allo-antigen presentation (see Figure 8.1) is relatively inefficient at triggering a rejection response. Furthermore, when a source of bystander help in the form of lymphokine producing T cells was deliberately provided immediately adjacent to an established cultured islet allograft, graft specific immunity was not activated.[54] That is, bystander T cell help could not replace the requirement for a donor-derived second signal *in vivo* for the activation of allograft immunity. Though local delivery lymphokines did not trigger allograft immunity *in vivo*, supernatants from the same activated T cells readily induced CTL activation in response to cultured allogeneic islet cells *in vitro* (Gill *et al.*, unpublished results). We would propose, then, that bystander help generated by the indirect pathway of allo-antigen recognition is much less efficient at triggering graft specific T cell immunity *in vivo* than is the direct pathway of activation. It should be noted that the CD4 cell activated by the indirect pathway *would* be able to interact with class II$^+$ B cells leading to the production of graft specific antibody production.

The nature of APCs for allo-immunity

The following is another fundamental question related to the passenger leucocyte model. If graft rejection is not due solely to MHC antigen but is triggered by specialised APCs within the graft, then what is the phenotype of these cells? That is, what constitutes a passenger leucocyte? We assumed above that an active APC is defined by the ability to elaborate the second signal, or co-stimulator, required for T cell activation and that this function is thought to be restricted to cells of lymphoreticular origin.[22] The exact nature of the co-stimulator(s) for T cell activation remains to be identified.

A major issue in defining the phenotype of the passenger leucocyte (S$^+$ cell) centres on the role of MHC class II$^+$ cells in triggering allograft rejection. Whereas elimination of Ia$^+$ cells/dendritic cells has led to graft prolongation in some studies,[34–36] such treatment has failed to produce graft prolongation in others.[55,56] The rationale for these studies was the assumption that class II MHC expression was a marker for passenger leucocytes. The failure to see allograft prolongation with anti-Ia treatment in some studies may be simply quantitative; studies by McKenzie *et al.*[57] suggested that more than 95% of donor Ia$^+$ must be eliminated from the graft before graft prolongation is observed. Another problem, however, is that class II MHC expression is not necessarily a reliable marker for the S$^+$ cell.

Though it is well documented that class II$^+$ cells are the main stimulators of the primary activation of alloreactive T cells, which particular class II$^+$ cells are required as APC for alloreactivity remains controversial. Inaba *et al.* have reported that class II$^+$ macrophages are not stimulatory for CD8+ cells and in fact may be suppressive;[58] dendritic cells appear to be the more potent cells for stimulating alloresponses.[59] Further, class II$^+$ small resting B cells cannot stimulate resting T cells[60] and in fact may be tolerogenic.[61] These observations indicate that class II per se is not sufficient as a marker for the S$^+$ cell. Further, studies by Sprent and Schaefer[62] have demonstrated the presence of Thy-1$^-$,Ia$^-$ APC in the spleen and bone marrow which are potent stimulators of CD8 T cells. This latter finding indicates that the expression of class II MHC is not necessary for the S$^+$ phenotype. It follows, then, that using class II MHC expression as a strict marker of APC function is not warranted.

Sprent and Schaefer[63] have proposed that the second signal for T cell activation is not an inductive molecule at all but a combination of cell surface properties, such as antigen density and accessory molecule expression, that affects the avidity of interaction between APC and the unprimed T cell. Thus APC function is a quantitative property of the presenting cell and not due to its ability to produce an inductive molecule (co-stimulator). Although cell surface properties may play an important role in defining APC function, other evidence suggests a role for soluble factors as the second signal for T cell activation. Experimental support for an inductive signal involved in T cell activation comes from the study of the immunogenicity of cloned tumour cell lines *in vitro*.[64] These studies demonstrated the existence of stimulating (S$^+$) and non-stimulating (S$^-$) tumour lines expressing the same MHC antigens. Ultraviolet (UV) irradiation of the S$^+$ tumour cells eliminated the ability of these cells to generate a T cell response. UV irradiation blocks metabolic functions of the cell such as RNA and protein synthesis.[65] Significantly, the response to S^- tumour cells or to UV inactivated cells could be reconstituted by the addition of exogenous cytokines to the cultures, indicating that these cells had recognisable antigens on the cell surface (Table 8.2). Since exogenous factors could not be expected to alter cell surface properties of the UV irradiated APC, the conclusion was that the second signal acted on the reactive T cell.

Clearly, the exact phenotype(s) of APCs for allo-immunity and the properties of APCs which confer the S^+ phenotype are crucial issues which need to be resolved. This understanding will facilitate developing strategies to better eliminate or inactivate these cells prior to grafting.

Table 8.2 Two signals are required for alloresponses

Stimulator cell	Cytotoxic activity (log CU/culture) Cytokine (−)	Cytokine (+)
P815 (γ)	5.4	6.0
P815 (UV)	<2.5	6.1
CaD2 (γ)	<3.7	6.0
None	<3.7	<3.7

C57Bl/6 lymph node cells were activated in primary cultures with the indicated stimulator cell. Cytokines were added where indicated in the form of supernatants from Con A-stimulated spleen cell cultures. P815(γ) (H-2^d) expresses the S^+ phenotype; γ-irradiated P815 tumour cells stimulate allogeneic lymphocytes in the absence or presence of exogenous cytokines[64]. UV irradiated P815 does not stimulate allogeneic lymphocytes in the absence of added cytokines; P815(UV) expresses the S^- phenotype. Although viable, the carcinoma CaD2(γ) (H−2^d) is constitutively S^-. S− cells do express recognisable allo-antigens in that the response can be restored by adding exogenous cytokines.

Implications of antigen presentation and allo-immunity

What implications can be drawn concerning allo-reactivity from current thinking on peptide presentation and the two signal model of T cell activation? Some degree of alloreactivity can be ascribed to the co-recognition of allogeneic MHC+peptide[17,18] – which would imply that the allograft response contains a degree of tissue specificity, since tissue specific peptides could be presented by MHC molecules. However, tissue specific allo-immunity is generally *not* the case. Does this mean that processed peptides do not play a role in allo-MHC recognition? The two signal model of T cell activation actually addresses this issue. The passenger leucocyte model (which is derived from the two signal hypothesis) proposes that only specialised APCs within the graft are responsible for the primary (direct) activation of responding T cells. Antigens presented on S^+ cells (active APCs) and *not* antigens presented by most tissue parenchymal (S^-) cells will be stimulatory for alloreactive T cells. Thus endogenous tissue specific peptides presented by tissue parenchymal cells would not be stimulatory to alloreactive T cells.

An elegant study by Ohashi *et al.*[66] supports this view of antigen presentation. These investigators examined the response of the developing immune system to a lymphocytic choriomeningitis virus (LCMV) glycoprotein gene product expressed in pancreatic islet β cells via a transgene. The transgenic animals expressed the viral gene product on the β cell surface but had no evidence of reactivity to the antigen, which would suggest that the animal was 'tolerant' to the viral antigen. However, when the animals were inoculated with live LCMV, a rapid and severe form of diabetes resulted from a response triggered by the live virus. In this study, the transgene product neither immunised nor tolerised the host animal but rather functioned as a 'null' antigen. This model of a 'tissue specific' antigen strongly supports the hypothesis that only antigens on an S^+ APC are capable of stimulating (or, under appropriate conditions, perhaps tolerising) responsive T cells. Thus antigens (processed peptides) presented in high enough density by the S^+ APC will be the most important in T cell activation, including allogeneic responses. Tissue specific peptides would only be important when processed and presented in unusually high degree by S^+ APCs. It is intriguing to speculate that allograft rejection may be mediated only by that proportion of T cells with specificity for allo-antigens (MHC + peptide) that are expressed both by S^+ APCs and by tissue parenchymal cells.

Acknowledgement

This work was supported by grant DK 33470 from the United States Public Health Service and by a grant from the Juvenile Diabetes Foundation International.

References

1. Batchelor JR, Welsh K, Burgos H. Transplantation antigens per se are poor immunogens within a species. *Nature* 1978; **273,** 54–56.
2. Flexner S, Jobling JW. On the promoting influence of heated tumor emulsions on tumor growth. *Proc Soc Exp Biol Med* 1907; **4,** 156.
3. Zinkernagel RM, Doherty PC. MHC-restricted cytotoxic T cells: studies on the biological role of polymorphic major transplantation antigens determining T-cell restriction – specificity, function and responsiveness. *Adv Immunol* 1979; **27,** 51–177.
4. Bjorkman PJ, Saper MA, Samraoui B, Bennett WS, Strominger JL, Wiley DC. The foreign antigen binding site and T cell recognition regions of class I histocompatibility antigens. *Nature* 1987; **329,** 512–518.
5. Brown JH, Jardetzky T, Saper MA, Samraoui B, Bjorkman PJ, Wiley DC. A hypothetical model of the foreign antigen binding site of class II histocompatibility molecules. *Nature* 1988; **332,** 345–850.
6. Townsend A, Ohlen C, Bastin J, Ljunggren H, Foster L, Karre K. Association of class I major histocompatibility heavy and light chains induced by viral peptides. *Nature* 1989; **340,** 443–448.
7. Van Bleek GM, Nathenson SG. Isolation of an endogenously processed immunodominant viral peptide from the class I H-2K^b molecule. *Nature* 1990; **348,** 213–216.
8. Rotzschke O, Falk K, Deres K *et al.* Isolation and analysis of naturally processed viral peptides as recognized by cytotoxic T cells. *Nature* 1990; **348,** 252–254.
9. Falk K, Rotzschke O, Rammensee H. Cellular peptide composition governed by major histocompatibility complex class I molecules. *Nature* 1990; **348,** 248–251.
10. Germain RN, Hendrix LR. MHC class II structure, occupancy and surface expression determined by post-endoplasmic reticulum antigen binding. *Nature* 1991; **353,** 134–139.
11. Rudensky AY, Preston-Hurlburt P, Hong S, Barlow A, Janeway Jr CA. Sequence analysis of peptides bound to MHC class II molecules. *Nature* 1991; **353,** 622–627.
12. Swain SL. T cell subsets and the recognition of MHC class. *Immunol Rev* 1983; **74,** 129–142.
13. Matzinger P, Bevan MJ. Why do so many lymphocytes respond to major histocompatibility antigens? *Cell Immunol* 1977; **29,** 1–5.
14. Lorenz RG, Allen PM. Thymic cortical epithelial cells can present self-antigens *in vivo*. *Nature* 1989; **337,** 560–562.
15. Kisielow P, Teh HS, Bluthmann H, von Boehmer H. Positive selection of antigen-specific T cells in thymus by resting MHC molecules. *Nature* 1988; **335,** 730–733.
16. MacDonald HR, Lees RK, Schneider R, Zinkernagel RM, Hengartner H. Positive selection of CD4$^+$ thymocytes controlled by MHC class II gene products. *Nature* 1988; **336,** 471–479.
17. Lombardi G, Sidhu S, Lamb JR, Batchelor JR, Lechler RI. Endogenous peptides contribute to the ligand recognized by anti-DR1 human alloreactive T cells. *Transplant Proc* 1989; **21,** 142–144.
18. Lechler RI, Lombardi G, Batchelor JR, Reinsmoen N, Bach FH. The molecular basis of alloreactivity. *Immunol Today* 1990; **11,** 83–88.
19. Schellekens PTA, Eijsvoogel VP. Lymphocyte transformation *in vitro*. III Mechanism of stimulation in the mixed lymphocyte culture. *Clin Exp Immunol* 1970; **7,** 229–239.
20. Lafferty KJ, Misko IS, Cooley MA. Allogeneic stimulation modulates the *in vitro* response of T cells to transplantation antigen. *Nature* 1974; **249,** 275–276.
21. Hardy MA, Lau H, Weber C, Reemtsma K. Pancreatic islet transplantation. Induction of graft acceptance by ultraviolet irradiation of donor tissue. *Ann Surg* 1984; **200,** 441–450.
22. Lafferty KJ, Prowse SJ, Simeonovic CJ. Immunology of tissue transplantation: a return to the passenger leukocyte concept. *Ann Rev Immunol* 1983; **1,** 143–173.
23. Bretscher P, Cohn M. A theory of self-nonself discrimination. *Science* 1970; **169,** 1042–1049.
24. Bach FH, Bach ML, Sondel PM. Differential function of major histocompatibility complex antigens in T-lymphocyte activation. *Nature* 1976; **259,** 273–281.
25. Snell GD. The homograft reaction. *Ann Rev Microbiol* 1957; **11,** 439–458.
26. Lafferty KJ, Bootes A, Dart G, Talmage DW. Effect of organ culture on the survival of thyroid allografts in mice. *Transplantation* 1976; **22,** 138–149.
27. Lacy PE, Davie JM, Finke ED. Effect of culture on islet rejection. *Diabetes* 1980; **29,** 93–97.
28. Bowen KM, Andrus L, Lafferty KJ. Successful allotransplantation of mouse pancreatic islets to nonimmunosuppressed recipients. *Diabetes* 1980; **29,** 98–104.
29. Haug CE, Gill RG, Babcock SK, Lafferty KJ, Bellgrau D, Weil R. Cyclosporine-induced tolerance requires antigens capable of initiating an immune response. *J Immunol* 1987; **139,** 2947–2949.
30. Prowse SJ, Bellgrau D, Lafferty KJ. Islet allografts are destroyed by disease occurrence in the spontaneously diabetic BB rat. *Diabetes* 1986; **35,** 110–114.
31. Simeonovic CJ, Prowse SJ, Lafferty KJ. Reversal of diabetes in outbred mice by islet

allotransplantation. *Diabetes* 1986; **35,** 1345–1349.
32. Lau H, Reemtsma K, Hardy MA. Prolongation of rat islet allograft survival by direct ultraviolet irradiation of the graft. *Science* 1984; **223,** 607–608.
33. Lacy PE, Davie JM, Finke EH. Prolongation of islet allograft survival following *in vitro* culture (24°C) and a single injection of ALS. *Science* 1979; **204,** 312–313.
34. Faustman D, Hauptfeld V, Lacy P, Davie J. Prolongation of murine islet allograft survival by pretreatment of islets with antibody directed to Ia determinants. *Proc Nat Acad Sci USA* 1981; **78,** 5156–5159.
35. Morrow CE, Sutherland DER, Steffes MW, Najarian JS, Bach FH. Lack of donor-specific tolerance in mice with established anti-Ia-treated islet allografts. *Transplantation* 1983; **36,** 691–694.
36. Faustman DL, Steinman RM, Gebel HM, Hauptfeld V, Davie JM, Lacy PE. Prevention of rejection of murine islet allografts by pretreatment with anti-dendritic cell antibody. *Proc Nat Acad Sci USA* 1984; **81,** 3864–3868.
37. La Rosa FG. Abrogation of mouse pancreatic islet allograft rejection by a four-day culture. *Transplantation* 1988; **46,** 330–333.
38. Hegre OD, Hickey GE, Marshall S, Serie JR. Modification of allograft immunogenicity in perinatal islets isolated and purified *in vitro*. *Transplantation* 1984; **37,** 227–233.
39. Hullett DA, Landry AS, Leonard DK, Sollinger HW. Enhancement of thyroid allograft survival following organ culture. *Transplantation* 1989; **47,** 24–27.
40. La Rosa FG, Talmage DW. The abrogation of thyroid allograft rejection by culture in acid medium. *Transplantation* 1987; **44,** 592.
41. Jacobs BB. Ovarian allograft survival. *Transplantation* 1974; **18,** 454.
42. Ramrakha PS, Sharp RJ, Yeoman H, Stanley MA. The influence of MHC-compatible and MHC-incompatible antigen-presenting cells on the survival of MHC-compatible cultured murine keratinocyte allografts. *Transplantation* 1989; **48,** 676–680.
43. Jacobs BB, Huseby RA. Growth of tumors in allogeneic hosts following organ culture explantation. *Transplantation* 1967; **5,** 410–419.
44. La Rosa FG, Talmage DW. Major histocompatibility complex antigen expression on parenchymal cells of thyroid allografts is not by itself sufficient to induce rejection. *Transplantation* 1990; **49,** 605–609.
45. Batchelor J, Welsh K, Maynard A, Burgos H. Failure of long surviving, passively enhanced kidney allografts to provoke T-dependent alloimmunity. I Retransplantation of (AS × AUG) F_1 kidneys into secondary AS recipients. *J Exp Med* 1979; **150,** 455–464.
46. Lechler RI, Batchelor JR. Restoration of immunogenicity to passenger cell-depleted kidney allografts by the addition of donor strain dendritic cells. *J Exp Med* 1982; **155,** 31–41.
47. Bowen KM, Prowse SJ, Lafferty KJ. Reversal of diabetes by islet transplantation: vulnerability of the established allograft. *Science* 1981; **213,** 1261–1262.
48. Vesole DH, Dart GA, Talmage DW. Rejection of stable cultured allografts by active or passive (adoptive) immunization. *Proc Nat Acad Sci USA* 1982; **79,** 1626–1628.
49. Markmann J, Lo D, Naji A, Palmiter RD, Brinster RL, Heber-Katz E. Antigen presenting function of class II MHC expressing pancreatic beta cells. *Nature* 1988; **336,** 476–479.
50. Lo D, Burkly LC, Widera G *et al.* Diabetes and tolerance in transgenic mice expressing class II MHC molecules in pancreatic beta cells. *Cell* 1988; **53,** 159–168.
51. Wagner H, Rollinghoff M. T-T-cell interactions during *in vitro* cytotoxic allograft responses. I Soluble products from activated Lyl^+ T cells trigger autonomously antigen-primed $Ly23^+$ T cells to cell proliferation and cytolytic activity. *J Exp Med* 1978; **148,** 1523.
52. Golding H, Singer A. Role of accessory cell processing and presentation of shed H-2 alloantigens in allospecific cytotoxic T lymphocyte responses. *J Immunol* 1984; **133,** 597–604.
53. Stock PG, Ascher NL, Chen S, Field J, Bach FH, Sutherland DER. Evidence for direct and indirect pathways in the generation of the alloimmune response against pancreatic islets. *Transplantation* 1991; **42,** 704–709.
54. Babcock SK, Gill RG, Bellgrau D, Lafferty KJ. Studies of the two signal model for T cell activation *in vivo*. *Transplant Proc* 1987; **19,** 303–306.
55. Gores PF, Sutherland DER, Platt JL, Bach FH. Depletion of donor Ia^+ cells before transplantation does not prolong islet allograft survival. *J Immunol* 1986; **137,** 1482.
56. Lloyd DM, Weiser MR, Kang RH, Buckingham M, Stuart FP, Thistlethwaite Jr JR. Does depletion of donor dendritic cells in an organ allograft lead to prolongation of graft survival on transplantation? *Transplant Proc* 1989; **21,** 482.
57. McKenzie JL, Beard MEJ, Hart DNJ. The effect of donor pretreatment on interstitial dendritic cell content and rat cardiac allograft survival. *Transplantation* 1984; **38,** 371–376.
58. Inaba K, Young JW, Steinman RM. Direct activation of $CD8^+$ cytotoxic T lymphocytes by dendritic cells. *J Exp Med* 1987; **166,** 182–194.
59. Steinman RM, Gutchinov B, Witmer MD, Nussenzweig MC. Dendritic cells are the principal

stimulators of the primary mixed leukocyte reaction in mice. *J Exp Med* 1983; **157,** 613–627.

60. Tetlay JP, Pure E, Steinman RM. Control of the immune response at the level of antigen-presenting cells: a comparison of the function of dendritic cells and B lymphocytes. *Adv Immuno* 1989; **47,** 45–116.
61. Eynon EE, Parker DC. Do small B cells induce tolerance? *Transplant Proc* 1991; **23,** 729–730.
62. Sprent J, Schaefer M. Antigen-presenting cells for Lyt-2^+ cells. I Stimulation of unprimed Lyt-2^+ cells by H-2 different Thy-1^-Ia$^-$ cells prepared from the spleen and bone marrow. *J Immunol* 1988; **140,** 3745–3750.
63. Sprent J, Schaefer M. Antigen-presenting cells for unprimed T cells. *Immunol Today* 1989; **10,** 17–23.
64. Talmage DW, Woolnough JA, Hemmingsen H, Lopez L, Lafferty KJ. Activation of cytotoxic T cells by nonstimulating tumor cells and spleen cell factor(s). *Proc Nat Acad Sci USA* 1977; **74,** 1610–1614.
65. Lafferty KJ, Andrus L, Prowse SJ. Role of lymphokine and antigen in the control of specific T cell responses. *Immunol Rev* 1980, **51,** 279–314.
66. Ohashi PS, Oehen S, Buerki K *et al.* Ablation of 'tolerance' and induction of diabetes by virus infection in viral antigen transgenic mice. *Cell* 1991; **65,** 305–317.

9

Transplantation antigens

S Koskimies and I Lautenschlager

Introduction

Graft rejection occurs when the host immune response against foreign tissue is induced by the antigens present in the graft but absent in the recipient. The antigens coded by the major histocompatibility complex (MHC) are the most important ones initiating an inflammatory cascade including the effector cells able to damage the graft.[1] The MHC antigens expressed on the cell surface may, in addition to the triggering of the anti-allograft response, also function as targets for the host immune response. Of the MHC antigens, the class II antigens are the most immunogenic.[2] In man, the class I (HLA-ABC) and class II antigens (HLA-DR/DQ/DP) are encoded by genes of the MHC on chromosome 6.

Other antigens also play a role in the anti-allograft response. The antigens coded by the minor histocompatibility loci are involved in rejection, as demonstrated in rodents.[3] Without immunosuppression, allografts from HLA identical siblings are rejected and even with immunosuppression, irreversible rejection may sometimes occur.[4] In addition, non-MHC antigens, detected on the cell surface of endothelial cells and monocytes,[5,6] or tissue specific antigens characteristic of particular cells, might be important in the mechanisms of rejection.[7] The significance of non-MHC antigens is, however, poorly understood.

Compatibility within the ABO blood group system has traditionally been a requirement for successful organ transplants. Hyperacute rejection has been recorded in hepatic allografts with ABO incombatibility[8] (see also Chapter 19). Transplantation across ABO blood groups or with a positive crossmatch, however, does not necessarily result in hyperacute rejection of liver grafts.[9,10]

In this overview, the genetic organisation and the molecular structure of the most important transplantation antigens are presented. In addition, the expression of MHC antigens in normal and pathological conditions of liver and the regulation of MHC expression are described. The role of transplantation antigens in the outcome of hepatic allografts is also discussed.

Transplantation antigens

During the 1950s it was observed that blood from multiparous women or transfused individuals contained antibodies which agglutinated leucocytes of other individuals. Identification of these human leucocytes antigens[11,12] was the first step towards the identification and characterisation of the major histocompatibility complex, MHC. Evidence for a functional role for MHC molecules in normal immune responses came from work where the genetic control of an immune response to simple synthetic peptides was studied. It was found that MHC molecules were involved in the production of antibodies only through collaboration between T and B lymphocytes and that with identity of MHC, an efficient immune response was achieved.

Genetic organisation of the major histocompatibility complex

The human MHC is located on the short arm of chromosome 6. The DNA of the MHC comprises 0.1% of the whole human genome, containing about 3.5×10^6 base pairs which is enough DNA to code at least 50 genes. A large number of genes have been mapped to this region of which several are non-functional pseudogenes or genes for which no expressed protein has thus far been found. The order of genes is shown in Figure 9.1. The MHC is divided into three regions; class I, class II and class III genes. The class I genes code for the classical major transplantation antigens: HLA-A, HLA-B and HLA-C. In addition, at least 14 other class I genes are found, for most of which the function is still unknown. Recently discovered class I genes, HLA-E, -F and -G, have been found to be functional. The gene products of HLA-E and -F genes have been detected by monoclonal antibodies both within the cells and in the supernatant of cultured cells but not on the cell surface, in contrast to the HLA-G protein which has been detected on the surface of trophoblasts in the human placenta.[13] Whether these genes play any role in allo-antigen recognition is not known.

Fifteen class II genes (6A and 9B genes) are mapped at the telomeric end of the MHC and comprise three major subregions: DR, DQ and DP. As shown in Figure 9.1, each of these subregions contains various numbers of A and B genes, of which some are pseudogenes. At least eight class II genes are functional; the function of DO and DN genes is unknown. A new gene family has been found recently between the DP and DQ regions.[14,15,16] These genes, called ABC transporter genes, encode proteins involved in membrane transport of different molecules, including peptides in the class I antigen presentation pathway.

The genes within the class III region have different functions. Genes coding complement C2, C4 and Bf proteins, genes for 21-hydroxylase, tumour necrosis factor, lymphotoxin, and heat shock proteins are all located in this region. A new gene cluster, the BAT genes, has been found in the class III region for which the gene products are not known.[17]

MHC genes are located very close together and are inherited as a block (a haplotype) consisting of a certain set of MHC genes. The inheritance follows Mendelian rules: 50% of children within a family are haplo-identical to each other which means that they share half the MHC genes which they inherited from one of the parents; 25% of children are HLA identical. Nearly all MHC genes express polymorphism, class I, class II

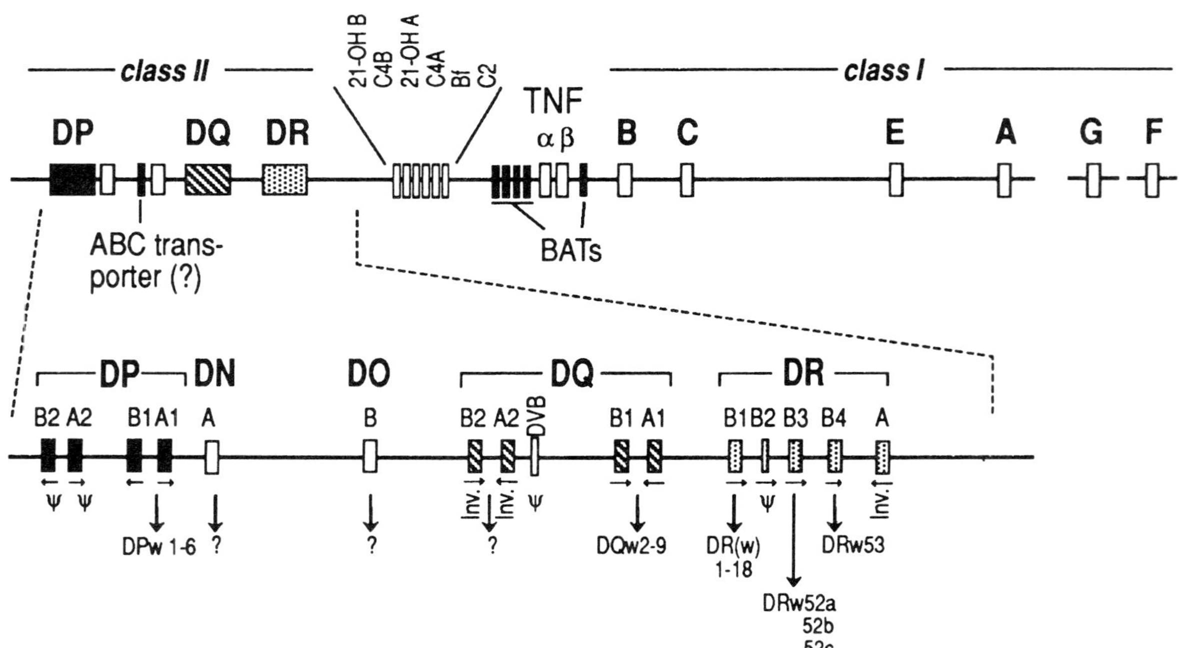

Fig. 9.1 Genetic organisation of MHC region in human chromosome 6 short arm. The centromere is towards the left. The pseudogenes are indicated by ψ. The alleles coded by class II A and B gene pairs are indicated below.

DRB, DQB, and DPB genes being the most polymorphic. The frequencies of different alleles of a particular gene locus vary between different races and ethnic groups. For example, HLA-B8 gene frequency doubles from Mediterranean countries to Northern Scandinavian and the frequency of HLA-B5 decreases to half. Some HLA alleles are found together in the same chromosome more often than would be expected from the gene frequency of the population. Such alleles are in linkage disequilibrium and forms called extended haplotypes.

From genes to molecules

MHC genes are the most polymorphic genes described and are co-dominantly expressed. Of the class I genes, at least 68 different HLA-A, B and C alleles have been sequenced and the number of serologically assigned alleles is over 80 (Table 9.1). HLA class I and class II molecules exist as heterodimers and are expressed on the surface of cells as integral membrane proteins. The class I molecule (HLA-A,B,C) consists of an MHC coded highly polymorphic heavy chain with a molecular weight of approximately 45 KDa which binds non-covalently with β_2-microglobulin (β_2m). The β_2m is a non-polymorphic molecule encoded on chromosome 15 which is essential for the expression of class I molecules. The heavy chain consists of three extracellular domains, each encoded by a separate exon, and the polymorphism resides mainly in the two outer domains $\alpha 1$ and $\alpha 2$ (Figure 9.2).

X-ray crystallography[18] has allowed the identification of a peptide binding site for MHC class I, a groove formed by two α-helices on top of a floor of β-pleated sheets. Several polymorphic residues are located in the part of the molecule that constitutes this groove.[19] Visualisation of the three dimensional structure of the HLA molecule has provided the framework for understanding the role of the MHC in the presentation of antigen to T cells and how this system can restrict immune reactivity to foreign antigens. One gene codes for one HLA class I molecule on the membrane. The

Table 9.1 Nomenclature for factors of the HLA system

HLA-A	HLA-B		HLA-C	HLA-DR	HLA-DQ	HLA-DP
A1	B5	Bw50(21)	Cw1	DR1	DQw1	DPw1
A2	B7	B51(5)	Cw2	DR2	DWw2	DPw2
A3	B8	Bw52(5)	Cw3	DR3	DWw3	DPw3
A9	B12	Bw53	Cw4	DR4	DDQw4	DPw4
A10	B13	Bw54(w22)	Cw5	DR5	DQw5(w1)	DPw5
A11	B14	Bw55(w22)	Cw6	DRw6	DQw6(w1)	DPw6
Aw19	B15	Bw56(w22)	Cw7	DR7	DQw7(w3)	
A23(9)	B16	Bw57(17)	Cw8	DRw8	DQw8(w3)	
A24(9)	B17	Bw58(17)	Cw9(w3)	DR9	DQw9(w3)	
A25(10)	B18	Bw59	Cw10(w3)	DRw10		
A26(10)	B21	Bw60(w40)	Cw11	DRw11(5)		
A28	Bw22	Bw61(w40)		DRw12		
A29(w19)	B27	Bw62(15)		DRw13(w6)		
A30(w19)	B35	Bw63(15)		DRw14(w6)		
A31(w19)	B37	Bw64(14)		DRw15(2)		
A32(w19)	B38(16)	Bw65(14)		DRw16(2)		
Aw33(w19)	B39(16)	Bw67		DRw17(3)		
Aw34(10)	B40	Bw70		DRw18(3)		
Aw36	Bw41	Bw71(w70)		DRw52		
Aw43	Bw42	Bw72(w70)		DRw53		
Aw66(10)	B44(12)	Bw73				
Aw68(28)	B45(12)	Bw75(15)				
Aw69(28)	Bw46	Bw76(15)				
Aw74(w19)	Bw47	Bw77(15)				
	Bw48	Bw4				
	B49(21)	Bw6				

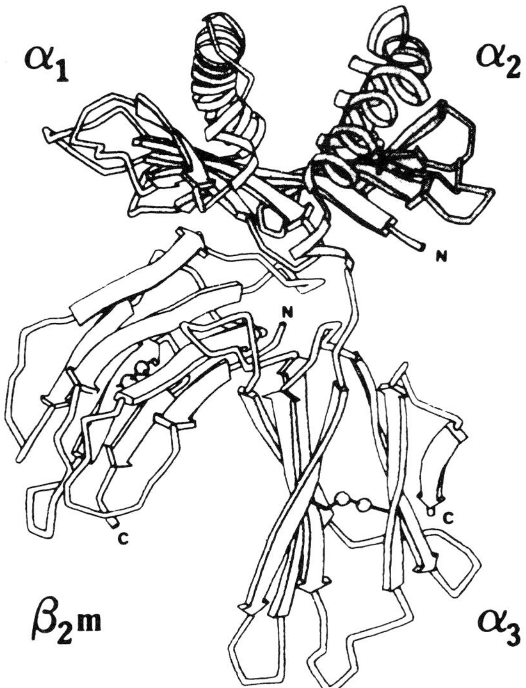

Fig. 9.2 The three-dimensional structure of a class I molecule. The domains of the class I heavy chain and β-2-microglobulin are indicated. The two α-helices and the β-pleated floor form the antigen peptide binding cleft (reproduced by kind permission of Macmillan Magazines).

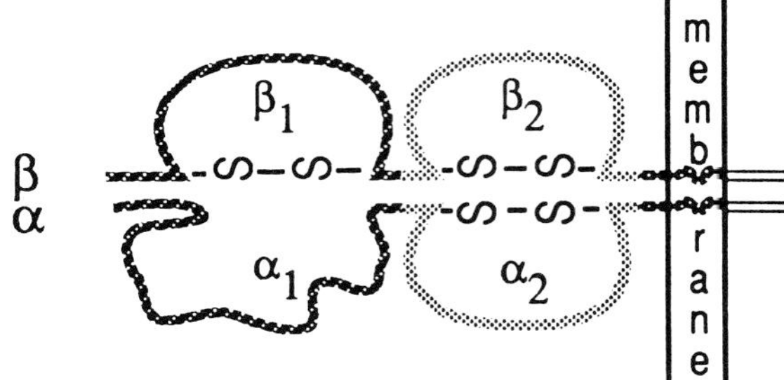

Fig. 9.3 Schematic diagram of class II molecule. Class II heterodimer is formed of α and β chains with two-domain structure.

allelic differences are very small, usually between one and ten amino acids difference.

Class II molecules HLA-DR, HLA-DQ and HLA-DP are composed of two α and β polypeptide chains, encoded by A and B genes respectively. Both polypeptides are integrated into the cell membrane where they form a dimer (Figure 9.3). The α chain has a molecular weight of 33 KDa and the β chain, 29 KDa. Biosynthetic intermediates of class II antigens, but not mature cell surface molecules, are associated with a non-polymorphic glycoprotein whose gene is encoded outside the MHC, referred to as the invariant chain.[20] Both α and β polypeptides contain two domains – α1, α2 and β1, β2 domains respectively (see Figure 9.3). The degree of polymorphism varies in DR, DQ or DP region genes. The DRB1 gene, coding for the DRβ polypeptide, is the most polymorphic; 34 alleles have been described. The corresponding number for DQB1 is 13, DQA1 8, DPB1 9 and DPA1 4. The DRA1 gene has very limited polymorphism. Most of the polymorphic sites are located in α1 and β1 domains which form the peptide binding groove and are thus implicated in peptide binding rather than T cell receptor interactions. Comparison of several class II sequences shows that the variability is not evenly distributed over the molecule but concentrated in the first domain and in particular in some hypervariable regions. In DRB gene 3 such regions have been identified whereas in DQB only two have been found. Class II MHC antigen domains share homology with class I MHC antigens and the constant region of immunoglobulins.

Allo-antigens

HLA allo-antigens express multiple serological specificities or allodeterminants. Several different antigens may share one or more cross-reactive specificities. Such cross-reactive groups are HLA-B7, B22, B27 specificities, and HLA-B5, e.g. B35 and B53 specificities. Using techniques that are more sophisticated than serology, such as iso-electric focusing (IEF) or cytotoxic T lymphocytes, even such alleles as HLA-B27 or HLA-A2 have shown structural variants. IEF analysis has revealed a greater degree of polymorphism (169%) than can be found by serological techniques. HLA-B27 has been extensively studied by IEF, yielding six variants for which the cDNA has been cloned and sequenced.[21,22] The variants differ by one to four amino acids in the α chain, which results from nucleotide substitutions in one to seven codons on positions 59–152. T cells can also recognise these variants which means that minimal structural differences may be functionally significant, and perhaps also relevant in transplantation. The first class II antigens, DR, were identified serologically in 1977. Subsequently the DQ series was defined. Serology is a poor technique for defining DP alleles which have been identified using cellular typing methods such as primed lymphocyte typing (PLT).[23] Serological typing for DQ is also unreliable because the $\alpha\beta$ polypeptide heterodimer expresses polymorphism in both polypeptide chains. The DQ molecule is encoded by two genes, DQA and DQB. Each individual has two sets of DQ genes, one in each chromosome 6, and thus these four DQ genes can generate heterodimers both in *cis* and *trans* complementation. This doubles the diversity of different antigen binding structures on the cell surface in heterozygous individuals,[24,25] but makes the typing complicated. The unreliability of current techniques has been emphasised by the application of recombinant DNA technology to tissue typing. The increasing availability of PCR suggests this will become the method of choice for tissue typing for Class II alleles.

Minor transplantation antigens, not controlled by MHC genes

The transplantation of organs or tissues between HLA identical siblings, fully matched for the entire MHC and usually matched for about half of the non-MHC (mH) transplantation antigens, leads to rejection unless immunosuppressive therapy is given. These reactions are serious and can be life threatening, particularly in bone marrow transplantation. They are believed to be due to incompatibilities at multiple non-MHC genes, which express polymorphism.

HLA class II disparate individuals induce strong primary immune response towards HLA antigens *in vitro* in mixed lymphocyte culture. In contrast, primary immune response to mH can only be induced *in vivo*, the *in vitro* response being generated only with primed cells. This difference is explained by the low number of specific T cells reactive to minor histocompatibility antigens.

Immune responses are obtained to small peptides presented by MHC molecules. We cannot yet identify the molecules that behave as mH antigens. The response towards mH *in vitro* is, however, highly MHC restricted; mH are recognised only in the context of self MHC molecules. The response is also under genetic control of immune response genes which have been best studied for Y chromosome controlled male specific mH antigen.[26]

The minor transplantation antigens have been most fully investigated in the mouse where over ten different gene loci coding allelic forms of mH have been described. The polymorphism, however, appears to be limited to a few alleles per locus. The mH antigens exhibit a wide range of immunogenic strengths; some antigen differences can cause rapid skin graft rejection but other differences are tolerated for long periods. Since MHC restricted recognition of mH antigens by T cells is required, mH antigen differences most often cause rejection in transplantation combinations where there is a degree of shared MHC, either class I or class II, between recipient and donor.

Immunogenicity for mH varies between different tissues and organs. In the mouse, skin, thyroid, heart, liver and lymphoid tissues all differ in their immunogenicity, skin grafts being rejected most rapidly. Females in general respond more strongly than males irrespective of parity, except for responses to H-Y to which multiparous female mice are tolerant.

When the recipient and the donor have different MHC haplotypes, the donor mH antigens are not recognised in the context of donor MHC unless they are processed by recipient antigen presenting cells. The immunity towards donor would not be directed at donor MHC/mH complex.[27] If the donor shares MHC molecules with the recipient, the donor cells can serve as antigen presenting cells for mH and anti-mH responses are initiated. This is likely to be the case in HLA identical transplants which are complicated by rejection.

Human minor histocompatibility antigens have not been well characterised. The clinical data of graft rejection and graft versus host disease in transplantation between HLA-identical siblings or HLA match unrelated persons provide some evidence for the presence of mH antigens in man. In some cases, T cell immunity to non-HLA antigens has been described.[28,29] HLA restricted cytotoxic T cells specific for male (H-Y) cells have been derived from a female patient who received a male bone marrow graft,[30] multitransfused female aplastic anaemia patients,[31,32] from multiparous women[33] and from a kidney grafted patient.[4] MHC restriction of T cell responses towards mH antigens involves HLA-A2 in a high frequency although examples of other restriction alleles such as HLA-B7, B27, B40, B44, and B62 have been described. The nature of the antigen, however, is still to be determined.

ABO blood groups

The antigenic determinants of the ABO system are the terminal sugars of carbohydrate chains. Most of the antigen on red cell surface is in the form of a glycoprotein but some is found as oligosaccharide attached to lipids. The terminal sugar of blood group A is N-acetylgalactosamine and in blood group B is galactose. When both sugars are lacking the rest of the carbohydrate chain is called H-antigen; thus blood group O red cells have this H-antigen on the cell surface. Red cells of A and B blood group also have H-antigen on the cell surface but the amount is smaller.

The inheritance of blood groups is determined by three allelic genes: A, B and O. A and B genes are codominant whereas the O gene is recessive. A and B genes code for transferase enzymes, which attach the terminal sugars to the backbone structure. The A gene codes for N-acetylgalactosamine transferase and the B gene codes for galactose transferase. The O gene does not code for any enzyme. A person of A blood group can be of a genotype AA or AO; of B blood group respectively BB or BO. The frequency of blood groups varies in different populations. The oriental races express much more blood group B than caucasoid populations. A, B and H antigens are also expressed in cells and tissues other than red cells. These antigens are found on leucocytes and in small amounts on thrombocytes, endothelial cells of most organs and blood vessels and on some epithelial cells. They are not found in the central nervous system or in connective tissue.

Blood group A can be subdivided into A1 and A2 groups. On A1 cells, the amount of A-antigen is higher than on A2 cells. The backbone structure of the carbohydrate chain is the same on both cells but on A2 cells a larger portion is in the H-antigen form. The A1 red cell has about 10^6 A determinants whereas A2 cells have only a quarter of a million instead. There are seven other rare A subtypes for which the frequency in all populations is very low.

Natural antibodies, iso-agglutinis, are found against blood group antigens; a person with blood group A has iso-agglutinis against blood group B and vice versa. Persons with blood group O have antibodies against both A and B but AB persons have no iso-agglutinis. The appearance of these antibodies is due to cross-reacting antigenic determinants present on bacteria and plants which enter the bloodstream via the gut and act as immunogens. Antibodies against a person's own blood group are not normally formed.

Anti-A and anti-B antibodies belong to the IgM immunoglobulin class; these antibodies do not cross the placenta and thus the newborn baby does not have blood group antibodies. These develop within the first six months. The amount of antibody increases until the age of 20 after which they decrease. Antibodies of IgG class can also be induced against A and B blood groups. A or B red cells given to B or A persons respectively are very potent immunogens and can cause the formation of IgG blood group antibodies. Due to the immunogenicity of different blood groups and the presence of iso-agglutinis, certain rules have to be followed in blood transfusions. In organ transplantation, particularly of heart or kidney, a rapid loss of the graft may occur when the donor ABO is incompatible with the recipient. This hyperacute rejection is mediated by the patient's blood group antibodies which combine with blood group antigens on the graft vascular endothelium, activating complement, causing vasospasm and platelet aggregation leading to rapid necrosis of the graft. Blood group antigens have also been found on hepatic cellular components.[34] In liver transplantation, however, successful transplantation with ABO incompatibility has been reported.[10]

Transplantation antigens in human liver

Expression of MHC antigens in normal liver

The expression of the two classes of MHC antigens on different cell types have a heterogeneous distribution in normal human tissues.[35,36] In general, the class I antigens are expressed on most nucleated cells, while class II antigens show a more restricted distribution, being limited mainly to the lymphoid system and accessory cells. In addition, some cells of parenchymal origin, e.g endothelial cells, may also express class II. However, the distribution of MHC class II in human tissues is quantitative rather than qualitative, and aberrant expression of class II molecules is a well-known phenomenon.

The early studies on human liver tissue demonstrated that in a normal liver the major parenchymal component, the hepatocytes, express no or only very low amounts of class I antigens.[37,38] Only slight expression, if any, is found on vascular endothelium and bile duct epithelial cells. More detailed subsequent analysis confirmed the early findings of low expression of class I in the liver parenchyma.[35,39] Thus, the remaining passenger cells, such as lymphocytes and mononuclear phagocytes including Kupffer cells, are the most antigenic components of the organ,[39] along with bone marrow derived dendritic cells in the liver parenchyma, which express both class I and class II strongly.[40]

The expression of class II molecules on the cell surface of human liver cells has been under intensive study for over a decade. In the early studies on disaggregated human liver cells, all parenchymal components were practically negative for class II, when analysed with polyclonal antibodies.[37] These results were subsequently confirmed on frozen sections.[39] However, some slight binding of monoclonal anti-HLA-DR antibodies was detected on endothelial cells and bile duct cells. In frozen sections, this minor expression of DR antigens was localised to the endothelium of sinusoids and portal tract bile ducts.[39] Using frozen material, others demonstrated some class II on vascular endothelium, but not on bile ducts.[36,41,42]

Although the parenchymal components of normal human liver do not express class II antigens in significant amounts, the passenger cells are strongly class II positive.[39] The tissue macrophages of liver, the Kupffer cells, are also considered to be passenger cells, and are replaced in a few weeks by cells of recipient origin.[43] Kupffer cells and the bone marrow derived dendritic cells are strongly class II positive,[39,40,43] and might act as antigen presenting cells (APC) in liver and initiate the anti-allograft response in the hepatic transplant.

Liver has been thought to be a privileged organ, which is not rejected as promptly as, for example, the kidney. One reason suggested to explain this is the antigenic anatomy of the organ. As the major component of liver parenchyma is not very antigenic, it is likely that only the passenger cells act as antigen presenting cells in the liver graft. The expression of MHC is inducible under various pathological situations, which might allow MHC antigens to act as targets of the anti-allograft response, even if they do not initiate it.

Expression of MHC antigens during rejection

The expression of MHC class I antigens in liver grafts before, during and after rejection has been intensively studied. In most studies, class I molecules have been demonstrated to be strongly expressed on hepatocytes and bile ducts during acute rejection.[43,44,45,46] The class I expression in the sinusoids represents not only expression on vascular endothelium but also on Kupffer cells which are localised in the sinusoids. It has also been demonstrated that HLA-A, HLA-B and HLA-C molecules are induced equally during rejection.[47] In addition to the class I molecules, an increase of the expression of beta-2-molecules, the light chain of class I, in the liver parenchyma has also been reported.[48,49]

The aberrant expression of class II molecules in liver has stimulated more interest than the class I antigens. The first study concerning expression of DR antigens on bile duct cells of rejecting liver was published in 1983.[50] In this first report, strong expression of DR antigens was demonstrated by immunofluorescence on liver graft frozen sections. This finding was confirmed by another immuno-labelling study,[51] which showed class II induction not only in bile ducts but also in portal and central vein and in hepatic artery endothelium. Several other groups have reported similar results on frozen section analysis and on fine needle aspiration biopsies of liver allografts.[43,45,51,52]

Most groups agree that there is inducible expression of class II in biliary and vascular structures of the liver. However, the expression of class II on hepatocytes seems still to be controversial. The first reports of class II induction on hepatocytes during rejection was demonstrated with fine needle aspiration biopsy (FNAB) monitoring of liver allografts.[52,54,55] The same phenomenon was then shown by the analysis of frozen sections of core biopsy material.[45,53] In our FNAB material, class II induction was recorded only during severe rejection with intense immune activation, while the bile duct cells were always strongly class II positive during acute rejection.[52]

Detailed analysis of induction of different class II molecules, HLA-DR, HLA-DQ and HLA-DP, has demonstrated that DQ or DP expression is less intensively induced than DR expression in the liver graft.[45,53] An elegant semi-quantitatively scored immuno histochemical staining analysis also demonstrated a correlation between increased class II expression and the importance of bile ducts and vascular endothelium as target structures during rejection.[53]

Induction of MHC antigen expression during other pathological conditions of liver allograft

Increased expression of MHC antigens in the liver may occur for several reasons. Liver diseases, such as cirrhosis of various aetiologies, are associated with increased class I expression on the hepatocytes.[56] Aberrant expression of class II molecules on bile duct epithelium was described in primary biliary cirrhosis[57,58] and hepatatis B viral infection.[59,60] Almost any injury or pathological process of the liver may be associated with increased membrane regulation of MHC antigens on the cell surfaces of parenchymal cells, and even cholestasis alone,[60] ischaemia or toxic reactions may enhance either class I or class II expression.[45,48]

Induction of class II expression resulting from viral infection is a common phenomenon observed in liver transplantation. In addition to hepatitis B virus,[60] other viruses especially CMV, cause expression of class II on the hepatocytes.[62] Because of the high incidence of viral infections in transplant patients, the diagnostic value of aberrant MHC expression is very limited and cannot be considered as a 'specific' diagnostic parameter for rejection.

The regulation of MHC antigen expression

MHC class I antigens may be upregulated by several cytokines, such as interferons and tumour necrosis factor, produced during various immunological processes. Interferon alpha and beta, produced by lymphoid cells and cells of parenchymal origin increase class I expression on the cell surfaces.[63] Of the cytokines studied, interferon gamma, which is produced by activated lymphocytes, is the most potent inducer for class II[64] but induces also class I.[63] Interferon gamma is produced in allograft rejection, where large numbers of alloreactive lymphocytes infiltrate the graft. In viral infections, lymphocyte activation occurs and large amounts of interferons are produced, which explains the upregulation of MHC antigens during such infections.[65]

The regulation of MHC gene transcription and the subsequent processing which leads to antigen expression under different circumstances is complex. The gene regulatory elements and factors, able to bind the response sequences of the MHC gene, control transcription. A model for the transcriptional regulation of MHC class II genes has been postulated.[66] In certain cell types such as B-lymphocytes, a high constitutive class II expression is the result of both the active tissue specific transcriptional enhancers and the transcriptionally active promoters. On the other hand, there are other type of cells such as T lymphocytes which express class II only when activated. In resting T cells, the transcriptional enhancer is active, but the promoter is blocked or inactive. With T cell, activation, the promoter becomes activated and the class II gene is transcribed. In some cells, class II expression is inducible by interferon gamma, although in the normal state the tissue specific enhancer and promoter elements are inactive and no gene transcription is seen. In the presence of interferon gamma, the promoter is activated and the gene is transcribed. The latter mechanism is observed in antigen presenting cells (APC) and in the tissue cells with aberrant inducible class II expression. In non-inducible cells, although MHC class II promoters are not inducible by interferon gamma, various additional stimuli have been suggested occasionally to result in MHC class II gene expression.

The up-regulation of class II molecules in human liver allografts, seen during rejection, viral infections and other pathological processes, probably results from T cell activation, interferon gamma production or other class II inducible factors. *In vitro*, interferon gamma has been demonstrated to induce HLA-DR on cultured hepatocytes.[67] Moreover, differences in cytokine regulation have been found between the different class II molecules, and cytokines other than interferon gamma may be important in the regulation process.[68]

The role of MHC expression, antigen presentation, T cell recognition of non-self MHC and the MHC bound peptides as well as the T cell activation cascade in the immunological mechanisms of allograft rejection are described elsewhere in this book (see Chapter 11).

Transplantation antigens and the outcome of hepatic allografts

The benefit of HLA matching in the outcome of renal allografts has been clearly demonstrated.[69] Both HLA-ABC and HLA-DR loci matches affect long term kidney graft survival.[69] In liver transplantation, the short graft preservation time has made pretransplant tissue typing impossible. Although the new preservation fluids and rapid HLA typing methods would make it possible to choose a graft of the appropriate HLA type, the shortage of donor organs remains a problem.

In spite of one year graft survival rates of 80–90%, acute rejection occurs in 60–80% of grafts and chronic rejection in up to 10% of grafts.[70,71,72] Acute rejection is a major cause of morbidity and hospitalisation of these patients and chronic rejection is usually an indication for retransplantation. In view of the high rejection rate in liver transplantation, the HLA matching could be of benefit. This is supported by demonstration of the alloreactivity of lymphocytes cultured from human liver biopsy material.[73]

Clinical data are, however, conflicting. In a retrospective study of 500 liver allografts, the HLA compatibility was associated with diminished graft survival, although a higher incidence of failure due to rejection correlated with a lower degree of HLA-DR compatibility.[74] Different features of liver allograft rejection and HLA compatibility have been published by others.[75,76] However, the limited clinical data and various immunosuppressive regimens may misrepresent the true role of HLA matching.

In chronic rejection (vanishing bile duct syndrome, VBDS) the role of matching is even less clear than in acute rejection. In some studies no significant effects of class I or class II mismatch have been seen,[77,78] although DQ mismatch seemed to be more related to VBDS than DR mismatch. Others described a correlation between DR mismatch and VBDS.[79] The role of viral infections is suggested by the findings that those with class I mismatch and class II match and CMV infection had an increased risk of developing VBDS.[78] Further work is required to confirm these observations and identify the mechanisms involved.

References

1. Bach FH, Sachs DH. Transplantation immunology. *N Eng J Med* 1987; **317,** 489–492.
2. Häyry P, von Willebrand E, Parthenais E *et al.* The inflammatory mechanisms of allograft rejection. *Immunol Rev* 1984; **7,** 85–142.
3. Snell GD, Dausset J, Natherson S. *Histocompatibility.* New York: Academic Press, 1976.
4. Pfeffer PF, Thorsby E. HLA-restricted cytotoxicity against male-specific (H-Y) antigen after acute rejection of an HLA-identical sibling kidney. *Transplantation* 1982; **33,** 52–56.
5. Cerilli J, Bay W, Brasilel. The significance of monocyte crossmatch in recipients of living related HLA-identical kidney grafts. *Human Immunol* 1983; **7,** 45–50.
6. Paul LC, Claas FH, van Es JA, Kalff MW, Graeff J. Accelerated rejection of a renal allograft associated with pretransplantation antibodies directed against donor antigens on endothelium and monocytes. *N Eng J Med* 1979; **300,** 1258–1260.
7. Steinmuller D. Tissue-specific and tissue-restricted histocompatibility antigens. *Immunol Today* 1984; **5,** 234–240.
8. Demitris AJ, Jaffe R, Tzakis A *et al.* Antibody mediated rejection in human orthotopic liver allografts: a study of liver transplantation across ABO blood group barriers. *Am J Path* 1988; **132,** 489–502.
9. Gordon RD, Iwatsuki S, Esquivel CO, Tzakis A, Todo S, Starzl TE. Liver transplantation across ABO blood groups. *Surgery* 1986; **100,** 342–348.
10. Gugenheim J, Samuel D, Reynes M, Bismuth H. Liver transplantation across ABO blood group barriers. *Lancet* 1990; **336,** 519–523.
11. Dausset J. Iso-leuco-anticorps. *Acta Haematol* 1958; **20,** 156–166.
12. Payne R, Rolfs MR. Fetomaternal leucocyte incompatibility. *J Clin Invest* 1958; **37,** 1756–1763.
13. Kovats S, Main EK, Librach C, Stubblebine M, Fisher SJ, DeMars R. A class I antigen, HLA-G expressed in human trophoblasts. *Science* 1990; **248,** 220–223.
14. Deversson EV, Grow IR, Coadwell WJ, Monaco JJ, Butcher GW, Howard JC. MHC class II region encoding proteins related to the multidrug resistance family of trans membrane transporters. *Nature* 1990; **348,** 738–741.
15. Spies T, Bresnahan M, Bahram S *et al.* A gene in the MHC class II region controlling the class I antigen presentation pathway. *Nature* 1990; **348,** 744–747.
16. Trowsdale J, Hanson I, Mochridge I, Beck S,

Townsend A, Kelly A. Sequences in the class II region related to the 'ABC' superfamily of transporters. *Nature* 1990; **348,** 741–744.

17. Spies T, Blanck G, Bresnahan M, Sands J, Strominger JL. A new cluster of genes within the human major histocompatibility complex. *Science* 1989; **243,** 214–217.
18. Björkman PJ, Saper MA, Samraoui B, Bennett WS, Strominger JL, Wiley DC. Structure of the human class I histocompatibility antigen, HLA-A2. *Nature* 1987; **329,** 506–512.
19. Björkman PJ. Structure, function and diversity of class I major histocompatibility complex molecules. *Ann Rev Biochem* 1990; **59,** 253–288.
20. Claesson-Welsh L, Barber PG, Larhammar D, Rask L, Ruddle FH, Petersson PA. The gene encoding the human class II antigen associated γ-chain is located on chromosome 6. *Immunogenetics* 1984; **20,** 89–93.
21. Choo SY, Antonelli P, Nisperos B. Six variants of HLA-B27 identified by isoelectric focusing. *Immunogenetics* 1986; **23,** 24–29.
22. Choo SY, John T, Orr HT. Molecular analysis of the variant alloantigen HLA-B27d (HLA-B*2703) identifies a unique single amino acid substitution. *Human Immunol* 1988; **21,** 209–219.
23. Shaw S, Johnson AH, Shearer GM. Evidence for a new sequential series of B cell antigen that are encoded in the HLA-D region and that stimulate secondary alloantigenic proliferative and cytotoxic responses. *J Exp Med* 1980; **152,** 565–580.
24. Kwak WW, Schwarz D, Nepom B, Hock RA, Thurtle PS, Nepom GT. HLA-DQ molecules from β heterodimers of mixed allotypes. *J Immunol* 1988; **141,** 3123–3127.
25. Lechler RI. MHC class II molecular structure permitted pairs. *Immunol Today* 1988; **9,** 76–78.
26. Fierz W, Brenan M, Mullbacher A, Simpson E. Non-H-2 and H-2 linked immune response genes control the cytotoxic T cell response to H-Y. *Immunogenetics* 1982; **15,** 261–270.
27. Silvers WC, Barlett ST, Chen HD, Fleming HL, Naji A, Barker CF. Major histocompatibility complex restriction and transplantation immunity. *Transplantation* 1984; **37,** 28–32.
28. Goulmy E, van Leeuwen A, Blokland E, van Rood JJ, Biddison WE. Major histocompatibility complex-restricted H-Y-specific antibodies and cytotoxic lymphocytes may recognise different self determinants. *J Exp Med* 1982; **155,** 1567–1572.
29. Telkolf WA, Shaw S. *In vitro* generation of cytotoxic cells specific for human minor histocompatibility antigens by lymphocytes from a normal donor potentially primed during pregnancy. *J Exp Med* 1983; **157,** 2172–2177.
30. Goulmy E, Termijtelen A, Bradley BA, van Rood JJ. Autoimmunity to human H-Y. *Lancet* 1976; **ii,** 1206.
31. Goulmy E, Bradley BA, Lansbergen Q, van Rood JJ. The importance of H-Y incompatibility in human organ transplantation. *Transplantation* 1978; **25,** 315–319.
32. Goulmy E, Hamilton JD, Bradley BA. Anti-self HLA may be clonally expressed. *J Exp Med* 1979; **149,** 545–550.
33. Singal DP, Wadia YJ, Naipaul N. *In vitro* cell mediated cytotoxicity to the male specific H-Y antigen in man. *Human Immunol* 1981; **2,** 45–53.
34. Rouger PH, Poupon R, Gane P, Mallisen B, Darnis F, Salmon CH. Expression of blood group antigens including HLA markers in human liver. *Tissue Antigens* 1986; **27,** 78–86.
35. Daar AS, Fuggle SV, Fabre JW, Ting A, Morris PJ. The detailed distribution of HLA-ABC antigens in normal human organs. *Transplantation* 1984; **38,** 287–292.
36. Daar AS, Fuggle SV, Fabre JW, Ting A, Morris PJ. The detailed distribution of MHC class II antigens in normal human organs. *Transplantation* 1984; **38,** 293–296.
37. Lautenschlager I, Häyry P. Expression of major histocompatibility complex antigens on different liver cellular components in rat and man. *Scand J Immunol* 1981; **14,** 241–426.
38. Barbatis C, Woods J, Morton JA, Fleming KA, McMichael A, McGhee JOD. Immunohistochemical analysis of HLA (A,B,C) antigens in liver disease using a monoclonal antibody. *Gut* 1981; **22,** 985–991.
39. Lautenschlager I, Taskinen E, Inkinen K, Lehto VP, Virtanen I, Häyry P. Distribution of the major histocompatibility complex antigens on different cellular component of human liver. *Cell Immunol* 1984; **85,** 191–200.
40. Prickett TCR, McKenzie JL, Hart DNJ. Characterisation of interstitial dendritic cells in human liver. *Transplantation* 1988; **46,** 754–761.
41. Koyama K, Fukunishi T, Barcos M, Tanigaki N, Pressman D. Human Ia-like antigens in non-lymphoid organs. *Immunology* 1979; **38,** 333–341.
42. Natali PG, de Martino C, Quanranta V *et al.* Expression of Ia-like antigens in normal non-lymphoid tissues. *Transplantation* 1981; **31,** 75–78.
43. Gouw ASH, Houthoff HJ, Huitema S, Beelen JM, Gips CH, Poppema S. Expression of major histocompatibility complex antigens and replacement of donor cells by recipient ones in human liver grafts. *Transplantation* 1987; **43,** 291–296.
44. So SKS, Platt Jl, Ascher NL, Snover DC. Increased expression of class I major histocompatibility complex antigens on hepatocytes in rejecting human liver allografts. *Transplantation* 1987; **43,** 79–85.
45. Steinhoff G, Wonigeit K, Pichlmayer R. Analysis of sequential changes in major histocompatibility

10

Tolerance

K Wood and O Farges

Introduction

In 1965, Garnier and his co-workers reported that liver grafts transplanted between pigs that were apparently genetically different survived spontaneously.[1] Subsequently, such acceptance of liver allografts was shown by Calne and his colleagues to be associated with the development of a state of specific unresponsiveness to the organ donor, such that skin, kidney or heart grafts from the same donor transplanted at a later time were not rejected.[2] These findings have since been reproduced successfully in other species, suggesting that this 'privileged status' of the liver with respect to tolerance is not species specific (for review see[3]). Furthermore, even in humans and other outbred species such as the dog or the baboon, where immunosuppression is required to prevent rejection of a liver allograft, anecdotal reports have suggested that the rejection response is usually easier to treat than that occurring in response to other organs, such as heart, kidney or skin grafts. These observations clearly highlight that there are two sides to the question of tolerance and liver transplantation: the development of spontaneous tolerance to the liver graft itself and the longer term induction of tolerance to donor allo-antigens presented by the transplanted liver.

The so-called privileged status of the liver is not unique; for example, grafts of cartilage or of the cheek pouch of the hamster also survive spontaneously for prolonged periods of time (for review see[4]). However, these tissues, in contrast to the liver, are heavily surrounded by connective tissue which is thought to limit their lymphatic drainage and therefore reduce the effectiveness of the afferent limb of the immune response to the graft. The term 'immunologically privileged' has also been applied to some sites in the body that inherently lack or have an abnormal lymphatic drainage. These include sites such as the anterior chamber of the eye, the cornea, the brain and again the cheek pouch of the syrian hamster. Each of these sites has been shown to be associated with the prolonged survival of a variety of allogeneic tissues. Lack of rejection at some sites in the body cannot be explained entirely on the basis of aberrant lymphatic drainage, as the thymus, which has efferent lymphatics, has also been reported to be a privileged site for transplantation.[5]

Other situations where prolonged graft survival occurs unexpectedly have been reported. For example, in some cases, very limited histo-incompatibility at either the class I or class II loci can result in spontaneous survival of fully vascularised grafts, such as kidney or heart.[6] The situation for liver grafts is not directly comparable, as spontaneous survival of liver grafts is also observed in many fully mismatched donor–recipient combinations.

The liver has been implicated as playing a central role in the induction of tolerance to other organ grafts; this is particularly so for tolerance induced following oral administration of allo-antigen[7] and other protein antigens (for review see[8]). Tolerance can also be induced by direct delivery of the antigen via the portal vein.[9] In some studies it has been suggested that this is a more potent route for the delivery of antigen than the more conventional intravenous route that is commonly used to induce tolerance to allo-antigen.[10] Tolerance to allografts other than the liver that are drained into the portal vein[11] and the prolongation of allograft survival by means of an extracorporeal hepatic haemoperfusion[12] have also been reported. All of these data suggest that the liver itself has an important function in the induction of tolerance.

Induction of tolerance or specific unresponsiveness to donor histocompatibility antigens in the longer term following orthotopic liver transplantation is another phenomenon not unique to liver grafts. The development of specific unresponsiveness has been documented in recipients with long surviving allografts in a variety of transplantation models. For example, in the rodent, tolerance to donor allo-antigens can develop after donor specific transfusion[13,14] or after treatment with anti-CD4 monoclonal antibody.[15,16] In experimental models using outbred animals and in humans, tolerance to donor histocompatibility antigens is more difficult to achieve. In general, recipients treated with the conventional immunosuppressive drugs do not become tolerant of their grafts. In other words, when the immunosuppressive therapy is withdrawn, often as a result of non-compliance, graft rejection occurs. However, it should be stated that the situation in relation to the development of tolerance to liver allografts in humans has not yet been fully explored and it may be that in some recipients, tolerance to the donor antigens does develop in the long term after transplantation. Unfortunately, *in vitro* assays that can be used to assess the degree to which tolerance to donor allo-antigens has been induced are still awaiting development.

To induce tolerance reliably in a high proportion of transplant patients, it may be necessary to use new strategies for immunosuppression, either alone or in combination with the immunosuppressive drugs that are currently available. Examples of strategies that could theoretically be employed to promote the induction of donor specific tolerance are:

1. by preventing donor antigens from coming into contact with the recipient's immune system, for example by introducing the donor tissue into an immunologically privileged site. As mentioned above, the liver may possess an inherent degree of privilege, resulting from properties of the organ itself or those associated with the site of implantation or portal drainage of the donor antigen after transplantation;
2. by reverting the immune system to a more immature state, such that the recipient's lymphoid cells encounter the donor allo-antigens when they first emerge from the thymus and therefore treat them as self molecules. This can be achieved in adult recipients in a number of ways; for example, using total lymphoid irradiation (TLI),[17,18] anti-lymphocyte globulin (ALG)[19] or anti-CD4 monoclonal antibody;[20]
3. by deleting donor reactive T cells from the recipient's T cell repertoire. If further investigation of the T cell receptor genes used by T cells to recognise allo-antigens reveals that it is possible to predict patterns of allorecognition, it may be possible to remove T cells that are capable of responding to the donor allo-antigen from the recipient's repertoire before transplantation. Preliminary analysis of panels of T cell clones with specificity for defined allo-antigens has not shown any predictable pattern of T cell receptor gene usage,[21–23] but only a limited number of analyses have been carried out thus far and more work remains to be done in this area. Analysis of T cells infiltrating allografts may be more informative,[24] but again the data in this area are very limited at present. Deletion of T cells from the repertoire can occur as a consequence of manipulations such as those described in (2) and has also been noted in some models of neonatal tolerance.[25] This may prove to be an important strategy in the future;
4. by making the alloreactive T cells impotent, so that when they encounter the donor allo-antigens they are unable to respond effectively; in other words, to induce anergy in the responding population. Several examples of this have been reported in the literature in the last few years,[26–28] but as yet a clear understanding of the molecular mechanisms involved has not been established;
5. by inducing a population of suppressor cells that are actively involved in suppressing the response to the transplanted tissue. The phenomenon of suppression has been extensively described in the transplant literature[29] but as yet, characterisation of the cell that mediates the suppression has not been completed.

The mechanisms responsible for the induction of tolerance to allo-antigens in adult recipients are still under investigation, but it is becoming clear that more than one mechanism may be involved. Indeed, in the case of liver grafts, the situation may be even more complex as the special status of the liver, in terms of site of transplantation and reduced susceptibility to rejection, may both contribute to the mechanisms involved both in inducing and maintaining tolerance to the graft.

The aim of the following sections is to consider the various experimental and clinical aspects of tolerance associated with liver transplantation and to review the hypotheses that have been put forward to explain the unusual behaviour of this organ graft. Tolerance to and resulting from liver grafts will be considered separately for reasons of clarity and because we believe that these two aspects may be largely independent. The rationale for this assumption is derived in particular from the following observations:

1. A liver graft is able to suppress rejection occurring in another organ graft transplanted into the same host, although it may itself occasionally be destroyed;[30]
2. Skin grafts are not or are seldom accepted when transplanted within one week of liver transplantation, whereas their acceptance is almost universal in recipients with long term surviving liver grafts;[31]
3. Donor specfic tolerance can be demonstrated in recipients with long term surviving liver allografts, but in the early post-transplant period tolerance is not donor specific.[30,32,33] Furthermore, tolerance cannot be demonstrated in every situation even though the liver graft is not destroyed.[34]

Tolerance to liver allografts in unsensitised recipients

Experimental observations

Most of the experimental studies have been performed in rats where inbred strains are available. In a number of fully allogeneic strain combinations, recipients of orthotopic liver grafts spontaneously accept the graft and become long term survivors, whereas in the same strain combination other types of organ graft are rejected acutely.[35,36] This pattern of reactivity is not found in all strain combinations; in some recipients the liver graft will be the subject of chronic rejection, leading to the death of the recipient in 1–2 months, whereas in others the graft will be destroyed acutely, resulting in death in 9–15 days. In the latter case, the time taken for the graft to be destroyed exceeds that usually found for acute rejection of other organs such as a heart or a kidney, although the reasons for this are unclear. Furthermore, in strain combinations where acute rejection does occur, it appears easier to induce long term survival of the liver graft with immunosuppressive than other types of organ graft. For example, Murase and colleagues[37] have shown in the ACI-RT1^{a} to LEW-RT1^{l} combination that indefinite survival of the liver graft can be induced with a short course of FK506 immunosuppressive therapy, but using the same protocol, survival of heart grafts is only increased. In the same strain combination, intravenous pretreatment with donor antigens was found to be much more effective in prolonging the survival of liver grafts as compared to the prolongation of cardiac, small bowel or skin allografts achieved following the same protocol.[38]

Clinical observations

Since all patients receiving a liver graft are immunosuppressed, it is difficult to study the spontaneous development of tolerance. There are also problems inherent in comparing the results for the survival of different organs, due to, for example, the unpredictable recurrence of many of the primary diseases; renal dialysis, that may limit the use of some very high risk immunosuppressive protocols; the variability of HLA matching requirements and pre-operative treatments such as a blood transfusion. Nevertheless, there are several observations which suggest that the stimulation of, or susceptibility to, an immune response directed towards allo-antigen in human liver transplant patients differs from that described in the recipients of heart or kidney grafts, although these differences are becoming less obvious since the introduction of cyclosporin A. Firstly, the survival curves for liver grafts tend to reach a plateau after the first post-operative year, whereas for kidney or heart grafts there is a steady attrition rate of the grafts beyond one year and therefore the survival curves continue to decrease. Secondly, although more than 80% of liver transplant recipients receiving conventional immunosuppressive therapy experience at least one rejection episode that is confirmed histologically, the majority of these episodes are not associated with evidence of significant liver dysfunction and the rejection episodes often resolve spontaneously (especially in the early post-operative period).[39]

As a result, in this study, only 30% of the patients required additional immunosuppressive treatment for this episode of acute rejection. Lastly, acute rejection seems less difficult to control in patients with liver transplants than in recipients of other types of organ grafts and in liver transplant patients, irreversible acute rejection is a very rare event, unlike the situation for heart or renal transplants where it is still a significant cause of acute graft loss.

We are not aware of any clinical studies investigating the effect of pre-operative blood on liver graft survival. It is interesting to speculate how the use of living related donors might pave the way for a more specific approach to the induction of tolerance to liver allografts in several areas. However, it should be remembered that a frequent complication of chronic liver disease warranting transplantation is portal hypertension and bleeding, which means that most patients will have been transfused for clinical reasons rather than as part of a specific transplant protocol before transplantation.

Genetic basis

Several experimental studies have attempted to correlate the lack of destruction of the liver graft with the type of MHC disparity between the donor and the recipient. There is evidence to suggest that tolerance may be partly MHC associated; however, many other observations show that MHC matching cannot fully account for the variable outcome of a liver graft:

1. PVG -RT1^c recipients are tolerant of DA-RT1^a liver grafts, whereas AUG -RT1^c recipients are not, although both PVG and AUG share the same MHC;[35,40]
2. AUG-RT1^c recipients reject a PVG-RT1^c liver with a mean survival time (MST) of 59 days;[41]
3. AO-RT1^u rats reject DA-RT1^a liver grafts,[40] but PVG-RT1^u recipients are tolerant of PVG-RT1;^{a} [35]
4. Backcross experiments do not always follow the pattern of reactivity observed for other types of organ grafts.[40]

All of these observations suggest that the minor histocompatibility genes are important in determining the fate of a liver allograft. The precise nature and role of these non-MHC antigens is unknown, but may include peptides derived from blood group antigens that are normally expressed in the liver[42] as well as cell or tissue specific antigens that can be presented by either donor or recipient MHC molecules.[43] In addition, immune response genes[44] or even immune suppression[45] genes may influence both the type and intensity of the immune response to specific antigens. An important observation in this respect is that the fate of the graft is mainly 'recipient' dependent[3] and with few exceptions, rat strains such as DA or PVG will accept fully incompatible grafts, whereas others such as LEW, BN or AUG will reject them.

It is too early for any definitive statements to be made on genetic influences in relation to the clinical data for a number of reasons, which include the limited number of studies available, incomplete data for HLA typing of donor and recipients, and only partial understanding of the mechanism of graft loss. This said, however, there are two clinical observations that are somewhat reminiscent of the experimental findings:

1. Preliminary results suggest that the clear effect of HLA haplotype matching on kidney, heart or cornea graft survival is not observed after liver transplantation and it has been suggested that matching may have an adverse effect;[46]
2. Some patients, known as the 'liver eaters', have a striking tendency to reject successive grafts and therefore may represent a group of high responders.

Mechanisms

The mechanisms responsible for the spontaneous survival of liver allografts in certain situations are not clearly understood but may be a combination of immunological and non-immunological factors and more work is needed to elucidate the factors involved.

The low expression of MHC antigens by liver cells has been implicated as possibly contributing to spontaneous induction of tolerance to liver allografts, which might result from 'weak' stimulation of the afferent limb of the immune response. This hypothesis is unlikely to be correct. For example, although hepatocytes (the preponderant cell type of the liver) do not express class II MHC antigens and express class I antigens very weakly, it should be noted that the cells of the portal tract, where any graft infiltrating cells are initially located, include dendritic cells which strongly express class II antigens in all species studied (whereas Kupffer cells, present in the sinusoids or endothelial cells, only express class II in some species) and bile duct cells which strongly express class I MHC antigens.[47,48] Furthermore, recent observations have suggested that primary stimulation of the immune response to donor antigen is mediated by donor derived dendritic cells migrating out of the graft[49] and there is little evidence to suggest that other cell types which express class II antigens are capable of stimulating primary immune responses.[50,51] It has also been shown that cells induced to express class II antigens are poor stimulators of a primary immune response,[52,53] but may amplify the response by presenting antigen to activated T cells. Therefore, one might expect that the level of MHC expression would remain low after transplantation in liver grafts that were spontaneously accepted. However, expression of both class I and II antigens is induced on all cell types of the liver after transplantation,[54,55] (Farges, Morris and Dallman, unpublished data). Induction of donor MHC antigens has also been reported on other types of organ grafts transplanted into tolerant recipients.[56] Probably the best evidence against this hypothesis is the observation that the development of spontaneous tolerance to rat liver allografts is associated with both a cellular and a humoral response. Evidence for this includes an early influx of recipient leucocytes,[57] the magnitude of which is, at least initially, similar to that observed in rejected grafts (Farges, Morris and Dallman, unpublished data). There is also a rise in the levels of antibodies directed against both donor class I and II antigens.[58] Thus liver grafts that survive spontaneously after transplantation are not overlooked by the immune system.

The immune response to a liver allograft may be complex, with two competing arms, one leading to the destruction of the graft, the other to tolerance. The most direct approach to address this issue has been to study the phenotype and function of the cells infiltrating liver grafts and to compare the events that are taking place in grafts that survive spontaneously with those occurring in grafts that reject acutely. There are a number of problems with this approach:

1. The proportion of the leucocytes present in the infiltrate that can specifically recognise the donor allo-antigens is very low, and as yet, there is no information on the exact number of cells required to mediate rejection of a liver graft;
2. Phenotypic studies reported to date have mainly documented the presence of leucocytes expressing classical phenotypes in the graft infiltrate, and these have clearly been shown as not necessarily reliable indicators of the functional properties of the cell identified.[59] More valuable information may be obtained by monitoring the appearance of graft infiltrating cells expressing activation markers, such as CD25, but the number of these present in the graft is still likely to be small;
3. The functional properties of graft infiltrating cells have been investigated either using cells freshly isolated from the graft or on clones grown in tissue culture for a number of generations. The conditions used to propagate cells *in vitro* are very different from the environment within the graft *in vivo*, where paracrine secretion of various mediators is thought to have a significant influence on the functional properties of the infiltrating cells. This approach has nevertheless proved valuable in the investigation of the mechanisms responsible for the induction of tolerance to organ grafts in a number of different models of transplantation tolerance.[28,56,60–63]

This approach has also been applied to liver grafts and some of the most interesting findings show that neither the number, the phenotype nor the donor specific cytotoxic potential of the graft infiltrating cells differs between rejected and spontaneously surviving liver grafts, at a time when significant differences in graft function are observed (Farges, Morris and Dallman, unpublished data). In particular, the IL-2 pathway of lymphocyte activation, that has been shown to be altered when tolerance to allo-antigens is induced in adult recipients by donor specific blood transfusion, appears unaffected in the tolerant animals. Taking these features into account, lack of destruction of liver allografts in these models appears to be a unique model of tolerance induction. So far, only a relatively limited number of parameters have been examined and these results do not rule out the possibility that other pathways of leucocyte activation could be specifically and differentially up- or down-regulated during rejection and the induction of tolerance thus leading to different outcomes as a result of the immunological challenge directed to a liver allograft.

Some of the anatomical or functional properties of the liver may help explain its capacity to resist immune destruction. In particular, the distribution of its blood supply and the synthesis of immunologically active products during hepatocyte metabolism have been proposed to play a role in this.

Vascularisation of hepatocytes is through a sinusoid network, whereas vascularisation of the parenchymal cells of other organs is of the terminal type. Damage to the vascular endothelium, which is thought to be one of the main targets of the rejection response,[64] might therefore more easily lead to the destruction of other types of organ graft, such as heart or kidney. It is interesting to note that vascularisation of bile duct cells is also of the terminal type and that these are frequently damaged specifically during both acute and chronic rejection of liver allografts. Finally the dual, portal and arterial, blood flow has also been suggested to play a protective role during rejection, by preventing the adhesion of the leucocytes to the sinusoidal wall. However, there is little evidence that this anatomical disposition has a protective effect; for example, in some models where spontaneous survival of liver grafts has been documented the livers have not been rearterialised.

Several functional properties of the liver could, at least theoretically, play a role in the spontaneous development of tolerance:

1. Hepatocyte cytosol, as well as alphafoetoprotein (AFP) and/or other liver derived substances secreted in several physiological or pathological conditions, have immunosuppressive properties;[65–67]
2. Mediators of the immune response are able to induce an acute phase response by the liver, one of the components of which is the secretion, at least in the rat, of α_2 macroglobulin which can participate in the regulation of immune responses as a result of its ability to bind various cytokines (for review see[68]);
3. The liver is able to regenerate.

Whether any or all of these properties play a role *in vivo* is under investigation. The evidence currently available suggests that the situation is not that straightforward and many other factors are also involved. For example, mRNA expression for AFP and other proteins of the acute phase response is comparable in rejected and non-rejected rat liver grafts (Farges, Morris and Dallman, unpublished data); hepatocytes in both experimental and clinical situations can be injured either by cellular[69] or humoral[70] mediators of the immune response and although regeneration does occur after liver transplantation, this feature does not appear to be specific to the rejection response,[71] although during rejection the degree of regeneration may be proportional to the severity of the lesions produced, being more intense in rejected than in non-rejected grafts.[72]

Finally, it has been noted that the site of transplantation may also play a role in the development of tolerance, as heterotopic liver grafts are rejected in strain combinations which are tolerance of orthotopic grafts.[73]

Tolerance of liver allografts in sensitised recipients and with liver xenografts

Experimental observations

Liver grafts also appear to be more resistant to rejection in the two situations where the humoral arm of the immune system is thought to play a predominant role – transplantation in sensitised recipients, and xenografts.

Experiments in sensitised rats have shown that not only will a liver allograft escape hyperacute rejection in some animals[74] but some grafts may spontaneously survive long term.[75] Thus protocols used to induce sensitisation which will lead to the hyperacute rejection of a liver graft need to be more aggressive than those used to initiate hyperacute rejection of other organs.[76] (It should be noted that it is difficult to induce hyperacute rejection in certain strains of rat.) Furthermore, when hyperacute rejection does develop, the onset occurs later than after transplantation of other organs and as well as the humoral response, a cellular response also appears to develop. Strain or genetic specificity of the resistance to hyperacute rejection has not been investigated and as yet no parallel can therefore be drawn with the observations in unsensitised recipients. Knechtle and co-workers have recently shown that a class I disparity is sufficient to mediate hyperacute rejection of rat liver grafts and they have suggested that non-MHC antigens may also play a role.[77] However, these requirements are not exclusive to the liver.

Experiments investigating responses to liver xenografts are limited but it has been documented that liver allografts survive for longer than other organs transplanted in the hamster to rat[78,79] and the pig to baboon[80] species combinations. In the former combination, spontaneous survival of liver grafts is not substantially different from that described for some allogeneic strain combinations.[78]

Clinical observations

Clinical liver transplantation across ABO blood group barriers is possible although graft survival may be reduced.[81] One in five recipients experiences no rejection episodes with conventional immunosuppressive therapy and in one in two, antibody mediated rejection is delayed, occurring more than four days after transplantation. Although high levels of panel reactivity have been associated with decreased survival of kidney or heart grafts, no such relationship has been demonstrated in liver transplant patients,[82] although this view has been challenged.[83,84] Interestingly, kidney transplantation can be performed successfully in a proportion of recipients despite a positive crossmatch following liver transplantation.[85,86]

Mechanisms

The ability of passively transferred hyperimmune serum to mediate hyperacute rejection of liver grafts, as well as the increased deposition of IgG and C3 in hyperacutely rejecting liver grafts as compared with grafts rejected by unsensitised animals, suggest that, in this model too, humoral events play a predominant role.[12,76,87,88] Some of the hypotheses put forward to account for the resistance of liver grafts to cellular rejection could at least theoretically account for its resistance to antibody mediated hyperacute rejection (see above). Additionally, the sinusoidal microvasculature of the liver lacks a basement membrane, which plays an important role in platelet aggregation after endothelial cell injury. This hypothesis is, however, controversial in view of the observations that there is no significant decrease in platelet counts during hyperacute rejection of liver grafts.[76]

A more specific hypothesis to explain the resistance of liver grafts to hyperacute rejection comes from the observation of an early decrease in the level of donor specific cytotoxic antibodies after revascularisation of the liver graft, as well as after donor specific extracorporeal liver haemoperfusion, a situation not observed after transplantation of other grafts or after haemoperfusion of non-donor specific livers.[12,87] The exact mechanisms of this decrease in the titre of specific cytotoxic antibodies is as yet unexplained. However, the lack of increased levels of circulating immune complexes in the effluent fluid from the haemoperfused liver,[12] or in the sera of the transplanted animals[87] could result from passive absorption of the cytotoxic antibodies by soluble class I antigens or by the organ itself. Kupffer cells have a high capacity to clear circulating immune complexes and massive deposition of IgG and C3, on sinusoidal cells and Kupffer cells respectively, was observed in the haemoperfused liver,[12] but paradoxically, deposition of IgG and C3 was not particularly striking in the transplanted livers.[87] Passive transfer experiments have also shown that this decrease in cytotoxic mediators correlates, *in vivo*, with the absence of destruction of heart grafts. Whether this is the only mediator of the resistance of the liver to hyperacute rejection may, however, be questioned in view of the recent report, in a porcine model, that in animals undergoing hyperacute liver allograft rejection there is also a rapid and complete disappearance of lymphocytotoxic antibodies.[89] This latter observation is in many ways analogous to the hyperacute or accelerated rejection of heart grafts in presensitised rats after immunosuppressive therapy despite reduced titres of anti-donor antibodies[90,91] and suggests a complementary role for cellular immune mechanisms in this process.

Tolerance to donor allo-antigens induced by long term surviving liver grafts

Experimental observations

Most of the work on tolerance induced by liver transplantation also comes from the study of the rat model, where spontaneous tolerance to liver allografts is associated with tolerance to donor allo-antigens that persists for the life of the animal. Donor specific tolerance also develops in strain combinations where tolerance to liver grafts has been induced by various immunosuppressive treatments[92] and even in presensitised animals.[30,40] This is reminiscent of tolerance that develops in rodents bearing a long term surviving heart or kidney graft, where long term graft survival has been induced with immunosuppressive therapy. Interestingly, tolerance does not develop in every recipient, even though the liver graft is not destroyed,[34,37] a situation that has also been reported in other models of tolerance.[93]

The time necessary for the development of this tolerance varies with the type of the secondary immune challenge. In the case of primarily vascularised grafts such as a kidney or a heart, tolerance to donor antigens appears to be induced almost as soon as liver transplantation is performed,[30,33] although at this stage the tolerance is not donor specific. On the contrary, tolerance to skin grafts, where revascularisation is delayed, is first detected in a small proportion of the animals on the fifth post-operative day and only appears as a reproducible event from day 15 onwards.[31]

Clinical observations

Some of these observations have been reproduced in transplant patients receiving, in addition to the liver, a renal graft from the same donor. An episode of rejection may occur selectively in the liver or the kidney.[94] Furthermore, the low rejection rate for kidneys that are transplanted simultaneously with a liver graft, even in patients that have a positive crossmatch, suggests that in this situation too the liver has the potential to protect a second graft transplanted simultaneously.[95]

Mechanism

Both cellular and humoral events have been suggested to play a role in this liver induced tolerance. Donor specific cytotoxicity disappears from the graft infiltrating cell population seven days after transplantation (Farges, Morris and Dallman, unpublished data). Kamada and his colleagues have shown, using adoptive transfer experiments, that thoracic duct lymphocytes obtained from rats which had received liver transplants more than 30 days earlier also lack cytotoxic potential.[96] It is, however, difficult to know whether assays which assess cytotoxic potential *in vitro* have any correlate with the ability of the graft infiltrating leucocytes to destroy the graft *in vivo*. Using adoptive transfer experiments, some groups[36,97] but not others[96] have witnessed suppressor cell activity in spleen cells from long term surviving recipients. However, no specific phenotype could be shown specifically to mediate this effect, and the mere existence of these cells has been questioned by other groups. Finally it has been observed experimentally, as well as clinically[98,99] that donor leucocytes present in the liver at the time of transplantation are replaced by leucocytes of recipient origin. It is possible that this process might reduce the likelihood of a persistent immune response[100] especially in view of the low expression of class I antigens by the liver.[101] However, direct experimental evidence to link these two ideas is lacking.

Conversely, a role for soluble class I antigens in the induction of long term tolerance in liver transplant recipients has been suggested, based on the observations that a soluble form of class I antigens is constitutively released by the liver and that after liver transplantation, expression rapidly switches to the donor type.[102] While a possible mechanism of action of these soluble class I molecules would be as competitive inhibitors with membrane bound class I antigens for class I restricted T cells or anti-class I antibodies, several observations suggest this is not the case:

1. Soluble class I antigens are also secreted by other tissues;[103]
2. Adoptive transfer experiments using serum from liver transplant recipients, shown to contain a high concentration of soluble donor class I antigen, have only been performed in the DA to PVG rat strain combination, and the DA liver is an especially high producer of these antigens;[103]
3. Secretion of the soluble class I antigen is increased during episodes of rejection.[102] If these molecules were important in inducing tolerance, they might therefore be expected to prevent damage to the graft;
4. Soluble class I antigens do not induce tolerance to the membrane bound ones nor do they inhibit the cytotoxicity directed against them;[104,105]
5. Continuous injection of these antigens only produces minimal prolongation of heart graft survival[106] and administration at doses conventionally used for the induction of specific

unresponsiveness had no immunosuppressive effect.[107,108]

Antibodies to MHC class II antigens are also possible candidates for the mechanism responsible for the induction of tolerance in liver transplant recipients. Serum from liver grafted rats is able to prolong the survival of allogeneic grafts in the same strain combination and the class II reactive IgG fraction of this serum can at least partly reproduce this effect,[3] although this has not been reproduced in another strain combination.[109]

From this discussion it is clear that the mechanism or mechanisms responsible for the induction of tolerance to donor allo-antigens in recipients of long term surviving liver allografts is still open to debate.

Conclusions

More information is clearly required before any definitive statements can be made regarding the mechanism or mechanisms that may be responsible for the induction of either spontaneous or long term tolerance to liver allografts. The liver itself obviously has an important role to play in both of these processes and much remains to be discovered regarding the capacity of the liver to resist attack during rejection and the special features of this site for implantation of tissue as a general route for the induction of tolerance to allo-antigens. Many of the observations that have been made concerning the events taking place in a liver allograft during either acceptance or rejection are reminiscent of observations reported during the induction of tolerance to other types of organ allografts. The functional inactivation of donor reactive cells, in other words the induction of anergy, rather than their deletion, may be part of the mechanism that is responsible for the induction of tolerance to liver grafts. This mechanism has recently been shown to be operating during the induction of tolerance to kidney, heart, islet and skin allografts in adult recipients either as a result of donor antigen pretreatment or anti-CD4 monoclonal antibody therapy.[26–28,110] The observations that donor specific cytotoxic T cells are present within surviving liver grafts clearly suggest that deletion of alloreactive cells, if it is occurring in recipients who become tolerant of a liver graft, is certainly not complete, if it is occurring at all, and that attempts to examine whether the donor reactive leucocytes are functionally inactivated may prove fruitful. The experimental evidence for inhibitors of anti-donor responses in liver graft recipients looked promising. However, recent data showing that soluble class I antigens do not have the capacity to induce tolerance in their own right and are ineffective when used as blocking agents, as well as data questioning the significance of blocking antibodies, would imply that these agents may not play a significant role in the induction of tolerance. The question of suppressor cells is still open. The phenomenon of suppression certainly exists, and suppressor cells have been demonstrated in recipients who either spontaneously accept or in whom tolerance to a liver graft develops in the long term. However, data describing the molecular properties of these cells is still awaited and until this information is forthcoming it is difficult to draw any conclusions as to the significance of these cells in the development of tolerance to a liver graft. It may prove interesting to explore the relationship between anergised cells and suppressor cells, but this work remains to be done.

A new area which needs to be explored in more detail is the regulation and relationship of the cytokine network during the induction of tolerance to liver grafts. The work that has already been carried out has produced some intriguing observations, but more information on the expression of the various cytokines within the graft is required before the significance of this complex network of soluble immune mediators can be assessed.

References

1. Garnier H, Clot JP, Bertrand M. Liver transplantation in the pig: surgical approach. *Seances Acad Sci (Paris)* 1965; **260,** 5621–5623.
2. Calne RY, Sells RA, Pena JR *et al.* Induction of immunological tolerance by porcine liver allografts. *Nature* 1969; **223,** 472–476.
3. Kamada N. *Experimental Liver Transplantation.* Boca Raton, Florida: CRC Press, 1988
4. Dallman MJ, Morris PJ. The immunology of rejection. In: *Kidney Transplantation Principles and Practice* (3rd edn), Morris J (ed). Philadelphia: WB Saunders, 1988.
5. Posselt AM, Barker CF, Tomaszewski JE, Markmann JF, Choti MA, Naji A. Induction of donor-specific unresponsiveness by intrathymic islet transplantation. *Science* 1990; **249,** 1293–1295.

6. Gracie JA, Bolton EM, Porteous C, Bradley JA. T cell requirements for the rejection of renal allografts bearing an isolated class I MHC disparity. *J Exp Med* 1990; **172,** 1547–1557.
7. Callery MP, Kamei T, Flye MW. The anatomic site-specificity of tolerance induction to alloantigen. *Transplantation* 1990; **49,** 230–233.
8. Thompson HSG, Staines NA. Could specific oral tolerance be a therapy for autoimmune disease? *Immunol Today* 1990; **11,** 396–399.
9. Squiers E, Salomon DR, Pickard LL, Howard RR, Pfaff WW. Abrogation of the induction of portal venous tolerance in a cardiac transplant model resulting from Kupffer cell inhibition by gadolinium. *Transplantation* 1990; **50,** 171–173.
10. Kennick S. Lowry RP, Forbes RDC, Lisbona R. Prolonged cardiac allograft survival following portal venous inoculation of allogeneic cells. What is hepatic tolerance? *Transplant Proc* 1987; **19,** 478–480.
11. Holman JM, Todd R. Enhanced survival of heterotopic rat heart allografts with portal venous drainage. *Transplantation* 1990; **49,** 229–230.
12. Gugenheim J, Charpentier B, Gigou M *et al.* Delayed rejection of heart allografts after extracorporeal donor-specific liver hemoperfusion. *Transplantation* 1988; **45,** 628–632.
13. Fabre JW, Morris PJ. The effect of donor strain blood pretreatment on renal allograft rejection in rats. *Transplantation* 1972; **14,** 608–617.
14. Wood KJ, Evins J, Morris PJ. Suppression of renal allograft rejection in the rat by class I antigen on purified erythrocytes. *Transplantation* 1985; **39,** 56–62.
15. Cobbold S, Waldmann H. Skin allograft rejection by L3T4$^+$ and LYT-2$^+$ T cell subsets. *Transplantation* 1986; **41,** 634–639.
16. Wood KJ, Pearson TC, Darby C, Morris PJ. CD4: a potential target molecule for immunosuppressive therapy and tolerance induction. *Transplant Rev* 1991; **5,** 150–164.
17. Myburgh JA, Meyers AM, Thomson PD *et al.* Total lymphoid irradiation: current status. *Transplant Proc* 1989; **21,** 826–828.
18. Strober S, Dhillon M, Schubert M *et al.* Acquired immune tolerance to cadaveric renal allografts: a study of three patients treated with total lymphoid irradiation. *N Eng J Med* 1989; **321,** 28–33.
19. Barber WH, Mankin JA, Laskow DA *et al.* Long-term results of a controlled prospective study with transfusion of donor-specific bone marrow in 57 cadaveric renal allograft recipients. *Transplantation* 1991; **51,** 70–75.
20. Pearson TC, Madsen JC, Morris PJ, Wood KJ. The induction of transplantation tolerance using donor antigen and anti-CD4 monoclonal antibody. *Transplant Proc* 1990; **22,** 1955–1956.
21. Sherman LA, Maleckar JR. Genetic and environmental regulation of the cytolytic T lymphocyte receptor repertoire specific for alloantigen. *Immunol Rev* 1988; **101,** 115–131.
22. Pierres M, Marchetto S, Naquet P *et al.* l-Aα polymorphic residues that determine alloreactive T cell recognition. *J Exp Med* 1989; **169,** 1655–1668.
23. Heath WR, Hurd ME, Murray R, Frelinger J, Sherman LA. Analysis of novel residues of class 1 involved in recognition by alloreactive T cells. *Immunogenetics* 1990; **32,** 138–141.
24. Miceli MC, von Hoegen P, Parnes JR. Adhesion versus coreceptor function of CD4 and CD8: role of the cytoplasmic tail in coreceptor activity. *Proc Nat Acad Sci* 1991; **88,** 2623–2627.
25. Streilein JW. Overview – neonatal tolerance of H-2 alloantigens: procuring graft acceptance 'the old-fashioned way'. *Transplantation* 1991; **52,** 1–10.
26. Qin S, Cobbold S, Benjamin R, Waldmann H. Induction of classical transplantation tolerance in the adult. *J Exp Med* 1989; **169,** 779–794.
27. Alters SE, Shizuru JA, Ackerman J, Grossman D, Seydel KB, Fathman CG. Anti-CD4 mediates clonal anergy during transplantation tolerance induction. *J Exp Med* 1991; **173,** 491–494.
28. Dallman MJ, Shiho O, Page TH, Wood KJ, Morris PJ. Peripheral tolerance to alloantigen results from altered regulation of the interleukin-2 pathway. *J Exp Med* 1991; **173,** 79–87.
29. Hutchinson IV. Suppressor T cells in allogeneic models. *Transplantation* 1986; **41,** 547–555.
30. Kamada N, White DGD. Antigen specific immunosuppression induced by liver transplantation in the rat. *Transplantation* 1984; **38,** 217–221.
31. Kamada N, Davies HS. Fully allogeneic liver grafting and the induction of donor-specific unreactivity. *Transplant Proc* 1981; **13,** 837–841.
32. Engemann R, Ulrichs K, Thiede A, Muller-Ruchholtz W, Hamelmann H. A mechanism of tolerance in arterialized rat liver transplantation. *Transplant Proc* 1983; **15,** 729–733.
33. Kamada N. A description of cuff techniques for renal transplantation in the rat. Use in studies of tolerance induction during combined liver grafting. *Transplantation* 1985; **39,** 93–95.
34. Hasuike Y, Monden M, Valdivia LA *et al.* Immunological unresponsiveness to hepatic allografts in rats. *Transplantation* 1989; **47,** 1043–1047.
35. Zimmermann FA, Davies HS, Knoll PP, Gokel JM, Scmid T. Orthotopic liver allografts in the rat. The influence of strain combination in the fate of the graft. *Transplantation* 1984; **37,** 406–410.

36. Tsuchimoto S, Kakita A, Uchino J *et al.* Mechanisms of tolerance in rat liver transplantation: evidence for the existence of suppressor cells. *Transplant Proc* 1987; **19,** 514–518.
37. Murase N, Kim DG, Todo S, Cramer DV, Fung JJ, Starzl TE. Suppression of allograft rejection with FK506. I Prolonged cardiac and liver survival in rats following short-course therapy. *Transplantation* 1990; **50,** 186–189.
38. Yamaguchi Y, Halperin EC, Harland RC, Wyble C, Bollinger RR. Orthotopic liver allografts in the rat. The influence of strain combination in the fate of the graft. *Transplantation* 1984; **37,** 406–410.
39. Samuel D, Gugenheim J, Saliba F, Castaing D, Bismuth H. Triple immunosuppression in liver transplantation. *Transplant Clin Immunol* 1989; **20,** 149–156.
40. Kamada N. Tolerance induced by liver transplantation in the rat. PhD thesis, University of Cambridge, 1982.
41. Ulrichs K, Engemann R, Thiede A, Muller-Ruchholtz W. Allograft tolerance in rats with orthotopic liver transplants: advantages of rearterialization. *Eur J Surg Res* 1981; **13,** 79.
42. Nakanuma Y, Sasaki M. Expression of blood group-related antigens in the intrahepatic biliary tree and hepatocytes in normal livers and various hepatobiliary diseases. *Hepatology* 1989; **10,** 174–178.
43. Ting A, Simpson E. Major and minor histocompatibility antigens. In: (eds). *Organ Transplantation: Current Clinical and Immunological Concepts*, Brent and Sells London: Baillère Tindall, 1989.
44. Loveland B, Simpson E. The non-MHC transplantation antigens: neither weak nor minor. *Immunol Today* 1986; **7,** 223–229.
45. Sasazuki T, Kikuchi I, Hirayama K, Matsushita S, Ohta N, Nishimura Y. HLA-linked immune suppression in humans. *Immunology* 1989; **2** (Suppl), 21–24.
46. Markus BH, Duquesnoy RJ, Gordon RD *et al.* Histocompatibility and liver transplant outcome. Does HLA exert a dualistic effect? *Transplantation* 1988; **46,** 372–377.
47. Daar AS, Fuggle SV, Fabre JW, Ting A, Morris PJ. The detailed distribution of HLA-A, B, C antigens in normal human organs. *Transplantation* 1984; **38,** 287–292.
48. Daar AS, Fuggle SV, Fabre JW, Ting A, Morris PJ. The detailed distribution of MHC class II antigens in normal human organs. *Transplantation* 1984; **38,** 293–298.
49. Austyn A, Larsen C. Migration patterns of dendritic cells. *Transplantation* 1990; **49,** 1–7.
50. Austyn JM, Steinman RM. The passenger leukocyte – a fresh look. *Transplant Rev* 1988; **2,** 139–176.
51. Sprent J, Schaefer M. Antigen presenting cells for unprimed T cells. *Immunol Today* 1989; **10,** 17–23.
52. Haltutten J. Immunogenicity of renal allograft nephron components *in vivo. Transplantation* 1990; **50,** 519–155.
53. La Rosa FG, Talmage DW. Major histocompatibility complex antigen expression on parenchymal cells of thyroid allografts is not by itself sufficient to induce rejection. *Transplantation* 1990; **49,** 605–609.
54. Settaf A, Milton AD, Spencer SC, Houssin D, Fabre JW. Donor class I and class II major histocompatibility complex antigen expression following liver allografting in rejecting and nonrejecting rat strain combinations. *Transplantation* 1988; **46,** 32–40.
55. Steinhoff G, Wonigeit K, Pichlmayr R. Analysis of sequential changes in major histocompatibility complex expression in human liver grafts after transplantation. *Transplantation* 1988; **45,** 394–401.
56. Wood KJ, Hopley A, Dallman MJ, Morris PJ. Donor major histocompatibility antigens are induced on non-rejected renal allografts in transfused rats. *Transplantation* 1987; **42,** 759–767.
57. Ishikura H, Tsuchimoto S, Misonou J, Natori T, Aizawa M. Leukocyte subsets infiltrating into fully allogeneic, long surviving rat liver allografts. *Transplantation* 1987; **43,** 709–714.
58. Kamada N, Shinomiya T. Serology of liver transplantation in the rat. I Alloantibody responses and evidence for tolerance in a nonrejector combination. *Transplantation* 1986; **42,** 7–13.
59. Swain SL. T cell subsets and the recognition of MHC class. *Immunol Rev* 1983; **74,** 129–142.
60. Armstrong HE, Bolton EM, McMillan I, Spencer SC, Bradley JA. Prolonged survival of actively enhanced rat renal allografts despite accelerated infiltration and rapid induction of both class I and class II MHC antigens. *J Exp Med* 1987; **165,** 891–907.
61. Dallman MJ, Wood KJ, Morris PJ. Specific cytotoxic T cells are not found in the non-rejected kidneys of blood transfused rats. *J Exp Med* 1987; **165,** 566–571.
62. Hamashima T, Yoshimura N, Matsui S, Lee CJ, Oshaka Y, Oka T. The effect of perioperative portal venous inoculation with donor lymphocytes on renal allograft survival in the rat. II Phenotypic and functional analyses of graft infiltrating cells. *Transplantation* 1990; **49,** 171–175.
63. Hancock WW, Distefano R, Braun P, Schweizer RT, Tilney NL, Kupiec-Weglinski JW. Cyclosporine and anti-interleukin 2 receptor monoclonal antibody therapy suppress accelerated

rejection of rat cardiac allografts through different effector mechanisms. *Transplantation* 1990; **49,** 416–421.
64. Adams DH, Wang L, Hubscher SG, Neuberger JM. Hepatic endothelial cell targets in liver allograft rejection? *Transplantation* 1987; **47,** 479–482.
65. Peck AB, Murgita RA, Wigzell H. Cellular and genetic restrictions in the immunoregulatory activity of a fetoprotein. *J Immunol* 1982; **128,** 1134–1140.
66. Eddington TS. Immune responses and liver disease, perhaps, but what about target organ defences? *Hepatology* 1983; **3,** 767–768.
67. Bumgardner GL, Billar T, So SK *et al. In vitro* immunosuppressive effects of murine haptocyte cytosol. *Transplant Proc* 1989; **21,** 1154–1155.
68. James K. Interactions between cytokines and a_2 macroglobulin. *Immunol Today* 1990; **11,** 163–166.
69. Ogawa M, Mori T, Mori Y *et al.* Inhibitory effects of prostaglandin E1 on T cell mediated cytotoxicity against isolated mouse liver cells. *Gastroenterology* 1989; **10,** 1024–1030.
70. Kurebyashi Y, Sato K, Ikeda T, Katami O, Ogawa H, Osada Y. Acute massive necrosis of the liver induced by an intravenous injection of monoclonal antibody to rat liver cell membrane in rats. *Igakunoayumi* 1988; **146,** 179–180.
71. Van Thiel DH, Gavalier JS, Kam I *et al.* Rapid growth of an intact human liver transplanted into a recipient larger than the donor. *Gastroenterology* 1987; **93,** 1414–1419.
72. Teramoto K, Shimizu K, Tsukada K, Kamada N. DNA synthesis in haptocytes during liver allograft rejection in rats. *Transplantation* 1990; **50**(2), 199–201.
73. Gugenheim J, Houssin D, Tamister D *et al.* Spontaneous long-term survival of liver allografts in inbred rats. Influence of the hepatectomy of the recipient's own liver. *Transplantation* 1981; **32,** 445–450.
74. Houssin D, Gugenheim J, Bellon B *et al.* Absence of hyperacute rejection of liver allografts in hypersensitised rats. *Transplant Proc* 1985; **17,** 293–295.
75. Kamada N, Davies HS, Roser BJ. Reversal of transplantion immunity by liver grafting. *Nature* 1981; **292,** 840–842.
76. Knechtle SJ, Kolbeck PC, Tsuchimoto S, Coundouriotis A, Sanfilippo F, Bollinger RR. Hepatic transplantation in sensitised recipients. Demonstration of hyperacute rejection. *Transplantation* 1987; **43,** 8–12.
77. Knechtle SJ, Yamaguchi Y, Coundouriotis A, Bollinger RR. Mediation of hyperacute rejection of rat hepatic allografts by RT-1 antigens. *Transplantation* 1989; **48,** 723–725.
78. Monden M, Valdivia LA, Gotch M *et al.* Hamster to rat orthotopic liver xenografts. *Transplantation* 1987; **43,** 745–746.
79. Settaf A, Merrigi F, van de Stadt J *et al.* Delayed hyperacute rejection of liver xenografts compared to heart xenografts in rats. *Transplant Proc* 1987; **19,** 1155–1157.
80. Calne RY, White DJ, Herbertson BM. Pig to baboon liver xenografts. *Lancet* 1968; **1,** 1176.
81. Gugenheim J, Samuel D, Reynes M, Bismuth H. Liver transplantation across ABO blood group barriers. *Lancet* 1990; **336,** 519–523.
82. Gordon RD, Fung JJ, Markus B *et al.* The antibody crossmatch in liver transplantation. *Surgery* 1986; **100,** 705–715.
83. Donaldson PT, Alexander GJ, O'Grady J *et al.* Evidence for an immune response to HLA class I antigens in the vanishing bile duct syndrome after liver transplantation. *Lancet* 1987; **1,** 945–951.
84. Kapprupan S, Ericzon BG, Moller E. Relevance of a positive crossmatch in liver transplantation. *Transplant International* 1991; **4,** 18–25.
85. Fung J, Griffin M, Duquesnoy R, Shaw B, Starzl TE. Successful sequential liver-kidney transplantation in a patient with preformed lymphocytotoxic antibodies. *Transplant Proc* 1987; **19,** 767.
86. Starzl TE, Demetris AJ, Todo S. Evidence for hyperacute rejection of human liver grafts: the case of the canary kidneys. *Clin Transplant* 1989; **3,** 37.
87. Houssin D, Bellon B, Brunaud MD, Gugenheim J, Meriggi F, Emond J. Interactions between liver allografts and lymphocytotoxic alloantibodies in inbred rats. *Hepatology* 1986; **6,** 994–998.
88. Knechtle SJ, Yamaguchi Y, Coundouriotis A, Sanfilippo F, Bollinger RR. Humoral rejection of rat hepatic transplants by passive transfer of serum. *Transplant Proc* 1987; **19,** 1072.
89. Merion RM, Colletti LM. Hyperacute rejection in porcine liver transplantation. I Clinical characteristics, histopathology and disappearance of donor-specific lymphocytotoxic antibodies from serum. *Transplantation* 1990; **49,** 861–868.
90. Hardy MA, Oluwole S, Fawwaz R, Satake K, Nowygrod R, Reemtsma K. Selective lymphoid irradiation. III Prolongation of cardiac xenografts and allografts in presensitised rats. *Transplantation* 1982; **33,** 237.
91. Schulak JA, Engelstad KM. Humoral presensitisation in rat heart allotransplantation. *J Surg Res* 1987; **42:** 454.
92. Engemann R, Gassel HJ, Lafrenz E, Stoffregen C, Thiede A. Transplantation tolerance after short-term administration of 15-deoxyspergualin in orthotopic rat liver transplantation. *Transplant Proc* 1987; **19,** 4241–4243.

93. Lim SML, White DJG. Long-term residence of a graft is an insufficient stimulus for the induction of tolerance. Investigating the role of cyclosporine in class I-disparate heart grafts in the rat. *J Exp Med* 1988; **168,** 807–810.

94. Gonwa TA, Nery JR, Husberg BS, Klintmalm GB. Simultaneous liver and renal transplantation in man. *Transplantation* 1988; **46,** 690–693.

95. Flye MW, Duffy BF, Phelan DL, Ratner LE, Mohanakumar T. Protective effects of liver transplantation on a simultaneously transplanted kidney in a highly sensitised patient. *Transplantation* 1990; **50,** 1051–1054.

96. Davies HS, Kamada N, Roser BJ. Mechanisms of donor-specific unresponsiveness induced by liver grafting. *Transplant Proc* 1983; **15,** 831–835.

97. Gassel HJ, Hutchinson IV, Engemann R, Morris PJ. Demonstration of donor specific T suppressor lymphocytes in rats accepting orthotopic liver allografts. *Transplant Proc* 1987; **19,** 4207–4209.

98. Gouw ASH, Houthoff HJ, Huitema S, Beelan JM, Gips CH, Poppema S. Expression of major histocompatibility complex antigens and replacement of donor cells by recipient ones in human liver grafts. *Transplantation* 1987; **43,** 291–296.

99. Baudot P, Capron-Laudereau M, Emond J, Gane P, Rouger P, Houssin D. Early disappearance of donor-specific immunofluorescence in spontaneously tolerated liver allografts in inbred rats. *Transplant Proc* 1987; **19,** 200–204.

100. Lechler RI, Batchelor JR. Restoration of immunogenicity to passenger cell-depleted kidney allografts by the addition of donor strain dendritic cells. *J Exp Med* 1982; **155,** 31–41.

101. Kawai M, Obata Y, Hamashima N. Differential involvement of CD4+ cells in mediating skin graft rejection against different amounts of transgenic H-2Kb antigen. *J Exp Med* 1991; **173,** 261–264.

102. Davies HS, Pollard SG, Calne RY. Soluble HLA antigens in the circulation of liver graft recipients. *Transplantation* 1989; **47,** 524–527.

103. Spencer SC, Fabre JW. Water soluble form of RT1-A class I MHC molecules in the kidney and liver of the rat. *Immunogenetics* 1987; **25,** 91–98.

104. Mann DW, Stroynowski I, Hood L, Forman J. Cytotoxic T lymphocytes from mice with soluble class I g10 molecules in their serum are not tolerant to membrane-bound g10[1]. *J Immunol* 1987; **138,** 240–245.

105. Arnold B, Messerle M, Jatsch L, Kublbeck G, Koszinowski U. Transgenic mice expressing a soluble foreign H-2 class I antigen are tolerant to allogeneic fragments presented by self class I but not to the whole membrane-bound alloantigen. *Proc Nat Acad Sci USA* 1990; **87,** 1762–1766.

106. Sumimoto R, Kamada N. Specific suppression of allograft rejection by soluble class 1 antigen and complexes with monoclonal antibody. *Transplantation* 1990; **50**(4), 678–682.

107. Priestley CA, Dalchau R, Sawyer GJ, Fabre JW. A detailed analysis of the potential of water soluble classical class I MHC molecules for the suppression of kidney allograft rejection and *in vitro* cytotoxic T cell responses. *Transplantation* 1989; **48,** 1031–1038.

108. Foster S, Cranston D, Wood KJ, Morris PJ. The effectiveness of pretreatment with soluble or membrane bound donor class I MHC antigens in the induction of unresponsiveness to a subsequent rat renal allograft. *Transplantation* 1992; in press.

109. Houssin D, Charpentier B, Gugenheim J *et al.* Spontaneous long-term acceptance of RT-1-incompatible liver allografts in inbred rats. Analysis of the immune status. *Transplantation* 1983; **36,** 615–620.

110. Wood KJ, Bushell AR, Darby CR, Pearson TC, West L, Morris PJ. Mechanism of induction of transplantation tolerance using donor antigen and anti-CD4 monoclonal antibody. *Transplant Proc* 1991; **23,** 133–134.

11

Mechanisms of liver transplant rejection

N Ascher

Introduction

Over the past 30 years, liver transplantation has become the preferred mode of treatment for most diseases causing end-stage liver disease. Although rejection was recognised histologically in both animal models[1,2] and clinically,[3] the full extent of liver allograft rejection in terms of incidence, patterns, outcome and implication has been realised only recently.[4–7] The recent appreciation of the importance of liver transplant rejection probably relates to the technical complications which challenged the field for some years. As liver transplant surgeons became more adept at treating complications effectively, and the incidence of complications decreased, the frequency and impact of rejection was recognised.

Much of what we assume regarding mechanisms of liver allograft rejection derives from the study of other transplanted solid organs and from a variety of animal models, many of which involve organs other than the liver. Although most principles regarding rejection apply to all organs, there are clearly features which are unique only to liver transplant rejection which will be discussed in this chapter.

Histological features of liver transplant rejection

In man, the histologic features of acute liver transplant rejection have been well described.[4] A mixed inflammatory cell infiltrate with lymphocytes, polymorphonuclear leucocytes (PMNs), eosinophils and plasma cells is seen within the portal tracts. However, the presence of inflammatory cells in the portal tract alone is not sufficient to make the diagnosis of liver transplant rejection; there must also be damage to the bile duct epithelium. This is manifest by inflammatory cell infiltration of bile duct wall. As a consequence, there is irregularity or absence of biliary epithelial cells. At times the inflammatory infiltrate may be so intense that bile duct architecture is difficult to discern. The endothelium of the central veins is often another site of inflammation with the appearance of endothelialitis and lymphocyte adherence to the endothelium. The endothelium may even be denuded. The portal tract infiltration may vary in intensity and the portal tract may be markedly disturbed, but the inflammation rarely extends into the adjacent parenchyma. The relative proportions of inflammatory cells are variable and depend on the treatment to which the patient has been subjected. Frequently, the heterogeneous nature of the infiltrate changes to a more homogeneous infiltrate as rejection therapy begins. Partially treated rejection may be manifest by lymphocytes or PMNs alone in the portal tracts. Acute liver allograft rejection may be difficult to differentiate from hepatitis if the rejection infiltrate is made up primarily of lymphocytes or if the parenchymal features of the hepatitic process are minimal. The key to differentiating acute rejection from acute hepatitis is the presence of bile duct injury in the former and the monotonous nature of the lymphocytic infiltrate and lack of bile duct damage in the latter. Parenchymal cell necrosis is more commonly seen in acute hepatitis. Staining for viral antigen may help make a diagnosis of acute hepatitis, but in the most difficult cases, the two processes – hepatitis and rejection – may co-exist. Acute liver allograft rejection shows many histologic features of acute graft-versus-host disease of the liver[8] – the lack of endothelialitis characterises graft-versus-host disease and the hepatic manifestations of graft-versus-host disease are never seen in the setting of liver transplantation. Hepatocyte drop-out or necrosis is rarely a feature of acute rejection; its presence necessitates documentation of the lack of ischaemic injury to the liver.

The histological features of chronic liver transplant rejection include the presence of chronic inflammatory cells in the portal region with varying degrees of bile duct damage. Another important feature is evidence of vascular ischaemia with central zone hepatocyte necrosis.[4,9] It is generally accepted that chronic rejection represents some component of vascular injury which may explain the ischaemic pattern. Occasionally, acute reversible liver transplant rejection is manifest solely by an ischaemic pattern of pericentral venous vacuolisation. Angiography in these circumstances may reveal intact arterial inflow but lack of normal arborisation of the arterial branches within the liver.

Another form of rejection which is a distinct clinical entity is the vanishing bile duct syndrome (VBDS).[4,10,11] This type of rejection is associated with disappearance of bile ducts on biopsy and a concomitant rise in alkaline phosphatase and bilirubin. It may occur early after transplantation but more commonly is a form of chronic rejection. Although most cases of VBDS lead to irreversible ductopenia and eventual liver failure, on occasion patients have been noted to develop restoration of ducts over time. Snover has correlated the recovery of ductopenic rejection with preservation of arterioles within the portal tracts; once these arterioles are destroyed in the rejection process, the ducts cannot recover.[4] An association has been made between cytomegalovirus infection and VBDS.

The distinction between acute and chronic rejection does not reflect the time of occurrence relative to transplantation but is associated with the chance for reversibility. An acute rejection episode may readily reverse with additional immunosuppression or a change in therapy. In contrast, a diagnosis of chronic rejection implies that the process is not amenable to treatment. There has not been a clear correlation between the type of rejection process or progression to chronic, irreversible pattern and the histological picture of liver transplant rejection. Acute rejection is basically a cellular process. VBDS and chronic rejection may result from a cellular process though the vascular component is felt to be based on humoral rejection. It is likely that these chronic processes reflect both cellular and humoral rejection.

The histological patterns of acute rejection seen in animal models of liver transplantation in the absence of immunosuppression are quite similar to the clinical situation in which immunosuppressive agents are utilised, though there are differences in the intensity and tempo of the inflammatory response. In rat liver allograft, a diffuse portal infiltrate can be seen within 4–5 days after grafting.[12,13] Depending on the donor – host combination, bile duct damage with increasing infiltrate is the common course for acute rejection. As this process continues the inflammation spills out into adjacent parenchyma and hepatocyte necrosis is seen. A similar pattern is seen in porcine and canine liver allograft.[1,2,14,15] The pattern of hepatocyte necrosis in human liver transplantation is only seen in severe or untreated rejection. Chronic rejection with evidence of ischaemic injury and vanishing bile duct syndrome are not recognised histological patterns seen in animal models of hepatic allograft rejection.

Although the rat liver allograft model has been used extensively, most of the data associated with it that concerns allograft rejection come from an earlier, non-arterialised model. More recently the arterialised rat liver allograft model has been employed;[16,17] histology of rejection must be considered in the light of the presence or absence of arterialisation – particularly if vascular rejection is to be studied.

MHC antigen expression in the hepatic allograft

It is presumed that expression of MHC antigens expressed on parenchymal and non-parenchymal cells dictates the pattern and severity of the rejection process. At the least, the expression of MHC antigens on these cells parallels the appearance and disappearance of the rejection response.[18,19,20] There are numerous examples in a variety of animal models examining expression of MHC antigens and their relation to rejection.[21–24] The relative importance of class I versus class II expression in eliciting a rejection response is also a matter of debate and intense examination. Faustman and Lacy delineated the importance of class II expression in islet transplantation;[25,26] treatment of islets using anti-class II antibody or culture conditions to decrease class II antigen expression led to marked prolongation of islet allografts. Stock examined the role of class I antigens in an *in vitro* model of murine islet rejection – mixed lymphocyte islet culture and found antibody to class I blocked development of cytotoxicity.[27,28] In a similar vein, Bumgardner demonstrated that antibody against class I expressed on hepatocytes abrogated the development of cytotoxic lymphocytes in mixed lymphocyte–hepatocyte culture.[29,30] Recent work by Faustman attests to the important role of class I antigen in islet and hepatocyte allograft rejection.[31]

The pattern of cellular infiltrate and damage seen in human and experimental models of allograft rejection appears to correlate with the expression of major histocompatibility antigens expressed within the graft.[18–20] Bile duct epithelium and central vein endothelium express both class I and II antigens. Class I and II antigens are also expressed on Kupffer cells. Hepatocytes, on the other hand, express relatively scant amounts of class I antigen and minimal class II antigen; most investigators have not detected class II expression even in the face of an acute rejection response.[18–20] We have studied human livers preserved in University of Wisconsin solution for the presence of MHC antigens in situ and confirm the presence of class I and II on bile duct epithelium and central vein endothelia and sole expression of class I antigens on hepatocytes.[32] Even after reperfusion of preserved livers, there is little up-regulation of major histocompatibility antigens. This may explain, in part, the relative resistance of the liver allograft to the immune response.

Hepatocytes isolated from human and mouse livers express only class I antigens,[29,32,33] even after culture with γ interferon, an agent known to induce class II expression on other parenchymal cells. The absence of class II on the surface of hepatocytes is documented by using immunoperoxidase straining and FACS sorting. Another aspect of class I antigen expression relates to the functional expression of antigens (i.e the ability of cells to stimulate an immune response). When used as simulators in mixed lymphocyte–hepatocyte co-culture systems, hepatocytes from class I and class II disparate mice induce a strong cytolytic response.[33] In contrast, hepatocytes from class I matched class II disparate donors fail to stimulate a cytolytic response. These findings support the notion of the lack of functional class II expression on the hepatocyte. In contrast, non-parenchymal cells from class I matched class II disparate mice can stimulate development of cytolytic cells in this *in vitro* model; consistent with functional class II expression on non-parenchymal cells such as bile duct epithelial cells and Kupffer cells. Hepatocytes from class II disparate mice also fail to sensitise when administered *in vivo*, in contrast to splenocytes from the same donor animals. In these experiments, sensitisation is reflected by second set skin graft rejection and/or *in vitro* proliferation. These data imply that cells having class II antigens stimulate the rejection response in hepatic allograft rejection. Taken together with the histological patterns seen in rejection, cells expressing class I and class II antigens appear to be the targets for the rejection reaction.

The presence of MHC antigen expression is not the sole determinant which dictates the target for liver transplant rejection. The Kupffer cell is rich in class I and II antigen expression, yet during rejection little inflammation is seen in proximity to the Kupffer cells. Possible explanations for the relative lack of inflammation around Kupffer cells during acute rejection, in spite of their rich MHC antigen expression, include (a) relative inaccessibility of Kupffer cells to infiltrating host cells; (b) limited MHC expression on Kupffer cells after liver transplantation; and (c) turnover of donor Kupffer cells. Donor Kupffer cells are gradually replaced by host Kupffer cells; this process may limit the ability of Kupffer cells to stimulate the rejection response, as well as limiting their role as targets of this rejection.

To date, there has been no attempt to match for HLA antigens in human liver transplantation. The emergent need, the paucity of organs, and the relatively short preservation time have all contributed to the lack of matching. Retrospective analysis of the effects of HLA matching on liver graft outcome has failed to show any beneficial effect.[34] It must be borne in mind that studies indicating the utility of HLA matching for cadaveric kidney transplantation involve thousands of patients. It may be that, with accumulation of additional data, a HLA matching effect will be apparent in liver transplantation.

An important issue that merits continued attention is whether some tissues and organs are more immunogenic than others. Certainly the skin has been recognised as highly immunogenic.[35] This attribute has been correlated with the presence of novel skin associated antigens. A recent study by Miller's group compared immunogenicity of canine liver and renal parenchymal cells to each other, and to lymphocytes using *in vitro* culture systems.[36] They found that the renal parenchymal and tubular cells were relatively more immunogenic than hepatocytes. Non-parenchymal liver cells, however, were highly immunogenic. These data are consistent with the murine studies showing increased functional antigen expression on non-parenchymal cells. The relative immunogenicity of a given cell must be evaluated in context: how accessible is that cell to the host responder cells *in vivo*? The accessibility of a cell *in vivo* relates to trafficking of responder cells, adhesive molecules associated with graft endothelium and the specific architecture of a given organ.

Cellular mechanisms of liver allograft effects

The exact cellular mechanisms by which the host reacts to and rejects the allografted liver are unknown. Much clinical information and most experimental models are incomplete in that they provide inferential evidence of involvement in rejection (i.e. we observe specific cells or cytokines in rejecting grafts and assign to them an important role in rejection). Furthermore, in the clinical situation the observation of specific cells and cytokines rests on the background of mainstream immunosuppression therapy. In spite of these limitations, we can construct a model of human liver rejection.

The lymphocytes apparent in light microscopic examination infiltrating the portal tracts and disrupting central vein endothelia in hepatic allografts appear to have a central role in graft rejection.[4–7,37] The host infiltrating cells can be monitored by surface antigenic markers; both CD4+ and CD8+ antigenic determinants mark the host cells present at the graft site when the diagnosis of acute rejection is made by histological findings and clinical manifestation. Examination of graft infiltrating cells according to these surface markers in sequential protocol biopsies reveal that CD4+ plus CD8+ cells infiltrating the portal tracts may be early predictors of rejection and precede biochemical and histological evidence of bile duct injury by several days.[38] Zeevis' group has been active in the study of infiltrating graft cells using *in vitro* propagation to expand the cell population.[39,40] They find that the cells which accumulate within liver allografts that can be expanded *in vitro* in the presence of donor allo-antigen are enriched for cells with cytotoxic potential directed against donor class I and class II antigens. When studied in a sequential fashion, cells with cytotoxic specificity for donor class I allografts were identified earlier after liver grafting than cytotoxic cells which were specific for class II. The concept of enrichment of cytotoxic cells locally at the allograft site is one that is generally accepted. The appearance of cells with cytotoxic activity against class I prior to cells with cytotoxic activity against class II is not understood. The potential limitation of Zeevis' work relates to the requirement for *in vitro* culture in the presence of donor allo-antigen to propagate host cells. Host cells with specificity against donor would be selected for enhanced growth in this culture system.

These data imply a central role for lymphocytes in the recognition and rejection response to the allograft. *In vitro* studies lend support to this idea.[29,30,31,41,42] The co-cultures of host spleen cells and either preferred hepatocytes or non-parenchymal cell simulators lead to the development of cytotoxic lymphocytes. When purified hepatocytes are used as simulators, the specificity of the cytotoxic lymphocytes is the class I expressed alone on the hepatocyte surface. On the other hand, when non-parenchymal cells are used alone as simulators in the presence of hepatocytes, the cytotoxic lymphocytes that develop have specificity for both class I and II. In both combinations (using either purified hepatocytes or non-parenchymal cell stimulators) the cytotoxic cells themselves are CD8+ though the original responder population must have CD4+ and CD8+ cells in order for cytotoxic cells to develop. Once cytotoxic cells have developed as a result of these *in vitro* culture systems, their specific cytotoxic efficacy can be demonstrated against tumour targets sharing MHC antigens with the stimulator cells, mitogen stimulated blast targets and against hepatocytes themselves. These hepatocyte stimulated cytotoxic lymphocytes have not yet been tested for their ability to injure bile duct cells *in vitro*. The injury to hepatocytes can be demonstrated by release of intracellular enzymes (transaminase) into the culture medium and by documentation of inhibition of protein synthesis by hepatocytes in the presence of cytotoxic lymphocytes (inhibition of leucine uptake). Since the hepatocyte appears to be mainly a late target of liver transplant rejection, inhibition of cellular function manifest by inhibition of protein synthesis may be more important in the pathogenesis of liver allograft injury than is direct hepatocyte lysis. Constitutional symptoms which may accompany clinical liver transplant rejection such as malaise and decreased level of consciousness may reflect the inhibition of normal hepatocyte function by sensitised lymphocytes. In spite of the enriched population of specific cytotoxic lymphocytes at the graft site, the majority of cells present are *not* specifically sensitised.[43] This indicates the presence of both specific and non-specific components of graft rejection.

The agents that are commonly used to treat liver transplant rejection underscore likely mechanisms of graft rejection and injury. Polyclonal and monoclonal anti-lymphocyte agents are known to be effective in the treatment of acute allograft rejection.[44,45] Their destruction of lymphocytes supports the central role of these cells in the acute rejection process. Cyclosporin[46,47,48] and FK506[49,50,51] inhibit IL-2 production; IL-2 is felt to play a central role in graft rejection in the expansion and maturation of sensitised cytotoxic lymphocytes. RS-61443[52,53] is an anti-metabolite which is particularly effective in inhibition of lymphocyte propagation.

Cytokines in the rejection response

Cytokines have been increasingly recognised as central to the allograft rejection process. Cytokines are molecules produced by cells which regulate activity of other cells (paracrine function) or cells of the same type (autocrine function). Cytokines are generally divided into two categories – inflammatory cytokines which have been identified at sites of inflammation, such as IL-1, IL-6 and tumour necrosis factor (TNF), and regulatory cytokines which have been associated with immune responses, such as IL-2, IL-4 and IL-5. The same cytokines may have stimulatory or inhibitory effects depending on the specific culture condition, the target cell and the state of activity of the target cell. Cytokines may also exhibit paradoxical effects when used in combination or in sequence.[54,55,56] A central role for IL-2 in graft rejection is assumed because it has been shown to be elaborated by T helper cells and one of its effects is to stimulate the proliferation and maturation of cytotoxic lymphocytes. Additionally, the agent cyclosporin is believed to exert its immunosuppressive effect by inhibition of IL-2 production and release and, as a consequence, inhibition of the development of cytotoxic lymphocytes. It is noteworthy that the cyclosporin effect can be overcome by addition of exogenous IL-2. Cyclosporin has little inhibitory effect on second set reactions. Antibodies to IL-2 and to the IL-2 receptor have been shown to be immunosuppressive in a number of animal models,[57,58,59] though the clinical trials using antibody to the IL-2 receptor have been disappointing.[60] It has been stated that the lack of clinical efficacy of anti-Tac antibody relates to relatively poor affinity to the IL-2 receptor. Using the sponge matrix allograft model, we have shown that administration of anti-IL-4 and anti-IL-2 antibodies into the sponge aborted the development of cytotoxicity;[61] supporting the role of these cytokines *in vivo*.

One approach to the study of cytokines in allograft rejection is to examine peripheral blood or other sites for the presence of cytokines. Simpson's group found increased IL-2 and IL-2 receptor levels in blood and urine of renal allograft recipients with acute rejection as compared to individuals with stable grafts.[62] These studies did not differentiate patients with cytomegalovirus infection who also displayed elevated IL-2 and IL-2 receptor levels. IL-1 has been followed in the serum of renal transplant recipients.[63] More recently, cytokine profiles have been obtained in liver transplant recipients.[64]

Tumour necrosis factor alpha or TNFα, an inflammatory cytokine which was described based on its inhibition of tumour growth, has also been implicated in the pathogenesis of rejection.[65] Busitil's group showed elevated peripheral TNF levels in liver transplant recipients with acute rejection;[66] patients with bacterial and viral infection also had elevated levels. These elevations seen in TNF levels preceded histological and biochemical evidence of acute rejection. In a parallel series of animal experiments, anti-TNF antibody treatment in rats prolonged hepatic allograft survival, providing further evidence for the role of TNF. These studies also implicated a role for lymphotoxin in allograft injury; treatment of animals with anti-lymphotoxin antibody prolonged hepatic allograft survival and the combination of antibodies to TNF and lymphotoxin had the greatest immunosuppressive effect.[67] These data indicate that both inflammatory as well as immunoregulatory cytokines have a role in liver allograft rejection.

Another approach to the study of the mechanisms of liver allograft rejection is the identification of cytokines which appear locally, at the site of allograft rejection. This can be accomplished by bio-assay of the specific cytokines in question or using polymerase chain reactions to provide the identification of message for production of a specific cytokine. This is possible since the sequence for specific cytokines is known and primers and probes for these genes can be readily synthesised. This approach has been used by our group in the study of biopsy specimens in patients undergoing hepatic allograft biopsy as a routine or in the setting of abnormal liver function tests. In the study of cytokines associated with rejection, biopsies from patients with documented viral infections were eliminated from consideration. None of the inflammatory cytokines tested, such as IL-1, TNFα and α-interferon, differentiated patients with rejection from those with hepatic abnormalities from other aetiologies. Study of immunoregulatory cytokines revealed that IL-4 failed to distinguish rejection from no rejection, but the presence of IL-5 was associated with rejection. Furthermore, a decrease in IL-5 was seen in hepatic biopsies as rejection resolved.[68]

IL-5 is known to be a growth factor for eosinophils and has been associated with the elaboration of eosinophil cytotoxic protein which has toxic potential.[69,70] IL-5 has also been associated with the development *in vitro* of cytotoxic lymphocytes.[72] The identification of IL-5 as a potentially important cytokine in liver allograft rejection may account for the previously observed but unexplained role of the eosinophils in graft rejection.[73,74] We hypothesise that IL-5 released at the site of the allograft may create harmful effects by stimulating eosinophils to elaborate a cytotoxic molecule which in turn damages the graft. Further studies of the interaction of IL-5 and eosinophils which accumulate at the site of the rejection response are underway. It must be kept in mind that the presence of message for production of a given molecule does not necessarily mean that the cytokine is present and/or that it is of biological importance. The identification of increased expression of message for a molecule and increased production manifest by presence of the cytokine itself is strong evidence for the importance of a given cytokine in the allograft response.

Early studies failed to discriminate between patients with or without rejection on the basis of presence of IL-2. It is commonly believed that the IL-2 is a central link between helper and cytotoxic lymphocytes interacting to effect graft injury; one would therefore expect message for IL-2 at the site of allograft rejection. All the patients in this study were maintained on immunosuppressive agents known to inhibit production of IL-2 (cyclosporin or FK506). One explanation is that in patients maintained on drugs which inhibit IL-2 production, alternate pathways exist to effect rejection. Another explanation is that increased message for IL-2 is associated with rejection but the message precedes histological changes so that the timing of assay for IL-2 is important. A kinetic study with serial determinations of cytokines message in a given patient will help elucidate this possibility. Alternatively, it may be that IL-2 is increased in association with hepatic allograft rejection and is an essential component of this response, but that PCR technology is too sensitive; minute amounts of message are assayed as being present in both non-specific inflammation and in instances of rejection. Recent studies using semiquantitative PCR indicate differential amounts of IL-2 in acute rejection.

Antibody related graft injury is a mechanism which assumes a major role in other solid organs but not a major role in liver transplant rejection. A positive pretransplant crossmatch; the presence of preformed anti-donor cytotoxic antibodies is an absolute contradiction to kidney transplantation. Though some investigators report a deleterious effect of a positive crossmatch on liver transplant outcome, many successful transplants have been done under these circumstances and most centres do not utilise the crossmatch prospectively to select donor – recipient indications.[75,76] Hyperacute rejection would be an expected outcome based on kidney transplant experience, but in actuality is an extremely rare phenomenon[77] and has been only recently reproduced in an animal model.[78] It is not known why the antibody response appears to have a less serious effect on liver transplant rejection. It is likely that the mechanism also relates to the ability to perform successful liver transplants in the face of donor – recipient ABO blood type incompatibility.[79] Our own success with ABO blood type compatibility demonstrates a vascular type rejection which may present as biliary tree damage (manuscript in preparation).

References

1. Starzl TE, Koupp HA, Brock DR, Linman JW. Studies on the rejection of the transplanted homologous dog liver. *Surgery, Gynaecology and Obstetrics* 1961; **112,** 135.
2. Starzl TE, Marduoro TL, Rowlands DT *et al.* Immunosuppression after experimental and clinical homotransplantation of the liver. *Annals of Surgery* 1964; **160,** 411.
3. Portmann B, Neuberger JM, Williams R. *Intrahepatic bile duct lesions.* In: Calne RV (ed). London: Greene and Stratton, 1983.
4. Snover DC, Freise DK, Sharp HL, Bloomer JR, Najarian JS, Ascher NL. Liver allograft rejection: an analyses of the use of biopsy in determining the outcome of rejection. *American Journal of Surgery* 1987; **11,** 1.
5. Demetris AJ, Lasky S, Van Thiel DH, *et al.* Pathology of hepatic transplantation; a review of 62 adult allograft recipients immunosuppressed with a cyclosporine/steroid regimen. *American Journal of Pathology* 1985; **118,** 151.
6. Vierling JM, Fennel RH Jr. Histopathology of early and late human hepatic allograft rejection: evidence of progressive destruction of interlobular bile ducts. *Hepatology* 1985; **5,** 1076.
7. Hubscher SG, Clements D, Elias E, McMaster. Biopsy findings in cases of rejection of liver allografts. *Journal of Clinical Pathology* 1985; **38,** 1366.
8. Snover DC, Weisdorf SA, Ramsay MKH *et al.* Hepatic graft-versus-host disease: A study of the productive value of biopsy in diagnosis. *Hepatology* 1984; **4,** 124.
9. Snover DC, Sibley RK, Freise DK, *et al.* Orthotopic liver transplantation: A pathological study. *Hepatology* 1984; **4,** 1212.
10. Demetris AJ, Markus BH. Immunology of liver transplantation CRC crit review. *Immunol* 1989; **2,** 67.
11. Ludwig J, Weisner RH, Butts KP *et al.* The acute vanishing bile duct syndrome. *Hepatology* 1987; **7,** 467.
12. Knechtle SJ, Wolfe JA, Burchette J, *et al.* Infiltrating cell phenotype and patterns associated with hepatic allograft rejection or acceptance. *Transplantation* 1987; **43,** 169.
13. Misumi M, Mori K, Yamaguchi Y *et al.* Immuno Autochemical characterisation of infiltrating macrophages in rejecting liver allograft in the rat. *Transplantation* 1991; **52,** 753–754.
14. I, Akoner J, *et al.* Fine needle aspiration cytology and histology of liver allografts in the pig. *Progress in liver transplantation* 1978;
15. Williams JD, Petters TG, Haggert R *et al.* Cyclosporine A in orthotopic canine hepatic transplants. *Journal of Surgery Research* 1982; **32,** 576.
16. Komaden W. *Experimental liver transplantation.* Boca Ranton FL: CRC Crit Press, 1988.
17. Liu T, Freise CE, Ascher NL, Roberts JP. A modified vascular 'sleeve' anastomoses for rearterialization in orthotopic liver transplantation in rats. *Transplantation,* In press.
18. Demetris AJ, Lasey S, Van Thiel DH, Starzl TE. Induction of DRI Ia antigen in human liver allografts. *Transplantation* 1985; **40,** 504.
19. Takais L, Szende B, Monostari E *et al.* Expression of HLA-DR antigen in bile ducts of rejecting liver transplants. *Lancet* 1985; **2,** 8365.
20. So SKS, Platt J, Ascher NL, Snover DC. Increased expression of Class I major histocompatibility complex antigens on hepatocytes in rejecting human liver allografts. *Transplantation* 1987; **43,** 79.
21. Haying P. MHC and rejection in common models: events in allograft destruction. *Transplantation* 1984; **38,** 1.
22. Tilney NL, Notis-McConatic J, Strom TB. Specificity of cellular migration into cardiac allografts in rats. *Transplantation* 1978; **26,** 181.
23. Skoskiewica MJ, Colven RB, Schneeberger EE, Russel RS: Inidispread and selection induction of MHC deterred antigens in vitro. *JE Medicine* 1985; **162.**
24. Warren HS, Simmeonociv CJ, Dison JE *et al.* Sensitised by 2+ cells trigger rejection of grafts expressing Class I major histocompatibility complex alloantigens. *Trans Proc* 1986; **18,** 310.
25. Faustman D, Hauptfeld V, Lacy P, Davie J. Prolomegation of murine islets allograft survival by pretreatment of islets with antibody directed to Ia determinant. *Proc National Academy Science* 1981; **78,** 5156.
26. Faustman D, Steinman RM, Geble HM, Hauptfeld V, Davie JM, Lacy PE. Prevention of rejection of murine islet allografts by pretreatment with antidendritic cell antibody. *Proc National Academy Science USA* 1984; **81,** 3864.
27. Stock PG, Meloche M, Ascher NL, Chen S, Bach FH, Sutherland DER. Generation of allospecific cytolytic T-lymphocytes stimulated by pure pancreatic B-cells in absence of Ia^+ dendritic cells. *Diabetes* (supplement 1) 1989; **161.**
28. Stock PG, Ascher NL, Chen S, Bumgardner G, Field MJ, Sutherland DER. The alloimmune response to murine islets occurs via indirect antigen presentation to lyT2+ and L3T4+ lympho-

cytes. *Trans Proc* 1990; **22**(2), 841.
29. Bumgardner GL, Chen S, Hoffman R *et al.* Afferent and efferent pathways in T-cell responses to MHC Class I, II, O hepatocytes. *Transplantation* 1989; **47,** 163.
30. So SK, Platt JL, Wilken LM *et al.* Cytolytic T lymphocyte – mediated injury of cultured hepatocytes is H-2 restricted, *Hepatology* 1985; **5,** 1017.
31. Faustman D, Coe C. Prevention of xenograft rejection by masking donor HLA Class I antigens. *Science* 1992; **252,** 1700.
32. So SK, Platt JL, Wilken LM *et al.* Cytolytic T lymphocyte – mediated injury of cultured hepatocytes is K-2 restricted. *Hepatology* 1985; **5,** 1017.
33. Clemming SM, Alan TK, Bumgardner GL, Ascher NL. Lack of Class II antigen expression on hepatocytes profoundly affect CTL development in vitro and in vivo. *Trans Proc* 1991; **(2)** 1, 817.
34. Morre SB, Wiesner RH, Perkins JK *et al.* A positive lymphocyte crossmatch and major histocompatibility complex mismatching do not predict early rejection of liver transplants in patients treated with cyclosporine. *Trans Proc* 1987; **19**(1), 2390.
35. Jakobisiok OF. Quantitative data concerning the development of the cellular infiltration of skin allograft in mice. *Transplantation* 1971; **12,** 364.
36. Ranjan D, Roth D, Esquenoz V *et al.* The effects of tissue associated and MHC Class II antigen presentation on in vitro lymphoproliferation response against canine liver and kidney cells subpopulation. *Transplantation* 1991; **51,** 480.
37. Lautenschleger I, Hockerstedt K, Akoner J *et al.* Cellular characteristics of liver allograft rejection. *Trans Proc* 1987; **19**(1), 2485.
38. Perkins JD, Wiesner RH, Banks DM, LaRusso NF. Immunohistologic labelling as an indication of liver allograft rejection. *Transplantation* 1987; **43,** 105.
39. Fung JJ, Zeevi A, Markins B *et al.* Dynamics of allospecific T lymphocyte infiltration in vascularised human allografts. *Immunol Research* 1986; **5,** 149.
40. Fung JJ, Zeevi A, Kaufman C *et al.* Interactions between bronchoalveolar lymphocytes and macrophages in heart-lung transplant recipients. *Immunol.* 1985; **14,** 287.
41. Bumgardner GL, Chen S, Hoffman RA, Ascher NL. Responder T cell subsets and antigenic stimulus in mixed lymphocyte hepatocyte culture. *Current Surgery* 1989; **46,** 20.
42. Bumgardner GL, Chen S, Almond S, Bach FH, Ascher NL, Matas AJ. Cell subsets responding to purified hepatocytes and evidence of indirect recognition of hepatocyte major histocompatibility complex Class I Antigen. *Transplantation* 1992; **33,** 857.
43. Orosz CG, Zinn NE, Sirinek C *et al.* In vivo mechanism of alloreactivity I frequency of donor reactive cytotoxic T lymphocytes in sponge matrix allografts. *Transplantation* 1986; **41,** 75.
44. Cosini AB, Cho SI, Delmonico FI *et al.* A randomised clinical trial comparing OKT3 and steroids for treatment of hepatic allograft rejection. *Transplantation* 1987; **43,** 91.
45. Fung JJ, Demetris AJ, Porter KA *et al.* Use of OKT3 with cyclosporine and steroid for reversal of acute kidney and liver allograft rejection. *Nephron* 1987; **46(1),** 19–33.
46. Borel JF, Fourer C, Magree C *et al.* Effects on the new antilymphocyte peptide cyclosporine A animals. *Immunology* 1977; **32,** 1017.
47. Hess AD, Tutschea PH, Pu Z, Santos GW. Effects of cyclosporine A on human lymphocyte response in vitro IV. Production of T-cell stimulatory growth factors and development of responsiveness to these growth factors in CSA treated primary MCK cultures. *J. Immunol* 1982; **128.**
48. Henderson DJ, Naya I, Bundick RV, Smith GM, Schmidt JA. Comparison of the effect of FK506, cyclosporine A and rapamycin on I1–2 production. *Immunology* 1991; **73,** 316.
49. Bierer BE, Schreiber SL *et al.* Mechanisms of immunosuppression by FK506. *Transplantation* 1990; **49,** 1168.
50. Kino T, Hatanaka H, Hashimoto M *et al.* FK506, a novel immunosuppressant isolated from a streptomycin: I. Fermentation, isolation and physical and chemical and biological characteristics. *J Antibiot* 1987; **40,** 1249.
51. Segal NH, Siekeirka JJ, Dumont FJ. Observations on the mechanisms of action of FK506. *Biochem Pharmacology* 1990; **40,** 2201.
52. Eugur EM, Mirkovich A, Allison AC. Lymphocyte – selective antiproliferative and immunosuppressive effect of mycophenolic acid in mice. *Second J Immunal* 1991; **33,** 175.
53. Platz KP, Sollinger HW, Hullett DA, Eckhoff DE *et al.* RS61443, a new potent immunosuppressive agent. *Transplantation* 1990; **51,** 27.
54. Mandrup-Pulson T, Bendtzen TK, Dinarello CA, Nerup J. Human tumor necrosis factor potentiates human interleukin 1 – mediated rat pancreatic beta cell cytotoxicity. *Journal Immunol* 1987; **139,** 4077.
55. Spits H, Yssel H, Paliard X *et al.* I1-4 inhibits I1–2 mediated induction of human lymphokine activated killer cells, but not the generation of antigen specific cytotoxic T lymphocytes in mixed leukocyte cultures. *Journal Immunol* 1988; **141,** 29.
56. Watman CF, Murray HW, Weiber M, Rubin BY. Identification of interferon γ as the lymphokine that activates human macrophage oxidative metabolism and antimicrobial activity. *Journal Experimental Medicine* 1983; **158,** 670.
57. Kupiec-Weglinski JW, Diamandstein T, Tilney

NL. Interleukin α and receptor targeted therapy – rationale and applications in organ transplantation. *Transplantation* 1988; **46,** 785.

58. Ueda H, Hancock WU, Cheun Y *et al.* The mechanism of synergeic interaction between anti-interleukin 2 receptor monoclonal antibody and cyclosporine therapy in rat recipients of organ allografts. *Transplantation* 1990; **50,** 545.
59. Hancock WW, Cord RH, Colby AJ *et al.* Identification of I1-2R+ T cells and macrophages within rejecting rat cardiac allografts and comparison of the effects of treatment with anti-I1-2 R monoclonal antibody or cyclosporine. *Journal Immunol* 1987; **138,** 164.
60. Soulillon JP, Cantorovich D, Le Mauff B *et al.* Randomised controlled trial of monoclonal antibody against the interleukin 2 receptor (33B3.1) as compared with rabbit antithymocyte globulin for prophylaxis against rejection of renal allografts. *N Eng J Med* 1990; **332,** 1175.
61. Martinez OM, Burke EC, Alan TJ, Ascher NL. Allogeneic hepatocytes stimulate the production of immunoregulatory molecules in mixed lymphocyte hepatocyte culture. *Trans Proc* 1991; **23,** 805.
62. Simpson MA, Madras PN, Coraby AJ *et al.* Sequential determinants of urinary cytology and plasma and urinary lymphkrines in the management of renal allograft recipients. *Transplantation* 1989; **47,** 218.
63. Mavry CPF, Tuppo. Serum immunoreactive interleukin 1 in renal transplant recipients. *Transplantation* 1988; **45,** 143.
64. Zilg H, Vogel W, Avlitzky WE *et al.* Evaluation of cytokines and cytokine induced secondary messages in sera of patients after liver transplantation. *Transplantation* 1990; **49,** 1074.
65. Maury CPF, Teppo AM. Raised serum level of cachetin/tumor necrosis factor and in renal allograft rejection. *Journal of Experimental Medicine* 1987; **166,** 132.
66. Imagawa DE, Millis JM *et al.* The role of tumor necrosis in allograft rejection. *Transplantation* 1990; **50,** 189.
67. Imagova DK, Millis JM, Olthoff KM *et al.* Antitumor necrosis factor antibody enhancer allograft survival in rats. *Journal Surgery Research* 1990; **48,** 355.
68. Martinez OM, Krams SM, Sterneck VF *et al.* Intragraft cytokine profile during human liver allograft rejection. *Transplantation* 1992; **53**(2), 449.
69. Fujusan T, Abu-Ghazaleh R, Kitn H *et al.* Regulatory effects of cytokine on eosinophil degranulation. *Journal Immunology* 1990; **144,** 642.
70. Valeruis T, Repp R, Kallen JR, Platter E. Effect of TFN on human eosinophil in comparison with other cytokines. *Journal Immunol* 1990; **45,** 2950.
71. Gilley WV, Holley KE *et al.* Identification of immunofluorescence of eosinophil granule major basic protein in living tissues of patients with bronchial asthma. *Lancet* 1982; **2,** 11.
72. Kormendi F, Amend WJC. The importance of eosinophil cells in kidney allograft rejection. *Transplantation* 1988; **45,** 537.
73. Foster PF, Sankary HN *et al.* Blood and graft eosinophil predictors of rejection in human liver transplantation. *Transplantation* 1989; **44,** 72.
74. Iwatsuski S, Iwasaki Y, Kane T *et al.* Successful liver transplantation from crossmatch positive livers. *Trans Proc* 1981; **13,** 286.
75. Fung JJ, Makor KA, Griffer L *et al.* Successful sequential liver-kidney transplantation-patients with preformed lymphocytotoxic antibodies. *Clinical Transplantation*. In press.
76. Hanto DW, Snover DC, Noreen HJ *et al.* Hyperacute rejection of human orthotopic liver allograft in a presensitised recipients. *Clinical Transplantation* **1,** 304–10.
77. Kynectle SJ, Kolbeck PS, Tsuchemntos *et al.* Hepatic transplantation into sensitised recipients. Demonstration of hyperacute rejection. *Transplantation* 1987; **43,** 8.
78. Gordon RD, Iwatsuki S, Esquire CO *et al.* Experience with primary liver transplantation across ABO blood groups. *Trans Proc* 1987; **19,** 4575.

12

Animal models of liver transplantation and their clinical relevance

N Kamada

Introduction

Background to liver grafting in animals

Progress in clinical liver transplantation has been built on extensive experimental liver grafting in animals.[1,2] A technique for liver transplantation was first described in the dog[3,4] using the extra or accessory heterotopic liver graft, and subsequently methods for orthotopic liver transplantation in that species were developed.[5–8] Thereafter, the pig was used as a model for orthotopic liver transplantation;[9–11] the porcine technique has been described in detail by Calne.[12] Among primates, both monkeys[13] and baboons[14] have been used. There is no doubt that these pioneering experimental series contributed greatly to the establishment of clinical liver grafting.

Rat liver transplantation was first established using the heterotopic method in which both donor and recipient livers were subjected to 70% hepatectomy.[15] Others also described modifed heterotopic (auxiliary) liver grafting in the rat.[16,17] Orthotopic liver transplantation was first performed in the rat by Lee and colleagues,[18,19] first using an extracorporeal shunt[18] and then without a shunt,[19] where the portal vein was anastomosed end-to-end using continuous suture methods and the donor bile duct was implanted directly into the recipient duodenum. The Lee orthotopic method, without a shunt, was then modified, the bile duct being anastomosed end-to-end using one tube[20] or two tubes.[21]

Recipient hyporeactivity in liver transplantation

Spontaneous prolonged survival of orthotopic liver allografts without immunosuppression was first reported in the pig;[22,23] some liver allografts were rejected in delayed fashion, whereas others underwent normal first set rejection.[23] Subsequently, independent reports of liver allograft survival in pigs were made.[10,11,24] Calne and coworkers[24] reported that out of 36 grafted animals, nine survived for between nine and 81 days and 11 were alive at the time of reporting; in none of the pigs subjected to post-mortem examination was there evidence of severe destruction due to rejection, though slight lymphocytic and other cellular infiltration was seen, while in similar pigs kidney and skin grafts were rejected acutely. Thus the liver as transplant appeared to have a favoured status in the pig; this was confirmed in the rat (below) but not found to be the case in the dog.

Liver allografts may not only survive indefinitely, but also protect subsequent transplants of donor-type organs from rejection. This has been observed in the pig and the rat. Calne *et al.*[24] first reported that auxiliary and orthotopic liver allografts in the pig prevented the rejection of subsequent donor-type skin, kidney and heart grafts (reviewed by Calne).[25] Subsequent results in the rat fully support these observations,[2] as described in this chapter.

Choice of an animal model

Large animals are of limited usefulness in liver transplantation studies because of the difficulty in obtaining defined and inbred strains. The rat, on the other hand, is ideally suited because of the ready availability of inbred strains, with well-defined MHC types, and because in certain strain combinations the phenomenon of non-rejection of liver grafts occurs, even though the MHC barrier is crossed and no immunosuppression is used. The development of surgical techniques for grafting of rat liver and other organs, together with the availability of inbred and congenic strains and an understanding of its MHC genes and immune system, have all contributed to the importance of the rat in transplantation research. For liver grafting in particular, the rat model has made it possible to examine in detail the immunological events which appear to be unique to this organ. These are (a) the often relatively weak rejection reactions against the liver compared with those against other organs; (b) the non-rejection of liver in some strain combinations despite a fully allogeneic MHC barrier and the absence of external immunosuppression; and (c) the ability of the liver to induce systemic transplantation tolerance, in which grafts of other organs of donor origin are also accepted.

A further advantage of the rat model has been the opportunity to investigate mechanisms of liver induced unresponsiveness in detail at the cellular and molecular levels. It has become clear that the tolerance which follows liver allografting in certain rat strain combinations is a complex phenomenon, involving alterations in cellular reactivity (such as clonal deletion of alloreactive T cells), a high level of serum antibody against class II transplantation antigens, and the presence of free class I antigens in the circulation.[2,26] The evidence for possible mechanisms of unresponsiveness are discussed in this chapter.

Rat liver grafting: technical considerations

For orthotopic liver grafting in the dog and the pig it is usually necessary to decompress the portal and caval systems by draining blood from the inferior vena cava and portal vein into the superior vena cava during the anhepatic phase. In the rat, external shunts are unnecessary[19] provided the anhepatic phase does not exceed 26 minutes.[21] However, it proved extremely difficult to establish the suture anastomosis of the portal vein within this time period, or to control the extracorporeal shunts in the rat, and these were the most frequent causes of failure in rat liver grafting. The introduction of cuff techniques was an important development which removed most of the difficulties encountered with the portal vein anastomosis and the anhepatic phase.[21,27] Most deaths in the early attempts were due to bleeding, infection and biliary complications; however, further modifications eliminated most of these problems and the orthotopic technique is now highly reliable. With the shortening of the time required for portal vein cross-clamping, made possible by the cuff technique, the success rate of the procedure improved greatly, so much so that it is now a reliable means of studying immunological problems of graft rejection and for analysing methods of organ preservation. In this laboratory, and previously in Cambridge, we have performed altogether over 3500 rat liver transplants; the techniques have been perfected to the extent that a success rate of 96–98% is always achieved. Our procedure for orthotopic rat liver transplantation has been described in detail elsewhere.[2,21]

Most workers in the field do not reconstruct the hepatic artery, though this was recommended by Ulrichs and co-workers.[28] The fact that, in our hands, over 95% of rats given fresh liver transplants survived indefinitely irrespective of whether arterial reconstruction was carried out[21] suggests that hepatic artery reconstruction is in fact unnecessary for successful orthotopic grafting. The study of Lee *et al.*[29] also supports this conclusion. Nevertheless, the question of whether arterialisation is of significant value in rat liver transplantation has excited some controversy.[30–35] Thus, three groups reported that the arterial blood supply to the donor bile duct was a crucial factor preventing biliary complications; their conclusions were based on anatomical considerations and on the dramatic improvement in recipient survival which accompanied hepatic artery anastomosis.[28,30–3] In their early experiments, Engemann and colleagues[30] showed that survival of LEW rats grafted with isogeneic liver improved from 45% to 80% with hepatic arterial anastomosis, while in the allogeneic non-rejector combination of BN into LEW, no rats survived for more than 22 days post-grafting without arterialisation. Moreover, biliary complications were almost completely eliminated when the graft was arterialised. Howden *et al.*[32] showed that establishment of the arterial circulation in orthotopic liver transplantation led to a significant improvement in 60 day survival rate (6/8 compared with 3/8), and also improved liver function and histology.

We recently re-examined the importance of hepatic artery reconstruction in the success of rat liver transplantation.[36] Orthotopic liver grafts were performed with or without re-anastomosis of the hepatic artery, in syngeneic donor/recipient combinations (DA into DA, PVG into PVG), allogeneic non-rejector combinations (DA into PVG, BN into LEW) and allogeneic rejector combinations (DA into WAG, LEW into BN). No significant improvement in recipient survival was found when arterialisation was performed and histological studies showed no differences in hepatocyte or bile duct architecture between arterialised and non-arterialised groups. Thus, in the syngeneic and allogeneic non-rejector combinations, survival was over 100 days in almost all cases in both arterialised and non-arterialised groups. Similarly, arterialisation produced no significant differences in survival time in the rejector combinations DA into WAG (13.7±2.5 versus 14.2±2.0 days) and LEW into BN (52±7.0 versus 46±7.1 days). In short, arterialisation does not make an important contribution to the outcome of liver transplantation in the rat; biliary complications associated with the non-arterialised method appear to be due mainly to technique related problems of bile duct anastomosis rather than a result of ischaemia.

The method for heterotopic non-auxiliary rat liver grafting, in which a 70% hepatectomised donor liver is implanted[37] has been used by French workers.[38] Although the liver is less disturbed by the anhepatic phase than orthotopic grafting, frequent bleeding from the hepatectomised donor liver and acute or subacute hepatic dysfunction result in a low success rate. At present it is generally recognised that bile duct reconstruction is the principal technical problem encountered with orthotopic liver transplantation in the rat as well as in man.

Transplantation antigens in rat liver

The distribution of MHC antigens on different liver cells might be a key to the unusual properties of the organ as an allograft, and there have been a number of studies in which liver sections or isolated liver cells have been stained with allo-antibodies, or in which the immunogenicity of cell populations has been assayed. Dendritic cells may play an important role in liver immunogenicity.

There has been considerable progress in recent years in understanding the genetic structure and allo-antigenicity of the rat MHC, RT1.[39,40] The loci are highly polymorphic and many different haplotypes have been identified; many inbred strains and a number of RT1 congenic lines have been developed. An outline map of the RT1 locus is shown in Figure 12.1. The principal class I antigens are coded in a single region, RT1A, while class II molecules are coded by two loci, RT1B and RT1D. All strong class I allo-antigenic activity derives from RT1A, which stimulates antibody, graft rejection and CTL responses.[41,42] RT1A antigens are expressed on most tissues, including red cells. Soluble RT1A antigen is found in the serum of DA rats, and RT1A antigen of donor type appears in recipient serum soon after liver grafting in the combination DA into PVG;[43,44] it is not known whether this results from shedding from the cell surface or secretion, but a separate mRNA species in mouse liver cells which may code for secreted antigen has been reported.[45] Two class II regions, B and D, are recognised; their products are stimulators of MLR and GVH response. As expected, class II antigen distribution is restricted to B cells, some macrophages, dendritic cells, etc.

Rat liver contains both class I and class II antigens, as demonstrated by absorption of allo-antibodies by liver homogenates,[46] elution of anti-RT1A antibodies from liver grafts,[20] and immunochemical staining of liver sections.[47–50] Following liver transplantation or injection of liver homogenate, antibodies to both classes appear in recipient serum.[20,51,52] Quantitative antibody absorption studies[46] showed that liver cell homogenates were rich in class I antigen, but much less so in class II. Binding of anti-RT1 antibodies to liver cells in suspension[53] showed that hepatocytes and

Locus/region	**A**	**B**	**D**	**C/E**
Class	I	II	II	I
Allo-antigenicity	Strong	Strong		Weak

Fig. 12.1 Outline map of the rat major histocompatibility complex, RT1.

vascular endothelial cells were negative for both class I and class II antigens, with some reactivity detectable on bile duct cells; Kupffer cells were more strongly positive for both and seemed to represent an important source of antigen. When frozen tissue sections were treated with radio-labelled anti-RT1A monoclonal antibody, localisation of class I antigen was predominantly in sinusoidal areas; after prolonged exposure, autoradiograms showed an intense, uniform staining, indicating an apparently wide distribution of RT1A.[50]

Immunohistological studies of the distribution of class II antigens in frozen sections of normal rat liver have given divergent results.[47,48] An RT1B specific monoclonal antibody reacted uniquely with dendritic cells concentrated around the portal tracts.[47] Liver dendritic cells are non-phagocytic, radiosensitive and replaced from the bone marrow via the bloodstream; they may be the major source of class II antigenic stimulation. It was suggested that they are the stimulatory 'passenger leucocytes'; their selective depletion could therefore profoundly influence the outcome of organ grafting.[54]

Indeed, evidence was provided that immunological enhancement results from opsonisation of dendritic cells by anti-MHC antibody.[55] In contrast, substantial amounts of class II antigen on normal Kupffer cells have been reported by immunofluorescent staining and rosetting, with lesser but significant staining of the endothelium of portal tract blood vessels.[48] One area of agreement among these reports is the absence of class II antigens on hepatocytes. An increase in class II antigen expression was observed during a GVH reaction;[49] while hepatocytes and portal vein endothelium remained class II negative, bile duct epithelium, hepatic (central) vein endothelium and large numbers of Kupffer cells became class II positive. Thus, a T cell mediated rejection reaction can increase the expression of MHC antigens over that in the normal tissue, which may provide the stimulus for a continuing response.[56]

Minor locus transplantation antigens can also cause liver rejection, though acute rejection has not been reported. Thus, in the MHC identical strains AUG and PVG (both RT16), AUG rejected PVG liver in delayed fashion (MST 59 days) while in the reverse direction (AUG into PVG) the grafts showed longterm survival (MST 179 days).[57]

The fact that donor lymphocytes remaining in the graft may be an additional source of antigen should not be ignored, as indicated by the high titres of antibodies to the lymphocyte (non-RT1) allo-antigen Pta found in the serum of a PVG recipient of DA liver.[20]

In conclusion, knowledge of the distribution of class I and class II antigens in rat liver is incomplete. There is an apparent absence of MHC antigens on hepatocytes, though this is evidently compensated for by a high density on other cells. Kupffer cells may be a major repository of class I antigen; however, few investigations on liver cells with monoclonal anti-class I antibodies have been reported and this is clearly an area where further work is needed. Class II antigen is present on dendritic cells of normal liver and on Kupffer cells during T cell mediated rejection; the reported class II antigenicity of normal Kupffer cells needs to be clarified. Finally, it is evident that the distribution and levels of MHC antigens are not static once rejection has commenced; a factor in determining rate of rejection may be the degree to which MHC antigens can be induced on liver cells by lymphokines from responding host T cells.

Genetics of liver graft rejection in the rat

Experience with liver transplantation in different species has consistently shown that, in appropriate donor–recipient combinations, the liver behaves as an immunologically favoured organ and survives without use of immunosuppressive agents where skin, renal or cardiac allografts in the same combinations would be rejected. This has been studied most thoroughly in the rat, where the availability of inbred and congenic lines, together with reliable surgical techniques, have made it possible to examine the genetics of rejection and non-rejection in detail (reviewed in[2]). It appears that while the antigenic difference between donor and recipient is one major factor in determining liver graft rejection, the inherited ability of the recipient to respond effectively to the difference is of equal importance.

The fate of liver grafts in the rat is genetically determined and strictly dependent on the particular combination of donor and recipient strains, as summarised in Table 12.1 (combinations arranged according to recipients) and Table 12.2 (combinations arranged according to donors). Three groups of donor–recipient combinations

Table 12.1 Survival times of liver allografts between different inbred rat strains (grouped according to recipients)

Recipient (MHC)	Donor (MHC)	MST (no.)	Reference
PVG ($RT1^c$)	DA ($RT1^a$)	>100 (70)	21
PVG ($RT1^c$)	PVG.$RT1^a$	321 (3)	53,53a
PVG ($RT1^c$)	LEW ($RT1^l$)	32 (5)	53,53a
		<81 (9); >218 (1)	26
PVG ($RT1^c$)	WAG ($RT1^u$)	<81 (9); <194 (1)	26
PVG ($RT1^c$)	BN ($RT1^n$)	210 (5)	53,53a
PVG ($RT1^c$)	AUG ($RT1^c$)	179 (4)	53,53a
AUG ($RT1^c$)	PVG ($RT1^c$)	59 (5)	53,53a
AUG ($RT1^c$)	DA ($RT1^a$)	11 (5)	53,53a
AUG ($RT1^c$)	LEW ($RT1^l$)	16 (5)	53,53a
AUG ($RT1^c$)	BN ($RT1^n$)	52 (4); 487 (1)	53,53a
AO ($RT1^u$)	DA ($RT1^a$)	17 (4)	2
PVG.$RT1^u$	PVG.$RT1^a$	231 (5)	53,53a
LOU ($RT1^u$)	DA ($RT1^a$)	16 (6)	2
WAG ($RT1^u$)	LEW ($RT1^l$)	<90 (5); >100 (4)	26
WF ($RT1^u$)	LEW ($RT1^l$)	>100 (5)	2
DA ($RT1^a$)	PVG ($RT1^c$)	>100 (4)	26
		224 (5)	53,53a
DA ($RT1^a$)	LEW ($RT1^l$)	197 (5)	53,53a
		11 (10)	27a
DA ($RT1^a$)	BN ($RT1^n$)	216 (5)	53,53a
DA ($RT1^a$)	AUG ($RT1^c$)	161 (5)	53,53a
LEW ($RT1^l$)	BN ($RT1^n$)	202 (4)	53,53a
		<22 (8)	61
		<35 (4); >90 (8)	62
LEW ($RT1^l$)	AUG ($RT1^c$)	18 (5)	53,53a
LEW $RT1^l$)	PVG ($RT1^c$)	16 (5)	53,53a
LEW ($RT1^l$)	DA ($RT1^a$)	11 (5)	53,53a
LEW ($RT1^l$)	(LEW×BN)F_1 ($RT1^l$/n)	>120 (7)	35
BN ($RT1^n$)	DA ($RT1^a$)	11 (6)	53,53a
		27 (7)	56
BN ($RT1^n$)	PVG ($RT1^c$)	36 (5)	53,53a
BN ($RT1^n$)	AUG ($RT1^c$)	45 (5)	53,53a
BN ($RT1^n$)	LEW ($RT1^l$)	48 (5)	53,53a
		<22 (13); <90 (3); >90 (7)	27a
BN ($RT1^n$)	(LEW×BN)F_1 ($RT1^{l/n}$)	>120 (7)	35

MST = mean survival time; (no.) = number of grafts.

can be recognised: namely (a) those in which acute rejection occurs, with MST of 11–18 days; (b) those in which rejection is delayed to between 30 and 50 days; and (c) those where liver survival is very prolonged or permanent. The third category (non rejection) is of particular interest because of the concurrent induction of tolerance.[43,44] Two recipient strains, DA ($RT1^a$) and PVG ($RT1^c$), show the longest survival times; DA appears to accept liver grafts from a wider range of allogeneic donors than any other.[57,58] Most immunological studies have been performed with the combination of DA liver into PVG recipient where, except for occasional surgical failures, permanent graft survival can be attained in 100% of cases.[2]

An extensive series of orthotopic liver grafts in different donor–recipient combinations was performed by Zimmermann and co-workers.[57,58] In six out of the seven non-rejector combinations discovered, the recipients were either PVG or DA: DA accepted liver grafts from all four allogeneic donors (PVG, AUG, BN and LEW), while PVG accepted DA and BN, but rejected LEW

Table 12.2 Survival times of liver allografts between different inbred rat strains (grouped according to donors)

Donor (MHC)	Recipient (MHC)	MST (no.)	Reference
DA (RT1^{a})	PVG (RT1^{c})	>100 (70)	21
DA (RT1^{a})	AUG (RT1^{c})	11 (5)	53,53a
DA (RT1^{a})	AO (RT1^{u})	17 (4)	2
DA (RT1^{a})	LOU (RT1^{u})	16 (6)	2
DA (RT1^{a})	LEW (RT1^{l})	11 (5)	53,53a
DA (RT1^{a})	BN (RT1^{n})	11 (6)	53,53a
		27 (7)	56
PVG.RT1^{a}	PVG (RT1^{c})	321 (3)	53,53a
PVG.RT1^{a}	PVG.RT1^{u}	231 (5)	53,53a
LEW (RT1^{l})	PVG (RT1^{c})	32 (5)	53,53a
		<81 (9); >218 (1)	26
LEW (RT1^{l})	AUG (RT1^{c})	16 (5)	53,53a
LEW (RT1^{l})	WAG (RT1^{u})	<90 (5); >100 (4)	26
LEW (RT1^{l})	WF (RT1^{u})	>100 (5)	2
LEW (RT1^{l})	DA (RT1^{a})	197 (5)	53,53a
		11 (10)	27a
LEW (RT1^{l})	BN (RT1^{n})	48 (5)	53,53a
		<22 (13); <90 (3); >90 (7)	27a
BN (RT1^{n})	PVG (RT1^{c})	210 (5)	53,53a
BN (RT1^{n})	AUG (RT1^{c})	52 (4); 487 (1)	53,53a
BN (RT1^{n})	DA (RT1$_{a}$)	216 (5)	53,53a
BN (RT1^{n})	LEW (RT1^{l})	202 (4)	53,53a
		<22 (8)	61
		<35 (4); >90 (8)	62
(LEW×BN)F$_{1}$(RT1$^{l/n}$)	LEW (RT1^{l})	>120 (7)	35
(LEW×BN)F$_{1}$(RT1$^{l/n}$)	BN (RT1^{n})	>120 (7)	35
PVG (RT1^{c})	DA (RT1^{a})	>100 (4)	26
		224 (5)	53,53a
PVG (RT1^{c})	LEW (RT1^{l})	16 (5)	53,53a
PVG (RT1^{c})	BN (RT1^{n})	36 (5)	53,53a
PVG (RT1^{c})	AUG (RT1^{c})	59 (5)	53,53a
PVG (RT1^{c})	WAG (RT1^{u})	<81 (9); >194 (1)	26
AUG (RT1^{c})	DA (RT1^{a})	161 (5)	53,53a
AUG (RT1^{c})	LEW (RT1^{l})	18 (5)	53,53a
AUG (RT1^{c})	BN (RT1^{n})	45 (5)	53,53a
AUG (RT1^{c})	PVG (RT1^{c})	179 (4)	53,53a

MST = mean survival time; (no.) = number of grafts.

liver grafts. The only other non-rejector was LEW grafted with BN liver. Clearly, non-rejection by any individual recipient strain is restricted to certain donor haplotypes and, vice versa, the rate of rejection of any particular donor depends on the recipient strain. There was no evidence for prolonged survival of grafts of other organs in the fully allogeneic combinations which accepted liver grafts. On the other hand, semi-allogeneic renal grafts have often been reported to survive in unmodified DA recipients,[59] and fully allogeneic LEW renal grafts are easily enhanced in DA, indicating a relatively weak rejection response. Thus, in some combinations at least, prolonged survival of liver grafts may be less anomalous than appears at first sight.

Serum assays of liver function were also performed (glutamate oxalacetate transaminase and alkaline phosphatase) and showed a good correlation with the fate of the graft, falling clearly into groups corresponding to acute, delayed and non-rejection patterns (see Figure 12.2). In acute

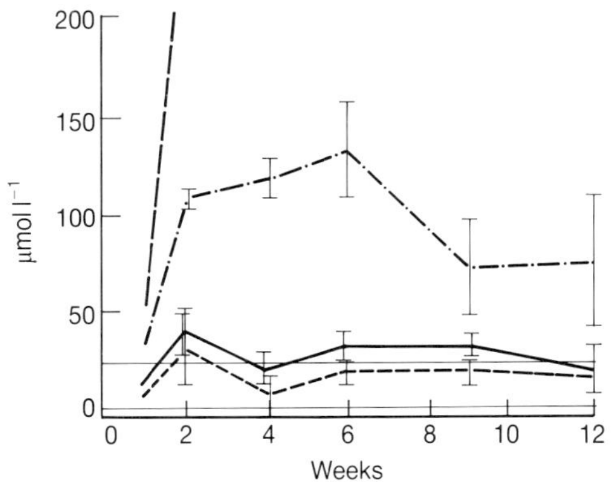

Fig. 12.2 Serum bilirubin levels in liver grafted rats. The recipients of DA liver grafts were PVG (———), BN (— — —, almost vertical), (BN × PVG)F_1 (–·–·–·), and PVG (------, lowermost line).[61]

rejection, serum enzyme levels increased rapidly, while in delayed rejection there were slower, progressive increases. In non-rejectors, an initial rise, attributable to operative trauma, was soon followed by a return to the normal range.

Kamada[2] performed orthotopic liver grafts using mostly DA as donors in a range of allogeneic recipients. While DA livers were accepted by PVG, they were rejected by LOU ($RT1^u$), AO ($RT1^u$) and BN ($RT1^n$). In this last combination, however, permanent DA liver graft acceptance could be obtained by short term use of cyclosporin A. Two animals received 15 mg CyA/kg/day by intramuscular injection for two weeks post liver grafting and another two received 5 mg/kg/day for one week; all survived for more than 100 days with no clinical sign of rejection, such as the loss in body weight invariably seen in rejection combinations.

A simple hypothesis to explain the variation in liver graft survival in different strain combinations would be that the rejection/non-rejection phenotype of a particular strain is the result of its genetically determined level of immune response against the allo-antigens of different donors.[60] Rejection of liver grafts across a whole haplotype barrier appears to be under multigenic control, with important roles both for classical MHC linked Ir genes and for non-MHC linked background genes.[2] However, further studies are required in this important area before definite conclusions can be reached.

Histology and functional competence of rat livers after transplantation

A detailed week-by-week investigation of the histological and biochemical events following grafting of livers from one particular donor strain (DA, $RT1^a$) into three different, fully allogeneic rejector and non-rejector recipient strains has been carried out.[61] The combinations chosen for this study were (1) DA liver grafted into BN ($RT1^n$) recipients (rejector); (2) DA liver into PVG ($RT1^c$) (non-rejector); and (3) DA liver into (BNxPVG)F_1 (non-rejector). Syngeneic controls were also included. The results showed that the non-rejection of DA liver by PVG and (BNxPVG)F_1 was not due to a failure of the host to initiate an anti-graft response, but rather to the termination of the rejection reaction at an early stage in PVG and at a more advanced stage in the F_1 hybrid.

All of 70 PVG and all of eight (PVGxBN)F_1 recipients of DA liver grafts survived for at least 100 days, whereas seven out of eight BN recipients were dead within 32 days (MST 16.7±7.1 days). Isografted DA and PVG rats survived normally. There was no evidence at any time for an immune response in isografted rats, but there was a gradual increase in bile ducts in the portal tracts. DA liver was acutely rejected by BN recipients, with marked swelling of portal tracts caused mainly by oedema and cellular infiltration. The cells were mononuclear and mostly of histiocytic origin, with occasional lymphocytes and large pyroninophilic cells. Concentrations of invading cells were seen in, and apparently migrating through the walls of, portal blood vessels; the latter also showed endothelial proliferation. Plasma cells were numerous at the limiting plates and mononuclear cells were present in large numbers in sinusoids, associated with a relative loss of hepatocytes. Surviving liver cells were shrunken, with dense eosinophilic cytoplasm and pyknotic nuclei. Although the degree of sinusoidal infiltration varied from one part of the liver to another, no part was completely spared. Occasional, randomly distributed foci of coagulative necrosis were also seen.

Although none of the PVG or (BNxPVG)F_1 recipients rejected DA liver grafts, there was histological evidence of a rejection reaction in both groups. The DA into PVG combination is the prototype for non-rejection and tolerance induction.[43] Nevertheless, at one and two weeks, mononuclear cells infiltrated the portal tracts, the infiltration being quite dense in some cases; sinusoids contained varying numbers of large mononuclear cells, but always fewer than in the DA to BN grafts. Hepatocytes showed numerous mitotic figures indicative of regeneration. By four weeks, sinusoidal mononuclear cells had virtually disappeared and those remaining in the portal tracts were mostly small lymphocytes. By 3–4 months, the histological appearance of the liver grafts had returned to normal, apart from residual bile duct proliferation and a slight increase in periportal connective tissue.

Although the rejector × non-rejector F_1 hybrids, (BNxPVG)F_1, accepted DA liver grafts, they displayed a more severe cellular reaction than PVG which was intermediate between that of the parental strains. Significant numbers of mononuclear cells accumulated in portal tracts by one week post-grafting, and extended into sinusoids. Occasional liver cells were shrunken with pyknotic nuclei. These changes were more advanced at two weeks, and of similar severity to those in livers undergoing acute rejection in BN recipients, though actual liver cell necrosis was milder and more focal. By four weeks, although there was still a dense cellular infiltrate in the portal tracts, many of the cells were small lymphocytes rather than pyroninophilic blasts. Limiting plates were well defined and there were few mononuclear cells remaining in the sinusoids. Liver cells showed widespread regenerative changes with twinning of liver cell plates and increased numbers of mitotic figures. At three and four months, resolution was complete with no residual inflammation, but again a varying degree of bile duct proliferation.

Serum samples from liver grafted rats were assayed for total bilirubin, serum alkaline phosphatase and serum alanine transaminase (Figure 12.2).[61] As would be expected, BN recipients undergoing acute rejection showed grossly abnormal liver tests that correlated well with the histological picture of widespread necrosis and cellular infiltration. In the DA to PVG non-rejector combination, values were consistently a little higher than in isografted animals, but returned to normal within 6–12 weeks. The liver grafted (BNxPVG)F_1 hybrids, in all three assays, showed abnormal levels that were intermediate in severity between the PVG and BN recipients, again correlating closely with the intermediate severity of the histological changes in their liver grafts. However, the biochemical values in the F_1s remained elevated throughout the 12 weeks of observation, and at times (such as at 12 weeks) where there was no longer any histological evidence of an immune response. The persistence of high levels of SGPT in these animals argues for an ongoing but microscopically undetectable process of hepatocellular damage, due to a form of chronic rejection. The absence of cellular infiltration suggests that liver damage in these animals might be due to a persistent antibody response.

Thus, it is evident that the non-rejection of DA liver grafts by PVG rats is not due to the absence of an immune response since transient mild rejection reaction occurred, which reached a peak at two weeks after grafting and subsequently disappeared. In the non-rejector (BNxPVG)F_1 hybrids there was a more vigorous host response, but this too disappeared and by 3–4 months liver architecture had been restored to normal, though the biochemical markers of liver function remained elevated. In the BN rats, the picture was one of acute rejection. The F_1 hybrid clearly shows an intermediate level of cellular response, but even this initially vigorous reaction gave way to almost complete resolution of the histological changes in the liver. These observations suggest competitive processes of rejection on the one hand and some form of liver induced immunosuppression on the other. Clearly, the liver has a remarkable natural capacity to suppress ongoing immune responses, such that neither the low responder (PVG) nor the intermediate responder (BNxPVG)F_1 can bring about complete rejection, despite initiation of a response.

Systemic tolerance induced by liver transplantation

The acceptance of a liver allograft is accompanied by two systemic effects which have attracted much interest from both theoretical and practical viewpoints. These are (a) the induction of donor specific transplantation tolerance, such that grafts of other organs from the liver donor strain are also accepted, and (b) donor specific immunosuppression, in which ongoing rejection responses in other grafted organs are terminated. Systemic unresponsiveness following liver grafting was first described in pigs by Calne and co-workers; renal grafts performed at the same time as liver grafts survived indefinitely, whereas non-liver grafted controls rejected kidney grafts promptly.[62] Rejection of skin grafts, on the other hand, could be delayed but not prevented altogether, even when performed two weeks after a successful liver transplant.

Liver induced tolerance has been extensively studied in the rat model.[2,26,63] PVG rats grafted orthotopically with a DA liver have been shown to be systemically tolerant of DA MHC antigens by the permanent acceptance of subsequent DA skin grafts[43] and simultaneous or subsequent grafts of DA heart[64] or kidney.[65] Survival of skin grafts is particularly impressive, as this is normally difficult to achieve across a fully allogeneic barrier either by antibody mediated enhancement[66] or by massive doses of cyclosporin A (60 mg/kg/day) (personal observation). There may be basic differences in mechanism between survival of skin grafts on liver grafted animals and survival of vascularised organs such as heart and kidney, since grafts of the latter organs can be applied on the same day as a liver graft and survive permanently,[64,65] whereas skin grafts only take when an interval of at least five days has elapsed after liver grafting.[44]

The first report of systemic tolerance following rat liver grafting was made in the DA–PVG combination,[43,44] in which it was shown that PVG rats carrying DA liver grafts would accept DA skin grafts but rejected third party (LEW) skin grafts. Skin grafting was performed 15 and 45 days after liver grafting; DA skin grafts survived permanently in perfect condition, with no suggestion of a rejection reaction. However, DA skin grafts placed immediately after liver grafting were acutely rejected (MST 13.5±2.6 days), though more slowly than on normal PVG rats (8.0±0.8 days); at five days after liver grafting, two out of six DA skin grafts were accepted permanently after an initial period of chronic rejection, while the other four were rejected (MST 16.0±4.0 days). Thus the time required to establish complete tolerance in this particular combination is between five and 15 days post-liver grafting. Similar acceptance of skin grafts has also been demonstrated in other rat strain combinations where liver grafts are accepted, namely (LEWxBN)F_1 into BN or LEW[38] and BN into LEW.[67,68] In all cases, tolerance was shown to be specific for antigens of the liver donor by the rejection of appropriate third party grafts. A phenomenon of a small but significant non-specific delay in rejection of third party skin grafts has often been noted, perhaps indicating a degree of non-specific immunosuppression in addition to specific unresponsiveness.

Skin grafting was also used in the DA to PVG combination to show that a liver graft can reverse an existing state of sensitisation (Figure 12.3). In the first experiments,[69] 12 PVG rats were sensitised to DA antigens by application of DA skin grafts; 28 days later they received orthotopic DA

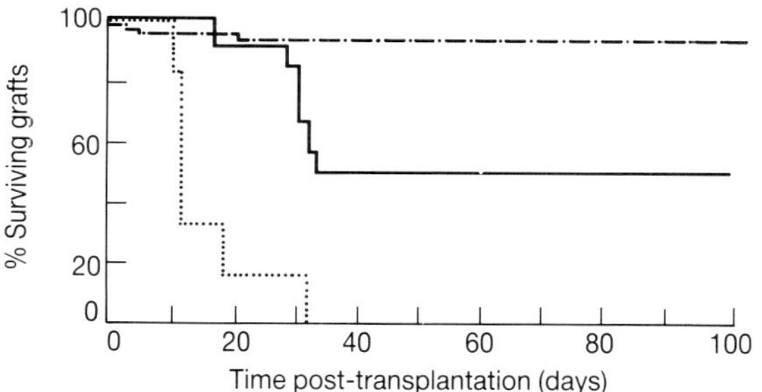

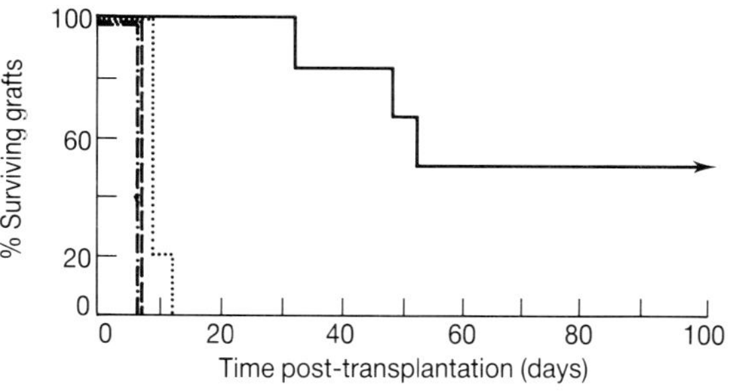

Fig. 12.3 Reversal of immunological memory by liver grafting. *Above* Survival of presensitised liver grafted rats. Normal PVG (non-rejector) rats grafted with DA livers survived indefinitely (–·–·–·) while BN (rejector) rats similarly grafted all died within 32 days (······). When PVG rats were presensitised by rejection of DA skin grafts 28 days before liver transplantation (———), 50% rejected and died within 34 days, while 50% failed to reject and survived indefinitely. *Below* Demonstration of systemic tolerance. The presensitised PVG recipients which survived DA liver grafting were challenged with another DA skin graft 28 days after liver grafting (———); second set skin grafts showed prolonged survival in all cases and remained permanently in 3/6, while third party (AO) skin grafts were rejected promptly (····). Control sensitised animals not liver grafted (–·–·–) or receiving a syngeneic (PVG) liver graft (------) rejected second set DA skin grafts rapidly.[63]

liver grafts. Six sensitised animals died 16–34 days after liver transplantation, with severe hepatocellular necrosis and intense mononuclear cellular infiltration of the liver; in contrast, the remaining six survived indefinitely and liver biopsies showed well-preserved architecture, normal liver cells, no significant excess of inflammatory cells in the portal tracts and no evidence of previous liver damage. Skin grafting was performed to investigate whether the long term surviving animals had become systemically tolerant of DA. Second set DA skin grafts applied 28 days after liver transplantation showed prolonged survival in three cases (32,48 and 52 days) and remained permanently in the other three; antigenic specificity of tolerance was demonstrated. These experiments have been repeated on a larger scale with essentially the same result,[70] using either DA skin or heterotopic DA heart grafts to demonstrate tolerance.

Thus, in half the rats under test, a liver graft was able to overcome the effect of presensitisation of the recipient, and in so doing converted a state of heightened reactivity characteristic of immune animals into one of specific hyporeactivity or complete unresponsiveness to DA antigens. Clearly, a liver graft can bring about the induction of tolerance in memory as well as normal cells, despite the fact that lymphocytes from DA primed PVG rats have an increased rejection activity of about 100-fold over normal in a quantitative adoptive transfer assay.[71] This experiment was earlier unsuccessful in the pig, where animals sensitised by previous rejection of renal transplants[62] or skin grafting[72] severely rejected subsequent liver allografts from the same donors. Indeed, this seems to have been the first time the specific conversion of a state of transplantation immunity against a full haplotype MHC difference into one of unresponsiveness had been achieved. It again shows that liver grafting can be more effective than cyclosporin A, which has been shown to be relatively ineffective in suppressing rejection of renal allografts in recipients previously sensitised by skin grafting.[73]

Through its ability to protect grafts of other organs from the same donor, the presence of a liver graft may in principle have clinically beneficial effects. A recent report of successful combined intestinal and liver grafting in a patient has exploited this potential.[74] The patient, who suffered from short gut syndrome, was treated by combined small bowel and liver grafting. In at least 20 previous patients who have undergone intestinal transplantation, rejection and sepsis have been serious complications and none have been able to resume a normal diet other than for short periods. However, in this patient, an enteral diet was resumed eight weeks post-grafting, the first time that small bowel transplantation has been successful. It is possible that the presence of the liver helped to lower the risk of intestinal rejection, though a thorough regime of immunosuppressive drugs and monoclonal antibody OKT3 was also employed.

The cellular basis of liver induced transplantation tolerance

Studies of the alloreactivity of T cells from tolerant, liver grafted rats indicate the selective clonal deletion of certain T cell activities. An informative approach has been the adoptive transfer assay, in which the graft rejection potential of lymphocytes from normal or tolerant rats is compared by transferring cells into heavily irradiated syngeneic hosts, which simultaneously receive allogeneic skin or heart grafts.[75] Without cell transfer, immunocompetence in the irradiated recipients gradually returns and skin allografts are rejected in 20–30 days and heterotopic heart grafts in 50–60 days. Adoptive transfer can distinguish three types of alloreactive T cell population: (a) normal T cells cause acute rejection of grafts in the irradiated host with the expected first set time course (10–12 days); (b) populations from which certain MHC specific clones have been deleted fail in varying degrees to reject grafts of the relevant MHC type in the irradiated host and in the extreme case the host eventually rejects the graft itself after recovering from the effects of irradiation; and (c) suppressor T cells cause graft survival to be prolonged beyond the normal recovery period of the host.[76]

In initial experiments,[77] thoracic duct lymphocytes (TDL) were obtained from PVG rats which had received orthotopic DA liver transplants more than 30 days earlier and in which liver induced tolerance of DA was well established. The cells were transferred into PVG hosts which one day before had been irradiated with 800 rad and grafted with DA skin; the skin grafts were rejected between 13 and 36 days later (MST 20.5±6.3 days), which was no different from irradiated PVG rats similarly skin grafted but receiving no cells (MST 21.2±5.7 days) (Figure 12.4). In contrast, irradiated animals receiving TDL from normal PVG donors rejected DA skin grafts 8–10 days after grafting (MST 9.4±0.8 days), close to the rejection time of non irradiated controls (MST 8.0±0.7 days). Antigen specificity was demonstrated with third party (AO) skin grafts on the irradiated PVG recipients, which were rejected at a normal tempo by DA tolerant TDL (MST 10.8±1.3 days). Thus, the behaviour of TDL from tolerant liver grafted rats is that expected of a population in which certain graft

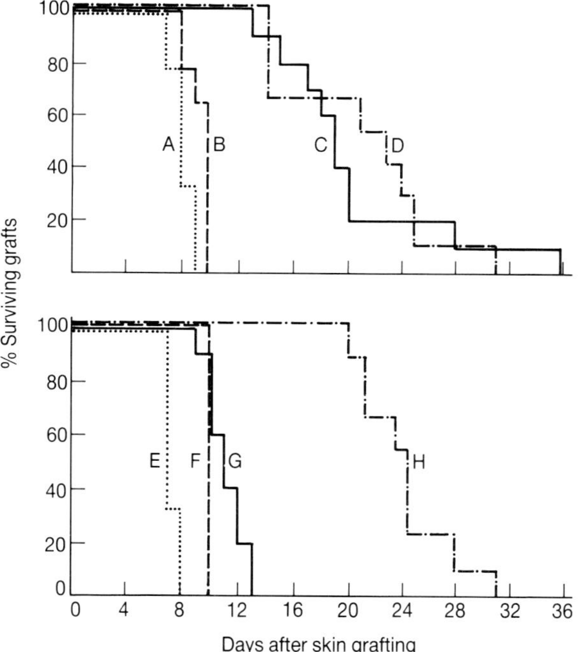

Fig. 12.4 Demonstration, by adoptive transfer assay, that liver transplantation leads to clonal deletion of graft reactive lymphocytes. Thoracic duct lymphocytes (TDL) from pVG rats bearing DA liver grafts for 30 days or longer were transferred to heavily irradiated PVG recipients, grafted on the same day with DA *(above)* or third party AO *(below)* skin. The behaviour of these skin grafts was compared with those on irradiated rats given either normal PVG cells or no cells. The irradiation controls given no cells (D, H) showed prolonged survival of both grafts compared with rats given normal cells (B, F) in which rejection was prompt and close to that of normal, non-irradiated animals (A, E). TDL from liver grafted rats failed to affect the survival of DA skin grafts (C) but restored prompt rejection of AO grafts (G), demonstrating the specific absence of clones responsible for DA graft rejection.[72]

reactive clones had been fully deleted;[77,78] the transferred cells neither accelerated nor delayed the rejection of DA skin grafts on the irradiated recipients, while still able to bring about the acute rejection of third party grafts. The inference is that tolerance involves the specific absence of DA reactive lymphocytes responsible for graft rejection from the recirculating pool with no indication that either suppressor T cells or soluble 'blocking' factors are required for the unresponsive state.

Further experiments showed that tolerance in TDL was established within the first two weeks after liver grafting.[77] During this period (six days post-liver grafting), it was also possible to recover alloreactive cells from the grafted liver itself after enzymatic digestion of the perfused organ (Figure 12.5). When the recovered cells were transferred into irradiated, skin grafted recipients, they showed the opposite characteristic from TDL of the same rats, namely DA specific enrichment in alloreactivity. Thus, in the first days after liver transplantation, DA reactive cells are apparently concentrated in the graft and selectively depleted from the recirculating pool; as already noted, they make a histologically detectable response at this time. Later, however, the liver shows no sign of cellular infiltration, and since cells capable of rejecting DA tissues are by then completely absent from TDL, it seems that they may well die within the liver. The mechanism of such 'clonal exhaustion' is unknown.

More recently, adoptive transfer was used to show that liver grafting can also bring about clonal deletion of effector memory cells in animals presensitised by skin grafting.[70] Heterotopic heart grafts rather than skin grafts were performed on the irradiated host animals. TDL from PVG rats in which immunological memory of DA priming had been abolished by DA liver grafting failed to increase the rate of rejection of DA heart grafts (MST 64.5±9.5 days); the same TDL caused efficient rejection of third party (WAG) heart grafts (MST 9.8±1.7 days). Thus, DA specific deletion of alloreactive T cells serves as one basis for tolerance in both normal and presensitised rats following DA liver transplantation.

The proliferative response of lymph node cells from long surviving (>100 days), liver grafted PVG rats tolerant of DA was investigated *in vivo* by the quantitative GVH reaction and *in vitro* by MLR.[77,78] Rather surprisingly, both the GVH and MLR reactivity of cells from liver grafted PVG rats were indistinguishable from those of normal

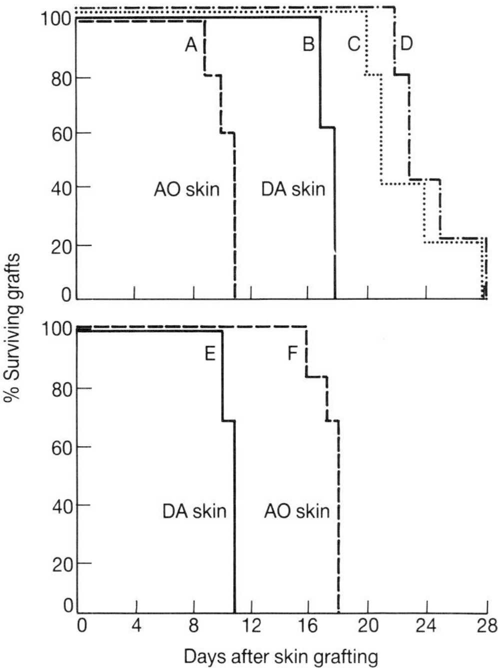

Fig. 12.5 Partial clonal deletion of DA reactive cells from TDL and their enrichment in the liver graft six days after liver transplantation. *Above* PCG recipients irradiated with 800 rad received DA or AO skin grafts followed by 5×10^7 TDL from pVG rats transplanted with DA liver six days earlier. In group A, rejection of third party (AO) skin grafts was prompt (MST 10.4 ± 0.8 days), while in B rejection of DA skin grafts was delayed (17.6 ± 0.5 days), showing specific deletion. Groups C and D show the rejection of AO and DA skin grafts respectively by rats receiving no restorative cells (22.8 ± 2.9 and 24.2 ± 2.1 days). *Below* The transferred cells were obtained from the liver graft. Group E show that 5×10^7 recovered cells rejected DA skin grafts promptly (10.7 ± 0.8 days), but in group F the rejection of third party grafts was delayed (17.3 ± 1.1 days), demonstrating enrichment of specific alloreactive cells within the liver graft.[77]

PVG. This was confirmed with TDL from PVG rats in which sensitisation against DA had been reversed by liver grafting.[70] However, cultures of tolerant cells developed much weaker cytotoxic activity against DA targets than did cells from normal PVG rats and this defect was specific for the tolerated allo-antigen.[77,78]

The normal proliferative responses of lymphocytes from rats tolerised by liver grafting stand in marked contrast to the deletion of alloreactive cells revealed by the adoptive transfer assay and weakened CTL responses *in vitro*. This situation can be described as partial or 'split' tolerance. It may be significant that a similar situation exists in rats following enhancement, where normal GVH responses are evoked by lymphocytes from rats carrying long term renal allografts; cytotoxic T cells could not be demonstrated in such animals *in vivo*, though they were generated *in vitro*.[66] One explanation for split tolerance would be that class I reactive CTL are selectively eliminated by liver grafting. The abundance of class I RT1 antigen in the liver and the relatively low level of class II antigens might well lead to a more effective trapping (and elimination?) of class I reactive T cells. However, the complexity of lymphocyte interactions in graft rejection[79,80] may make this explanation oversimplified.

Immunosuppression by liver transplantation

In contrast to skin grafting, cardiac or renal allografting in the DA to PVG combination can be carried out on the same day as liver transplantation with permanent acceptance of both grafted organs. This suggests that the non-rejection of vascularised organs when co-transplanted with a liver is not due, in the first instance, to systemic tolerance but to a donor specific immunosuppression. The distinction between the two is made here on the basis of whether a central cellular alteration in the recipient alloreactive repertoire can be demonstrated. This is clearly the case a few days after liver transplantation, when specific clonal deletion occurs. The speed with which a liver graft can affect cardiac and renal allografts appears to preclude a central effect and is more likely to be due to circulating suppressive agents. Moreover, a liver graft has the ability to reverse well-established rejection reactions in distant organs and is more powerful in this respect than cyclosporin A.

Heart grafts were implanted heterotopically into the neck of rats using the cuff method;[64] rejection was assessed by daily palpation of the graft, with histological examination if the heart stopped beating or the host died. Combined DA heart and orthotopic liver transplantation was carried out on the same day in PVG recipients. In animals receiving a heart graft alone, rejection was indicated by an increase in graft size on day three or four with decreased strength of beat, and confirmed histologically. All the grafted hearts ceased beating between days 7–9, with active cellular rejection (Table 12.3). In contrast, when combined with a DA liver graft, the hearts did not enlarge and maintained a healthy beat throughout the life of the recipients. More than three months later, the grafted heart structure was normal, with no evidence of existing or earlier rejection. The liver transplants showed only minor structural changes, but no signs of ongoing rejection. The specificity of the protective effect of liver grafting was demonstrated with third party (WAG) heart grafts; all were rejected, but DA liver grafting did induce a significant prolongation of survival from 7.6±0.74 days to 15.0±7.43 days suggesting an element of partial non-specific suppression.

In further experiments, liver transplantation was delayed until five or six days after heart grafting (see Table 12.3). By day five, all heart grafts showed significant swelling and poor beat, signs of impending rejection. Following liver transplantation on days five or six, these signs gradually disappeared in every case, and both heart size and strength of beat returned to normal within three days, indicating reversal of the rejection reaction. Seven out of 13 recipients died 18–25 days after liver grafting with signs of liver failure, presumably due to sensitisation induced by the cardiac allograft. Nevertheless, in all these animals the heart grafts were clinically normal at the time of death with no cellular infiltration, interpreted to be the result of resolution of the rejection reaction. The liver grafts, in contrast, were in an advanced state of acute cellular rejection. In the remaining six recipients, the heart and liver grafts both continued to function normally for over 100 days after the operation. Histologically, the heart grafts were identical in appearance to those in the rats which died earlier, while the livers showed architectural distortion with some portal scarring, bile duct proliferation and lymphocytic infiltration. These changes were more severe than normally seen in a DA into PVG liver graft, suggesting that a rejection reaction had occurred in the liver but had almost wholly resolved. Specificity was again demonstrated using WAG heart grafts as third party controls. Interestingly, massive doses of cyclosporin A (30 mg/kg IM at daily intervals) completely suppressed rejection when started on the same day as heart grafting, but had no effect when started five or six days later. In this respect, CyA is thus less effective than a liver transplant.

In order to see whether another highly vascularised organ could be similarly protected from rejection by a liver transplant, combined DA liver and kidney transplantations were performed on PVG rats.[65] The mean rejection time of DA renal allografts alone was 9.5±0.5 days, but when renal grafting was followed immediately by DA liver transplantation in the same operation, the kidney grafts were fully protected. Third party WAG kidneys were all rejected even if accompanied by DA liver grafts, but their survival was slightly prolonged by the latter (MST 15±5.5 days compared with 9.1±0.7 days). Thus it appears that for kidney as well as for heart grafts, the protective effect of liver transplantation requires no lag period.

Thus, heart or kidney grafts are immediately protected by a liver graft, with no requirement to have the liver graft in place first, whereas with skin grafting 5–15 days must elapse between liver and skin grafts to ensure survival of the latter.[43]

Table 12.3 Suppression of heart graft rejection by liver transplantation

Strain of donor heart	DA liver graft	Heart graft survival (days)	MST (days ± SD)
DA	none	7,7,8,8,8,8,9,9,9	8.1 ± 0.78
DA	day 0	>100 (6)	>100
DA	day 5	19,20,21,25;	20.3 ± 2.27*
		remainder >100(3)	>100
DA	day 6	18,20,23;	20.3 ± 2.05*
		remainder >100(3)	>100
WAG	none	7,7,7,7,8,8,8,9	7.6 ± 0.74
WAG	day 0	10,10,11,11,20,28	15.0 ± 7.43
WAG	day 6	8,9,9,10,11,24	11.8 ± 6.05

PVG rats received a heterotopic DA or WAG heart graft in the neck either alone or with a DA liver graft performed at the same time (day 0) or five or six days later.

*There was no histological evidence of rejection in the heart in these grafts; the recipients died following rejection of liver graft.

Data from [58].

A crucial difference is the vascularity of the test graft: heart and kidney are vascularised as soon as implanted, whereas skin grafts are not vascularised for several days in the technique used here. Particularly impressive was the ability of a liver graft to terminate a vigorous rejection reaction already well advanced in a distant organ.[64] This effect is unique and could not be reproduced by massive doses of cyclosporin A. In half the rats receiving a DA heart graft followed by a DA liver graft 5–6 days later, the liver itself was rejected while the heart recovered. This was perhaps the least predictable result, since under normal circumstances the liver survives, and rejection in the heart was already in progress at the time of liver grafting. The rejection of the liver can be explained by the sensitisation produced by heart grafting.

The rate of suppression of rejection, its specificity and occurrence in vascularised grafts only, suggest the involvement of a soluble, antigen specific suppressive agent released by the transplanted liver and carried in the bloodstream. A likely candidate is free RT1 donor antigen (see below). However, this does leave unresolved the problem of why the apparently powerful suppressive effect is not exerted locally in the liver itself. An alternative possibility is that alloreactive cells are in fact regularly leaving the sites of rejection to recirculate; this would make it possible for them to become trapped in the larger liver graft and depleted from other sites of rejection.

Serology of liver transplantation in the rat

Allo-antigens and allo-antibodies both appear in the serum of liver grafted rats and it is quite likely that either or both contributes to the survival of the liver itself or subsequent tissue grafts. Certainly they would have the necessary specificity for such a role. Soluble class I antigen may be responsible for rapid, reversible immunosuppression, while class II antibody may mediate permanent survival of allografts by a process of enhancement, to which the rat is particularly susceptible. Soluble mechanisms could therefore make an important contribution to liver graft survival, transplantation tolerance and suppression in this rat model, and may have potential clinical applications.

Allo-antibody responses

Antibodies against class I and class II donor antigens in sera of DA grafted PVG rats are detected by a binding assay using red cells or lymph node cells of the congenic strain PVG.RT1^a and radiolabelled sheep anti-rat immunoglobulin.[52] The antibody response against class I (RT1A^a) allo-antigens in this non-rejector combination reached a peak during the first two weeks after liver grafting, but the titre was at all times low, with an endpoint of less than 1:50 serum dilution. Thereafter, the serum anti-class I level declined and by six weeks had returned to pretransplantation levels (Figure 12.6). In PVG rats sensitised against DA antigens by skin grafting and surviving for more than 100 days after DA liver grafting, the effect of a liver graft was first to restimulate and then to depress very significantly the anti-class I response.

In contrast, the response to class II RT1B^{a}D^a antigens in normal PVG recipients of a DA liver graft was slow to start, but then rose over a period of several weeks to titres of over 1:1000 (Figure 12.7 *above*). Thereafter, the anti-class II level remained high for some time, and only started to decline after three months. In presensitised PVG recipients with long term survival after DA liver grafting, a typical secondary response was seen, with a more rapid appearance and higher peak levels; serum titres were again maintained at a

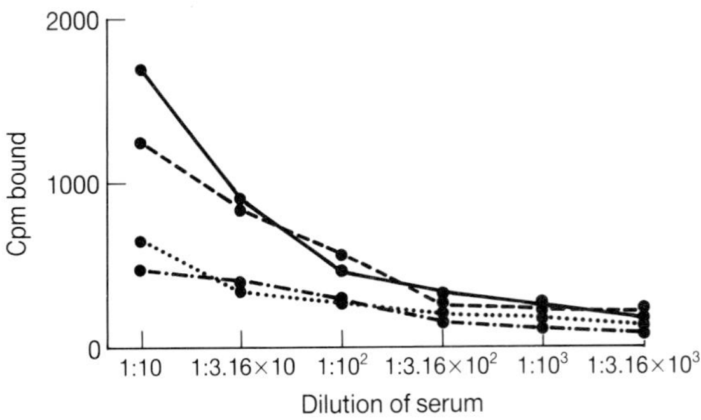

Fig. 12.6 Antibody response to class I RT1^a antigens in a normal PVG recipient of a DA liver graft (rat 976). Sera were taken one week (———), two weeks) (– – –), four weeks (····) and six weeks (–·–·–) after liver transplantation and assayed by titration against PVG.RT1^a red cells, with detection by ^{125}I-labelled sheep anti-rat Ig. Bar indicates background of assay.[52]

high level much longer than the anti-class I antibodies (Figure 12.7 *below*).

A drawback of using serum titres as an indicator of response is that the grafted liver will act as an antigen adsorbent and remove an amount of antibody from the circulation which may be hard to quantitate. Nevertheless, it seems clear that class I and class II antigens in DA liver are both immunogenic in PVG and can stimulate primary and secondary responses, but with major differences in strength and duration of response against the two classes of molecule. The anti-class I response is the weaker of the two and shows a close correlation with the establishment of transplantation tolerance, while the anti-class II response is considerably greater both in level and duration. The fall-off in anti-class I response might indicate loss of RT1A antigens from the graft or their blocking by antibody; however, the failure to detect any trace of a secondary anti-class I response after skin grafting liver transplanted rats[52] indicates the induction of tolerance or specific immunosuppression. In contrast, primary antibody responses to $RT1B^a/D^a$ antigens after liver grafting reach considerably greater serum titres and start to decline only in the fourth month after transplantation.

These serological findings mirror the state of split or partial tolerance seen in T cell mediated responses. Thus, to judge from the disappearance of antibody, tolerance in the anti-class I response seems to occur about three weeks after liver grafting; in contrast, the anti-class II response continues to increase. One can speculate that T cells responsible for delivering help to B cells in the antibody response to class I allo-antigens may be among those deleted by the liver graft. The high levels of anti-class II antibody which follow liver grafting in this combination may contribute to the survival of the liver graft itself, or to that of subsequent tissue grafts, by enhancement mechanisms (see below).

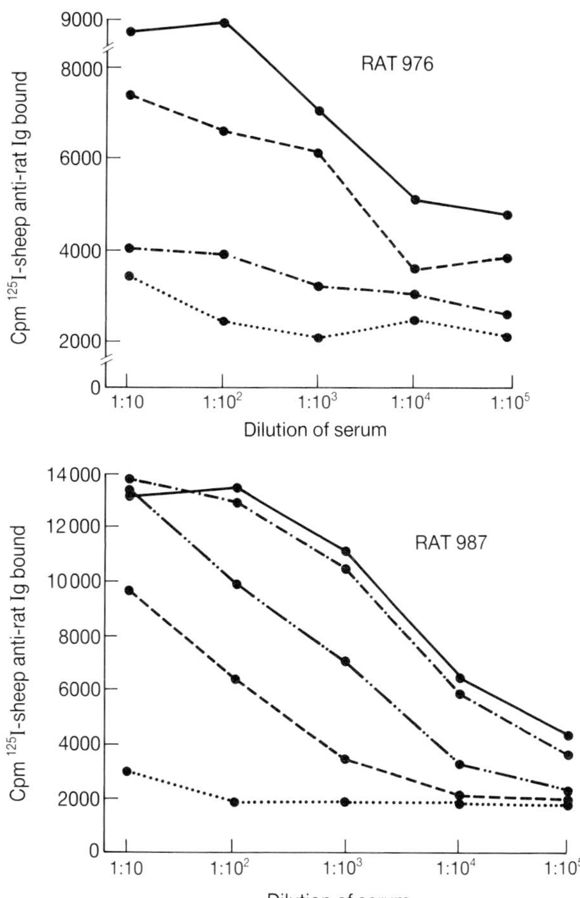

Fig. 12.7 *Above* Antibody response to class II $RT1^a$ antigens in a normal PVG recipient of a DA liver graft (rat 976). Sera were taken one week (· · · ·), two weeks (–·–·–), four weeks (– – – –) and six weeks (———) after liver transplantation and assayed by titration against PVG.$RT1^a$ lymph node cells, with detection by ^{125}I-labelled sheep anti-rat Ig. (The background in this assay, indicated by bar, is due to binding of the labelled anti-Ig reagent to rat B cells.) *Below* Antibody response to class II $RT1^a$ antigens in a PVG rat (987) sensitised by DA skin grafting and transplanted with a DA liver four weeks later. Sera shown were taken immediately before (· · · · ·) and one week (— ——), two weeks (–···–···), six weeks (———) and ten weeks (–·–·–) after liver grafting. Assay as above.

Donor transplantation antigen in recipient serum after liver grafting

A soluble form of class I antigen has been found in serum, lymph and urine of different animal species and man.[81–86] The heavy chain of the soluble form is smaller by some 5 KDa than that of the membrane molecule and is also associated with β_2-microglobulin.[85] Soluble class I antigen with these properties has been isolated in quantity from aqueous rat liver extracts[87] and it seems that the liver may be one principal source of the serum antigen. The origin of the molecule is uncertain;[88] alternative splicing of the class I mRNA may remove the transmembrane and cytoplasmic anchoring domains[89] or it may be derived by proteolytic cleavage of the membrane bound form. The level of soluble class I in the circulation is low (about 350 ng/ml in DA serum) and its half-life short (2.5 hours).[85] The physiological role of such material is unclear. The fact that the liver is a major source of soluble class I[87] has suggested that it may be involved in the immunosuppressive properties of liver grafting (see below), and more generally in establishment of self tolerance.[90]

The presence of free RT1A antigen in the serum of DA liver grafted PVG rats was demonstrated by inhibition of binding of a labelled monoclonal anti-RT1A^a antibody (R3/13)[91] to DA red cells or lymphocytes.[43,44] Inhibitory activity at a level comparable with that of normal DA serum was present within a few days after grafting (Figure 12.8). In the example shown, the binding of labelled R3/13 was specifically blocked

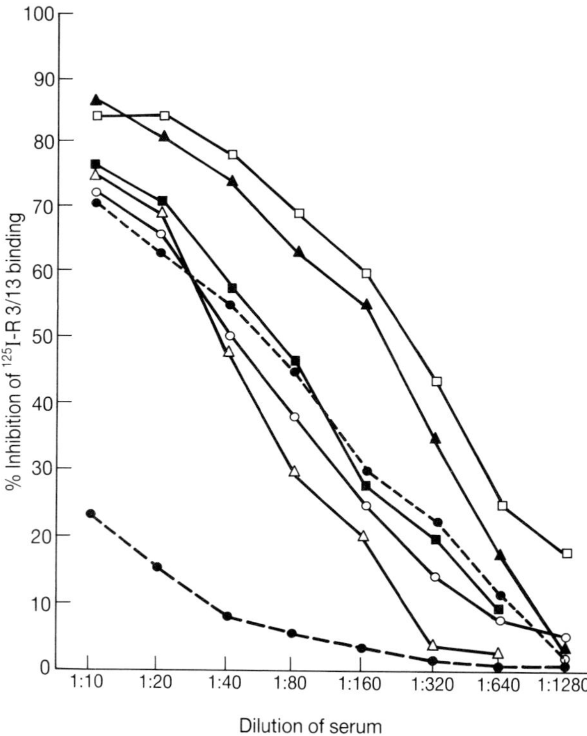

Fig. 12.8 Class I blocking activity of liver graft sera. Inhibition of binding of ^{125}I-labelled R3/13 to DA red cells by normal DA (·-------) or PVG serum (·—·—) and by sera of PVG rat 976 taken one week (○—○—), two weeks (△—△—), four weeks (▲—▲—), six weeks (□—□—) and 14 weeks (■—■—) after receiving a DA liver graft.

by normal DA serum with an endpoint of 1:50–1:100; the same inhibitory endpoint was achieved by one week after liver transplantation and never fell significantly below this level during 14 weeks of observation. Molecular sizing of the inhibitor in normal DA serum by gel filtration was consistent with it being the free, monomeric form of RT1A^a, while in liver graft sera some of the antigen was self-aggregated or complexed with antibody. Since inhibitory material was removed by passage through columns of R3/13, but not by anti-rat Ig, antibody and immune complexes do not seem to play a major part in the inhibition.[44,78]

Free circulating class I RT1 antigen could play an important role in the complex picture of immunosuppression and tolerance which follows liver grafting in the DA–PVG combination. Recently, we investigated a role for soluble class I antigen in suppression of cardiac allograft rejection, by *in vivo* administration of donor serum before and after removal of class I antigen.[92–94]

Soluble class I antigen was demonstrated in normal DA serum by RIA to an end point of 1:16. Passage through an anti-RT1A^a monoclonal antibody (mAb) column (YR1/100) was found to be effective in removing all class I activity. The material eluted from this column at pH 11.5 was highly enriched in class I activity (endpoint 1:128) (Figure 12.9). Class I antigen was also purified from DA liver homogenates by papain digestion of the membrane fraction, followed by affinity chromatography on the mAb anti-class I column.

In the first experiment, PVG rats received a graft of PVG.RT1^a heart in the neck with continuous infusion from day O of Hartman's solution (control), normal DA serum or DA serum depleted of class I antigen (Table 12.4).[93] In control animals, grafts were rejected in nine days or less (MST 8.2±0.7 and 8.0±0.4 days respectively). Continuous infusion of normal DA serum (2 ml per day) from day O led to prolongation of graft survival in all animals, with rejection delayed up to day 13 (MST 11.4±1.5 days). In contrast, serum depleted of class I antigen had no effect on graft survival (MST 8.0±0.7 days). Continuous serum infusion was then delayed until four days after grafting, a time at which rejection would be in progress. Once again, normal DA serum was able to prolong survival in most animals (7/11), two carrying a beating graft for 15 days (MST 10.9±2.5). The effect of DA serum was allo-antigen specific, as third party grafts (WAG) were not significantly prolonged. Re-

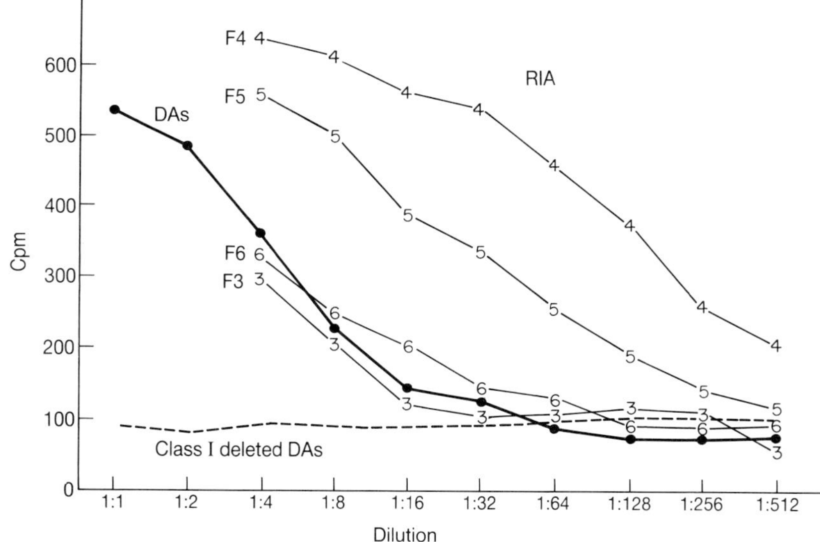

Fig. 12.9 Purification of class I antigen from DA serum and liver homogenates. Fractions were eluted from the YR1/100 anti-RT1a[a] mAb column after the passage of DA serum or DA liver homogenates. The level of class I antigen in different fractions (3–6) was determined by two-site radio-immunoassay (RIA). Fraction 4 (from liver homogenate) contained a class I concentration 30–40 times that of DA serum. Passage of DA serum through the column completely removed class I material.[94]

Table 12.4 Effect of donor serum, class I antigen and monoclonal anti-class I antibody on survival of allogeneic (PVG.RT1[a]) heart grafts in PVG rats

Group	Treatment	Starting day	Survival of individual rats (days)	MST ± S.D.	P
1	Untreated control	–	7,7,8,8,8,8,8,8,9,9	8.1 ± 0.7	
2	Hartman's solution by continuous infusion, 4 ml/day	0	7,8,8,8,8,9	8.0 ± 0.4	ns
3	Normal DA serum, daily injection of 2 ml	0	8,8,8,8,9,9	8.3 ± 0.5	ns
4	Normal DA serum, continuous infusion, 2 ml/day	0	10,10,10,11,13,13,13	11.4 ± 1.5	<0.01
5	Normal DA serum, continuous infusion, 2 ml/day	4	8,8,8,9,10,11,11,12,13,15,15	10.9 ± 2.5	<0.01
6	Normal DA serum after removal of class I antigen, continuous infusion, 2 ml/day	0	7,8,8,8,9	8.0 ± 0.7	ns
7	Normal DA serum after removal of class I antigen, continuous infusion, 2 ml/day	4	8,8,8,9,9,11	8.8 ± 1.1	ns
8	Purified soluble class I antigen from DA liver, continuous infusion, 700 ng/day	4	8,8,11,11,11,11	10.0 ± 1.5	0.05
9	Monoclonal anti-class I antibody R3/13, 10 μg/day, continuous infusion	4	8,8,8,8,9,11	8.6 ± 1.2	ns
10	Normal DA serum, 2 ml/day, and R3/13, 10 μg/day	4	12,13,13,15,16,23,24	15.6 ± 3.0	<0.001

No prolongation of survival of third party (WAG) grafts was obtained. Data from [78].

moval of class I antigen from DA serum again abolished its ability to prolong survival of PVG.RT1[a] heart grafts (MST 8.8±1.1 days).

The effect of purified soluble class I antigen was investigated by infusion, from day four after grafting, at an estimated equal concentration to that of DA serum (see Table 12.4).[93] This induced a modest but significant prolongation of graft survival (MST 10.0±1.5 days). The effect of complexing class I antigen with anti-class I mAb was particularly striking; infusion of DA serum from day four in combination with mAb R3/13 was the most effective graft prolonging regimen (MST 15.6±3.0 days).

These results directly support a role for soluble class I antigen in MHC specific immunosuppression. With the amount of antigen used the suppression was temporary, leading to a significant delay in rejection rather than permanent acceptance. The levels of class I antigen achieved in the recipient may be at about the threshold of effectiveness; alternatively, the fact that the graft combination was fully MHC incompatible leaves open the possibility of rejection via recognition of class II antigens. It is noteworthy that class I antigen administration could be delayed until rejection was already initiated, four days after grafting, and remained almost as effective as when infused from the outset. The explanation we favour for the phenomenon is blocking of the recognition of class I antigen on the graft by class I reactive CTL; recent experiments in this laboratory have demonstrated inhibition of T cell cytotoxicity by affinity purified class I antigen *in vitro*. The possibility that free antigen contributes to the elimination of class I reactive T cells in liver graft recipients should also be considered, for example, by opsonisation of alloreactive T cells by complexes of RT1A antigen and anti-RT1A antibody.[95]

In contrast, Spencer and Fabre[87] failed to find any evidence that soluble class I liver antigen administered as a single injection at the time of grafting or at intervals thereafter prolonged graft survival, using the same DA–PVG combination as here. The short half-life of the class I molecule in the circulation (about 1.5–2.5 hours) may well explain the ineffectiveness of this mode of antigen administration. The use of continuous pumped infusion of donor serum, rather than bolus inoculation, probably played a significant part in revealing the effect of class I antigen in our experiments and will make it possible in future to explore further the suppressive effect of purified MHC antigen *in vivo*.

In summary, soluble liver derived antigen is likely to be a mediator of the striking immunosuppressive effects of liver grafting described above and perhaps of the induction of systemic tolerance as well. The observation that complexes with monoclonal antibody are more potent than class I alone suggests a practical means whereby class I tolerance might be induced. Soluble MHC antigens may contribute to the goal of securing donor specific unresponsiveness in human graft recipients.

Immunosuppression by lymph from liver grafted rats

In these experiments, the effect on graft rejection of passive transfer of lymph from liver grafted rats was studied.[96] In contrast to the permanent enhancement brought about by liver graft serum (see below), the results with lymph transfer indicated a reversible interference with early stages of sensitisation of the recipients.

Thoracic duct lymph was taken from PVG rats 30–60 days after grafting of DA liver (OLT lymph), when tolerance of DA was fully established. Inoculations of 2–3 ml daily were given to PVG recipients via the tail vein, starting on the day of grafting with skin, kidney or heart. When lymph was injected for 28 days into skin grafted PVG rats, DA grafts but not third party (AO) grafts had a considerably prolonged survival; MST were 38.9±2.0 days (DA skin, lymph inoculated), 8.4±0.5 days (AO skin, lymph inoculated) and 8.2±0.4 days (DA skin, no lymph inoculation). The DA grafts remained intact for as long as OLT lymph was administered, but acute rejection commenced a few days after lymph transfer was terminated, with a time course similar to a first set reaction. There were some signs of destructive attack on the graft – loss of hair and atrophy – during the period of lymph administration, but the epithelium remained intact. Controls of lymph from isografted rats (PVG liver into PVG) had no effect on survival of skin grafts. Essentially the same results were obtained with fully allogeneic DA renal or heterotopic heart grafts, which also survived until lymph treatment was terminated, when they were rejected with a first set time course.

Thus, lymph from liver allografted PVG rats transfers suppression of graft rejection to normal PVG recipients which is specific for the antigens of the liver donor, short term and reversible, lasting for the period of lymph administration. Such suppression may be due to prevention of sensitisation of the recipient (afferent inhibition). Lymph did not induce the tolerance which follows liver transplantation itself or enhancement by OLT serum, as described below. Antibody, antigen and complexes are candidates as specific immunosuppressive agents; antibody (anti-MHC or anti-idiotypic) would seem to be the most likely in lymph, though the presence of free or complexed DA antigens cannot be discounted. However, as noted above, the effects of lymph differ markedly from the enhancement produced by anti-class II antibody. Free antigen is unlikely to be the sole agent since repeated attempts to prolong survival of DA grafts with lymph from DA isografted rats were unsuccessful. Thus at present the nature of the immunosuppressive agent in lymph is unresolved.

Graft enhancement by serum from liver grafted rats

The strong anti-class II allo-antibody response which follows liver grafting in the DA–PVG combination may be central to the survival of the liver graft and transplantation tolerance, since anti-class II antibodies are potent mediators of enhancement in the rat.[66,97,98] We have investigated the enhancing effects of liver graft serum, notably its ability to bring about permanent survival of allogeneic heart grafts in PVG recipients and induce systemic transplantation tolerance.

Immunological enhancement: background

The prolongation of the survival of foreign grafts by the action of antibody[97–99] can be achieved in two ways. In passive enhancement, the recipient is given antibodies against the MHC incompatibilities of the graft at the time of transplantation or soon afterwards; in active enhancement, the recipient is immunised with donor cells or tissue extracts some time before transplantation. Passive enhancement can suppress graft rejection to varying degrees in different models and has generated much interest in its possible clinical application as a means of donor specific immunosuppression. The rat is the species in which most enhancement work has been carried out, especially since the microsurgical techniques for organ grafting in that species were developed. However, understanding of the mechanisms is still incomplete and research in suitable animal models is vital to the potential future promise of enhancement as a clinically viable technique.

In the current picture of the immunology of passive enhancement, two phases are distinguished.[97,99] During an early 'induction phase', antibodies against the MHC antigens of the graft effectively suppress the development of a primary immune response, including antibody production and CTL, either by masking donor antigens, removing passenger lymphocytes, especially dendritic cells,[55] or opsonising host lymphocytes by antibody/antigen complexes.[95] The later, prolonged maintenance phase of enhancement is characterised by development of specific unresponsiveness in the host, such that further grafts from the same donor may be accepted without further treatment.[97] CTL responses seem to be selectively inhibited, while MLR and GVH reactivity can remain intact. IgG antibodies against class II antigens are effective in enhancement induction[98,100] and it is doubtful whether enhancement can be brought about without such antibodies where a class II incompatibility exists. The reason they are so effective reflects the role of class II antigens in induction of rejection reactions. Interaction of helper and cytotoxic T cell (CTL) subsets seems to be required in generating rejection. CTL recognise class I antigens on the graft, followed by killing of graft cells. Helper T cells are required for CTL induction; they recognise class II antigens on dendritic cells and release the IL-2 required for CTL proliferation. Thus, in this scenario, the action of enhancing antibody is to prevent recognition of class II antigens by helper T cells, inhibiting IL-2 release and CTL development. The mechanisms suggested for the maintenance phase include antibody blocking factors, clonal deletion of host T cell subsets, suppressor T cells, and loss of graft antigenicity.

Enhancement by serum of liver grafted rats

A model for enhancement of heart allografts in the rat using serum from PVG rats tolerised by DA liver grafts has been established.[101] PVG rats received semi-allogeneic or fully allogeneic heart grafts from (DAxPVG)F_1 or PVG.RT1[a] donors respectively and were treated with varying amounts of serum from liver graft recipients (OLT serum) or its purified IgG fraction. The serum came from PVG recipients of DA liver grafts sacrificed 2–4 months after liver transplantation. In initial experiments, (PVGxDA)F_1 heart grafts were rejected by PVG rats in 10.9±2.4 days, but inoculation of 0.5 ml OLT serum immediately after heart grafting led to permanent acceptance of the graft in 5/7 recipients.

In the fully allogeneic combination of PVG.RT1[a] hearts grafted into PVG, the behaviour of PVG.RT1[a] grafts is identical to that of DA, with which they share RT1 haplotype. Different amounts of OLT serum were inoculated intravenously into heart graft recipients immediately after grafting. The effect on graft survival was dose dependent (Figure 12.10). Thus, permanent survival in 11/11 animals was produced by 1 ml of serum; 0.5 ml caused permanent acceptance of the heart graft in 10/14 recipients, the MST in the remaining four being 21±7.1 days; with 0.25 ml serum, no heart grafts were accepted permanently but all showed significantly increased survival times (MST 16.3±1.8 days compared with control of 8.4±0.5 days). The specific nature of the effect was shown by third party (WAG) heart grafts, the survival of which on PVG recipients was not improved by 1 ml liver graft serum. Enhancement was not induced by normal DA serum or serum taken from PVG rats four weeks after DA skin grafting. IgG from the OLT serum pool showed the same enhancing properties as whole serum. Removal of anti-class I antibodies did not alter the result, supporting the view that class II antibodies present in OLT serum in high titre are the principal agents of enhancement.[101] OLT serum was also highly effective in enhancing survival of renal allografts in the same combination, 1 ml of serum given at the time of grafting causing long term survival of PVG.RT1[a] kidney grafts in eight out of eight PVG recipients.[102]

The responsiveness of PVG rats with permanently surviving PVG.RT1[a] heart grafts after enhancement by OLT serum was tested by grafting PVG.RT1[a] and WAG skin (Figure 12.11). PVG.RT1[a] skin grafts were accepted permanently by all the enhanced rats, while third party skin grafts on the same rats were rejected acutely. Thus, enhancement leads to specific, systemic transplantation tolerance.

Antibody levels against class I and class II RT1[a] antigens were assayed in normal and enhanced PVG recipients of PVG.RT1[a] heart grafts 80 days after grafting.[101] In normal recipients, where heart grafts were rejected within nine days, good alloantibody responses to class I and class II antigens were still present at 80 days, the titres for both being in the range of 1:100–1:1000 serum dilution. In rats in which heart graft survival was enhanced by OLT serum, the class I response was markedly reduced, being barely detectable in some cases and with a maximum endpoint of about 1:10 in others; the anti-class II response was seemingly unaffected and was maintained at a high level after enhancement. Thus, the tolerant state of

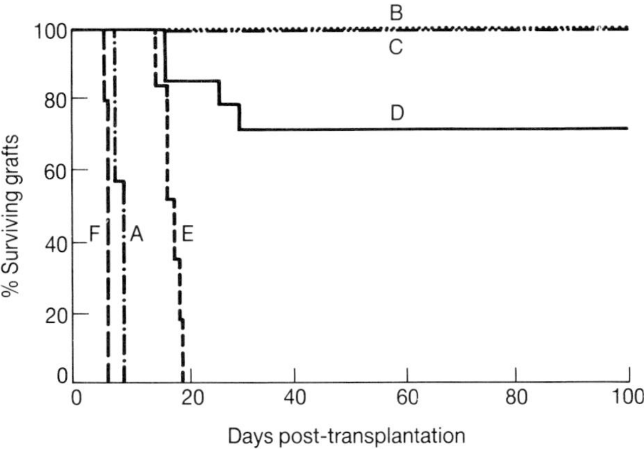

Fig. 12.10 Enhancement of survival of PVG.RT1[a] heterotopic heart grafts on PVG recipients by liver graft serum. Survival of PVG.RT1[a] heart grafts (A) on untreated PVG recipients; (B) on PVG rats given 1 ml liver graft serum immediately after grafting; (C) on PVG rats given 0.5 ml liver graft serum immediately after grafting and 0.5 ml two days later; (D) on PVG rats given 0.5 ml liver graft serum immediately after grafting; and (E) on PVG rats given 0.25 ml liver graft serum immediately after grafting. (F) Survival of WAG (third party) heterotopic heart grafts on PVG rats given 1 ml liver graft serum immediately after grafting. The same pool of serum, from PVG rats carrying DA liver transplants, was used throughout.[101]

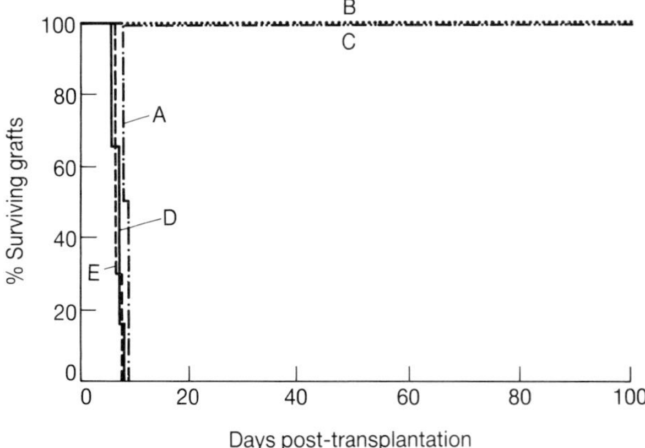

Fig. 12.11 Survival of skin grafts on PVG rats carrying long term surviving PVG.RT1[a] heterotopic heart grafts. Survival of PVG.RT1[a] heterotopic heart grafts for 80 days, the survival of the heart grafts having been enhanced by 1 ml liver graft serum; (c) on PVG rats carrying PVG.RT1[a] heterotopic heart grafts for 80 days, the survival of the hearts having been enhanced by 12 mg liver graft IgG. Survival of WSG skin grafts (d) on normal PVG rats and (e) on PVG rats carrying PVG.RT1[a] heterotopic heart grafts for 80 days, the survival of the heart grafts having been enhanced by 1 ml liver graft serum.[101]

these animals is also reflected in their anti-class I, but not in their anti-class II allo-antibody responses.

These experiments demonstrated that passive transfer of OLT serum or its purified IgG fraction enhances survival of allogeneic PVG.RT1^{a} heart and kidney grafts in PVG recipients. At the highest doses of serum used (1 ml per recipient), heart and kidney grafts took permanently. The anti-class II antibody content of the serum was 50–100 μg per ml; thus, to secure permanent acceptance of a heart graft in this combination requires about 50 μg of antibody, while 25 μg produces a significant prolongation. This indicates that a circulating level of 5–10 μg anti-class II antibody per ml leads to permanent acceptance of a PVG.RT1^{a} heart graft in a PVG rat. The effectiveness of anti-class II antibodies in enhancement of allografts in the rat is well recognised.[98,100] The unresponsiveness associated with enhancement was not confined to the grafted heart; PVG rats with long term surviving PVG.RT1^{a} heart grafts were systemically tolerant of RT1^{a} antigens, as demonstrated by permanent specific acceptance of RT1^{a} skin grafts. Transplantation tolerance has been demonstrated in several rat combinations following enhancement[98,103] and is regarded as part of the maintenance phase.[98,99]

Cellular mechanisms of enhancement by OLT serum

We have recently demonstrated a direct effect of exposure to OLT serum on alloreactive TDL. Normal PVG lymphocytes were incubated with PVG anti-DA OLT serum *in vitro*, followed by transfer into irradiated, skin grafted PVG recipients (Table 12.5).[104] A specific reduction in allograft reactivity against DA was seen in the prolongation of survival of DA skin grafts (MST 15.3±2.1 days) but not of WAG grafts (9.3±0.9). This represents a highly significant, though partial, deletion of DA reactive cells, possibly through opsonisation by class I antigen/antibody complexes.

Recently, we have attempted to evaluate further the cellular basis of unresponsiveness during enhancement using the adoptive transfer assay (Table 12.6).[102] TDL were obtained from normal PVG rats ('normal TDL') or PVG recipients carrying a PVG.RT1^{a} heart graft for more than 60 days following inoculation of 1 ml OLT serum ('enhanced TDL'). Cells were injected into irradiated PVG recipients which also received a heterotopic heart graft from PVG.RT1^{a} or WAG donors. Irradiated recipients without TDL administration did not reject heart grafts over a 60 day period, but transfer of 5x10^{7} normal TDL restored the time to rejection to 11.3±0.8 days and 10.6±0.5 days for PVG.RT1^{a} and WAG grafts respectively. When the same number of enhanced TDL were injected, no rejection of PVG.RT1^{a} grafts occurred over the 60 day observation period (6/6 recipients), whereas WAG grafts were again rejected rapidly (10.7±0.5 days). Thus, enhanced TDL behaved as though functionally and specifically unresponsive to RT1^{a} antigens.

Irradiated recipients were also given a mixture of 5x10^{7} normal and 5x10^{7} enhanced TDL, and

Table 12.5 Adoptive transfer assay: survival of DA and WAG skin grafts on irradiated PVG rats following transfer of PVG TDL treated with normal or OLT sera

TDL transferred	Skin graft	Graft survival times in individual rats (days)	MST ± SD
None	DA	21,23,23,25,25,26,27,27,30,31,34	26.5 ± 3.7
	WAG	20,21,22,24,25,25,28,29,30,32,33	26.2 ± 4.2
PVG, normal untreated	DA	8,9,9,9,10,10,10	9.2 ± 0.7
	WAG	8,8,9,9,9,10,10	9.0 ± 0.7
PVG, pre-incubated in normal PVG serum	DA	8,8,9,9,10	8.8 ± 0.7
	WAG	8,8,9,9,9	8.6 ± 0.5
PVG, pre-incubated in OLT serum	DA	12,13,14,14,14,16,16,17,18,19	15.3 ± 2.1
	WAG	8,8,9,9,9,9,10,10,10,11	9.3 ± 0.9
PVG, pre-incubated in normal DA serum	DA	8,8,9,9,11	9.0 ± 1.1
	WAG	8,8,8,9,10	8.6 ± 0.8

PVG thoracic duct lymphocytes (TDL) were incubated at a concentration of 2.5 × 10^{7}/ml in either normal PVG serum, serum from PVG recipients of DA liver grafts (OLT serum) or normal DA serum, prior to adoptive transfer into irradiated (850 rad) PVG recipients. The latter were given grafts of DA or WAG skin and the rate of skin graft rejection was recorded. Data from [96].

Table 12.6 Adoptive transfer assay of TDL from recipients of cardiac allografts enhanced by OLT serum

Group	TDL transferred	Heart graft donor	Graft survival times in individual rats (days)	MST ± SD
1	None	PVG.RT1[a]	33, >60 (10 animals)	>60
		WAG	>60 (6 animals)	>60
2	5×10^7 normal TDL	PVG.RT1[a]	10,10,11,11,12,12,12,12	11.3 ± 0.8
		WAG	10,10,10,11,11,11	10.6 ± 0.5
3	5×10^7 enhanced TDL	PVG.RT1[a]	>60 (6 animals)	>60
		WAG	10,10,11,11,11,11	10.7 ± 0.5
4	5×10^7 normal TDL plus 5×10^7 enhanced TDL	PVG.RT1[a]	10,17,21,22	17.5 ± 4.7
			>60, >60	>60
		WAG	10,10,11,11	10.5 ± 0.5

Normal TDL = cells from normal PVG rats. Enhanced TDL = cells from PVG rats carrying PVG.RT1[a] cardiac allografts for more than 60 days following enhancement by 1 ml OLT serum. Animals were observed for 60 days. Data from [92].

either PVG.RT1[a] or WAG heart grafts. In 5/6 animals given a PVG.RT1[a] graft, survival was significantly prolonged compared with rats given normal TDL alone: grafts in 2/6 survived for over 60 days, in three others for 17 days or more and only one was rejected within the period of animals given normal TDL. This effect was donor specific, since 4/4 WAG heart grafts were rejected at the normal tempo. This result suggests an active, donor specific suppression of rejection by enhanced TDL acting on normal TDL.

Enhancement and liver graft survival

A possible effect of passively transferred anti-class II antibodies would be to mask class II antigens in the graft and prevent recognition by helper T cells; alternatively, the antibodies might lead to removal of class II bearing interstitial dendritic cells,[55] a major immunogenic source of class II antigen in organ grafts, or to opsonisation of the class II reactive lymphocytes.[95] These last two hypotheses are difficult to accept in view of the strength of the anti-class II response in the enhanced recipients. The masking hypothesis would seem to accord best with the observations, since eventual disappearance of the enhancing antibody by shedding or metabolism would allow the anti-class II response to occur. During the period when class II antigens on the heart graft are not available, tolerance of RT1A[a] antigens is evidently induced. While it might be entirely brought about by the high level of anti-class II antibody, i.e. 'auto-enhancement', the long term survival of allogeneic skin grafts on the enhanced recipients is more compatible with cellular unresponsiveness against class I antigens, since survival of skin grafts is generally difficult to prolong to this extent by antibody alone.

When TDL from rats carrying enhanced cardiac grafts were analysed in the adoptive transfer assay (see above), they behaved as if functionally deleted for alloreactivity against RT1[a], that is, they failed to accelerate rejection of heart grafts on the irradiated hosts. They also had the ability to suppress rejection by normal TDL.[102] Suppression was specific for the RT1[a] donor type, suggesting the presence of an antigen specific suppressor cell population in enhanced TDL. Recent evidence from other groups, using similar adoptive transfer assays, indicates that donor specific T cell mediated suppression is a common feature of enhancement.[105–106] The fact that suppression of normal cells was only partial whereas enhanced TDL alone failed to reject any grafts suggests that the suppressor mechanism may be superimposed on clonal deletion of alloreactive cells. As already noted, the latter is a characteristic of TDL from tolerant liver graft recipients themselves.[70,77] We have also shown elsewhere that direct action of OLT serum on normal TDL *in vitro* leads to specific partial elimination of alloreactivity on adoptive transfer.[104]

It is clear that in many respects, the phenomena associated with enhancement after administration of OLT serum are closely similar to those in the PVG recipient of a DA liver graft. These include the induction of systemic tolerance; the presence of high levels of serum class II antibody which persist for long periods; the clonal deletion of alloreactivity from TDL; and the existence of suppressor cells. The resemblance between the serological findings following enhancement and liver grafting raises the question of whether unresponsiveness associated with the latter is perhaps antibody induced. The finding that relatively small amounts of OLT serum cause enhancement supports a role for anti-class II antibody in the maintenance of unresponsiveness after liver grafting, and possibly in its induction as well. Anti-class II antibody, presumably through interference with class II recognition by T cells of the graft recipient, is thus a key element in the maintenance both of liver graft induced tolerance and serum induced enhancement.

References

1. Calne RY (ed). *Liver Transplantation. The Cambridge King's College Hospital Experience.* London: Grune and Stratton, 1983.
2. Kamada N. *Experimental Liver Transplantation.* Boca Raton, Florida: CRC Press, 1988.
3. Welch CS. A note on transplantation of the whole liver in dogs. *Transpl Bull* 1955; **2,** 54.
4. Goodrich EO, Welch HF, Nelson JA *et al.* Homotransplantation of the canine liver. *Surgery* 1956; **39,** 244.
5. Moore FD, Smith LL, Burnap TK *et al.* One stage homotransplantation of the liver following total hepatectomy in dogs. *Transplant Bull* 1959; **6,** 103.
6. Moore FD, Wheeler HB, Demissianos HV *et al.* Experimental whole organ transplantation of the liver and of the spleen. *Ann Surg* 1960; **152,** 374.
7. Starzl TE, Bernhard VM, Cortes N, Benvenuto R. A technique for one-stage hepatectomy in dogs. *Surgery* 1959; **46,** 880.
8. Starzl TE, Kaupp HA, Brock DR *et al.* Reconstructive problems in canine liver homotransplantation with special reference to the postoperative role of hepatic venous flow. *Surg Gyn Obstet* 1960; **111,** 733.
9. Garnier H, Clot JP, Chomette G. Orthotopic transplantation of the porcine liver. *Surg Gynec Obstet* 1970; **130,** 105.
10. Peacock JH, Terblanche J. Orthotopic homotransplantation of the liver in the pig. In: *The Liver*, Read AE (ed). London: Butterworths, 1967.
11. Calne RY, White HJO, Yoffa DE *et al.* Observation of orthotopic liver transplantation in the pig. *Br Med J* 1967; **2,** 478.
12. Calne RY. Technique in the pig. In: *Liver Transplantation: The Cambridge–King's College Hospital Experience*, Calne RY (ed). London: Grune and Stratton, 1983.
13. Calne RY, Davis DR, Pena JR *et al.* Hepatic allografts and xenografts in primates. *Lancet* 1970; **i,** 103–108.
14. Myburgh JA, Smit JA, Mieny CJ, Mason JA. Hepatic allotransplantation in the baboon. III The effects of imunosuppression and administration of donor-specific antigen after transplantation. *Transplantation* 1971; **12,** 202.
15. Lee S, Edgington TS. Heterotopic liver transplantation using inbred rat strains. *Am J Path* 1968; **52,** 649.
16. Korto WJ, Wolff ED, Eastham WN. Heterotopic auxiliary liver transplantation in rats. *Transplantation* 1971; **12,** 415–420.
17. Hess F, Jerusalem C, van der Heyde NM. Advantages of auxiliary liver homotransplantation in rats. *Arch Surg* 1972; **104,** 76.
18. Lee S, Charter AC, Chandler JG, Orloff MJ. A technique for orthotopic liver transplantation in the rat. *Transplantation* 1973; **16,** 664–667.
19. Lee S, Charter AC, Orloff MJ. Simplified technique for orthotopic liver transplantation in the rat. *Am J Surg* 1975; **130,** 38–40.
20. Zimmermann FA, Butcher GW, Davies HS *et al.* Techniques for orthotopic liver transplantation in the rat and some studies of the immunologic responses to fully allogeneic liver grafts. *Transplant Proc* 1979; **11,** 571–577.
21. Kamada N, Calne RY. A surgical experience with 530 liver transplants in the rat. *Surgery* 1983; **93,** 64–69.
22. Cordier G, Garnier H, Clot JP *et al.* La greffe de foie orthotopique chez le porc; premiers resultats. *Mem Acad Chir* 1965; **92,** 27.
23. Garnier H, Clot JP, Bertrand M *et al.* Liver transplantation in the pig: surgical approach. *Seances Acad Sci* (Paris) 1965; **260,** 5621–5623.
24. Calne RY, White HJO, Yoffa DE *et al.* Prolonged survival of liver transplants in the pig. *Br Med J* 1967; **4,** 645–648.
25. Calne RY. Allografting in the pig. In: *Immunological Aspects of Transplantation Surgery*, Calne RY (ed). Lancaster: MTP, 1973.
26. Kamada N. The immunology of experimental liver transplantation in the rat. *Immunology* 1985; **55,** 369.
27. Limmer J, Herbertson BM, Calne RY. Orthotopic rat liver transplantation using different combinations of four inbred strains. *Eur Surg Res* 1980; **12,** 343–348.
28. Ulrichs K, Engemann R, Thiede A, Muller-Ruchholtz W. Allograft tolerance in rats with orthotopic liver transplants: advantages of rearterialization. *Eur Surg Res* 1981; **13,** 79.
29. Lee S, Skivolocki WP, Fernande-Cruz L *et al.* Influence of portal vein arterialisation on liver regeneration in a double liver rat biopsy model. *Eur Surg Res* 1981; **13,** 17.
30. Engemann R, Ulrichs K, Thiede A *et al.* Value of a physiological liver transplant model in rats. Induction of specific graft tolerance in a fully

allogeneic strain combination. *Transplantation* 1982; **33,** 566–568.
31. Hasuike Y, Monden M, Valdivia LA *et al.* A simple method for orthotopic liver transplantation with arterial reconstruction in rats. *Transplantation* 1988; **45,** 830.
32. Howden B, Jablonski P, Grossman H, Marshall VC. The importance of the hepatic artery in rat liver transplantation. *Transplantation* 1989; **47,** 428.
33. Gassel HJ, Engemann R. Preservation of rat liver grafts. *Transplantation* 1987; **44,** 726–727.
34. Isai H, Miyata M, Miyakawa A *et al.* Angiographic evidence of collateral rearterialisation of the grafted liver in the rat. *Transplant Proc* 1989; **21,** 2463–2465.
35. Hickman R, Engelbrecht GHC, Duminy FJ. A technique for liver transplantation in the rat. *Transplantation* 1989; **48,** 1080.
36. Kamada N, Sumimoto R, Kaneda K. The value of hepatic artery reconstruction as a technique in rat liver transplantation. *Surgery* 1991; in press.
37. Hess F. Liver transplantation. In: *Microsurgery Experimental Techniques in the Rat and Clinical Applications*, Marguart, Hess F, Kort, Botckx (eds). Ghent: European Press, 1976.
38. Houssin D, Gigou M, Franco D *et al.* Specific transplantation tolerance induced by spontaneously tolerated liver allograft in inbred strains of rat. *Transplantation* 1980; **29,** 418–419.
39. Cortese Hassett AL, Misra DN, Kunz HW, Gill TJ III. The major histocompatibility complex of the rat. In: *Immunogenetics of the Major Histocompatibility Complex*, Srivastava R, Ram BP, Tyle P (eds). New York: VCH Publishers, 1991.
40. Butcher GW, Howard JC. The MHC of the laboratory rat, Rattus norvegicus. In: *Handbook of Experimental Immunology*, Weir DM (ed). Oxford: Blackwell Scientific Publications, 1985.
41. Butcher GW, Licence DR, Roser BJ. The genetics of the graft-versus-host reaction in rats: strength of reaction against RT1A and RT1B antigens alone and in combination. *Transplant Proc.* 1981; **13,** 1375.
42. Gunther E, Stark O. At least two loci of the major histocompatibility complex can determine mixed lymphocyte stimulation in the rat. *Tissue Antigens* 1978; **11,** 465.
43. Kamada N, Brons G, Davies HS. Fully allogeneic liver grafting in rats induces a state of systemic nonreactivity to donor transplantation antigens. *Transplantation* 1980; **29,** 429–431.
44. Kamada N, Davies HS, Roser BJ. Fully allogeneic liver grafting and the induction of donor-specific unreactivity. *Transplant Proc* 1981; **13,** 837–841.
45. Kress M, Cosman D, Khoury G, Jay G. Secretion of a transplantation-related antigen. *Cell* 1983; **34,** 189–196.
46. Hart DNJ, Fabre JW. Quantitative studies on the tissue distribution of Ia and SD antigens in the DA and Lewis rat strains. *Transplantation* 1979; **27,** 110–119.
47. Hart DNJ, Fabre JW. Demonstration and characteristics of Ia-positive cells in the interstitial connective tissues of rat heart and other tissues but not brain. *J Exp Med* 1981; **154,** 347.
48. Lautenschlager I, Nyman N, Vaananen H, Lehto VP, Virtanen I, Hayry P. Antigenic and immunogenic components in rat liver. *Scand J Immunol* 1983; **17,** 61.
49. Suitters AJ, Lampert IA. Class II antigen induction in the liver of rats with graft-versus-host disease. *Transplantation* 1984; **38,** 194–196.
50. Weinberg WC, Deamant FD, Iannaccone PM. Patterns of expression of class I antigens in the tissues of congenic strains of rat. *Hybridoma* 1985; **4,** 27–36.
51. Hart DNJ, Fabre JW. Antibodies to liver-specific auto- and alloantigens after alloimmunisation with liver tissue in the rat. *Transplantation* 1981; **31,** 178–182.
52. Kamada N, Shinomiya T. Serology of liver transplantation in the rat. I Alloantibody responses and evidence for tolerance in a nonrejector combination. *Transplantation* 1986; **42,** 7.
53. Lautenschlager I, Hayry P. Expression of the major histocompatibility complex antigens on different liver cellular components in rat and man. *Scand J Immunol* 1981; **14,** 421–426.
54. Pegg DE, Taylor MJ. Immunological modification of grafts during preservation. In: *Transplantation Immunology, Clinical and Experimental*, Calne RY (ed). Oxford: Oxford University Press, 1984.
55. Hart DNJ, Fabre JW. Mechanism of induction of passive enhancement. Evidence for an interaction of enhancing antibody with donor interstitial dendritic cells. *Transplantation* 1982; **33,** 319–322.
56. Mason DW, Dallman MJ, Arthur RP, Morris PJ. Mechanisms of allograft rejection: The roles of cytotoxic T cells and delayed type hypersensitivity. *Immunol Rev* 1984; **77,** 167–184.
57. Zimmermann FA, Knoll PP, Davies HS *et al.* The fate of orthotopic liver allografts in different rat strain combinations. *Transplant Proc* 1983; **25,** 1272–1275.
58. Zimmermann FA, Davies HS, Knoll PP *et al.* Orthotopic liver allografts in the rat. The influence of strain combination in the fate of the graft. *Transplantation* 1984; **37,** 406–410.
59. McKenzie JL, Fabre JW, Morris PJ. Studies on the cross-reactivity of allosera for kidney graft enhancement in rats. *Transplantation* 1980; **30,** 9–15.

60. Butcher GW, Howard JC. Genetic control of transplant rejection. *Transplantation* 1982; **34,** 161–166.
61. Kamada N, Davies HS, Wight D *et al.* Liver transplantation in the rat: biochemical and histological evidence of complete tolerance induction in nonrejector strains. *Transplantation* 1983; **35,** 304–311.
62. Calne RY, Sells RA, Pena JR *et al.* Induction of immunological tolerance by porcine liver allografts. *Nature* 1969; **223,** 472–476.
63. Kamada N. Transplantation tolerance and immunosuppression following liver grafting in rats. *Immunol Today* 1985; **6,** 336.
64. Kamada N, Wight DGD. Antigen-specific immunosuppression induced by liver transplantation in the rat. *Transplantation* 1984; **38,** 217–221.
65. Kamada N. A description of cuff techniques for renal transplantation in the rat. Use in studies of tolerance induction during combined liver grafting. *Transplantation* 1985; **39,** 93–95.
66. Stuart FP, Weiss A, Fitch FW. Induction and maintenance of immunological enhancement. In: *Immunological Tolerance and Enhancement*, Stuart FP, Fitch FW (eds). Lancaster: MTP, 1979.
67. Engemann R, Ulrichs K, Thiede A *et al.* Value of a physiological liver transplant model in rats. Induction of specific graft tolerance in a fully allogeneic strain combination. *Transplantation* 1982; **33,** 566–568.
68. Engemann R, Ulrichs K, Thiede A *et al.* A mechanism of tolerance in arterialized rat liver transplantation. *Transplant Proc* 1983; **15,** 729–733.
69. Kamada N, Davies HS, Roser BJ. Reversal of transplantation immunity by liver grafting. *Nature* 1981; **292,** 840–842.
70. Kamada N, Shinomiya T. Clonal deletion as the mechanism of abrogation of immunological memory following liver grafting in rats. *Immunology* 1985; **55,** 85.
71. Hall BM, Dorsch SE, Roser BJ. The cellular basis of allograft rejection *in vivo*. II The nature of memory cells mediating second set heart graft rejection. *J Exp Med* 1978; **149,** 890.
72. Galmarini D, Vercesi G, Fassati LR *et al.* The value of skin allografts in the evaluation of the rejection of liver allotransplants in pigs. *Eur Surg Res* 1971; **3,** 340.
73. Homan WP, Fabre JW, Millard PR, Morris PJ. Effect of cyclosporin A upon second-set rejection of rat renal allografts. *Transplantation* 1980; **30,** 354–357.
74. Grant D, Wall W, Mimeault R *et al.* Successful small-bowel/liver transplantation. *Lancet* 1990; **335,** 181.
75. Dorsch SE, Roser BJ. The adoptive transfer of first-set allograft responses by recirculating small lymphocytes in the rat. *Aust J Exp Biol Med Sci* 1974; **52,** 33.
76. Roser BJ, Dorsch SE. The cellular basis of transplantation tolerance in the rat. *Immunol Rev* 1979; **46,** 54.
77. Davies HS, Kamada N, Roser BJ. Mechanisms of donor-specific unresponsiveness induced by liver grafting. *Transplant Proc* 1983; **15,** 831–835.
78. Roser BJ, Kamada N, Zimmermann F, Davies HS. Immunosuppressive effects of experimental liver allografts. In: *Liver Transplantation: The Cambridge–King's College Hospital Experience*, Caln RY (ed). London: Grune and Stratton, 1983.
79. Hall BM, Dorsch SE. Cells mediating allograft rejection. *Immunol Rev* 1984; **77,** 31.
80. Mason DW, Dallman MJ, Arthur RP, Morris PJ. Mechanisms of allograft rejection: the roles of cytotoxic T cells and delayed type hypersensitivity. *Immunol Rev* 1984; **77,** 167–184.
81. Van Rood JJ, van Leeuwen A, van Santen MCT. Anti-HLA-A2 inhibitor in normal human serum. *Nature* 1970; **226,** 366.
82. Callahan GN, Ferrone S, Allison JP, Reisfeld RA. Detection of H-2 antigens in serum. *Transplantation* 1975; **20,** 431.
83. Vincent C, Revillard JP. Characterisation of molecules bearing HLA determinants in serum and urine. *Transplant Proc* 1979; **11,** 1301.
84. Devlin JJ, Lew AM, Flavell RA, Coligan JE. Secretion of a soluble class I molecule encoded by the Q10 gene of the C57BL/10 mouse. *EMBO J* 1985; **4,** 369.
85. Singh PB, Brown RF, Roser BJ. Class I transplantation antigens in solution in body fluids and in the urine. *J Exp Med* 1988; **168,** 195.
86. Davies HS, Pollard SG, Calne RY. Soluble HLA antigens in the circulation of liver graft recipients. *Transplantation* 1989; **47,** 524.
87. Spencer SC, Fabre JW. Bulk purification of a naturally occurring soluble form of RT1-A class I major histocompatibility complex antigens from DA rat liver, and studies of specific immunosuppression. *Transplantation* 1987; **44,** 141.
88. Gussow D, Ploegh H. Soluble class I antigens: a conundrum with no solution? *Immunol Today* 1987; **8,** 220.
89. Krangel MS. Unusual RNA splicing generates a secreted form of HLA-A2 in a mutagenised B lymphoblastoid cell line. *EMBO J* 1985; **4,** 1205.
90. Kress M, Cosman D, Khoury G, Jay G. Secretion of a transplantation-related antigen. *Cell* 1983; **34,** 189.
91. Howard JC, Butcher GW, Licence DR *et al.* Isolation of six monoclonal antibodies against rat histocompatibility antigens: clonal competition. *Immunology* 1980 **41,** 131.

92. Sumimoto R, Kamada N. Evidence that soluble class I antigen in donor serum induces the suppression of heart allograft rejection in rats. *Immunol Letts* 1990; **26,** 81–84.
93. Sumimoto R, Kamada N. Specific suppression of allograft rejection by soluble class I antigen and complexes with monoclonal antibody. *Transplantation* 1990; **50,** 678–682.
94. Sumimoto R, Kamada N. Immunosuppressive effect of soluble class I antigen and its complexes with monoclonal antibody on advanced heart graft rejection in rats. *Transplant Proc* 1991; **23,** 86–88.
95. Hutchinson IV. Antigen-reactive cell opsonisation (ARCO) and its role in antibody-mediated immune suppression. *Immunol Revs* 1980; **49,** 167.
96. Kamada N. Transfer of specific immunosuppression of graft rejection using lymph from tolerant, liver-grafted rats. *Immunology* 1985; **55,** 241.
97. Morris PJ. Suppression of rejection of organ allografts by alloantibody. *Immunol Rev* 1980; **49,** 93.
98. Davies DAL. Enhancement. In: *Transplantation Immunology, Clinical and Experimental*, Calne RY (ed). Oxford: Oxford University Press, 1984.
99. Batchelor JR. Immune mechanisms responsible for the prolonged kidney allograft survival in immunological enhancement. *Transplant Proc* 1981; **13,** 562–565.
100. Davies DAL, Alkins BJ. What abrogates heart transplant rejection in immunological enhancement? *Nature* 1974; **247,** 294.
101. Kamada N, Shinomiya T, Tamaki T, Ishiguro K. Immunosuppressive activity of serum from liver-grafted rats. Passive enhancement of fully allogeneic heart grafts and induction of systemic tolerance. *Transplantation* 1986; **42,** 581.
102. Yamaguchi A, Kamada N. Mechanisms in passive enhancement of cardiac and renal allograft by serum from liver-grafted rats. *Immunology* 1991; **72,** 79–84.
103. Batchelor JR, Welsh KI, Burgos H. Immunological enhancement. *Transplant Proc* 1977; **9,** 931.
104. Kamada N, Sumimoto R, Baguerizo A *et al.* Mechanisms of transplantation tolerance induced by liver grafting in rats: involvement of serum factors in clonal deletion. *Immunology* 1988; **64,** 315.
105. Hall BM. Mechanisms maintaining enhancement of allografts. I Demonstration of a specific suppressor cell. *J Exp Med* 1985; **161,** 123.
106. Padberg WM, Lord RHH, Kupiec-Weglinski JW *et al.* Two phenotypically distinct populations of T cells have suppressor capabilities simultaneously in the maintenance phase of immunologic enhancement. *J Immunol* 1987; **139,** 1751.

13

The immunology of hepatic xenotransplantation

KI Welsh and TDH Cairns

Introduction

To the clinician, xenotransplantation offers an opportunity to control organ donation, in terms of availability of organs and circumstances of donation (including details of tissue antigens, etc.). To the immunologist, xenotransplantation offers the possibility of elective control over the immune response to a transplanted organ, including specific, non-toxic methods of abrogating or pre-empting that response. For both the clinician and the immunologist, key issues of physiological compatibility, ethics, and public acceptability have still to be resolved.

The immunologist requires precise determination of the response to xenografts, defined both by species and organ type. To date in experimental hepatic xenotransplantation, only a few species combinations have been investigated, but it is very likely that a number of different and disparate mechanisms will be found to contribute to similar macroscopic appearances in xenograft loss, as is the case with renal and cardiac xenotransplantation. This chapter is concerned with a description of the possible immune responses to a vascularised solid organ xenograft, including speculation on what those responses may be in the case of hepatic xenografts, and drawing where possible on existing evidence. It is also concerned with the immunophysiological and immunopathological consequences of the grafting of a liver from one species into another (what one could call graft *vs* host interactions): notably hepatic constituents and products with immune function (donor leucocytes, complement, acute phase reactants, etc.), and their interactions with recipient cells and other immune components; and the role of the liver in the metabolism of both immunoglobulin (IgG, IgA) and immune complexes.

Experience of hepatic xenotransplantation (in humans and in various animal models), and of *ex vivo* hepatic perfusion across species, has been extensively reviewed recently.[1] The relevant histological studies allow direct comparison to the circumstances of hepatic allotransplantation.

In hepatic allotransplantation the presence of donor specific antibodies (such as anti-ABO, anti-HLA) prior to transplantation does not carry the same catastrophic implication that pertains so consistently to renal allotransplantation. It is now apparent that such antibodies do, however, confer a substantial risk of graft loss within the first 30 days for anti-ABO[2], and within the first year for anti-HLA[3]. The histological features are of antibody mediated destruction, although they are different from those typical of hyperacute rejection in renal allografts lost to IgM anti-ABO (intense microvascular coagulopathy) or to IgG anti-HLA. In renal xenotransplantation the presence of IgM anti-species antibody is associated with a microvascular coagulopathy which destroys the graft,[4] while IgG anti-species antibody appears to be associated with direct endothelial and tubular epithelial destruction.[5] It has also been suggested that endothelial luminal surface in a xenograft may augment[6] or directly activate[7] recipient species complement. These patterns of rejection have been called the xenograft reaction, and xenograft loss of this timescale (minutes to hours) is used to classify the species combination as discordant.[8] A parallel is drawn therefore between allograft rejection due to pretransplant donor specific antibody, and the xenograft reaction. Just as in allotransplantation there is a difference in timescale of graft loss to pretransplant antibody between renal grafts (minutes to hours) and hepatic grafts (within 30 days), so in the few discordant combinations used in experimental hepatic xenotransplantation there is a difference between renal xenografts (minutes to hours) and hepatic (hours to days), although it is less pronounced.[9] In a discordant combination of particular interest (pig to human), isolated pig kidneys artificially perfused with human blood complete a microvascular coagulopathy within one hour.[10] In contrast, isolated pig livers, either perfused artificially[11] or connected to the circulation of patients with hepatic failure,[12] do not demonstrate a xenograft reaction within the limited period of the perfusion ($\leqq$ 8 hours). Hepatic xenotransplantation therefore offers a window through which two areas of interest can be looked at:

1. What are the effects of pretransplant donor specific antibody, if not causing a xenograft reaction or allograft hyperacute rejection?
2. How is the rest of the immune response engaged by a hepatic xenograft?

For the purposes of discussion we have divided the response into a number of stages:

Stage 1	Initial events:	Ischaemic damage Pretransplant donor specific antibody
Stage 2	Adhesion	Leucocyte/platelet adhesion to: endothelium extracellular matrix
Stage 3	Specific recognition	
Stage 4	Maturation of recipient response	
Stage 5	Effectors of the cell mediated response	
Stage 6	Effectors of the humoral response	

Stage 1: initial events

Between the taking of an organ and its transplantation, endothelium is damaged. The relationship between reperfusion, endothelium, up-regulation of surface molecules and cytokine production is

Table 13.1 Hepatic xenotransplantation: the immunological balance

For	Against
Increased resistance to: (a) cellular responses b) humoral responses c) preformed antibody	(100)n peptide a) cellular response b) humoral response c) function
Polymorphism decrease of: a) tethering/adhesion b) migration c) maturation d) targeting	(10)n carbohydrate a) cellular b) humoral c) function GVHD

now well established.[13] A major advantage of a xenotransplantation will be the ability (through elective organ retrieval) to minimise ischaemic damage. In addition, reagents which inhibit ischaemic damage (such as superoxide dismutase[14]) can be tested very easily and directly on species donor organs using *in vitro*/*ex vivo* systems.

Pretransplant donor specific antibodies, however, are likely both to enhance the process of ischaemic damage (even if not involved in immediate rejection) and to show enhanced binding to damaged/up-regulated endothelium. As an example of the latter effect, it is known that in human renal allotransplantation, IgM against the carbohydrates i/I can cause damage to the graft only in the period immediately following reperfusion.[15]

In the discordant combinations looked at, the intensity of the reaction due to pretransplant donor specific antibodies seems to vary. The results from the early years of experimental and clinical hepatic transplantation are difficult to interpret because they were dominated by problems of haemostasis and sepsis. Nevertheless the effects of antibody in pig to primate (including human) transplantation or *ex vivo* perfusion do seem to be less intense than in the various guinea pig to rat xenograft experiments that have been performed. In the latter case, grafts are lost within minutes.[16] In contrast, pig livers into baboons have survived for up to 3.5 days when transplanted without immunosuppression.[17] There was no gross immunologically mediated damage in the pig to human perfusion experiments referred to above. These observations lead to a first key point in discordant models that involve anti-species antibody: the target antigen specificities and immunoglobulin isotypes vary from one species combination to another.

Important in discussions of xenotransplantation are IgM anti-species antibodies. All mammals investigated have IgM antibodies against some other species. Such IgM is regarded as being a natural antibody, inasmuch as it is found in all normal species members tested, without apparent immunisation. It was suspected by analogy with many other natural antibodies, especially IgM anti-blood group, that the target antigens are carbohydrate. A good deal of evidence now exists to support this proposition. We have established that human IgM anti-pig binds to determinants in glycoconjugate fractions of homogenised pig kidneys, including notably glycolipids (work in collaboration with Professor Samuelsson, Gothenberg, Sweden). Other groups have also demonstrated binding of human anti-pig to pig glycoconjugate fractions.[18,19]

The xenograft reaction is centred on vascular endothelium. It has also been proposed by a number of groups that donor endothelium is activated by recipient blood, and again there is now some support for this.[20] If IgM anti-species antibody is indeed specific for carbohydrate, it is certainly possible to imagine how such antibody could result in endothelial activation, especially in light of other protein/carbohydrate interactions that trigger endothelial/haemostatic activation–bacterial endotoxins (*E. coli* verotoxins).

Glycosylation patterns contribute to cell differentiation, determining cell/cell and cell/matrix interactions, contributing to hormone/receptor binding, signal transduction, etc. Vascular endothelium in different tissues may be distinguished by the pattern of glycosylation, for example the constitutive expression of the carbohydrate ligand for the L-selectin on the high endothelial venules of peripheral lymph nodes.[21] This ligand is involved in lymphocyte traffic. CD44 is another determinant of preferential migration of lymphocytes to specific sites that has a carbohydrate ligand.[22] There is, therefore, differential glycosylation of vascular endothelium between and within tissues. It is also apparent that glycosylation varies between species. Although there may be considerable homology of protein sequence between species, glycosylation may be very different, for instance as seen with complement, the component of which has C1q the carbohydrate residues of functional significance.

So there are good reasons to suppose that carbohydrate ligands might be involved in endothelial/haemostatic activation as they are involved in immune cell activation (mitogens) and interactions (selectins), complement/immunoglobulin interactions, and haemostatic events (the heparin proteoglycans, platelet activation, etc.). In addition, we have isolated two EBV transformed human B cell lines that produce IgM antibodies;[23] both are cytotoxic to pig lymphocytes and both bind to the same carbohydrate, galactose-3-sulphate, in sulphatides of different origin and chain length. It is thought that sulphatide is the ligand for endothelial and platelet P-selectin (CD62).[24]

Two further key points can be extracted from the above discussion: the xenograft reaction may involve induction of donor endothelium as a trigger for the events of rejection; and differences in glycosylation patterns between species may explain how such induction occurs.

For hepatic xenotransplantation two further points should be borne in mind. Because of the differential glycosylation of vascular beds it may not be possible to extrapolate from effects in one organ to another; there may be no expression of the relevant carbohydrate target, or it may be expressed but have different functional significance (in the latter case, rejection might be of a different mechanism and time course). Secondly, in addition to expecting different events to follow antibody binding, the liver, as discussed above, has properties that appear to offer partial protection against antibody mediated damage immediately after transplantation.

Stage 2: adhesion

The passage of leucocytes into the graft, the synergy of endothelial, platelet and leucocyte effects at the endothelial surface, and the direct toxic effects to endothelium are all dependent on the adhesion molecules these elements express. An active role for endothelium has emerged with translocation of P-selectin from secretory granules to endothelial cell surface within seconds of exposure to thrombin or histamine.[25] P-selectin will transiently tether unactivated polymorphonucleocytes (PMN). The same stimuli result within minutes in endothelial synthesis of platelet activating factor (PAF) which, at the luminal surface, will bind PMNs and activate PMN β2-integrin expression. β2-integrins mediate binding to endothelial ICAM-1 and 2. T cells likewise are tethered, even when not activated, by selectins – E-selectin expressed on endothelium, L-selectin on lymphocyte.[26] Activation results in integrin expression by the T cell, further adhesion and then migration, partly through transience of integrin expression, and partly through shedding of, for instance, L-selectin. The T cell migrates, therefore, in an activated state. It is what has been called the cascade of adhesion molecules that results in the specificity of the response – the molecules that may be expressed are restricted to certain leucocyte subsets and to specific vascular endothelia. Memory T cells, for instance, tend to home to the region of original stimulation, perhaps reflecting the specialisation of T cell subsets for particular tissues.

It is expected, therefore, that as there are a variety of regional responses for each species, so the responses to specific endothelia from other species will vary. *In vitro* models of human monocyte and neutrophil migration have successfully used pig endothelium, and human neutrophils have been observed to adhere in various xenotransplantation models. However, only limited inferences can be drawn from this work, which does not exclude some failure of integrin/extracellular matrix interaction (laminin, etc.) later in migration. Much more detailed consideration of cross-reactivity of adhesion events between species may of course reveal that this stage of the response is restricted compared to allotransplantation.

An alternative possibility is that some parts of the response are enhanced or even induced by xeno-endothelium. Two components of arterial platelet adhesion, platelet glycoprotein Ib (GPIb) and von Willebrand factor (vWF), only develop specific affinity for each other in the presence of shear force.[27] Implied is an exposure of ligand or receptor site only in those circumstances, a principle that has been suggested for other components of haemostasis and complement; that is, the receptor and its respective ligand are already present at the appropriate cell surface/matrix, etc., but that binding is dependent on conformational change, exposing necessary residues. This provides a possible circumstance in xenotransplantation for enhancement or even induction of adhesion, and other components of the immune response, with constitutive expression of the key residues on xeno-endothelium reacting with recipient species molecules, or vice versa. Again, there is regional variation in haemostatic mechanisms that may be reflected in the xenograft responses: platelet adhesion in veins does not appear to involve GPIb/vWF but rather other integrins that are not shear dependent, and coagulation is dominated less by platelets and more by fibrin deposition. In the species combinations that involve marked haemostatic activation, the character of the events (which do vary between combinations) may well be determined by whether xeno-endothelium has arterial molecular configuration or venous.

Stage 3: specific recognition

Adhesion events continue to play a role in specific recognition, which is partially blocked by inhibitors such as anti-ICAM.[28,29] Nevertheless there is a more important ligand – target interaction which contributes both adhesion and specificity to the recognition process. The ligand is CD4 which targets the helper/inducer T cell subset to class II MHC and this recognition of 'self' is essential for the polymorphic alpha and beta chains of the T cell receptor to bind and be triggered by the peptide/MHC complex.

We have no direct published data to tell us how efficient the human CD4 molecule is in recognising xeno MHC class II. Indirect data from mixed lymphocyte culture reactivities between species and our knowledge of CD4 and class II sequences imply that human CD4 will react with the class II of both pigs and baboons, for instance. However, subtleties involving the relative reactivities with individual specificities, alpha and beta chains, or even with individual loci remain to be determined. In allografting, CD4 and not CD8 is the important directional molecule at the specific recognition stage, and we speculate that the major effect of the cross-species reactivity of CD8 will be at the specific targeting stage.

The influence of absolute HLA matching in allotransplantation is undisputed for bone marrow transplants and for live related renal allografts. For other forms of transplantation the influence of HLA matching is centre, organ, and patient dependent. It has been shown that the number of rejection episodes observed is related to the degree of mismatch.[30] We assume that, unless the species difference causes a block in a critical step in the process, a xenograft will be equivalent to a fully mismatched graft and hence that, on conventional immunosuppression, repeated MHC activated rejection episodes will be expected to occur.

In renal and cardiac alloresponses individual peptides bound in the MHC groove are mostly identical between individuals. Polymorphism generated differences do occur and can in rare cases lead to allograft rejection. Despite the high degree of polymorphism of peptides and glycopeptides produced by the liver, the increase in polymorphism of alloresponse that one would expect does not occur in hepatic xenotransplantation. This is true both in terms of rejection and of functional effects on the transplanted liver. The putative reasons for this lack of response have different implications for hepatic xenotransplantation, where one would expect the differences to be greater. It is possible that conventional immunosuppression limits the response. Another possibility is the apparent requirement in alloresponses for there to be at least two differences from self for a non-MHC molecule to be stimulatory. In other words, the polymorphisms act as haptens or non-immunogenic carriers. If this latter effect does contribute to limiting the response then liver xenotransplants will be very difficult indeed to maintain because hundreds of liver produced proteins will have multiple sequence/conformational differences to the native products. We expect that functional impairment of both molecules and grafts will be considerable.

The immunogenicity of carbohydrate determinants in allotransplantation is limited in different ways. It is partly governed by Landsteiner's Law[31] – natural IgM antibodies are produced only to those determinants that the individual does not express, and not to those that are expressed. This law appears to be dynamic in that antibody production is actively dependent on absence of host expression of the target carbohydrate. The clue as to why this law operates is being sought by many groups interested in xenotransplantation. The Landsteiner law operates for carbohydrate determinants on glycolipids, glycoproteins and possibly for soluble oligosaccharides. While this may operate in allotransplantation, in xenotransplantation one of the questions is whether it works if the core molecule of a glycoconjugate is changed as well as the carbohydrate. Is the law broken such that the carbohydrate can be responded to (perhaps with an IgG response), or does the law extend itself to protein such that response to the protein is decreased? A process which may be related to the Landsteiner law is termed accommodation. Here an anti-carbohydrate antibody can co-exist in the presence of its target without damage occurring. Accommodation is not simple but can be partly explained by access. Without damage to vascular endothelium, an IgM antibody will not escape the vasculature, so that its target remains unaffected.

Although consideration of the anti-carbohydrate response is very important for xenotransplantation, we still do not know how such responses occur at a mechanistic level. Without any direct evidence for T cell receptor involvement, we nevertheless presume that there must be involvement in some cases because IgG antibodies are made.

Stage 4: maturation of the recipient response

After recognition of the xeno-organ, T cells leave as part of a maturation process. Further to this, donor antigen, lost from the graft tissue, is picked up and presented by host antigen presenting cells (APCs). This latter route, often minor in allograft models, may assume a major rule in xenotransplantation. It might be expected that the T cell maturation process is the same for all T cells which have recognised antigen, either within the graft or in host lymphoid tissue. Cell maturation basically occurs through receipt of signals, and usually a minimum of two are needed per step. One is absolutely specific (peptide presentation) and a second is partially specific (a lymphokine). The cell then up-regulates receptor (e.g. IL-2R) and waits for the next set of signals, one of which in this example must be IL-2. Most of this process will occur quite normally in a xenograft recipient unless some critical signal is of mainly hepatic manufacture, and will not operate on the host species. At present there appears no evidence for such a factor. We assume therefore that although the epitopes that activate the cellular and hence the T dependent humoral response will be more varied in a xeno situation, the actual response mechanism itself will be unaffected.

In addition, donor APCs leave the graft, migrate to the lymphoid organs and present donor antigens to a new set of T cells. The donor APC migration step may be impaired or enhanced in the new species. Since the molecules which stimulate and direct migration within a species are not well understood, it is perhaps a little premature to consider what might happen in a cross-species combination.

B cell maturation pathways will probably remain unaffected, but the greatly increased number of stimulatory determinants and the fact that modern immunosuppressives target T cells predominantly tell us that humoral responses will be very important in xenotransplantation.[32,33] One additional factor which may be critical to the response, especially if the response is to lead to antibody formation, is the dual ligand interaction (CDLA-4 and CD28) with the B7 determinant on APC and activated B cells. Again these interactions have not been investigated between species.

Stage 5: effectors of the cell mediated response

The major allotarget is MHC class I. As with class II and CD4, knowledge of the importance and cross-species reactivity of the CD8 molecule with its MHC class I target is still in its infancy. Further, the actual methods by which the killing event occurs may be impaired. For example, the perforin–granzyme system of activated T cells and NK cells, whereby perforin punches the hole in the target cell and granzyme I carries through the effector process, may be affected. Perforin shows considerable sequence homology with C9 and granzyme 1, and is, like C2 and C4, a serine protease.[34,35] Complement *in toto* is known to function very differently in a xeno situation, a subject we will return to in the next section.

So far we have assumed in stages 1–5 that the rules of T cell engagement observed for allotransplants apply (albeit in a modified form) to xenotransplants. The substantial work carried out in the 1970s on cross-species rosettes suggests that additional interactions occur at the surface of specialised cells. Adhesion between an activated recipient cell and a non-specific target can lead to cell death. NK cells, which have a minor role in allotransplantation,[36] may be included in this category.

Stage 6: effectors of the humoral response

Following the consideration of antibody in Stage 1, complement remains to be discussed. It has long been known that the lytic process is considerably enhanced for both allo- and xeno-antibodies when xenocomplement is used. Indeed, standard serological tissue typing methods exploit the enhanced lysis of human cells achieved by using rabbit complement. There are several possible explanations for this effect. Those components of complement that are enzymes may simply have greater activity in one species than another. Those involved in regulation of the response, such as membrane co-factor protein (MCP) and decay accelerating factor (DAF), may have diminished efficacy across species. This possibility forms the basis for a number of initiatives in developing strategies to overcome the humoral response in xenotransplantation. It is thought that rendering the donor transgenic to human MCP and DAF, for instance, will abrogate complement mediated damage. Finally, there is evidence to suggest that xeno-endothelium may actively promote non-proteolytic C3 (alternative) pathways in certain species combinations.

The liver has immune functions, including central roles in immune complex metabolism and the IgA 'economy'. It can be imagined that these functions might serve either to protect it from damage or to expose it to an enhanced response. The potential dangers of these functions to the recipient will be considered in the final section.

Graft versus host interactions

Following a xenograft, liver derived host components will slowly be replaced to a greater or lesser extent by donor components. At the same time donor lymphocytes will be mounting a graft versus host response and the recipient immune system will be kicked into activation. Even those complement components whose function would otherwise be identical between species might be affected by differential glycosylation. The final complication stems from the fact that, at least in some species combinations, complement binding alone (as discussed above in stage 6) is quite sufficient to reject the organ rapidly by a process temporally distinct from hyperacute rejection.[37] In hepatic xenotransplantation the donor complement components could cause massive host endothelial cell damage in relevant combinations.

Summary

Hepatic xenotransplantation is a long term goal. Initial experiments were encouraging, but the problems in going from a few days' survival to graft survival approaching that which can be achieved by allotransplantation are immense. We conclude that liver xenograft success will be harder to achieve than kidney and heart and that a combination of several strategies will be necessary. These will probably include:

1. Removal or inactivation of natural antibody;
2. Induction of tolerance pretransplant involving the use of liver antigen and monoclonal therapy;
3. An inbred donor species incorporating genes coding for selected human complement components;
4. Pretransplant perfusion with selected reagents designed to decrease both GVH induction and stage 1 of the immune response.

These strategies have to be tried separately and in combination, together with newer immunosuppressives, against a background of allograft success. This necessitates the development of an animal model closely related to the human, e.g. pig to baboon. We need from such animal models a reliable method of proving that tolerance is induced before a transplant proceeds, as well as the information necessary to refine our pretreatment regimes individually and in combination.

References

1. Cramer DV, Sher L, MaKowa L. Liver xenotransplantation: clinical experience and future considerations. In: *Xenotransplantation: The Transplantation of Organs and Tissues Between Species*, Cooper D, Kemp E, Reemtsma K *et al.* (eds). Berlin: Springer-Verlag, 1991.
2. Demetris A, Jaffe R, Tzakis A *et al.* Antibody-mediated rejection of human liver allografts. Transplantation across ABO blood group barriers. *Am J Pathol* 1988; **489,** 132–137.
3. Sheil AG, McCaughan GW, Thompson JF *et al.* Liver transplantation – an Australian experience. In: *Clinical Transplantation 1990*, Terasaki P. (ed). Los Angeles: UCLA, 1991.
4. Larsen S, Starklint H. Histopathology of kidney xenograft rejection. In: *Xenotransplantation: The Transplantation of Organs and Tissues Between Species*, Cooper D, Kemp E, Reemtsma K *et al.* (eds). Berlin: Springer-Verlag, 1991.
5. Marino I, Celli S, Ferla G. Histopathological, immunofluorescent, and electron-microscopic features of hyperacute rejection in discordant renal xenotransplantation. In: *Xenotransplantation: The Transplantation of Organs and Tissues Between Species*, Cooper D, Kemp E, Reemtsma K *et al.* (eds). Berlin: Springer-Verlag, 1991.
6. Horstmann R, Pangburn M, Muller-Eberhard H. Species specificity of recognition by the alternative pathway of complement. *J Immunol* 1985; **134,** 1101.
7. Edwards J. Complement activation by xenogeneic red blood cells. *Transplantation* 1981; **31,** 226.
8. Calne R. Organ transplantation between widely disparate species. *Transplant Proc* 1970; **2,** 550.
9. Wight DGD. Hisopathology of liver xenograft rejection. In: *Xenotransplantation: The Transplantation of Organs and Tissues Between Species*, Cooper D, Kemp E, Reemtsma K *et al.* (eds). Berlin: Springer-Verlag, 1991.
10. Welsh KI, Taube DH, Thick ME *et al.* Human antibodies to pig determinants and their association with hyperacute rejection of xenografts. In: *Xenotransplantation: The Transplantation of Organs and Tissues Between Species*, Cooper D, Kemp E, Reemtsma K *et al.* (eds). Berlin: Springer-Verlag, 1991.
11. Lim SML, Heng KK, Wee A. A study of the xenogeneic response in an isolated liver perfusion circuit. *Transplant Proc* 1992 (in press).
12. Dubernard JM, Bonneau M, Latour M. *Heterografts in Primates*. Villeurbanne, France: Sinep Editions, 1974
13. Stern DM. An overview of endothelial cell biology. Proceedings of the First International Congress on Xenotransplantation. *Transplant Proc* 1992 (in press).
14. Hasuoka H, Sakagami K, Orita K. A new slow delivery type of superoxide dismutase prevents warm ischaemia damage in swine orthotopic liver transplantation. *Transplant Proc* 1991; **51,** 693–697.
15. Belzer FO, Reed TW, Pryor JP, Kountz SL, Dunphy JE. Red cell cold agglutinins as a cause of failure in renal allotransplantation. *Transplantation* 1971; **11,** 422–424.
16. Setaff A, Meriggi F, van de Stadt J *et al.* Delayed rejection of liver xenografts compared to heart xenografts in the rat. *Transplant Proc* 1987; **19,** 1155–1158.
17. Calne RY, White DJO, Herbertson BM, Millard PR, Davis DR, Salaman JR, Samuel JR. Pig to baboon liver xenografts. *Lancet* 1968; **1,** 1176.
18. Ratner AJ, Canhui H, Pepino P *et al.* Lymphocyte xenoantigens recognised by preformed antibodies. *Transplant Proc* 1992 (in press).
19. Platt JL, Lindman BJ, Chen H, Spitalnik SL, Bach FH. Endothelial cell antigens recognised by

xenoreactive human natural antibodies. *Transplantation* 1990; **50,** 817–821.
20. Platt JL, Bach FH. The barrier to xenotransplantation. *Transplantation* 1991; **52,** 937–947.
21. Bevilacqua MP, Butcher EC, Furie B *et al.* Selectins: a family of adhesion receptors *Cell* 1991; **67,** 233.
22. Aruffo A, Stamenkovic I, Melnick M, Underhill CB, Seed B. CD44 is the principal cell surface receptor for hyaluronate. *Cell* 1990; **61,** 1303–1313.
23. Breimer ME, Samuelsson BE, Holgersson J, Cairns TDH, Taube DH, Welsh KI. Carbohydrate specificity of pig lymphocytotoxic IgM antibodies produced by two EBV transformed human B cell lines. Proceedings of the First International Congress on Xenotransplantation. *Transplant Proc* 1992 (in press).
24. Aruffo A, Kolanus W, Walz G, Fredman P, Seed B. CD62/P-selectin recognition of myeloid and tumor cell sulfatides. *Cell* 1991; **67,** 35–44.
25. Zimmerman GA, Prescott SM, McIntyre TM. Endothelial cell interactions with granulocytes: tethering and signaling molecules. *Immunol Today* 1992; **13,** 93–100.
26. Shimizu Y, Newman W, Tanaka Y, Shaw S. Lymphocyte interactions with endothelial cells. *Immunol Today* 1992; **13,** 106–112.
27. Roth GJ. Platelets and blood vessels: the adhesion event. *Immunol Today* 1992; **3,** 100–105.
28. Moses RD, Auchincloss H Jr. Defects in accessory molecules and other cell surface molecule interactions are responsible for weak mouse helper T-cell responses to xenoantigens. *Transplant Proc* 1991; **23,** 883–885
29. Wee SI, Cosimi AB, Preffer FI, Rothelin R, Faanes R, Conti D, Colvin RB. Functional consequences of anti-ICAM (CD54) in cynomolgus monkeys with renal allografts. *Transplant Proc* 1991; **51,** 279–281.
30. Salmela K, von Willebrand E, Kyllonen L, Koskimies S, Isoniemi B, Eklund B, Hockerstedt K, Ahonen J. The association on HLA-DR antigens with acute steroid reistant rejection and poor kidney graft survival. *Transplantation* 1991; **51,** 768–772.
31. Landsteiner K. *Specificity of Serological Reactions*. New York: Dover, 1962.
32. Grailer A, Nichols J, Hullet D, Sollinger HW, Burlingham WJ. Inhibition of human B cell responses *in vitro* by RS-61443, cyclosporin A and DAB486 IL-2. *Transplant Proc* 1991; **51,** 314–316.
33. Tepper MA, Petty B, Bursuker I, Pasternak RD, Cleaveland J, Spitalny GL, Schacter B. Inhibition of antibody production by the immunosuppressive agent, 15-deoxyspergualin. *Transplant Proc* 1991; **51,** 328–332.
34. Berke G., Lymphocyte-triggered internal target disintegration. *Immunol Today* 1991; **12,** 396–399.
35. Krahenbuhl O, Tschopp J. Perforin-induced pore formation. *Immunol Today* 1991; **12,** 399–404.
36. Markus PM, van den Brink M, Harnaha XCJ, Palomba L, Hiserodt JC, Cramer DV. Effect of selective depletion of natural killer cells on allograft rejection. *Transplant Proc* 1991; **51,** 178–179.
37. Forty J, Watson CJ, Carey N, White DJG, Wallwork J. Perfusion of rabbit hearts with human blood results in immediate graft thrombosis which is temporally distinct from hyperacute rejection. Proceedings of the First International Congress on Xenotransplantation. *Transplant Proc* 1992 (in press).

SECTION III

Clinical Aspects of Rejection

14

Acute rejection of human liver allografts

R Ayres and D Adams

Introduction

Rejection was not considered to be a major problem in early series of human liver transplants, a view supported by animal studies.[1–3] However, the clinical features of rejection were not understood and a reluctance to carry out liver biopsy because of perceived risks to the graft meant that rejection was underdiagnosed. Furthermore, technical and septic complications dominated the early years so rejection was comparatively less of a problem. The marked improvement in survival which has occurred in recent years as a consequence of technical advances and a better understanding of immunosuppression has allowed rejection to be put in its true perspective.[4] The clinical and histological features have been documented and there is now broad agreement about the characteristic findings, allowing the diagnosis of graft rejection to be made with confidence.[5] This process has been greatly aided by the increasing use of protocol and serial liver biopsies to document histological progression of graft rejection.[6–10]

At least 50% of patients will develop histological features of acute, reversible rejection and between 5% and 10% develop chronic rejection,[11–14] which is usually irreversible and requires retransplantation.[10,15–17] Rejection contributes to mortality and morbidity both directly and through infection related to immunosuppression.[4,8,16] In a series of 129 adult liver transplants carried out in Pittsburgh, 21 of 40 deaths were due to infection. Rejection was present in 29% of autopsies although in only 9.6% of these (7.5% overall) was it considered to be the cause of death[18] (Table 14.1). A recent study from the same unit demonstrated that the indication for retransplantation was acute rejection in 11% of patients and chronic rejection in 11.3%. The most frequent causes of graft failure in this study were primary non-function (30%) and vascular complications (27%)[4] (Table 14.2). Acute rejection is therefore a significant cause of both morbidity and mortality following liver transplantation.

Table 14.1 Principal cause of death in 40 consecutive adult patients studied who survived at least 24 hours but ultimately died after liver transplantation[18]

Principal cause of death	n
Infection	21
Multi-organ failure	8
Rejection	3
Massive GI bleeding	3
Massive CNS haemorrhage	2
Massive pulmonary bleeding	1
Pulmonary thrombo-embolism	1
Hyperkalaemia	1
TOTAL	40

Definitions

Rejection can be defined as graft damage arising from the response of the recipient immune system to the transplanted liver and may take several forms resulting in different clinical patterns. Problems arise from the lack of accepted definitions of the different types of rejection. The terms 'acute' and 'chronic' rejection rightly relate to the clinical course of the rejection episode but are often based on histological findings with inflammatory infiltrates, cholangitis and endotheliitis indicating 'acute rejection' and arteriopathy and ductopenia

Table 14.2 Causes of retransplantation in 177 consecutive liver transplant patients[4]

Diagnosis	n	%	Timing of failure in days (mean ± SEM)	Comments
Primary non-function	53	30.0	3.4 ± 0.3	
Ischaemic graft injury	17	9.6	17.5 ± 1.9	
Acute rejection	19	10.7	30.4 ± 6.4	
Vascular complication	47	26.6	59.6 ± 24.1	
Chronic rejection	20	11.3	496.3 ± 136.0	
Recurrent primary liver disease	12	6.8	550.5 ± 172.1	Hepatitis B (7), hepatocellular carcinoma (1), probable auto-immune CAH (2), NANBH (2)
Miscellaneous	9	5.0	300.0 ± 110.6	Non-recurrent hepatitis B (2), herpes hepatitis (1), acute hepatitis, cause unknown, with chronic rejection (1), suppurative cholangitis (1), severe acute cholangitis with ischaemia (1), bile duct necrosis with bile leak and CMV hepatitis (1), unknown (2)

indicating 'chronic rejection'.[19] However, the histological features characteristically associated with chronic rejection may occur 'acutely' and those features associated with acute rejection may develop insidiously. Moreover, the association of acute rejection with reversibility and chronic rejection with irreversibility does not always hold.[20] Clinically acute rejection may be unresponsive to treatment and cases of reversible ductopenia have been described.[20,21] It has been suggested that the terms 'cellular', 'ductopenic' and 'arteriopathic' be used to describe the histological features of rejection; that, pre-treatment, 'responsive/reversible' and 'unresponsive/irreversible' be used to describe response to therapy, leaving the terms 'acute', 'persistent' (or unresolved) and 'chronic' to describe the clinical course.[19,21] For reasons of clarity, the terms acute/reversible and chronic/irreversible rejection will be used to describe the main syndromes, fulminant rejection will be used to describe the rare syndrome of fulminant or hyperacute graft rejection. The acute vanishing bile duct syndrome will be discussed in the next chapter.

Acute/reversible rejection

Clinical features

Significant acute rejection requiring treatment affects between 30% and 80% of patients following liver transplantation usually within the first two weeks[14,16,17,22] (Figure 14.1). Common but no means invariable symptoms are fever, malaise and jaundice and bile becomes thin and pale with reduced flow.[23,24,25] Serum liver function tests frequently show a sharp rise in serum bilirubin which may be followed by more modest increases in alkaline phosphatase and aspartate transaminase levels. The prothrombin time is usually unaffected.[11,26] These features are not specific to rejection and other causes of graft dysfunction need to be excluded before rejection can be diagnosed with confidence. The main differential diagnoses are ischaemia due to vascular thrombosis, preservation injury, biliary obstruction and infection. Hepatic artery thrombosis may present acutely with high transaminase levels and a lengthening prothrombin time or more insidiously with the development of an ischaemic hepatic abscess, bacteraemia or breakdown of biliary anastomosis. If suspected, hepatic artery thrombosis should be excluded by angiography or Doppler ultrasound. Biliary obstruction, either due to mechanical causes related to the biliary anastomosis or to biliary sludge, presents as a rising serum bilirubin and alkaline phosphatase often associated with bacterbilia or sometimes overt cholangitis. If a T tube is in place cholangiography is indicated, otherwise HIDA scanning provides an alternative way of assessing the biliary tract but may lack sufficient sensitivity and specificity. Recent improvements in surgical technique and management have resulted in reduced morbidity related to the biliary anastomosis.[27] Infection must be excluded since it will be exacerbated by inappropriate treatment with high dose immunosuppression. Bacterial colonisation of bile is common and can result in overt cholangitis and

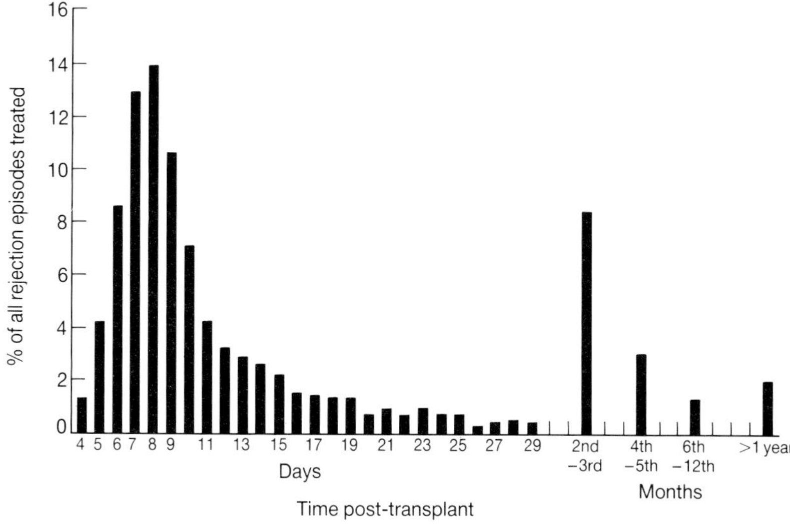

Fig. 14.1 Time post-transplant of treated episodes of acute allograft rejection (first 500 patients receiving a primary liver graft in Birmingham).

septicaemia, particularly in the presence of biliary obstruction. If suspected, bile and blood culture should be taken and appropriate antibiotic therapy instigated. Viral infections usually occur after the first three weeks and include recurrent hepatitis B and D, as well as recurrent and *de novo* hepatitis C and A.[28-31] The most common serious viral infection, however, is CMV[32,33] which can be due either to reactivation of latent infection or a *de novo* primary infection. When symptomatic, CMV infection is associated with a high swinging fever (several degrees higher than that usually seen with rejection) and occurs later than the majority of acute rejection episodes, around the end of the first month following transplantation.[16,34] It is crucial to differentiate between CMV infection and rejection since successful treatment of CMV infection requires a reduction in immunosuppression. The diagnosis should be suspected by the timing and nature of the fever and by the finding of leucopenia, thrombocytopenia or atypical lymphocytosis. A diagnosis can be confirmed by serology or culturing the virus from urine, or by histology of the liver using either immunohistochemistry to detect viral antigens or *in situ* hybridisation to detect viral DNA. Conventional histological examination of liver biopsy may detect diagnostic findings of CMV such as viral inclusions or neutrophil clusters. Duodenal and/or rectal biopsies often show features of tissue invasive CMV in cases of CMV hepatitis. Infection of the graft by other viruses such as herpes simplex, Epstein Barr virus and adenovirus is less common but should be considered.[33-35] Viral infections are discussed in more detail elsewhere (Chapter 21).

Another potential cause of graft dysfunction is drug toxicity and both azathioprine and cyclosporin have been associated with cholestasis and liver dysfunction.[8,36,37]

Diagnosis of rejection

Biochemical tests

The clinical and biochemical features of rejection are non-specific and suspicion of rejection is based upon the timing of graft dysfunction, usually around the end of the first week, and the associated biochemical abnormalities.[11,23,24,25] Conventional biochemical tests are sensitive markers of rejection but lack specificity[38] and liver biopsy should be used wherever possible to confirm the diagnosis (Table 14.3). The earliest and most significant biochemical abnormality is a rise in serum bilirubin which usually precedes a rise in transaminase levels.[11,14,38] However, a subset of patients present with a sudden and marked rise in serum transaminase levels. This 'hepatitic' rejection pattern has been associated with a more severe clinical course in some studies.[22,25] Dynamic liver function tests which measure the clearance of factors such as aminopyrine, indocyanine green, caffeine or lidocaine have been studied but offer no benefit over conventional liver biochemistry.[39]

Table 14.3 Sensitivity and specificity of conventional liver function tests in the diagnosis of acute allograft rejection[38]

	Predysfunction				Peak dysfunction			
	BILI	ALP	AST	ALT	BILI	ALP	AST	ALT
Sensitivity	89	78	79	63	94	84	57	84
Specificity	4	50	15	48	7	31	31	15

Histology

The gold standard for diagnosing rejection remains histological examination of liver biopsy. Although fine needle aspiration biopsy is used routinely by a few centres,[40] the majority rely on conventional core needle biopsy. A recent study from the Mayo Clinic has confirmed that liver biopsy is a safe procedure after liver transplantation since complications requiring treatment developed in only 17 out of a total of 950 transplant liver biopsies. The complications were bleeding in 11 and infection in six patients; all the patients recovered.[41] The realisation that liver biopsy is a relatively safe procedure has encouraged the routine use of both diagnostic and protocol liver biopsy following liver transplantation, allowing the development of a consensus about the histological features.[5,19] Acute rejection is characterised by a triad of histological findings:

1. A mixed inflammatory cell infiltrate in portal tracts consisting of not only lymphocytes and monocytes but also neutrophils and eosinophils;
2. Infiltration and damage to the biliary epithelium of intrahepatic bile ducts;
3. Inflammation of venous endothelium within portal tracts, the so-called venous endotheliitis[7,8,42,43] (Figure 14.2).

In severe cases all three features are present throughout the biopsy but in milder cases the changes may be patchy. Endotheliitis is the least common but most specific histological feature. Bile duct damage is functionally more important but less specific, being present in viral and drug hepatitis as well as extrahepatic obstruction and early preservation injury.[4,7,8,42] Arteritis or arteriolitis may be present in some patients[42,43] and this, together with paucity of bile ducts and evidence of ischaemic damage, is indicative of progression to chronic rejection.[10,15] Following successful treatment, the histological features of rejection usually resolve rapidly, although there

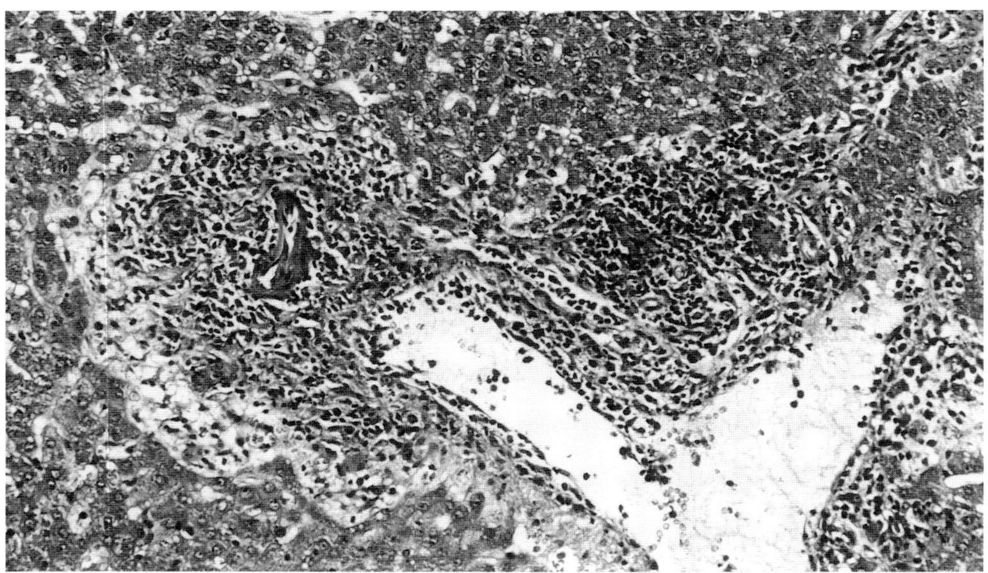

Fig. 14.2 Acute rejection – portal tracts contain a dense mixed inflammatory infiltrate. There is inflammatory infiltration of the small bile ducts and subendothelial infiltration of a portal venule.

may be a period of cholestasis before graft function returns to normal. Rejection is associated with an increase in the expression of both MHC antigens and adhesion molecules[44,45] on liver components and it has been suggested that such immunohistochemical techniques might provide additional diagnostic information. However the diagnosis of rejection can usually be made successfully by conventional staining techniques alone.

Whereas rejection episodes associated with severe histological changes nearly always require treatment with increased immunosuppression, the clinical significance of milder histological findings can be difficult to assess. Protocol biopsies at the end of the first week frequently reveal characteristic histological changes of mild rejection in patients without clinical and biochemical dysfunction.[8,10,17,42,43] Such changes will usually resolve without the need for anti-rejection treatment. Cases of spontaneously resolving acute rejection associated with biochemical dysfunction are less common but have been reported.[46] Experience in our unit includes eight patients with mild or moderate histological features of rejection and biochemical abnormalities in whom rejection resolved completely without additional immunosuppressive treatment. The clinical implications of these findings are unclear at present but as experience increases the tendency in most units has been to reserve treatment with increased immunosuppression for patients with biochemical dysfunction and characteristic findings on liver histology.[14,46] Such policies have resulted in a fall in the incidence of treated rejection episodes from 70% previously to between 30% and 50% in most units now.[14,17,46] There is no evidence that such changes in policy have resulted in an increased progression to chronic irreversible rejection; indeed, the incidence is falling in some units[47] (Table 14.4). The use of less high-dose immunosuppression to treat acute rejection episodes is likely to result in a reduction in serious infectious complications, such as aspergillosis and CMV, which are directly related to the amount of increased immunosuppression used to treat rejection episodes.[33,34,48]

Table 14.4 Proportion of patients treated for acute rejection and proportion developing vanishing bile duct syndrome in 1st–4th cohort of 100 patients grafted

	Patients treated for acute rejection. Percentage treated of first grafts surviving >7 days	**Percentage of grafts developing VBDS**
1st 100 patients	76	13.3
2nd 100 patients	78	12.2
3rd 100 patients	67	5.4
4th 100 patients	64	2

Fine needle aspiration biopsy

The technique of fine needle aspiration biopsy was originally described by Hayry and von Willibrand[49,50] and is used routinely in the Helsinki program.[40] Several studies have demonstrated a close correlation between cytological and histological findings in both animal and human liver transplants and rejection can be differentiated from other causes of post-transplant graft dysfunction, including CMV infection.[51,40,52,53,54] Kirby and co-workers demonstrated a close association between aspiration cytology and histology in the first eight weeks, allowing rejection to be diagnosed with a sensitivity of 81.3% and a specificity of 90%. This fell after eight weeks to 53.3% and 71.4% respectively.[52] The technique is safe and easy to perform but requires skill and experience in interpretation. In a series of 691 aspiration biopsies performed in 35 liver grafts, representative samples were obtained in 598 (86.5%) and no complications were observed. Failure of the technique was due to insufficient sample or contamination with blood, lymph or ascites in 13% of cases. Other studies have confirmed the major difficulty of non-representative samples (28%) due to too few parenchymal cells.[55]

Imaging

Doppler ultrasound is of value in excluding hepatic ischaemia due to hepatic artery or portal vein occlusion[56] and has also been suggested as a diagnostic test in rejection.[57] In a series of paediatric liver transplants 78% of biopsy proven rejection episodes were associated with abrupt damping of the normally pulsatile hepatic venous blood flow. However, similar findings were noted following perioperative ischaemia and in cholangitis. In eight patients Doppler changes preceded clinical and biochemical evidence of rejection. There was no episode of biopsy proven rejection with normal hepatic vein Doppler signals.

Is there a role for immunological monitoring of patients following liver transplantation?

A serological marker of acute rejection which could be measured in patients on a daily basis would be of great benefit in the management of graft dysfunction and much attention has focused on the potential of various immunological tests to fill such a role.[58] The rejection process is an inflammatory cascade[59–62] and the immunological events which accompany each step of the process can potentially be monitored as indices of immune activation and rejection. The recognition of donor transplant antigens by the host immune system results in the activation of host helper T cells. Lymphocyte activation is accompanied by the expression of activation markers on the cell membrane and the secretion of an array of cytokines. These cytokines are then responsible for the recruitment, activation and control of other arms of the immune response.[63–65] Such a process might be reflected by phenotypic changes in circulating lymphocyte subsets and several workers have attempted to determine whether such changes are specific to the rejection process.[66–69]

However whilst it is generally agreed that lymphocyte counts increase during rejection, this is non-specific. No study has reported a pattern in lymphocyte subset composition of peripheral blood which is a reliable indicator of graft rejection. The measurement of soluble lymphocyte products is an alternative way of monitoring lymphocyte activation. Tilg and co-workers[71] measured a number of cytokines in serum after liver transplantation. Whilst they found that gamma interferon, beta-2-microglobulin and neopterin were elevated, they were not specific for rejection.[70–71] Other studies have confirmed a lack of specificity for serum β2M and neopterin.[72,73] Activated lymphocytes release soluble forms of many of their surface antigens in addition to cytokines. These include the receptor for interleukin 2 (CD25) which is expressed on the cell surface in increased amounts during lymphocyte activation[74] and also shed in a stable, soluble form which can be measured by enzyme linked immunosorbent assay.[75] Two studies have reported elevated plasma levels of SIL2R during both rejection episodes and also infective complications in the absence of detectable rejection.[76,77]

Since the inflammatory response of rejection is centred on small bile ducts, bile sampling offers direct access to the site of the rejection process. In those patients whose transplant involves the use of an externally draining T tube there is easy access to bile for daily monitoring. Several studies have now shown that the analysis of bile provides a more accurate reflection of immune activation within the liver allograft than does the analysis of serum. Biliary levels of both SIL2R and β2M were far more sensitive and specific markers of rejection than the corresponding serum levels.[76–78] In addition, the study of another surface molecule which is shed on activation, soluble intercellular adhesion molecule-1 (CD54), shows similar results[79] (Table 14.5). Lymphocytes accumulate at the site of rejection by a combination of proliferation *in situ* and recruitment from the periphery in response to locally secreted chemotactic factors.[80,81] Specific lymphocyte chemotactic factors are secreted into bile early in the rejection process.[69,82,83] Although the studies published to date have been concerned with the mechanisms of rejection rather than the development of a diagnostic test, a simplified *in vitro* chemotaxis assay,

Table 14.5 Sensitivity, specificity and convenience of experimental immunological tests for rejection

	Sensitivity	Specificity	Convenience
Bilirubin	+	−	+++
T cell subsets (peripheral blood)	−	−	−
IL2R (serum)	+++	+	++
sIL2R (bile)	++	+++	+
β2M (serum)	+++	+	++
β2M (bile)	+++	++	++
sICAM-1 (serum)	++	+	+
sICAM-1 (bile)	++	+++	+/−
TNFα (serum)	+	++	++
Neopterin	+	+	++
Secretory component (bile)	++	++	+/−
Hyaluronic acid (serum)	+++	++	+
Neutrophil activation	++	+	−
Lymphocyte chemotaxis (bile)	+++	+++	−
Eosinophil count (blood)	+++	++	++

using micro-well chambers, can produce a semi-quantitative result within six hours and has potential as a monitor of immune activation.

Graft damage during rejection is mediated by different effector mechanisms including cytotoxic T cells, antibody secretion and the activation of eosinophils, neutrophils and monocytes.[12,59,62] Lymphocyte mediated cytotoxicity to donor spleen cells can be detected *in vitro* after transplantation although the development of such responses occurs in the absence of clinical rejection and is therefore not specific enough to be used in diagnosis.[84] Activated cytotoxic T cells with specificity for donor class I HLA antigens have been isolated from liver biopsies during rejection and CD8 positive cells are seen on liver biopsies infiltrating target structures such as bile ducts.[85–87] The isolation of T cell clones from liver biopsies takes several days and cannot be used for daily monitoring. However, activated CD8+ T cells shed a soluble form of the CD8 receptor which can be measured in biological fluids. Plasma levels of soluble CD8 rise before episodes of rejection whereas no rise is seen in patients who fail to develop rejection (Hathaway and Adams, unpublished observations) (Figure 14.3). Whether soluble CD8 is also elevated in viral and bacterial infections after transplantation is yet to be determined but seems likely. Studies demonstrating increased levels of circulating donor specific antibodies provide evidence for the involvement of humoral mechanisms.[88,89] During episodes of acute rejection, local secretion into bile of immunoglobulins (particularly IgM and IgG)

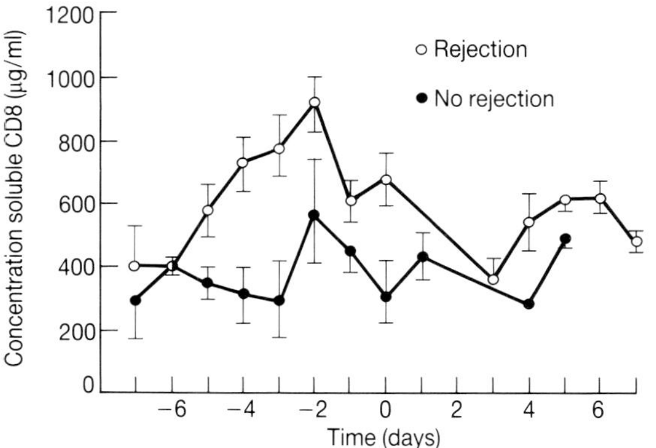

Fig. 14.3 Concentration of soluble CD8 before and after acute allograft rejection in patients who did (n = 6) and did not (n = 6) develop acute cellular rejection of the liver allograft on day 0.

occurs although the low specificity and sensitivity of such findings precludes their use as diagnostic tests.[90] Peripheral blood neutrophils become activated during episodes of acute rejection when they show increased chemotactic responses and an enhanced secretion of superoxide radicals and proteolytic enzymes *in vitro*.[91] These findings are in keeping with the histological observations that large numbers of neutrophils are present within the portal infiltrate during rejection.[42,43,92] However, it is likely that neutrophils will also be activated during infective episodes, particularly bacterial cholangitis, reducing the diagnostic specificity of neutrophil function tests. Likewise large numbers of eosinophils are seen in the portal tract inflammatory infiltrate during rejection episodes and Sankary *et al.* used multivariate analysis to demonstrate that their presence was a strong histological indicator of rejection.[92] In addition the same group has shown that peripheral blood eosinophil counts rise prior to episodes of rejection and that this rise is both sensitive and specific for rejection.[93,94] Thus a simple differential white cell count might be a powerful diagnostic tool to differentiate rejection from other causes of graft dysfunction. Activated macrophages, which are also present in the inflammatory infiltrate,[42,43,95] secrete many cytokines including tumour necrosis factor α (TNFα) and three studies have reported elevated serum levels of TNFα during rejection.[70,96,97] However, the specificity of TNFα is poor which reflects the release of this cytokine in response to a wide variety of stimuli.

The important targets for the inflammatory response in acute rejection are the biliary epithelium, venous endothelium and, less importantly, hepatocytes.[42,43,98] In man, secretory component is confined to the biliary epithelium where it binds to monomeric IgA or IgM to form the secretory forms of IgA and IgM. Although free secretory component is shed into bile during rejection, similar elevated levels are detected during infective complications such as bacterial cholangitis, reducing its specificity as a diagnostic tool.[99,100] Lymphocyte mediated bile duct damage is probably directed at HLA class 1 molecules which are expressed strongly on bile ducts after transplantation.[44] Studies have demonstrated release of soluble class I antigens into serum during rejection and into bile after transplantation, although the numbers of patients studied were too small to assess their use as a diagnostic test.[101] Elevated serum levels of hyaluronic acid, a prote-

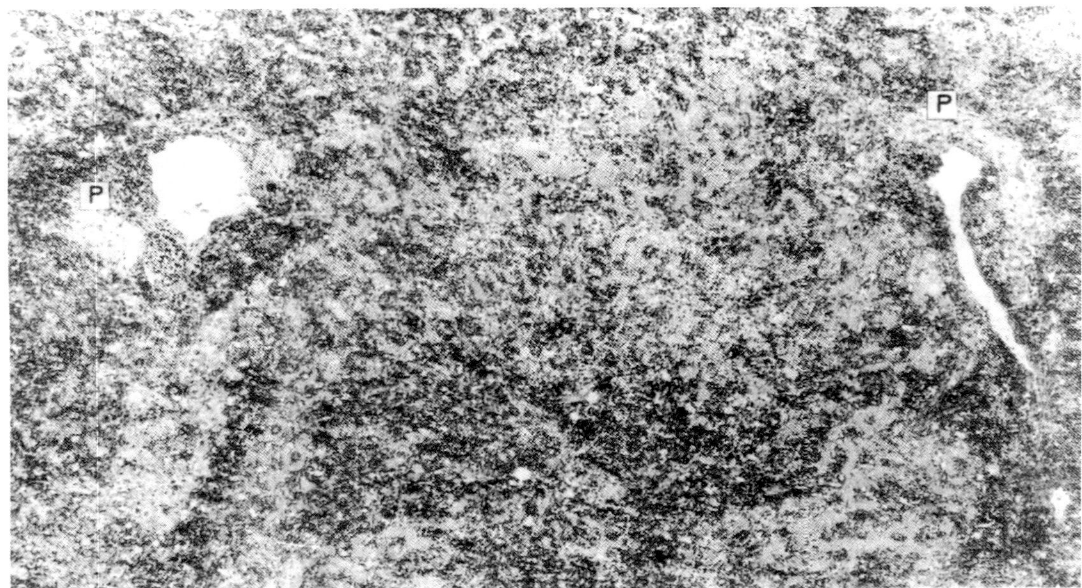

Fig. 14.5 Massive haemorrhagic necrosis – hepatectomy specimens taken nine days after liver transplantation showing panacinar haemorrhage and hepatocyte necrosis. Focal haemorrhage is also seen in two surviving portal tracts.

similar histological picture, although in hepatic artery thrombosis, haemorrhage is not extensive. The paucity of cellular infiltrate in this syndrome suggests that cell mediated mechanisms are not primarily involved and it is likely that such cases represent a delayed form of hyperacute, humoral rejection.[124] Other groups have described similar findings which they have attributed to a fulminant form of humoral rejection.[124,125] Furthermore, the reporting of widespread MHC antigen induction associated with antibody and complement deposition further supports the idea that this syndrome is a fulminant form of graft rejection.[123–125]

Association of fulminant rejection with ABO incompatible transplants

There is increasing evidence that fulminant rejection is more commonly seen in patients who are transplanted with an ABO incompatible liver. In one series of 234 liver transplants, six patients out of 17 who received ABO incompatible liver allografts developed fulminant rejection, characterised by haemorrhagic infiltration of portal tracts and deposition of IgM and fibrinogen on sinusoidal endothelial cells[125] (Table 14.6). There is no evidence that patients with this syndrome respond to increased immunosuppression and the only effective treatment is rapid retransplantation.

Table 14.6 Incidence of fulminant rejection in Birmingham and Villejuif[125]

	Villejuif	Birmingham
Incidence	3.7% (6/224)	3.2% (8/250)
ABO incompatible	100% (6/6)	25% (2/8)

Immune mechanisms of acute rejection

Graft antigens

Rejection occurs when the host immune system recognises allogeneic histocompatibility determinants expressed on the transplanted liver. The most important of these are coded for by the major histocompatibility complex[126,127] and act as recognition signals in lymphocyte reactions.[128] The expression of MHC antigens varies between different tissues. In human liver, HLA class I (ABC) and class II (DR, DP, DQ) are strongly expressed on sinusoidal lining cells, HLA-DR and weak class I expression is seen on vascular endothelium, and class I and occasionally class II antigen expression on biliary epithelium. Hepatocytes are usually negative for both class I and class II expression.[44,129–131] The expression of HLA be of benefit. The use of new therapies for rescue treatment, such as FK506[109] or antibodies to the adhesion molecule ICAM-1 or the IL-2 receptor show promise, but need confirming in larger studies before they can be recommended for routine use (Figure 14.4).

Fulminant/hyperacute rejection

Evidence for hyperacute rejection of liver allografts

Hyperacute rejection as described in renal and cardiac transplantation occurs within hours of transplantation in patients with preformed cytotoxic antibodies. These antibodies bind to endothelial antigens within the graft leading to complement activation, vasospasm and platelet aggregation with rapid loss of the graft.[110] The causative antibodies are thought to be anti-A and anti-B red cell iso-agglutinins and some groups of lymphocytotoxic antibodies directed against T lymphocytes.[111] Until recently it was thought that true hyperacute rejection did not occur following liver transplantation. A number of theories were suggested to explain the resistance of the liver to rejection, including clonal deletion of alloreactive lymphocytes by soluble MHC antigens and Kupffer cell removal of immune complexes.[112,113] Early animal and clinical studies supported the notion that the liver was protected from hyperacute rejection.[2,114] No decrease in graft survival was reported for transplants carried out in the presence of a positive donor–recipient lymphocytotoxic crossmatch or panel reactive antibodies, and transplants were successful even in the face of ABO incompatibility and a positive crossmatch.[2,3,115,116] Later studies reported a modest advantage of ABO matched adults at one year and five years.[117] Animal studies produced conflicting results. Houssin reported induction of high pre-operative lymphocytotoxic antibodies in rats which was associated with a reduction in graft survival compared with unsensitised animals, although post-mortem liver histology did not show classical features of hyperacute rejection.[118] Other reports with rats[119] and rhesus monkeys[120] have demonstrated hyperacute rejection associated with high cytotoxic antibody levels. Perhaps the most persuasive evidence for the existence of hyperacute rejection in liver transplants comes from Starzl and co-authors. They described two patients who received liver and kidney transplants from the same donor in whom hyperacute rejection of the kidney was associated with severe coagulopathy and the development of necrosis of the liver within hours of implantation. They felt it was likely that the same mechanism affected both kidney and liver.[121] The pre-operative cytotoxic crossmatch was negative in one of these patients, suggesting that crossmatching will not always prevent this complication.

In 1989 Bird and co-workers reported a 47 year old woman transplanted with an ABO identical liver who developed a syndrome compatible with hyperacute rejection.[122] Six hours after a technically uneventful operation and initial graft function, PT and AST rapidly rose, the former being unrecordable at 40 hours. Vascular integrity was confirmed angiographically and retransplantation was undertaken at 44 hours. Histology of the graft revealed massive eosinophilic necrosis with a predominantly polymorphonuclear infiltrate of portal tracts and parenchyma. No venous endotheliitis was seen. Small and medium sized arterial branches were intact. Pre- and post-operative sera had high titres of panel reactive antibodies. Six of the first 85 patients who received the first 100 liver transplantations in the Birmingham series developed a similar syndrome of fulminant hepatic failure with distinctive clinical and pathological features[123] (Figure 14.5). After an uneventful initial post-operative period of between three and 20 days, sudden deterioration in graft function developed with markedly increased serum transaminase levels, lengthening prothrombin time and rapid progression to liver failure and grade IV coma. All six patients died. At autopsy the graft was swollen, and congested and histological examination revealed massive haemorrhage and hepatocyte necrosis most severe in acinar zones 2 and 3. Only mild inflammatory changes were evident without occlusive lesions in large arteries or veins. Two cases showed portal inflammation and bile duct loss (90% in one case). Although the main hepatic arterial and venous branches were normal microscopically and radiologically, subendothelial foam cell proliferation in large and medium sized arteries was seen in the two cases with associated bile duct loss. Small arteries and arterioles were consistently normal unless destroyed by haemorrhagic necrosis. There was no evidence of infection either from cultures or histologically.

Both vascular thrombosis and infection must be rigorously excluded since either may produce a

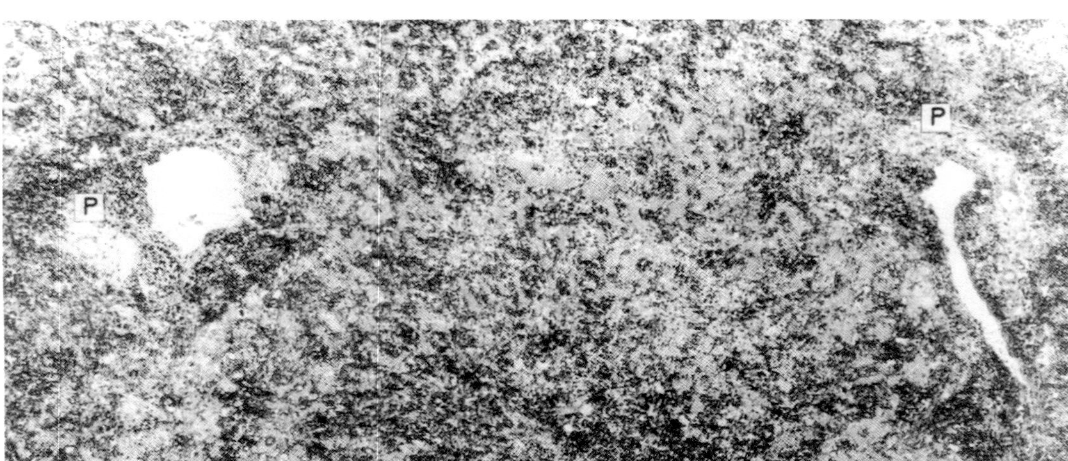

Fig. 14.5 Massive haemorrhagic necrosis – hepatectomy specimens taken nine days after liver transplantation showing panacinar haemorrhage and hepatocyte necrosis. Focal haemorrhage is also seen in two surviving portal tracts.

similar histological picture, although in hepatic artery thrombosis, haemorrhage is not extensive. The paucity of cellular infiltrate in this syndrome suggests that cell mediated mechanisms are not primarily involved and it is likely that such cases represent a delayed form of hyperacute, humoral rejection.[124] Other groups have described similar findings which they have attributed to a fulminant form of humoral rejection.[124,125] Furthermore, the reporting of widespread MHC antigen induction associated with antibody and complement deposition further supports the idea that this syndrome is a fulminant form of graft rejection.[123–125]

Association of fulminant rejection with ABO incompatible transplants

There is increasing evidence that fulminant rejection is more commonly seen in patients who are transplanted with an ABO incompatible liver. In one series of 234 liver transplants, six patients out of 17 who received ABO incompatible liver allografts developed fulminant rejection, characterised by haemorrhagic infiltration of portal tracts and deposition of IgM and fibrinogen on sinusoidal endothelial cells[125] (Table 14.6). There is no evidence that patients with this syndrome respond to increased immunosuppression and the only effective treatment is rapid retransplantation.

Table 14.6 Incidence of fulminant rejection in Birmingham and Villejuif[125]

	Villejuif	Birmingham
Incidence	3.7% (6/224)	3.2% (8/250)
ABO incompatible	100% (6/6)	25% (2/8)

Immune mechanisms of acute rejection

Graft antigens

Rejection occurs when the host immune system recognises allogeneic histocompatibility determinants expressed on the transplanted liver. The most important of these are coded for by the major histocompatibility complex[126,127] and act as recognition signals in lymphocyte reactions.[128] The expression of MHC antigens varies between different tissues. In human liver, HLA class I (ABC) and class II (DR, DP, DQ) are strongly expressed on sinusoidal lining cells, HLA-DR and weak class I expression is seen on vascular endothelium, and class I and occasionally class II antigen expression on biliary epithelium. Hepatocytes are usually negative for both class I and class II expression.[44,129–131] The expression of HLA antigens on liver components is increased during episodes of rejection. Hepatocytes display a membranous pattern of focal staining for HLA class I and class II (HLA-DR, DP) and biliary epithelium and vascular endothelium show intense staining for class I and II (DR and DP but not DQ).[44,132–134] This presumably occurs in response to locally produced cytokines (particularly gamma–interferon) which are known to be capable of increasing tissue expression of MHC products[135,136] thereby rendering the tissue more susceptible to T cell mediated cytolytic damage. Lymphocytes isolated from human liver grafts show alloreactivity towards cells bearing donor MHC class I antigens.[85,86] Furthermore, soluble class I antigen and β2M (which is part of the class I complex on the cell surface) are shed into bile during episodes of acute rejection[78,101] suggesting that damage is directed towards MHC antigens on the biliary epithelium.

However, this increase in MHC expression is not specific for rejection and is also seen in other forms of graft dysfunction and in patients in whom rejection has resolved, although the intensity of expression tends to be less in these groups. Other factors must therefore be involved. T cells must adhere to apposing cells before they can react with MHC antigens, a process mediated by lymphocyte adherence receptors such as CD2 which interacts with lymphocyte function associated antigen 3 (LFA-3) and LFA-1 which interacts with the ligands ICAM-1, ICAM-2 and ICAM-3.[137,138] ICAM-1 expression is a prerequisite for antigen presentation *in vitro*[139] and the interaction of ICAM-1/LFA-1 and LFA-3/CD2 is an important co-stimulus in T cell activation.[140] The ICAM-1/LFA-1 pathway is of particular interest in this context since expression of ICAM-1 is up-regulated *in vitro* and *in vivo* by pro-inflammatory cytokines consistent with a regulatory role in inflammatory reactions.[137] In normal liver there is little ICAM-1 expression; however, during graft rejection ICAM-1 expression is induced on target structures (bile ducts, endothelium and focally on hepatocytes). This expression persists or increases in patients who fail to respond to pulse immunosuppression whereas it is rapidly abolished in responders.[45,141]

Pro-inflammatory cytokines are produced within the liver during rejection[95] (Figure 14.6) and probably induce both MHC antigens and ICAM-1 expression on structures such as the biliary epithelium, allowing increased lymphocyte adherence, interaction with graft antigens and

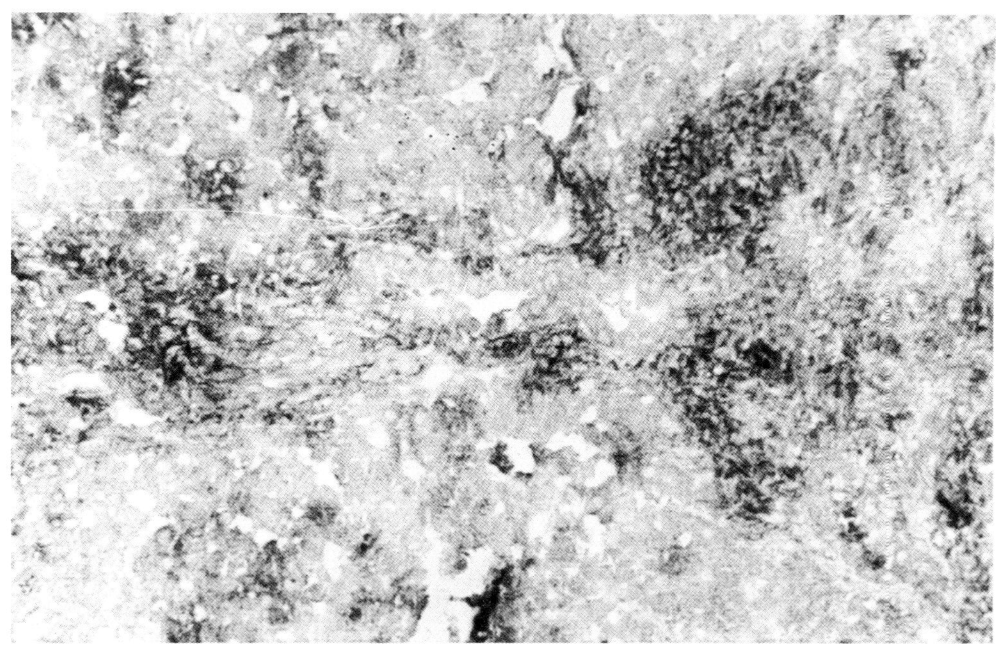

Fig. 14.6 Portal tract in a case of acute allograft rejection. Several areas show cells containing positive immunohistochemical staining for TNF. Scattered TNF containing cells are also present in adjacent hepatic sinusoids.

ultimately cytotoxicity. Corticosteroids do not down-regulate ICAM-1 expression on cell lines *in vitro* and their *in vivo* effect might be mediated by suppression of the secretion of such pro-inflammatory cytokines from infiltrating mononuclear cells. There is also evidence that the expression of LFA-3, which reacts with the CD2 T cell receptor, is marginally increased on hepatocytes, endothelia and bile duct cells.[141]

Minor transplantation antigens and blood group antigens may also act as targets for rejection. The expression of blood group antigens occurs on biliary epithelium and can be increased by infection and cholestasis and it has been claimed recently that bile duct lesions are more common in ABO incompatible liver transplants.[142]

Antigen presentation

Transplant antigens can be recognised by the recipient immune system either directly, without the need for processing, or after processing by host antigen presenting cells (APCs). The former is probably the most important since it provokes the strongest allogeneic response *in vitro*.[143,144] Cells of the macrophage lineage are usually associated with antigen presentation and the liver is particularly rich in these cells. Dendritic cells in portal tracts and Kupffer cells which line liver sinusoids are both able to present antigens efficiently.[145] Dendritic cells have been implicated in the pathogenesis of the obliterative arteriopathy of VBDS.[146] Following human transplantation, donor Kupffer cells are replaced by cells expressing the host phenotype. In patients with severe rejection this process occurs rapidly, within the first few weeks, whereas it occurs gradually in patients who accept their grafts. It is not known how this dynamic alteration in the balance of Kupffer cells expressing host and donor MHC affects the allogeneic response.

Animal studies have shown that vascular endothelial cells and possibly also biliary epithelial cells (although not hepatocytes) are capable of presenting antigen. Class II antigens are induced on these structures during episodes of rejection and therefore they may be involved in 'secondary' presentation of antigen, resulting in continued immune stimulation.[147]

Cellular events in liver allograft rejection

The presentation of allogeneic MHC antigens to the host immune system results in the activation of T cells capable of releasing lymphokines which initiate and orchestrate the effector arm of rejection. This role has traditionally been ascribed to CD4+ T cells although there is evidence that CD8+ T cells may also be involved. The effector response involves the generation of cytotoxic lymphocytes and delayed-type hypersensitivity reactions, the recruitment of other inflammatory cells and probably the secretion of antibody.[60,61,148]

The role of T cells in human liver allografts

T cells are the most common cell type infiltrating human liver transplants during rejection.[4,42,87] Although the majority of these T cells express the alpha/beta T cell receptor, between 5–25% express the gamma/delta T cell receptor.[149] The relative importance of these subsets is not known. Both helper (CD4+) and suppressor (CD8+) T lymphocytes accumulate in portal tracts during rejection and infiltrate biliary epithelium and endothelium, the principal targets of the rejection process.[87] The presence of a predominantly CD4+ T cell infiltrate has been associated with reversible rejection episodes, whereas a predominantly CD8+ infiltrate is associated with more severe rejection and progression to vanishing bile duct syndrome.[87,104] The majority of infiltrating T cells express the CD45 RO antigen and are therefore functionally primed or memory cells (Adams and Hathaway, unpublished observations) and many also express activation markers such as HLA-DR and IL-2 receptors[150] which are shed locally into bile during episodes of rejection.[76] Functional analysis of T cell clones from rejecting human liver tissue has demonstrated proliferative and cytotoxic activity directed at donor MHC class I antigens during acute rejection.[85,86] *In vivo* these cells probably adhere to biliary epithelial cells and endothelial cells via adhesive molecules such as ICAM-1 and then interact with transplantation antigens resulting in cell lysis. A different mechanism of CTL mediated liver damage has been demonstrated by So *et al.*[151] who used a murine mixed lymphocyte/hepatocyte culture system to demonstrate that cytolytic lymphocytes can inhibit hepatocyte functions, such as protein synthesis, without causing cell lysis. This might be due to the release of cytokines such as transforming growth (factor β (TGFβ) which can inhibit hepatocyte growth.

T cells may accumulate at the site of rejection either by continual migration in response to locally secreted chemotactic factors or by proliferation *in situ* in the presence of T cell growth factors. In man, circulating T cell counts increase prior to rejection of liver allografts and there are increased numbers of CD8+ and CD4+ cells within the liver during rejection[87,104] suggesting that T cells move preferentially from the periphery to accumulate within the graft. *In situ* proliferation of T cells has been demonstrated in experimental models[80] and is supported by the studies of Lautenschlager *et al.* Using fine needle aspiration biopsy, they demonstrated that intragraft lymphocytes expressed the activation markers HLA-DR and IL-2 receptors during episodes of rejection whereas peripheral blood lymphocytes harvested at the same time did not.[150]

The detection of chemotactic activity in bile samples from patients during rejection episodes suggests that locally active chemotactic factors are involved in the selective recruitment of leucocytes to human liver allografts.[69,82,83] Lymphocyte chemotactic factors with selective activity for CD8+ T cells, which include IL-6, are released into bile, probably by graft infiltrating CD4+ T cells, prior to episodes of rejection.

Other leucocytes

Although T cells are required for graft rejection there is increasing evidence that other leucocytes may act as effector cells.[12,62,91] The inflammatory infiltrate of human liver rejection consists of large numbers of monocytes, neutrophils and eosinophils and these cells may have important effector functions. The presence of the latter two cell types in liver biopsies is a reliable predictor of rejection[92] and neutrophils appear in bile during episodes of graft rejection.[152] Neutrophils isolated from patients after liver transplantation become activated shortly before the onset of clinical rejection and release increased amounts of superoxide radicals and proteolytic enzymes, both of which may cause tissue damage.[91] This neutrophil activation may occur in response to activating factors secreted by lymphocytes since peripheral blood lymphocytes (PBL) cultured from patients during episodes of rejection secrete a neutrophil activating factor. Neutrophil activation is suppressed in those patients who respond to treatment with high-dose corticosteroids.[91] In man, rejection of the liver is associated with both graft and peripheral blood eosinophilia and eosinophilic basic protein is released locally within the liver during rejection.[93,94]

The detection of increased circulating levels of monokines such as TNFα and IL-1 and their immunohistochemical detection within the portal infiltrate during rejection[95–97] suggest an effector role for activated monocytes/macrophages. Delayed type hypersensitivity, involving activation of macrophages with surface Fc receptors, has been implicated in animal studies but not so far in human liver rejection.

Humoral mechanisms

Although liver allografts are much less susceptible to damage from preformed lymphocytotoxic antibodies when compared with kidney or heart grafts, there is increasing evidence to implicate humoral mechanisms in the pathogenesis of fulminant rejection[153] as discussed above. Humoral mechanisms may play a more widespread role in rejection. Two studies have reported increased levels of anti-class I cytotoxic antibodies in patients with rejection[88,89] and significant amounts of immunoglobulin, particularly IgM, are deposited in arterial walls of rejected livers.[153] There is also evidence that IgG and particularly IgM are secreted within the liver during episodes of acute rejection.[90]

The cellular events leading to the development of acute rejection in liver transplantation are possibly as follows (Figure 14.7):

1. Antigen presenting cells (which may include dendritic cells and Kupffer cells and subsequently possibly biliary epithelial cells and hepatic endothelial cells) present transplant antigens to CD4+ (and possibly also CD8+) T helper cells in the presence of co-stimulatory factors such as interleukin 1;
2. These T cells become activated and release IL-2 and other cytokines which result in the clonal proliferation, differentiation and recruitment of T cells. Some of these T cells will have immunoregulatory functions whilst others have cytotoxic potential;
3. The escalating immunological reaction results in an intense inflammatory response during which pro-inflammatory cytokines induce increased graft MHC antigen and adhesion

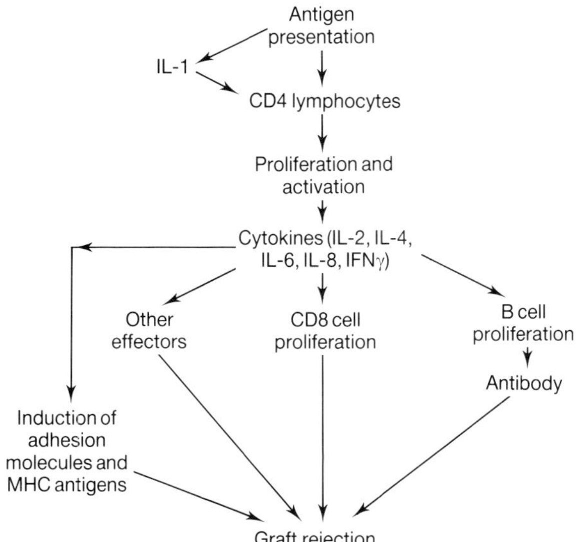

Fig. 14.7 Mechanisms of liver allograft rejection.

molecule expression and attract and activate other effector cells;

4. Graft damage results from T cell cytotoxicity directed at MHC products and a more generalised inflammatory cascade involving eosinophils, macrophages and neutrophils.

The factors which determine whether this process is self-limiting or relentlessly progressive are poorly understood.

References

1. Calne RY, White HJ, Yoffa DE *et al.* Observations of orthotopic liver transplantation in the pig. *Br Med J* 1967; **2,** 478–480.
2. Starzl TE (ed) *Experiences in Hepatic Transplantation*. Philadelphia: W. B. Saunders, 1969.
3. Starzl TE, Koep LJ, Halgrimson CG *et al.* Fifteen years of clinical liver transplantation. *Gastroenterology* 1979; **77,** 375–388.
4. Quiroga J, Colina I, Demetris JA, Starzl TE, van Thiel DH. Cause and timing of first allograft failure in orthotopic liver transplantation: a study of 177 consecutive patients. *Hepatology* 1992; **14,** 1054–1062.
5. Demetris JA, Belle SH, Hart J *et al.* Intraobserver and interobserver variation in the histological assessment of liver allograft rejection. *Hepatology* 1991; **14,** 751–755.
6. Eggink HF, Hofstee N, Gips CH *et al.* Histopathology of serial graft biopsies from liver transplant recipients. *Am J Pathol* 1984; **114,** 18–31.
7. Snover DC, Sibley RK, Freese DK *et al.* Orthotopic liver transplantation: a pathological study of 63 serial liver biopsies from 17 patients with special reference to diagnostic features of rejection and natural history of rejection. *Hepatology* 1984; **4,** 1212–1222.
8. Williams JW, Peters TG, Vera SR, Britt LG, van Voorst SJ, Haggit RC. Biopsy-directed immunosuppression following hepatic transplantation in man. *Transplantation* 1985; **39,** 689–696.
9. Hubscher SG, Clements D, Elias E, McMaster P. Biopsy findings in cases of rejection of liver allografts. *J Clin Pathol* 1985; **38,** 1366–1373.
10. Snover DC, Freese DK, Sharp HL, Bloomer JR, Najarian JS, Ascher NL. Liver allograft rejection. An analysis of the use of biopsy in determining the outcome of rejection. *Am J Surg Pathol* 1987; **11,** 1–10.
11. Adams DH, Neuberger JM. Patterns of graft rejection following liver transplantation. *J Hepatol* 1990; **10,** 113–119.
12. Vierling JM. Immunologic mechanisms of hepatic allograft rejection. *Sem Liver Dis* 1992; **12,** 16–27.
13. Klintmalm GBG, Nery JR, Husberg BS *et al.* Rejection in liver transplantation. *Hepatology* 1989; **10,** 978–985.
14. Mor E, Solomon H, Gibbs JF *et al.* Acute cellular rejection following liver transplantation: clinical pathological features and effect on outcome. *Sem Liver Dis* 1992; **12,** 28–38.
15. Ludwig J, Weisner RH, Batts KP, Perkins JP, Kromn RAF. The acute vanishing bile duct syndrome (acute irreversible rejection) after orthotopic liver transplantation. *Hepatology* 1987; **7,** 476–483.
16. Ascher N, Stock PG, Bumgardner GL, Payne WD, Najarian JS. Infection and rejection of primary hepatic transplantation in 93 consecutive patients treated with triple immunosuppressive therapy. *Surg Gynaecol Obstet* 1988; **167,** 474–484.
17. Saliba F, Gugenheim J, Samuel D, Ciardullo M, Reynes M, Bismuth H. Orthotopic liver transplantation in humans: monitoring by serial graft biopsies. *Transplant Proc* 1987; **19,** 2454–2456.
18. Cuervas-Mons V, Martinez AJ, Dekkar A *et al.* Adult liver transplantation: an analysis of the early causes of death in 40 consecutive cases. *Hepatology* 1986; **6,** 495–501.
19. Ludwig J. Classification and terminology of hepatic allograft rejection: whither bound? *Mayo Clin Proc* 1989; **64,** 676–679.
20. Hubscher SG, Buckels JAC, Elias E, McMaster P, Neuberger JM. Reversible vanishing bile duct syndrome after liver transplantation: report of six cases. *Transplant Proc* 1991; **23,** 1415–1416.
21. Wiesner RH, Ludwig J, van Hoek B, Krom

RAF. Current concepts in cell-mediated hepatic allograft rejection leading to ductopenia and liver failure. *Hepatology* 1991; **14,** 721–729.
22. Pichlmayr R, Gubernatis G. Rejection of the liver and review of current immunosuppressive protocols. *Transplant Proc* 1987; **19,** 4367–4369.
23. Esquivel CO, Jaffe R, Gordon RD *et al.* Liver rejection and its differentiation from other causes of graft dysfunction. *Sem Liver Dis* 1985; **5,** 369–374.
24. Ascher NL, Freese DK, Paradis K *et al.* Rejection of the transplanted liver. In: *Transplantation of the Liver*, Maddrey WC (ed). New York: Elsevier, 1988.
25. Gubernatis G, Kemnitz J, Tusch G, Pichlmayr R. HLA compatibility and different features of liver allograft rejection. *Transplant Int* 1988; **1,** 155–160.
26. Maddrey WC, van Thiel DH. Liver transplantation: an overview. *Hepatology* 1988; **8**(4), 948–959.
27. Klein AS, Savader S, Burdick JS *et al.* Reduction of morbidity and mortality from biliary complications after liver transplantation. *Hepatology* 1991; **14,** 818–823.
28. Demetris AJ, Todo S, van Thiel DH *et al.* Evolution of hepatitis B virus liver disease after hepatic replacement: practical and theoretical considerations. *Am J Pathol* 1990; **137,** 667–676.
29. Rizzetto M, Macagno S, Chiaberge E *et al.* Liver transplantation in hepatitis delta virus disease. *Lancet* 1987; **ii,** 469–471.
30. Martin P, Munoz SJ, Di Bisceglie AM *et al.* Recurrence of hepatitis C after liver transplantation. *Hepatology* 1991; **13,** 719–721.
31. Fagan E, Yousef G, Brahm J *et al.* Persistence of hepatitis A virus in fulminant hepatitis and after liver transplantation. *J Med Virol* 1990; **30,** 1313–1316.
32. Bronsther O, Makowka L, Jaffe R *et al.* Occurrence of cytomegalovirus hepatitis in liver transplant patients. *J Med Virol* 1988; **24,** 423–434.
33. Singh N, Dummer JS, Kusne S, Breinig MK, Armstrong JA, Makowka L, Starzl TE, Ho M. Infections with cytomegalovirus and herpesviruses in 121 liver transplant recipients: transmission by donated organ and the effect of OKT3 antibodies. *J Infect Dis* 1988; **158,** 124–131.
34. Drummer JS. CMV infection after liver transplantation: clinical manifestations and strategies of prevention. *Rev Inf Dis* 1990; **12,** 767–775.
35. Koneru B, Jaffe R, Esquivel CO *et al.* Adenoviral infections in paediatric liver recipients. *J Am Med Assoc* 1987; **258,** 489–492.
36. Sterneck M, Wiesner R, Ascher N *et al.* Azathioprine toxicity after liver transplantation. *Hepatology* 1991; **14,** 806–810.
37. Klintmalm GBG, Iwatsuki S, Starzl TE. Cyclosporin A hepatotoxicity in 66 renal allograft recipients. *Transplantation* 1981; **32,** 488–489.
38. Sankary HN, Williams HN, Foster PF. Can serum liver function tests differentiate rejection from other causes of liver dysfunction after hepatic transplantation? *Transplant Proc* 1988; **20,** 669–670.
39. Clements D, McMaster P, Elias E. Indocyanine green clearance in acute rejection after liver transplantation. *Transplantation* 1987; **46,** 383–385.
40. Lautenschlager I, Hockerstedt K, Salmela K, Isoniemi H, Holmberg C, Jalanko H, Hayry P. Fine-needle aspiration biopsy in the monitoring of liver allografts. *Transplantation* 1990; **50,** 798–803.
41. Bubak ME, Porayko MK, Krom RAF, Wiesner RH. Complications of liver biopsy in liver transplant patients: increased sepsis associated with choledochojejunostomy. *Hepatology* 1992; **14,** 1063–1065.
42. Hubscher SG. Histological findings in liver allograft rejection: new insights into the pathogenesis of hepatocellular damage in liver allografts. *Histopathology* 1991; **18,** 377–383.
43. Wight DGD, Portman B. Pathology of liver transplantation. In: *Liver Transplantation*, Calne RY (ed). London: Grune and Stratton, 1987.
44. Steinhoff G. Major histocompatibility antigens in human liver transplants. *J Hepatol* 1990; **11,** 9–15.
45. Adams DH, Hubscher SG, Shaw J, Rothlein R, Neuberger JM. Intercellular adhesion molecule-1 on liver allograft during rejection. *Lancet* 1989; **ii,** 1122–1124.
46. Adams DH, Neuberger JM. Treatment of acute rejection. *Sem Liver Dis* 1992; **12,** 80–89.
47. Pirsch JD, Kalayoglu M, Hafez GR *et al.* Evidence that the vanishing bile duct syndrome is vanishing. *Transplantation* 1990; **49,** 1015–1018.
48. Boon AP, O'Brien D, Adams DH. Ten year review of invasive aspergillosis detected at necropsy. *J Clin Pathol* 1991; **44,** 452–455.
49. Hayry P, von Willibrand E. Monitoring of organ allograft rejection by transplant aspiration cytology. *Ann Clin Res* 1981; **13,** 264–287.
50. Hayry P, von Willibrand E. Practical guidelines for fine needle aspiration biopsy of human allografts. *Ann Clin Res* 1981; **13,** 288–306.
51. Lautenschlager I, Hockerstedt K, Teskinen E *et al.* Fine needle aspiration cytology of liver allograft in the pig. *Transplantation* 1984; **38,** 330–334.
52. Kirby RM, Young JA, Hubscher SG, Elias E, McMaster P. The accuracy of aspiration cytology in the diagnosis of rejection following orthotopic

liver transplantation. *Transplant Int* 1988; **1,** 119–126.
53. Schlitt HJ, Nashan B, Ringe B, Bunzendah H, Wittekind C, Wonigeit K, Pichlmayr R. Differentiation of liver graft dysfunction by transplant aspiration cytology. *Transplantation* 1991; **51,** 786–792.
54. Kubota K, Ericzon BG, Reinholt FP. Comparison of fine-needle aspiration biopsy and histology in human liver transplants. *Transplantation* 1991; **51,** 1010–1013.
55. Carbonnel F, Samuel D, Reynes M, Benhamou JP, Bismuth H, Bach JF, Chatenoud L. Fine-needle aspiration biopsy of human liver allografts. *Transplantation* 1990; **50,** 704–707.
56. Flint EW, Sumkin JH, Zajko AB, Bowen A. Duplex sonography of hepatic artery thrombosis after liver transplatation. *Am J Roentgenol* 1988; **151,** 481–483.
57. Coulden RA, Britton PD, Farman P, Noble-Jamieson G, Wight DGD. Preliminary report: hepatic vein doppler in the early diagnosis of acute liver transplant rejection. *Lancet* 1990; **336,** 273–275.
58. Adams DH. Immunological indices of liver allograft rejection. In: *Immunologic, Metabolic and Infectious Complications of Liver Transplantation*, Vuitton DA, Balabaud C, Houssin D, Dheumeux D (eds). Paris: John Libbey Eurotext, 1991.
59. Sanfilippo F. Immunology of liver transplantation. In: *Transplantation of the Liver*, Maddrey WC (ed). New York: Elsevier, 1988.
60. Ascher NL, Hoffman RA, Hanto DW, Simmons RL. Cellular basis of allograft rejection. *Immunol Rev* 1984; **77,** 217–232.
61. Hayry P, von Willibrand E, Parthenais E, Nemlander A, Soots A, Lautenschlager I, Alfoldy P, Renkonen R. The inflammatory mechanisms of allograft rejection. *Immunol Rev* 1984; **77,** 85–142.
62. Adams DH. Mechanisms of human liver allograft rejection. *Clin Sci* 1990; **78,** 343–350.
63. Raulet DH, Bevan MJ. A differentiation factor required for the expression of cytotoxic T cell function. *Nature* 1982; **296,** 754–757.
64. Heidecke CD, Kupiec-Weglinski JW, Lear DA *et al.* Interactions between T lymphocyte subsets supported by IL2 rich lymphokines produce acute rejection of vascularised cardiac allografts in T cell deprived rats. *J Immunol* 1984; **133,** 582–588.
65. Nathan C, Sporn MB. Cytokines in context. *J Cell Biol* 1991; **113,** 981–986.
66. Herrod HG, Williams JW, Valenski WR, Vera S. Serial immunologic studies in recipients of hepatic allografts. *Clin Immunol Immunopath* 1986; **40,** 298–304.
67. Herrod HG, Williams JW, Dean PJ. Alteration in immunologic measurements in patients experiencing early hepatic allograft rejection. *Transplantation* 1988; **45,** 923–925.
68. Munn SR, Tominaga S, Perkins JD, Hayes DH, Weisner RH, Krom RAF. Increasing peripheral T lymphocyte counts predict rejection in human liver allografts. *Transplant Proc* 1988; **20** (suppl 1), 674–675.
69. Hathaway M, Adams DH, Burnett D, Elias E. Recruitment of lymphocytes to human liver allografts during rejection. *Transplant Proc* 1990; **22,** 2306–2307.
70. Tilg H, Vogel W, Aulitzky WE, Herold M, Knigsrainer A, Margreiter R, Huber C. Evaluation of cytokines and cytokine-induced secondary messages in sera of patients after liver transplantation. *Transplantation* 1990; **49,** 1074–1080.
71. Tilg H, Vogel W, Aulitzky WE, Schnitzer D, Margreiter R, Dietze O, Judmaier G, Wachter H, Huber C. Neopterin excretion after liver transplantation and its value in differential diagnosis of complications. *Transplantation* 1989; **48,** 594–599.
72. Maury CPJ, Hockerstedt K, Tepo AM, Lautenschlager I, Scheinin TM. Changes in serum amyloid A protein and beta-2-microglobulin in association with liver allograft rejection. *Transplantation* 1984; **38,** 551–553.
73. Oldhafer KJ, Schaefer O, Wonigiet K, Ringe B, Pichlmayr R. Monitoring of serum neopterin levels after liver transplantation. *Transplant Proc* 1988; **20,** 671–673.
74. Uchiyama T, Broder S, Waldmann TA. A monoclonal antibody (anti-TAC) reactive with activated and functionally mature human T cells. *J Immunol* 1981; **126,** 1393–1397.
75. Rubin LA, Kurman CC, Fritz ME *et al.* Soluble interleukin-2 receptors are released from activated human lymphoid cells *in vitro*. *J Immunol* 1985; **135,** 3172–7.
76. Adams DH, Wang L, Hubscher SG, Elias E, Neuberger JM. Soluble interleukin-2 receptors in serum and bile of liver transplant recipients. *Lancet* 1989; **i,** 469–472.
77. Perkins JD, Nelson DL, Rakela J, Grambasch PM, Krom RAF. Soluble interleukin-2 receptor level as an indicator of liver allograft rejection. *Transplantation* 1989; **47,** 77–81.
78. Adams DH, Burnett D, Stockley RA, McMaster P, Elias E. Biliary beta-2-microglobulin in liver allograft rejection. *Hepatology* 1988; **8,** 1565–1570.
79. Adams DH, Mainolfi E, Elias E, Neuberger JM, Rothlein R. Detection of circulating ICAM-1 after liver transplantation: evidence for local release within the liver during graft rejection.

Transplantation 1992 (in press).

80. Ascher NL, Chen S, Hoffman RA *et al.* Maturation of cytotoxic T cells within sponge matrix allografts. *J Immunol* 1983; **131,** 617–621.

81. Kupiec-Weglinski JW, de Sousa M, Tilney NL. The importance of lymphocyte migration patterns in experimental organ transplantation. *Transplantation* 1985; **40,** 1–6.

82. Adams DH, Burnett D, Stockley RA, Elias E. Patterns of leucocyte chemotaxis following liver transplantation. *Gastroenterology* 1989; **97,** 433–438.

83. Hathaway M, Adams DH, Burnett D, Elias E. Secretion into bile of chemotactic factors for CD8+ lymphocytes during rejection of human liver allografts. *Transplant Proc* 1991; **23,** 1424–1425.

84. Grant D, Wall W, Stiller C, Keown P, Duff J, Ghent C. Immunologic monitoring for rejection after liver transplantation. *Transplant Proc* 1986; **18,** 171–173.

85. Fung JJ, Zeevi A, Starzl TE, Iwatsuki S, Duquesnoy RJ. Functional characterization of infiltrating T lymphocytes in human hepatic allografts. *Hum Immunol* 1986; **16,** 182–199.

86. Markus BH, Demetris AJ, Saidman S, Fung JJ, Zeevi A, Starzl TE, Duquesnoy RJ. Alloreactive T lymphocytes cultured from liver transplant biopsies: associations of HLA specificity with clinicopathological findings. *Clin Transplant* 1988; **2,** 70–75.

87. McCaughan GW, Davies JS, Waugh JA, Bishop GA *et al.* A quantitative analysis of T lymphocyte populations in human liver allografts undergoing rejection; the use of monoclonal antibodies and double immunolabelling. *Hepatology* 1990; **12,** 1305–1313.

88. Donaldson PT, Alexander GJM, O'Grady J *et al.* Evidence of an immune response to HLA class 1 antigens in the vanishing bile duct syndrome after liver transplantation. *Lancet* 1987; **i,** 945–948.

89. Bryan CF, Newman JT, Tilquist RL, Husberg B, Klintmalm GB, Stone MJ. Development of class I-directed lymphocytotoxic antibodies after liver transplantation. *Transplant Proc* 1987; **19,** 2392–2393.

90. Adams DH, Hubscher SG, Burnett D, Elias E. Immunoglobulins in liver allograft rejection: evidence for deposition and secretion within the liver. *Transplant Proc* 1991; **22,** 1834–1835.

91. Adams DH, Wang LF, Burnett D, Stockley RA, Neuberger JM. Neutrophil activation: an important cause of tissue damage during liver allograft rejection? *Transplantation* 1990; **50,** 86–91.

92. Sankary S, Foster P, Hart M *et al.* An analysis of the determinants of hepatic allograft rejection using step-wise logistic regression. *Transplantation* 1989; **47,** 74–77.

93. Foster P, Sankary S, Hart M, Ashmann M, Williams JW. Blood and graft eosinophilia as predictors of rejection in human liver transplantation. *Transplantation* 1989; **47,** 72–74.

94. Foster PF, Bhattacharyya A, Sankary HN, Coleman J, Ashmann M, Williams JW. Eosinophil cationic protein's role in human hepatic allograft rejection. *Hepatology* 1991; **13,** 1117–1125.

95. Hoffman MW, Wonigeit K, Steinhoff M, Behrend M *et al.* Tissue necrosis factor alpha and interleukin beta in rejecting liver grafts. *Transplant Proc* 1991; **23**C11: 1421–1423.

96. Adams DH, Garner C, Neuberger JM. Serum tumour necrosis factor alpha in liver transplantation. *Transplant Proc* 1990; **22,** 2310.

97. Imagawa DK, Millis JM, Olthoff KM, Derus LJ, Chia D, Sugich LR, Ozawa M, Dempsey RA, Iwaki Y, Levy PJ, Terasaki PI, Busuttil RW. The role of tumor necrosis factor in allograft rejection. *Transplantation* 1990; **50,** 219–225.

98. Vierling JM, Fennell RH. Histopathology of early and late human hepatic allograft rejection: evidence of destruction of interlobular bile ducts. *Hepatology* 1985; **5,** 1076–1082.

99. Adams DH, Burnett D, Stockley RA, McMaster P, Elias E. Markers of biliary epithelial damage in liver allograft rejection. *Transplant Proc* 1987; **19,** 3820–3821.

100. Bresson-Hadne S, Rossel M, Seilles E *et al.* Serum and bile secretory immunoglobulins and secretory component during the early postoperative course after liver transplantation. *Hepatology* 1992; **14,** 1046–1053.

101. Pollard SG, Davies HFFS, Calne RY. Soluble class I antigen in human bile. *Transplantation* 1989; **48,** 712–714.

102. Adams DH, Wang L, Hubscher SG, Neuberger JM. Hepatic endothelial cells: targets in liver allograft rejection? *Transplantation* 1989; **47,** 479–482.

103. Forbes GM, Oliveira DBG, Hughes RD, O'Grady JG, Calne RY, Williams R. Serum F protein estimation in liver allograft recipients with graft dysfunction. *Transplantation* 1989; **48,** 995–997.

104. Perkins JD, Rakela J, Sterioff S, Banks PM, Weisner RH, Krom RAF. Results of treatment in hepatic allograft rejection depend on the immunohistologic pattern of the portal T-lymphocyte infiltrate. *Transplant Proc* 1988; **20,** 223–225.

105. Lasky S, Demetris AJ, Dekker A *et al.* Glutamyl transpeptidase as a marker for rejection following liver transplantation. *Hepatology* 1984; **4,** 1045.

106. White DJG, Friend PJ. Immunosuppression. In:

Liver Transplantation, Calne RY (ed). London: Grune and Stratton, 1987.

107. Cosimi AB, Cho SI, Delmonico FC, Kaplan MM, Rohrer RJ, Jenkins RL. A randomised trial comparing OKT3 and steroids for the treatment of hepatic allograft rejection. *Transplantation* 1987; **43,** 91–95.
108. Renard TH, Andrews WS, Foster ME. Relationship between OKT3 administration, EBV seroconversion and the lymphoproliferative syndrome in paediatric liver transplantation. *Transplant Proc* 1991; **23,** 1473–1476.
109. Fung JJ, Todo S, Tzakis A *et al.* Conversion of liver allograft recipients from cyclosporin to FK506-based immunosuppression: benefits and pitfalls. *Transplant Proc* 1991; **23,** 14–21.
110. Starzl TE, Lerner RA, Dixon FS *et al.* Schwartzmann reaction after human renal transplantation. *N Eng J Med* 1968; **278,** 642–648.
111. Ting A. The lymphocytotoxic crossmatch test in clinical renal transplantation. *Transplantation* 1983; **35,** 403–407.
112. Wardel EN. Kupffer cells and their function. *Liver* 1987; **7,** 63–75.
113. Roser BJ, Kamada N, Zimmerman F, Davies HS. Immunosuppressive effect of experimental liver allografts. In: *Liver Transplantation*, Calne RY (ed). New York: Grune and Stratton, 1987.
114. Calne RY, Sells RA, Pena YR *et al.* Induction of immunological tolerance by porcine liver allografts. *Nature* 1969; **223,** 472–476.
115. Gordon RD, Fung JJ, Markus B *et al.* The antibody crossmatch in liver transplantation. *Surgery* 1986; **100,** 705–715.
116. Gordon RD, Esquivel CO, Iwatsuki S, Starzl TE. Liver transplantation across ABO blood groups. *Surgery* 1986; **100,** 342–348.
117. Iwatsuki S, Rabin BS, Shaw BW, Starzl TE. Liver transplantation against T cell-positive warm crossmatches. *Transplant Proc* 1984; **16,** 1427–1429.
118. Houssin D, Bellon B, Brunaud MD, Gugenheim J, Settaf A, Meriggi F, Emond J. Interactions between liver allografts and lymphocytotoxic alloantibodies in inbred rats. *Hepatology* 1986; **6,** 994–998.
119. Knechtle SJ, Kolbeck PC, Tsuchimoto S, Coundouriotis A, Sanfilippo F, Bollinger RR. Hepatic transplantation into sensitized recipients. *Transplantation* 1987; **43,** 8–12.
120. Gubernatis G, Lauchart W, Jonker M, Steinhoff G, Bornscheuer A, Neuhaus P, van Es AA, Kemnitz J, Wonigeit K, Pichlmayr R. Signs of hyperacute rejection of liver grafts in rhesus monkeys after donor-specific presensitization. *Transplant Proc* 1987; **19,** 1082–1083.
121. Starzl TE, Demetris AJ, Todo S *et al.* Evidence for hyperacute rejection of human liver grafts. The case of the canary kidney. *Clin Transplant* 1989; **3,** 37–45.
122. Bird G, Friend P, Donaldson P, O'Grady J, Portmann B, Calne R, Williams R. Hyperacute rejection in liver transplantation: a case report. *Transplant Proc* 1989; **21,** 3742–3744.
123. Hubscher SG, Adams DH, Neuberger JM, Buckels JAC, McMaster P, Elias E. Massive haemorrhagic necrosis of the liver following transplantation. *J Clin Pathol* 1989; **42,** 360–370.
124. Gubernatis G, Kemnitz J, Bornscheuer A, Kuse ER, Pichlmayr R. Potential various appearances of hyperacute rejection in human liver transplantation. *Langenbecks Arch Chir* 1989; **374,** 240–244.
125. Gugenheim J, Samuel D, Reynes M, Bismuth H. Liver transplantation across ABO blood group barriers. *Lancet* 1990; **336,** 519–523.
126. Bach FH, van Rood JJ. The major histocompatibility complex – genetics and biology. *N Eng J Med* 1976; **295,** 806–813.
127. Halloran PH, Wadgymar A, Autenreid P. The regulation of expression of major histocompatibility complex products. *Transplantation* 1986; **41,** 413–420.
128. Bach FH, Bach ML, Sondel PM. Differential function of major histocompatibility complex antigens in T lymphocyte activation. *Nature* 1976; **259,** 273–281.
129. Daar AS, Fuggle SV, Fabre JW, Ting A, Morris PJ. The detailed distribution of HLA A B and C antigens in normal human organs. *Transplantation* 1984; **38,** 287–292.
130. Daar AS, Fuggle SV, Fabre JW, Ting A, Morris PJ. The detailed distribution of MHC class 2 antigens in normal human organs. *Transplantation* 1984; **38,** 293–298.
131. Lautenschlager I, Hayry P. Expression of major histocompatibility complex antigens on different liver cellular components in rat and man. *Scand J Immunol* 1981; **14,** 421–426.
132. Gouw ASH, Houthoff HJ, Huitema S, Beelen JM, Gips CH, Poppema S. Expression of major histocompatibility antigens and replacement of donor cells by recipient ones in human liver allografts. *Transplantation* 1987; **43,** 291–294.
133. Hubscher SG, Adams DH, Elias E. Beta-2-microglobin expression in the liver after liver transplantation. *J Clin Pathol* 1988; **41,** 1049–1057.
134. SG Hubscher, DH Adams, Elias E. Changes in the expression of MHC class II antigens in liver allograft rejection. *J Pathol* 1990; **22,** 1828–1829.
135. Rosa F, Hatat D, Abadie A, Fellous M. Regulation of histocompatibility antigens by interferon. *Ann Inst Pasteur (Immunol)* 1985; **136C,** 103–105.
136. Skoskiewicz MJ, Colvin RB, Schneeberger EE,

Russel PS. Widerpread and selective induction of major histocompatibility complex-determined antigens *in vivo* by gamma-interferon. *J Exp Med* 1985; **162,** 1645–1664.

137. Springer TA. Adhesion receptors of the immune system. *Nature* 1990; **346,** 425–433.
138. Shaw S, Luce GEG, Quinones R *et al.* Two antigen independent adhesion pathways used by human cytotoxic T cell clones. *Nature* 1986; **323,** 262–264.
139. Altman DM, Hogg N, Trowsdale J, Wilkinson D. Cotransfection of ICAM-1 and HLA-DR reconstitutes human antigen-presenting cell function in mouse cells. *Nature* 1989; **338,** 512–514.
140. Van Seventer GA, Shimizu Y, Horgan KJ, Shaw S. The LFA-1 ligand ICAM-1 provides an important costimulatory signal for T cell receptor-mediated activation of resting T cells. *J Immunol* 1990; **11, 144**(12), 4579–4586.
141. Behrend M, Steinhoff G, Wonigeit K, Pichlmayr R. Patterns of adhesion molecule expression in human liver allografts. *Transplant Proc* 1991; **23,** 1419–1420.
142. Sterioff S, Sanchez L, Rosen C, Schwerman L, Noack K. Increased bile duct complications in ABO incompatible liver transplants. *Transplant Proc* 1991; **23,** 1440–1441.
143. Lechler RI, Lombardi G, Batchelor JR, Reinsmoen N, Bach FH. The molecular basis of alloreactivity. *Immunol Today* 1990; **11,** 83–88.
144. Sherwood RA, Brent L, Rayfield L. Presentation of alloantigens by host cells. *Eur J Immunol* 1986; **16,** 569–572.
145. Rubinstein D, Roska AK, Lipsky PE. Antigen presentation by liver sinusoidal lining cells after antigen exposure *in vivo*. *J Immunol* 1987; **138,** 1377–1380.
146. Oguma S, Banner B, Zerbe T, Starzl T, Demetris AJ. Participation of dendritic cells in vascular lesions of chronic rejection of human allografts. *Lancet* 1988; **ii,** 933–935.
147. Lautenschlager I, Nyman N, Vaananen H, Lehto VP, Virtanen I, Hayry P. Antigenic and immunogenic components in rat liver. *Scand J Immunol* 1983; **17,** 61.
148. Steinmuller D. Which T cells mediate allograft rejection?. *Transplantation* 1989; **40,** 229–233.
149. Kabelitz D, Da Silva Lobo ML, Schurmann G, Hofmann WJ, Otto G. Presence of gamma/delta T cell receptor-expressing T cells in liver biopsies following liver transplantation. *Hum Immunol* 1990; **28,** 167–169.
150. Lautenschlager I, Hockerstedt K, Hayry P. Activation markers in acute liver allograft rejection. *Transplant Proc* 1988; **20,** 646–647.
151. So SKS, Wilkes LM, Platt JL, Ascher NL, Simmons RL. Purified hepatocytes can stimulate allospecific cytolytic T cells in a mixed lymphocyte-hepatocyte culture. *Transplant Proc* 1987; **19,** 251–252.
152. Kubota K, Ericzon BG, Barkholt L, Reinholt FP. Bile cytology in orthotopic liver transplantation. *Transplantation* 1989; **48,** 998–1003.
153. Demetris AJ, Jaffe R, Tzakis A *et al.* Antibody mediated rejection of human orthotopic liver allografts: a study of liver transplantation across ABO blood barriers. *Am J Pathol* 1988; **132,** 489–493.

15

Chronic rejection of the liver allograft

S Hubscher and J Neuberger

Introduction

Chronic rejection of liver allograft is generally considered to be an irreversible condition, characterised by immune mediated destruction of bile ducts and an obliterative vasculopathy involving large and medium sized arteries.[1–5] This results in a syndrome of progressive cholestasis which is usually unresponsive to immunosuppression and results in graft failure.

The subdivision of rejection into acute and chronic forms is based principally on time of occurrence, but also on behaviour and characteristic histological features. Various other terms have been advocated to describe rejection in the liver allograft on the basis of these three main features (Table 15.1). Whilst each of these alternatives offers theoretical advantages in classifying rejection, a point which will be considered again later, none is entirely satisfactory. Despite their limitations, acute and chronic rejection remain the most widely used terms and will be used here.

Although the subdivision of rejection into 'acute' and 'chronic' forms remains of considerable clinical value, there are overlapping features for each of the three main components that characterise these two patterns of graft damage. Individual cases are often difficult to classify. Most cases of chronic rejection are preceded by episodes of acute rejection but this is not always so. It is still not clear whether acute and chronic rejection are fundamentally different processes which happen to have overlapping clinicopathological features, or whether they represent different ends of a broad spectrum of immune mediated damage in the liver allograft.

Table 15.1 Terms used to describe the two main patterns of rejection in the liver allograft (VBDS = vanishing bile duct syndrome)

Time of occurrence	Acute (Early)	Chronic (Late)
Behaviour	Reversible	Irreversible
Main histological features	Cellular	Ductopenic (VBDS) Vascular

Incidence

The reported incidence of chronic rejection (CR) varies from centre to centre. In 11 series recently reviewed by Wiesner *et al.*[6] the incidence ranged from 2.4% to 16.8%. Out of a total of 1401 allografts transplanted in these 11 centres, 111 developed chronic rejection, giving an overall incidence of 7.9%. In our programme, 36 out of 441 grafts (8.2%) have failed as a result of chronic rejection over a minimum follow-up period of 12 months.

Chronic rejection is the most common cause of graft failure in patients who survive the early post-operative period after liver transplantation, resulting in up to 50% of late graft failures.[7,8] In our programme, chronic rejection accounts for 33% (21/64) of all retransplant operations and for 75% (18/24) of regrafting procedures carried out more than two months post-transplant.

Two main factors are responsible for producing a wide variation in the reported incidence of CR. Firstly, not all of the figures quoted are directly comparable. Some studies refer to the incidence of CR in primary grafts, others to the incidence in all grafts (including second and subsequent ones in which a higher incidence has been reported). Some studies exclude cases of rejection resulting in graft failure within the first three months of transplantation, while others only give figures for patients who have survived more than three months post-transplant.

In addition to the reasons for apparent differences in incidence noted above, there is some evidence to suggest that the incidence of chronic rejection may be genuinely declining as a result of changes in immunosuppressive therapy. Three recent studies have shown a lower incidence of rejection (acute and chronic) in patients treated with triple or quadruple immunosuppression compared with those on double therapy[9–11] – this is discussed later.

Clinical features

The typical clinical presentation is one of progressive jaundice associated with severe biochemical cholestasis; for instance, the median serum bilirubin level at the time of retransplantation in our programme is 720 μmol/l (range 255–990).[12] Minor elevations of serum transaminases are also commonly observed. These clinical and biochemical features are non-specific and cannot be reliably distinguished from other causes of cholestasis in liver allografts, including biliary obstruction, sepsis, viral infection and, possibly, drug toxicity. Accurate diagnosis is still dependent on histological examination.

The time of presentation and natural history of chronic rejection are very variable.[13] Terms such as 'accelerated' CR (presenting less than two months post-transplant), 'delayed' CR (2–6 months post-transplant) and 'late' CR (more than six months post-transplant) may be used to describe different patterns of presentation of chronic rejection. The peak incidence of CR in our series is 2–6 months post-transplant. However, several patients have presented at a time when distinction from 'acute' (potentially reversible) rejection is difficult and three have progressed to end-stage disease requiring retransplantation within six weeks of the initial transplant operation. The term 'acute vanishing bile duct syndrome' has been used to describe cases developing graft failure within the first 100 days of liver transplantation.[14] However, in all other respects these are indistinguishable from 'typical' CR and the distinction is, therefore, somewhat artificial. Chronic rejection is rare more than 12 months post-transplant. Only three patients in our programme have presented with features of CR at this time. Other centres have also reported occasional cases of 'late' chronic rejection, occurring more than one year post-transplant.[3,9,15,16] There is some evidence to suggest that these late cases have a more insidious presentation and prolonged course than those with 'typical' CR. Histologically they tend to have cholestasis and ductopenia without conspicuous cellular infiltrates.

In most patients, cholestatic features gradually progress over a period of several weeks or months and result in graft failure. Response to immunosuppression is poor and retransplantation represents the only effective method of treatment for these cases. In some patients cholestatic features evolve more rapidly while in others there is a static period following by gradual recovery ('reversible VBDS').

Histological features

Two main features are generally regarded as diagnostic of chronic rejection. The first is destruction of intrahepatic bile ducts, hence the terms vanishing bile duct syndrome (VBDS) and ductopenic rejection (DR). The second is an obliterative vasculopathy involving large and medium sized arteries – vascular rejection. Characteristic changes are also seen in the liver parenchyma in the form of perivenular cholestasis and hepatocyte drop-out.

Bile duct lesions

Bile duct loss in CR typically occurs gradually and can be seen as a progressive lesion in serial needle biopsy specimens. During the early stages, there is usually a prominent portal inflammatory infiltrate associated with bile duct damage (Figure 15.1). Ducts may be present in normal numbers at this stage, making distinction from 'acute', potentially reversible rejection difficult. Portal inflammatory changes tend to subside as bile ducts are destroyed, giving rise to a characteristic 'burnt out' appearance in end-stage livers (Figure 15.2). Bile ductular proliferation is not a feature of chronic rejection, in contrast with other syndromes associated with a vanishing bile duct syndrome such as primary biliary cirrhosis or sclerosing cholangitis.

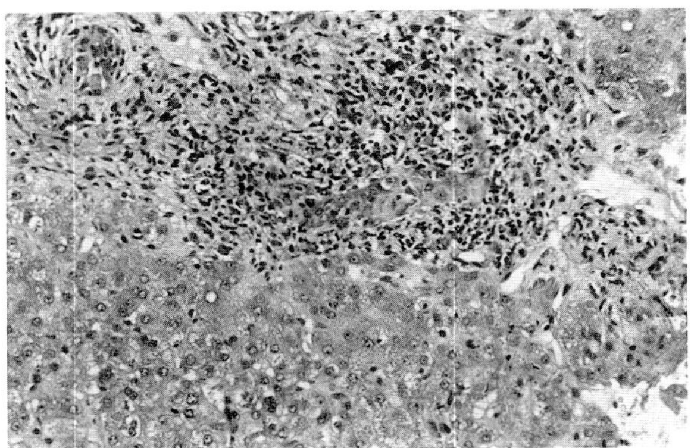

Fig. 15.1 Early chronic rejection. Portal tract contains a dense inflammatory infiltrate associated with bile duct damage. Ducts are still present in normal numbers and distinction from acute (potentially reversible) rejection cannot be made at this stage (Haematoxylin and Eosin ×220).

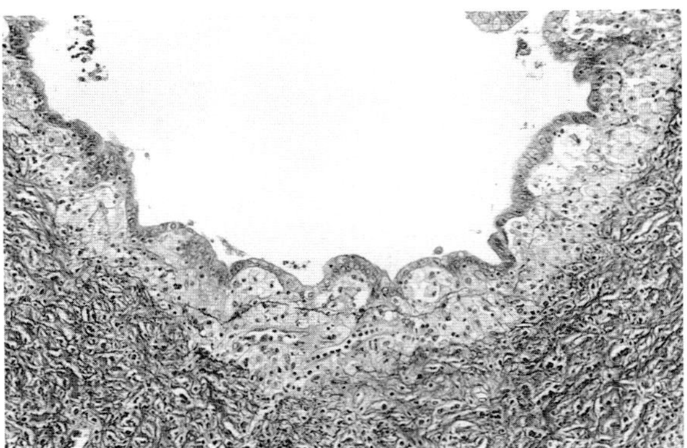

Fig. 15.3 Large (hilar) bile duct shows focal infiltration by lymphocytes and is surrounded by a cuff of foam cells (Elastic Haematoxylin van Gieson ×140).

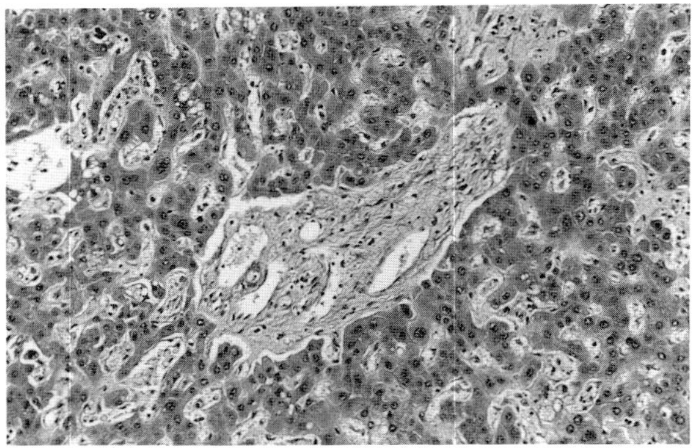

Fig. 15.2 End-stage chronic rejection in a liver obtained at retransplantation. Portal tract has a characteristic 'burnt-out' appearance. Several small vessels are present, but there is no accompanying bile duct and no significant inflammation. Several foamy histiocytes are present in the adjacent hepatic sinusoids (Haematoxylin and Eosin ×140).

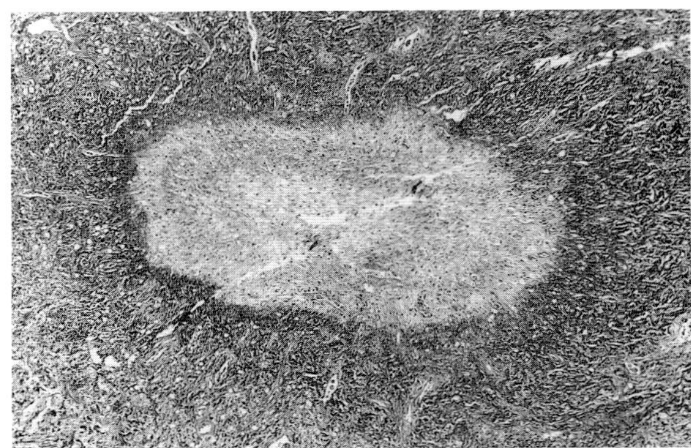

Fig. 15.4 Large (hilar) bile duct shows luminal obliteration by loose fibrous tissue admixed with scattered lymphocytes and foamy histiocytes. No residual epithelium was identified in any bile ducts from this case (Elastic Haematoxylin van Gieson ×60).

The pattern of bile duct damage is variable, but in general small ducts are more severely affected than larger ones. In the great majority of end-stage livers obtained at retransplantation, bile ducts are present in less than 20% of small portal tracts. Medium sized (septal) ducts are sometimes also reduced in number, although to a lesser degree than small (interlobular) ducts. Inflammatory aggregates including foamy histiocytes are seen around some larger ducts (Figure 15.3) which occasionally show a characteristic pattern of luminal obliteration by loose fibrous tissue admixed with inflammatory cells (Figure 15.4). Three patients in our programme have shown a complete absence of epithelium in ducts of all sizes throughout the liver.

Vascular changes

Arterial lesions usually take the form of foam cell aggregates which are present in large and medium sized arteries (Figure 15.5). Foam cells are thought to be of macrophage origin,[2] are predominantly intimal in location and result in varying degrees of luminal obliteration. Foam cells are

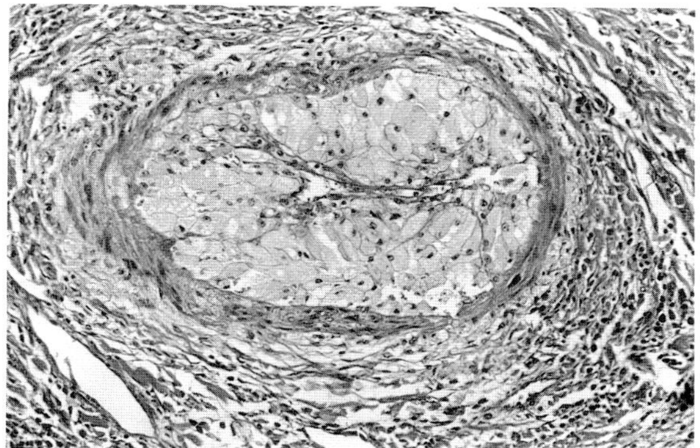

Fig. 15.5 Typical vascular lesion of chronic rejection. A medium sized artery contains numerous intimal foam cells resulting in marked luminal narrowing. Occasional foam cells are also present in the media (Haematoxylin and Eosin ×175).

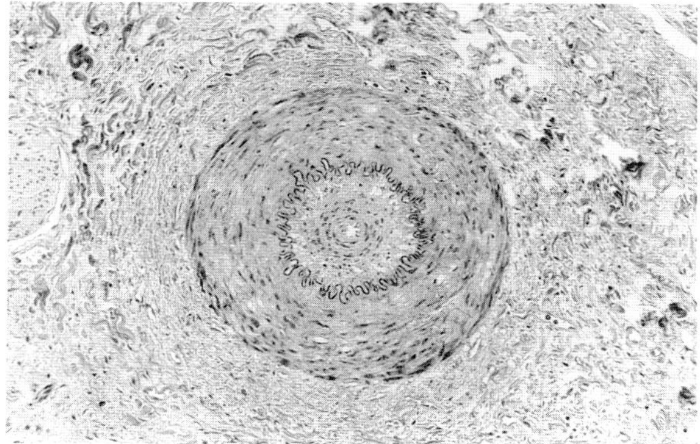

Fig. 15.6 Medium sized artery showing intimal fibrosis and myo-tintimal hyperplasia. This is a less common pattern of chronic vascular rejection in the liver allograft (Elastic Haematoxylin van Gieson ×140).

sometimes also seen in the media of affected vessels. Less commonly, arteries show myointimal hyperplasia and intimal fibrosis (Figure 15.6); these changes probably reflect more longstanding damage. Foam cell lesions are rarely seen in small arteries. However, a paucity of arteriolar branches may accompany ductopenia in small portal tracts.[8] Although venular damage tends to be regarded as a diagnostic feature of acute rejection (see p. 200), mild degrees of venous endothelial inflammation are sometimes also observed in chronic rejection (Figure 15.7). Foam cells may also be present in the walls of portal venules.

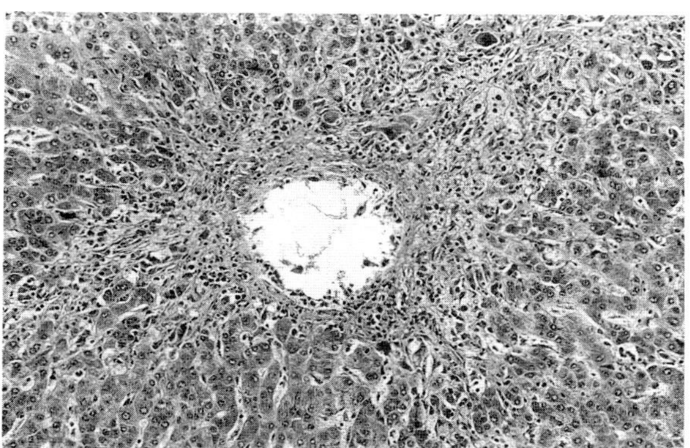

Fig. 15.7 Hepatic venular endothelial inflammation in a liver removed for end-stage chronic rejection. Surrounding the hepatic venule there is an area of inflammation and hepatocyte necrosis (Haematoxylin and Eosin ×140).

Relationship between bile duct and vascular lesions in CR

The great majority of end-stage livers obtained at retransplantation for CR have both ductopenia and characteristic vascular changes. Morphometric studies have shown a parallelism between the severity of these two lesions.[8] However, in some cases there may be an advanced vanishing bile duct syndrome with minimal or no vascular lesions.[14] Conversely, arterial foam cell lesions are sometimes encountered in hepatectomy specimens without any accompanying bile duct loss.[3] In one recent study, it was suggested that patients with a 'pure' vanishing bile duct syndrome had a more favourable outcome than those in whom ductopenia was combined with ischaemic parenchymal lesions of centrilobular necrosis.[15] However, this interesting observation requires confirmation by other studies.

Other portal tract lesions

Portal tracts show variable fibrous expansion, generally mild but sometimes associated with bridging fibrosis.[4] A few studies have reported the occasional development of true cirrhosis.[5,15,17] In addition to deposition in vessels and bile ducts, foamy histiocytes may also be observed in hilar nerve branches and lying free within portal connective tissue.

Parenchymal damage

Perivenular cholestasis and hepatocyte necrosis are also characteristic findings in chronic rejection. Cholestasis is usually prominent, even at an early stage, and is invariably severe in end-stage disease. Sinusoidal aggregates of foam cells are sometimes seen in association with severe cholestasis. Hepatocyte necrosis usually has a lytic pattern in the early stages, and is associated with varying degrees of congestion and inflammation (Figure 15.8). Areas of hepatocyte necrosis are gradually replaced by fibrous tissue as the disease progresses (Figure 15.9). In more severe cases there are larger areas of confluent and bridging necrosis involving peripheral acinar zones, producing a picture similar to that observed in severe acute hepatitis. Cholestasis is most probably related to the duct loss which characterises chronic rejection, although ischaemia cannot be excluded as an aetiological factor. The pathogenesis of hepatocyte necrosis is uncertain – both ischaemia and direct immune mediated damage may be involved.[18]

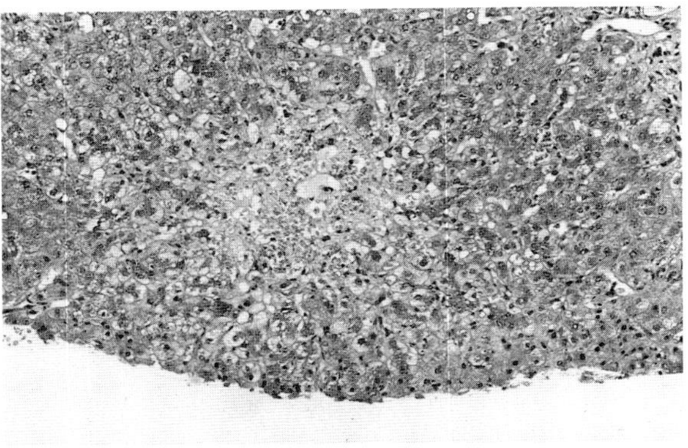

Fig. 15.8 Parenchymal damage in a case of early chronic rejection. Surrounding the terminal hepatic venule there is a zone of congestion and lytic hepatocyte necrosis. Extensive bile plugging is present in the adjacent hepatocytes (Haematoxylin and eosin ×140).

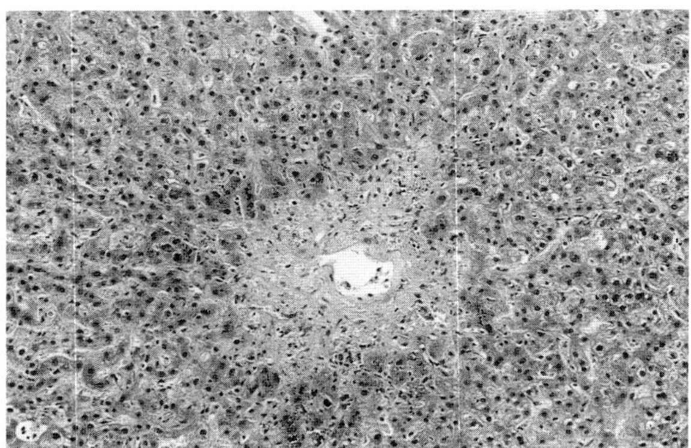

Fig. 15.9 Parenchymal damage in a case of 'late' chronic rejection, immediately prior to retransplantation. An area of perivenular hepatocyte necrosis has undergone fibrous scarring. Severe cholestasis is present in the adjacent hepatocytes (Haematoxylin and eosin ×140).

Problems with the histological diagnosis of chronic rejection

The diagnosis of chronic rejection is straightforward in end-stage livers obtained at regrafting where the full range of characteristic lesions can be readily appreciated. Histological diagnosis is less easy in earlier needle biopsy specimens where one or more of the typical features may not be present. In particular, arterial lesions are rarely seen in biopsy specimens, which sample smaller vessels.

There are three main practical problems in the histological diagnosis of chronic rejection:

1. *Early diagnosis* – features *predictive* of irreversible damage

During the early stages of chronic rejection, when bile ducts are present in normal numbers, distinction from cases of 'acute', potentially reversible rejection is very difficult (see Figure 15.1). Although most cases of chronic rejection are preceded by episodes of 'acute' rejection, this is not always so. In our experience, the incidence and severity of acute rejection are greater in patients who develop irreversible rejection than in those who do not. In the series reported by the group from Minnesota, patients who developed chronic rejection experienced acute rejection earlier than those who did not.[15] However, there is a considerable overlap and these quantitative differences are not reliable in assessing prognosis in individual cases. Other features which have been suggested as being predictive of chronic rejection include:

(a) Paucity of bile ducts;[4]
(b) Bile duct atypia;[19]
(c) Arterial lesions (foam cells or inflammatory);[4,20]
(d) Foam cells in hepatic sinusoids[2] and/or portal tracts; and

(e) Perivenular hepatocyte ballooning or hepatocyte necrosis.[4,21]

Of these, bile duct loss is best regarded as a diagnostic rather than a predictive feature of chronic rejection, arterial lesions are rarely observed in biopsy specimens, and sinusoidal foam cells are probably a non-specific manifestation of severe cholestasis.[22] Portal tract foam cells, although characteristic, are rarely seen in the absence of advanced duct loss. The presence of bile duct atypia in the form of nuclear pleomorphism, cytoplasmic vacuolation and disordered polarity (Figure 15.10) often in the absence of significant inflammation, is probably the best sign of impending CR. Perivenular hepatocyte ballooning and drop-out may be a reflection of ischaemia due to factors other than rejection.[18,23–26] However, persistent centrilobular necrosis has been associated with an increased risk of developing CR and may be present before diagnostic duct lesions are seen.[4,21]

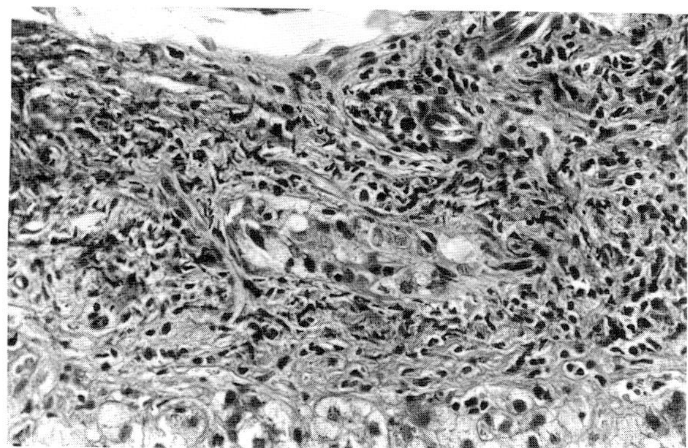

Fig. 15.10 Bile duct in a case of early chronic rejection showing a characteristic pattern of 'dysplastic' damage, with nuclear pleomorphism, disordered polarity and cytoplasmic vacuolation. Ducts were still present in normal numbers in this biopsy, but subsequently disappeared (Haematoxylin and eosin ×350).

2. *Diagnosis of end-stage disease* – features *indicative* of irreversible damage

It is often difficult to determine a point at which irreversible damage due to rejection has occurred. The most important diagnostic feature in needle biopsy specimens is duct loss. The degree of certainty of irreversible damage should increase in proportion to the number of bile ducts which have been destroyed. Clearly there are problems with sampling variation in small biopsy specimens and there is no clear guide as to what level of duct loss constitutes irreversible damage.

A small proportion of portal tracts (up to 20–30%) may be devoid of bile ducts as part of a normal variation.[8,12,27,28] In our view, a biopsy containing bile ducts in fewer than 50% of portal tracts should be regarded as suggestive of irreversible rejection, especially if the characteristic parenchymal lesions are also present. However, some patients who appear to be suffering from an irreversible rejection (with clinical, biochemical and histological features) have recovered either spontaneously or with conventional immunosuppression.[12,15,29] The six patients we reported with 'reversible VBDS' are all currently well with normal biochemistry.[12] However, three have had follow-up biopsies showing a paucity of bile ducts, but without any other histological features of chronic rejection. We have also seen ductopenia as an incidental finding in liver biopsies taken as part of annual review in patients who are clinically well, with no previous biopsies to suggest chronic rejection. These observations suggest that some patients may suffer permanent duct loss as a result of rejection, but that sufficient ducts remain to enable the graft to function normally. As regards a definite histological diagnosis of irreversible rejection on needle biopsy specimens, we have never seen recovery from a biopsy showing no ducts in ten or more portal tracts.

In view of the difficulties which may be encountered in diagnosing irreversible damage according to the degree of bile duct loss, it has been suggested that the diagnosis of chronic rejection should be based instead on the characteristic arterial lesions and the resultant ischaemic damage which they produce.[15,17] This approach is also fraught with problems, as already discussed. Firstly, arterial lesions are rarely seen in small biopsy specimens and the perivenular damage which they produce may be due to other vascular problems. Secondly, in some livers which clearly have undergone irreversible rejection with severe cholestasis and an advanced vanishing bile duct syndrome, only mild vascular lesions are seen. It is difficult to imagine that these have contributed significantly to graft failure. Thirdly, in some cases arterial foam cell lesions may be observed as an incidental finding without any other features to suggest irreversible rejection.

3. *Differential diagnosis of chronic rejection*

Chronic rejection can be readily distinguished histologically from most other cholestatic syndromes occurring in the liver allograft, including biliary obstruction, viral hepatitis, sepsis and drug jaundice.[3,5]

In cases where chronic rejection occurs in a patient initially transplanted for primary biliary cirrhosis, there are potential problems in distinguishing CR from recurrent disease.[30] However, although histological similarities exist between CR and PBC, there are many differences.[16,31,32] These differences apply not only to histological appearances but also to clinical features including time of occurrence, speed of progression and association with other auto-immune phenomena.

Problems with the terminology of chronic rejection

In terms of therapeutic and prognostic considerations, the subdivision of rejection into 'acute' and 'chronic' forms is of considerable importance. However, as mentioned earlier, there is an overlap for each of the three main criteria used to distinguish these two patterns of rejection (see Table 15.1). 'Acute' is generally regarded as synonymous with 'early' or 'reversible' rejection, and chronic with 'late' or 'irreversible' rejection. However, acute rejection can occur any time after transplantation, while features of chronic rejection are sometimes seen within the first month of transplantation. Similarly, up to 20% of patients with acute cellular rejection will develop graft failure due to chronic rejection while 20–30% of people with chronic rejection may recover spontaneously.[12,15,29]

In view of the problems associated with classifying acute and chronic rejection in terms of time of occurrence and behaviour, a purely histological classification has been advocated. Terms such as 'cellular', 'ductopenic' and 'vascular' could be used individually or together without having connotations for timing or prognosis.[6] However, there are also problems with this approach. A broad spectrum of histological appearances exists between classic early 'acute' cellular rejection and end-stage, burnt-out 'chronic' rejection. There are problems with sampling variation in counting bile ducts, especially in small specimens, and fluctuating levels of duct loss may be seen in serial biopsies. Vascular lesions are rarely seen in biopsy specimens. No account is taken of the early changes which may predict the likely development of chronic irreversible/ductopenic rejection before ductopenia has occurred.

For these reasons we still prefer to use the terms 'acute' and 'chronic' in classifying rejection. However, the term CR can be modified according to the clinical and histological features present (Table 15.2). The distinctions made are arbitrary but serve to illustrate the broad spectrum of clinicopathological changes that are embraced by the term chronic rejection.

Table 15.2 Terms which may be used to classify chronic rejection according to time of presentation and degree of ductopenia

Time of presentation	
Accelerated CR	<2 months
Delayed/typical CR	2–6 months
Late CR	>6 months
Degree of duct loss	**% of portal tracts with bile ducts**
Early CR	>50%
Established CR	<50%
Irreversible CR	0

Diagnosis

The diagnosis of chronic rejection is based on a combination of the clinical, biochemical and histological features described above. Of these, histology is the most specific in identifying that rejection is the *cause* of graft dysfunction. The clinical status and biochemical progression are used to determine the point at which irreversible damage has taken place. Various other approaches to the diagnosis of CR have been suggested, although none of these has gained widespread acceptance.

The arterial lesions may produce areas of narrowing on angiography.[33] Changes in hepatic venous blood flow have also been identified by Doppler ultrasound in acute rejection.[34] The specificity of these changes remains to be determined but they could be a useful adjunct to the diagnosis of CR.

Fine needle aspiration (FNA) cytology is useful as an adjunct to conventional histology in the diagnosis of acute rejection, where there are large numbers of infiltrating lymphoid cells which can be aspirated.[35–39] FNA is an unreliable method for diagnosing chronic rejection, which is characterised by a diminishing cellular infiltrate as bile ducts are lost.[40] The presence of large numbers of monocytes or macrophages in liver aspirates may be a pointer to the development of chronic rejection,[35,41] but histology is still required to make a definitive diagnosis.

In addition to the non-specific biochemical changes of cholestasis, other more specific immunological markers of rejection may be detected in serum and bile. Serum levels of hyaluronic acid (HA), a marker of hepatic endothelial cell function,[42] interleukin-2 receptor (IL-2R) and circulating intercellular adhesion molecule-1 (CICAM-1), markers of lymphocyte activation[43,44] are elevated during allograft rejection. Biliary levels of HA, IL-2R and CICAM-1 are also elevated, possibly reflecting immune events in portal areas. There is a suggestion that persistently elevated levels of these markers may be useful in the early diagnosis of chronic rejection, before characterstic histological changes have occurred, but further studies are required to confirm this.

Immunohistochemical staining may be used as an adjunct to conventional histology in assessing cellular infiltrates and damage to target structures in rejecting liver allografts. Similar techniques have also been applied to lymphoid cells obtained from peripheral blood and bile. Studies employing these methods are discussed further in the aetiology and pathogenesis of chronic rejection. Although such approaches have provided a valuable insight into the pathogenesis of chronic rejection, none has been established in routine diagnosis.

Aetiology and pathogenesis

Immune mechanisms

The immunopathogenetic mechanisms involved in liver allograft rejection are discussed in detail elsewhere. Here, a brief consideration will be given to the main changes occurring in chronic rejection which may be of diagnostic and/or prognostic value.

MHC antigens

Several studies have shown that the expression of MHC antigens is increased on various structures in the liver after transplantation, rendering these structures more susceptible to immune mediated damage.[45–51] In particular, there is 'aberrant' expression of class I antigens on hepatocytes and class II antigens on bile ducts. Increased expression of class I and II antigens is also observed on vascular endothelium. These changes probably occur in response to locally produced cytokines released by activated T lymphocytes. Increased expression of MHC antigens is also seen in other post-transplant syndromes including ischaemia, biliary obstruction and viral infection. However, the degree of expression, at least as judged by the intensity of immunohistochemical staining, is significantly greater in rejection than in the other non-rejection complications. Furthermore, in cases of acute rejection responding to increased immunosuppression, expression of MHC antigens returns towards baseline levels whereas in cases progressing to CR enhanced expression of MHC antigen persists on target structures. The possibility that enhanced MHC expression is simply an epiphenomenon still cannot be entirely excluded. However, the above observations strongly suggest that it is likely to be an important pathogenetic mechanism in the ongoing damage to bile ducts, vascular endothelium and hepatocytes which occurs in CR.

Although HLA matching is of proven benefit in reducing the incidence of chronic rejection and increasing graft survival in kidney allografts, the status of HLA matching in liver transplantation is less certain.[52,53] In the study of O'Grady *et al.*, the combination of a complete mismatch of class I antigens with a partial or complete match of class II antigens was significantly associated with the development of VBDS.[54] However a similar study by Batts *et al.* failed to confirm these findings.[55] Further studies are clearly required to resolve these conflicting results.

Cell mediated immunity

Immunohistochemical studies have shown that the majority of lymphocytes present in portal tracts during acute rejection have the T cell phenotype.[46,56] Similar studies on lymphocytes obtained by fine needle aspiration also show a predominance of T lymphocytes.[38] This includes a mixture of CD4+ and CD8+ cells, which are present in varying proportions, and infiltrate bile ducts and portal venular endothelium. These changes parallel the enhanced MHC expression which occurs in these target structures.

Relatively little is known about the role of cell mediated immunity in chronic rejection. The presence of a predominantly CD8+ infiltrate has been associated with a higher risk of progression to irreversible rejection[57,58] and may be associated with direct cytotoxic destruction of biliary epithelium. CD8+ cells are also present in the lobules of chronically rejecting liver allografts and may in part be responsible for the hepatocellular damage which characteristically occurs in chronic rejection. The lack of inflammation seen in end-stage disease may reflect a diminishing antigen challenge as bile ducts have been largely destroyed. Nevertheless, cellular infiltrates around surviving bile ducts in livers obtained at retransplantation are still composed largely of T lymphocytes.

Humoral mechanisms

Although humoral factors are implicated in hyperacute rejection, there is some evidence to suggest that they may also play a role in chronic rejection. The study of Donaldson *et al.* revealed an association between donor specific class I antibodies and the development of VBDS.[59] These antibodies could be directed against donor bile ducts which strongly express class I antigens. Immunoglobulins, especially IgM, are deposited in arterial walls of chronically rejected livers.[60] Increased numbers of IgM containing plasma cells have also been noted in the portal tracts of rejecting liver allografts.[61] If humoral mechanisms were important in the pathogenesis of CR, one might anticipate an increased incidence in patients receiving ABO incompatible grafts. The group from the Mayo Clinic have reported an association between positive lymphocyte crossmatch and the development of acute VBDS.[14,55] Ductopenia was also noted in two out of six cases of acute massive haemorrhagic necrosis,[62] a pattern of graft damage which is characteristically seen in accelerated humoral mediated rejection of human and animal hepatic allografts.[63–65] Two studies have shown a high incidence of biliary complications occurring in ABO incompatible grafts.[65,66] Although an immune mediated mechanism has been postulated for these, there is no clear evidence that they are related to chronic rejection.

Other immune mechanisms

Adhesion molecules

There is increasing evidence to suggest that other non-MHC associated molecules are important in enabling lymphocytes to interact with each other and with other target cells. These molecules are principally involved with cell adhesion and augment the interaction between MHC antigens and other lymphoid receptors. An increased expression of the intercellular adhesion moecule-1 (ICAM-1) has been observed on target structures in rejecting liver allografts.[67,68] ICAM-1 is the ligand for the leucocyte receptor LFA-1, which is expressed on many lymphoid cells infiltrating portal tracts during liver allograft rejection. The pattern of enhanced expression closely parallels that observed for MHC antigens and is probably also induced by pro-inflammatory cytokines such as gamma interferon.[69] Strong expression of ICAM-1 persists in cases progressing to chronic rejection whilst returning rapidly to baseline levels in cases of acute rejection which respond to immunosuppression. This again suggests that enhanced adhesion molecule expression is important in the pathogenesis of ongoing immune damage to target structures which occurs in CR.

Cytomegalovirus infection

An association has been noted between CMV infection and chronic rejection.[54] The evidence for this is based principally on serological studies, although viral culture, immunohistochemical staining and *in situ* DNA hybridisation have also been used to detect CMV in various tissues The mechanisms whereby CMV infection should predispose to CR are poorly understood. Although the virus binds to beta-2-microglobulin[70] and may thus be able to use class I as a receptor for entry into cells, it is only rarely demonstrable within biliary epithelium. Direct immune mediated destruction of bile ducts is thus unlikely. Studies on mice have suggested that CMV infection may augment cytotoxic T cell responses against allogeneic histocompatibility antigens[71,72] possibly by up-regulating the expression of HLA class 1 antigens. However, an alternative explanation for the reported association between CMV infection and VBDS could be that a reduction in immunosuppression consequent upon CMV infection might predispose to more severe episodes of rejection.

Data from other studies have given conflicting results regarding the possible role of CMV infection in chronic rejection. Most have shown no definite association[6,9,11,15] although the numbers of cases studied in some are small. In our programme, a higher incidence of chronic rejection has been observed in patients with proven CMV infection[73] but the precise relationship between these two events remains uncertain.

Non-immune damage

Ischaemia

Although it is generally accepted that bile duct damage in chronic rejection is caused largely by immune mediated mechanisms, other factors may be involved. Loss of bile ducts may, in part, be an ischaemic response related to the obliterative arteriopathy which characterises chronic rejection. In support of this, morphometric studies have shown that the degree of bile duct loss parallels the severity of vascular damage in end-stage grafts with chronic rejection.[8]

Disease association

Early studies failed to show any association between the original disease for which transplantation was carried out and the development of chronic rejection.[74] Two recent studies have reported a high incidence of chronic rejection in patients transplanted for primary sclerosing cholangitis.[9,11] Another study reported a higher incidence of CR in patients transplanted for primary biliary cirrhosis.[31] Differences in the incidence of CR between biliary and non-biliary disease are generally fairly small and further studies are required to determine if there is a genuine association. The problem of distinction from recurrent disease clearly has to be considered when ductopenic rejection occurs against a background of chronic biliary disease, although in most cases this distinction is not difficult.

Treatment

Immunosuppression

Chronic rejection is regarded as an irreversible condition unresponsive to immunosuppresion. However, as mentioned earlier, some 20–30% of cases appear to resolve spontaneously or with conventional immunosuppression.

Prevention is clearly better than cure and, in this regard, it is encouraging to note three recent studies in which a lower incidence of irreversible rejection was obtained using triple therapy (cyclosporin, prednisone, azathioprine)[9,11] or quadruple therapy (as above with anti-lymphoblast globulin).[10] Data from our programme suggest that aggressive immunosuppression is only required during the first few months, when patients are at most risk of developing chronic rejection. Withdrawal of corticosteroids at three months, in patients who are clinically well, has not been associated with a high risk of developing late chronic rejection.

Recent studies have suggested that FK506 may be useful as a 'rescue therapy' in treating cases of severe rejection unresponsive to conventional therapy and likely to proceed to irreversible damage.[19,75] Claims for the efficacy of new drugs, such as FK506, in treating presumed cases of 'early' chronic rejection need to be treated with caution. Clearly, in order for these drugs to be effective, they need to be used at a time when bile ducts are present in normal or near-normal numbers, since there is little evidence to suggest that bile ducts (as opposed to ductules) can regenerate once they are destroyed. However, there are problems in defining 'early' chronic rejection histologically and little is known about its natural history. By the time a diagnosis of CR can be made with a high degree of confidence, that is when very few ducts are left, there is little chance of regaining normal function.

Retransplantation

Most cases of chronic rejection will progress to graft failure and require retransplantation. In view of the potential for spontaneous recovery in some patients who appear to have advanced chronic rejection and the risks associated with undertaking a second transplant operation,[7] the decision to regraft should be delayed until a confident diagnosis of irreversible damage can be established.

Although survival following retransplantation is reduced compared to primary transplant operations, 11 of 19 patients who have been regrafted for CR in our programme are currently alive at intervals of 12 months to seven years post-transplant.

Disease recurrence

The question of whether the development of chronic rejection in one graft predisposes to recurrent CR in subsequent grafts is controversial. Anecdotally, many transplant centres have noted occasional patients who have suffered repeated episodes of chronic rejection, sometimes occurring with increasing rapidity in successive grafts –

so-called 'liver eaters'. One recent study reported a 90% recurrence rate of chronic rejection following retransplantation.[76] In our series the incidence of recurrent chronic rejection resulting in graft failure following retransplantation is 33% (7/21 grafts) as compared with an incidence of 7.2% (27/377) in the initial grafts and 4.7% (2/43) in new livers inserted for complications other than chronic rejection.

Conclusion

Chronic rejection remains an important cause of graft failure during the first year following liver transplantation and, rarely, thereafter. The diagnosis is based on a combination of clinical, biochemical and histological features, of which histology remains the 'gold standard'.

There are still problems in the diagnosis and management of chronic rejection. In particular, it is not possible to be certain, at an early stage, which cases are likely to develop chronic rejection, nor is it easy to determine a point at which irreversible damage has occurred. There are areas which require further study if the currently available therapeutic options are to be used optimally and the efficacy of new treatments is to be assessed properly.

References

1. Vierling JM, Fennell RH. Histopathology of early and late human hepatic allograft rejection: evidence for progressive destruction of interlobular bile ducts. *Hepatology* 1985; **5,** 1076–1082.
2. Grond J, Gouw ASH, Poppema S, Sloof MJH, Gips CH. Chronic rejection in liver transplants: a histopathologic analysis of failed grafts and antecedent serial biopsies. *Transplant Proc* 1986; **18,** 128–135.
3. Wight DGD, Portmann B. Pathology of liver transplantation. In: *Liver Transplantation*, Calne RY (ed). London: Grune and Stratton, 1987; 385–435.
4. Snover DC, Freese DK, Sharp HL, Bloomer JR, Najarian JS, Ascher NL. Liver allograft rejection. An analysis of the use of biopsy in determining outcome of rejection. *Am J Surg Pathol* 1987; **11,** 1–18.
5. Demetris AJ, Jaffe RK, Starzl TE. A review of adult and paediatric post-transplant liver pathology. *Pathol Ann* 1987; **22,** 347–386.
6. Wiesner RH, Ludwig J, van Hoek B, Krom RAF. Current concepts in cell-mediated hepatic allograft rejection leading to ductopenia and graft failure. *Hepatology* 1991; **14,** 721–729.
7. Shaw BW, Gordon RD, Iwatsuki S, Starzl TE. Retransplantation of the liver. *Sem Liver Dis* 1985; **5,** 394–401.
8. Oguma S, Belle S, Starzl TE, Demetris AJ. A histometric analysis of chronically rejected human liver allografts: insights into the mechanisms of bile duct loss: direct immunologic and ischaemic factors. *Hepatology 1989*; **9,** 204–209.
9. Klintmalm GBG, Nery JR, Husberg BS, Gonwa TA, Tillery GW. Rejection in liver transplantation. *Hepatology* 1989; **10,** 978–985.
10. Pirsch JD, Kalayoglu M, Hafez GR, d'Alessandro AM, Sollinger HW, Belzer FO. Evidence that the vanishing bile duct syndrome is vanishing. *Transplantation* 1990; **49,** 1015–1018.
11. Van Hoek B, Wiesner RH, Ludwig J, Gores GJ, Moore B, Krom RAF. Combination immunosuppression with azathioprine reduces the incidence of ductopenic rejection and vanishing bile duct syndrome after liver transplantation. *Transplant Proc* 1991; **23,** 1403–1405.
12. Hubscher SG, Buckels JAC, Elias E, McMaster P, Neuberger JM. Vanishing bile duct syndrome following liver transplantation – is it reversible? *Transplantation* 1991; **51,** 1004–1010.
13. Adams DH, Neuberger JM. Patterns of graft rejection following liver transplantation. *J Hepatol* 1990; **10,** 113–119.
14. Ludwig J, Wiesner RH, Batts KP, Perkins JD, Krom RAF. The acute vanishing bile duct syndrome (acute irreversible rejection) after orthotopic liver transplantation. *Hepatology* 1987; **7,** 476–483.
15. Freese DK, Snover DC, Sharp HL, Gross CR, Savick SK, Payne WD. Chronic rejection after liver transplantation: a study of clinical histopathological and immunological features. *Hepatology* 1991; **13,** 882–891.
16. Polson RJ, Portmann B, Neuberger J, Calne RY, Williams R. Evidence for disease recurrence after liver transplantation for primary biliary cirrhosis. *Gastroenterology* 1989; **97,** 715–725.
17. Snover DC. Liver transplantation. In: *The Pathology of Organ Transplantation*, Sale GE (ed.). Boston: Butterworths, 1990; 385–435.
18. Hubscher SG. Histological findings in liver allograft rejection – new insights into the pathogenesis of hepatocellular damage in liver allografts. *Histopathology* 1991; **18,** 377–383.
19. Demetris AJ, Fung JJ, Todo S *et al.* Pathologic observations in human allograft recipients treated with FK506. *Transplant Proc* 1990; **22,** 25–34.
20. Porter KA. The pathology of rejection in human liver allografts. *Transplant Proc* 1988; **20,** 483–485.
21. Ludwig J, Gross JB, Perkins JD, Moore SB. Per-

sistent centrilobular necrosis in hepatic allografts. *Hum Pathol* 1990; **21,** 656–661.

22. Wight DGD. Differential diagnosis of cholestasis in liver allografts. *Transplant Proc* 1986; **18** (suppl 4), 152–156.
23. Williams JW, Vera S, Peters TG *et al.* Cholestatic jaundice after hepatic transplantation: a non-immunologically mediated event. *Am J Surg* 1986; **151,** 65–70.
24. Ray RA, Lewin KJ, Colonna J, Goldstein LI, Busuttil RW. The role of liver biopsy in evaluating acute allograft dysfunction following liver transplantation. *Hum Pathol* 1988; **19,** 835–848.
25. Goldstein NS, Hart J, Lewin KJ. Diffuse hepatocyte ballooning in liver biopsies from orthotopic liver transplant patients. *Histopathology* 1991; **18,** 323–330.
26. Ng IOL, Burroughs AK, Rolles K, Belli IS, Scheuer PJ. Hepatocellular ballooning after liver transplantation: a light and electron microscopic study with clinicopathologic correlation. *Histopathology* 1991; **18,** 331–338.
27. Alagille D, Odievre M, Gautier M, Dommergues JP. Hepatic ductular hypoplasia associated with characteristic facies, vertebral malformations, retarded physical, mental and sexual development and cardiac murmur. *J Paediatr* 1975; **86,** 63–71.
28. Nakanuma Y, Ohta G. Histometric and serial section observations of the intrahepatic bile ducts in primary biliary cirrhosis. *Gastroenterology* 1979; **76,** 1326–1332.
29. Noack KB, Wiesner RH, Batts K, van Hoek B, Ludwig J. Severe ductopenic rejection with features of vanishing bile duct syndrome: clinical biochemical and histological evidence for spontaneous resolution. *Transplant Proc* 1991; **23,** 1448–1451.
30. Jones EA. Primary biliary cirrhosis and liver transplantation. *N Eng J Med* 1982; **306,** 41–43.
31. Demetris AJ, Markus BH, Esquivel C *et al.* Pathologic analysis of liver transplantation for primary biliary cirrhosis. *Hepatology* 1988; **8,** 939–947.
32. Neuberger J, Hubscher S. Does primary biliary cirrhosis recur after liver transplantation? In: *Immunological, Metabolic and Infectious Aspects of Liver Transplantation*, Vuitton DA, Balabaud C, Houssin D, Dhumeaux D (eds). Paris: John Libbey Eurotext, 1991.
33. White RM, Zajko AB, Demetris AJ, Bron KM, Dekker A, Starzl TE. Liver transplant rejection: angiographic findings in 35 patients. *Am J Roentgenol* 1987; **148,** 1095–1098.
34. Coulden RA, Britton PD, Farman P, Noble-Jamieson G, Wight DGD. Preliminary report: hepatic vein doppler in the early diagnosis of acute liver transplant rejection. *Lancet* 1990; **336**(II), 273–275.
35. Kirby RM, Young JA, Hubscher SG *et al.* The accuracy of aspiration cytology in the diagnosis of rejection following orthotopic liver transplantation. *Transplant Int* 1988; **1,** 119–126.
36. Lautenschlager I, Hockerstedt K, Ahonen J *et al.* Fine-needle aspiration in the monitoring of liver allografts II. Application to human liver allografts. *Transplantation* 1988; **46,** 47–53.
37. Carbonnel F, Samuel D, Reynes M *et al.* Fine-needle aspiration biopsy of human liver allografts. Correlation with liver histology for the diagnosis of acute rejection. *Transplantation* 1990; **50,** 704–707.
38. Lautenschlager I, Hockerstedt K, Salmela K. Fine-needle aspiration biopsy in the monitoring of liver allografts. Different cellular findings during rejection and cytomegalovirus infection. *Transplantation* 1990; **50,** 798–803.
39. Kubota K, Ericzon BG, Reinholt FP. Comparison of fine-needle aspiration biopsy and histology in human liver transplants. *Transplantation* 1991; **51,** 1010–1013.
40. Schlitt HJ, Nashan B, Ringe B *et al.* Differentiation of liver graft dysfunction by transplant aspiration cytology. *Transplantation* 1991; **51,** 786–796.
41. Lautenschlager I, Hockerstedt K, Taskinen E. Fine needle aspiration cytology of liver allografts in the pig. *Transplantation* 1984; **38,** 330–334.
42. Adams DH, Wang L, Hubscher SG, Neuberger JM. Hepatic endothelial cells. Targets in liver allograft rejection? *Transplantation* 1989; **47,** 479–482.
43. Adams DH, Wang L, Hubscher SG, Elias E, Neuberger JM. Soluble interleukin-2 receptors in serum and bile of liver transplant recipients. *Lancet* 1989; **1,** 469–471.
44. Adams DH, Mainolfi E, Neuberger JM, Elias E, Rothlein R. Secretion of circulating ICAM-1 into bile during human liver allograft rejection. *Gut* 1991; **32,** A576.
45. Nagafuchi Y, Hobbs KEF, Thomas HC, Scheuer PJ. Expression of beta-2-microglobulin on hepatocytes after liver transplantation. *Lancet* 1985; **i,** 551–554.
46. Demetris AJ, Lasky S, Van Thiel DH, Starzl TE, Whiteside T. Induction of DR/IA antigens in human liver allografts. *Transplantation* 1985; **40,** 504–509.
47. So SKS, Platt JL, Ascher NL, Snover DC. Increased expression of class 1 major histocompatibility antigens on hepatocytes in rejecting human liver allografts. *Transplantation* 1987; **43,** 79–85.
48. Gouw ASH, Houthoff HJ, Huitema S, Beelen JM, Gips CH, Poppema S. Expression of major histocompatibility complex antigens and replacement of donor cells by recipient ones in human liver grafts. *Transplantation* 1987; **43,** 291–296.

49. Hubscher SG, Adams DH, Elias E. Beta-2 microglobulin expression in the liver following liver transplantation. *J Clin Pathol* 1988; **41,** 1049–1057.
50. Steinhoff G, Wonigeit K, Pichlmayr R. Analysis of sequential changes in major histocompatibility complex expression in human liver grafts after transplantation. *Transplantation* 1988; **45,** 394–401.
51. Hubscher SG, Adams DH, Elias E. Changes in the expression of major histocompatibility complex class II antigens in liver allograft rejection. *J Pathol* 1990; **162,** 165–171.
52. Neuberger JM, Adams DH. Is HLA matching important for liver transplantation? *J Hepatol* 1990; **11,** 1–4.
53. Steinhoff G. Major histocompatibility complex antigens in human liver transplants. *J Hepatol* 1990; **11,** 9–15.
54. O'Grady JG, Alexander GJM, Sutherland S *et al.* Cytomegalovirus infection and donor/recipient HLA antigens: interdependent co-factors in pathogenesis of vanishing bile duct syndrome after liver transplantation. *Lancet* 1988; **ii,** 302–305.
55. Batts KP, Moore SB, Perkins JD, Wiesner RH, Grambsch PM, Krom RAF. Influence of positive lymphocyte crossmatch and HLA mismatching on vanishing bile duct syndrome in human liver allografts. *Transplantation* 1988; **45,** 376–379.
56. Perkins JD, Wiesner RH, Banks PM, Larusso NF, Ludwig J, Krom RAF. Immunohistologic labelling as an indicator of liver allograft rejection. *Transplantation* 1987; **43,** 105–108.
57. Perkins JD, Rakela J, Sterioff S, Banks PM, Wiesner RH, Krom RAF. Results of treatment in hepatic allograft rejection depend on the immunohistologic pattern of the portal T lymphocytic infiltrate. *Transplant Proc* 1988; **20,** 223–225.
58. McCaugan GW, Davies JS, Waugh JA *et al.* A quantitative analysis of T lymphocyte populations in human liver allografts undergoing rejection: the use of monoclonal antibodies and double immunolabelling. *Hepatology* 1990; **12,** 1305–1313.
59. Donaldson PT, Alexander GJM, O'Grady J *et al.* Evidence for an immune response to HLA class 1 antigens in the vanishing bile duct syndrome after liver transplantation. *Lancet* 1987; **1,** 945–948.
60. Demetris AJ, Markus BH, Burnham J *et al.* Antibody deposition in liver allografts with chronic rejection. *Transplant Proc* 1987; **19,** 121–125.
61. Adams DH, Hubscher SG, Burnett D, Elias E. Immunoglobulins in liver allograft rejection: evidence for deposition and secretion within the liver. *Transplant Proc* 1990; **22,** 1834–1835.
62. Hubscher SG, Adams DH, Neuberger JM, Buckels JAC, McMaster P, Elias E. Massive haemorrhagic necrosis of the liver following liver transplantation. *J Clin Pathol* 1989; **42,** 360–370.
63. Knechtle SJ, Kolbeck PC, Isuchimoto S *et al.* Hepatic transplantation into sensitised recipients. Demonstration of hyperacute rejection. *Transplantation* 1987; **43,** 8–12.
64. Demetris AJ, Jaffe R, Tzakis A *et al.* Antibody mediated rejection in human orthotopic liver allografts: a study of liver transplantation across ABO blood group barriers. *Am J Pathol* 1988; **132,** 489–502.
65. Gugenheim K, Samuel D, Reynes M, Bismuth H. Liver transplantation across ABO blood group barriers. *Lancet* 1990; **ii,** 519–523.
66. Sanchez-Urdazpal L, Sterioff S, Janes C, Schwerman L, Rosen C, Krom RAF. Increased bile duct complications in ABO incompatible liver transplant recipients. *Transplant Proc* 1991; **23,** 1440–1441.
67. Adams DH, Hubscher SG, Shaw J, Rothlein R, Neuberger JM. Intercellular adhesion molecule 1 on liver allografts during rejection. *Lancet* 1989; **2,** 1122–1125.
68. Steinhoff G, Behrend M, Wonigeit K. Expression of adhesion molecules on lymphocytes/monocytes and hepatocytes in human liver grafts. *Hum Immunol* 1990; **28,** 123–127.
69. Rothlein R, Czajkowski, O'Neil MM, Martin SD, Mainolfi E, Merluzzi VJ. Indiction of intercellular adhesion molecule-1 on primary and continuous cell lines by pro-inflammatory cytokines. *J Immunol* 1988; **14,** 1665–1669.
70. Grundy JE, McKeating JA, Ward PJ, Sanderson AR, Griffiths PD. Beta-2 microglobulin enhances the infectivity of cytomegalovirus and when bound to the virus enables class I HLA molecules to be used as a virus receptor. *J Gen Virol* 1987; **68,** 793–803.
71. Grundy JE, Reid MF. The effect of primary and secondary infection with cytomegalovirus on the host response to alloantigens. *Transplant Proc* 1985; **17,** 592–594.
72. Grundy JE, Ayles HM, McKeating JA, Butcher RG, Griffiths PD, Poulter LW. Enhancement of class 1 HLA antigen expression by cytomegalovirus: role in amplification of virus infection. *J Med Virol* 1988; **25,** 483–495.
73. Umana JP, Neuberger JM, McMaster P, Elias E, Buckels JAC, Mutimer DJ. Cytomegalovirus infection following liver transplantation. *J Hepatol* 1991; **13,** S76.
74. Fennell RH, Shikes RH, Vierling JM. Relationship of pretransplant hepatobiliary diesease to bile duct damage occurring in the liver allograft. *Hepatology* 1983; **3,** 84–89.
75. Starzl TE, Todo S, Fung J, Demetris AJ, Venkatarmamman R, Jain A. FK 506 for liver, kidney

and pancreas transplantation. *Lancet* 1989; **2,** 1000–1004.

76. Van Hoek B, Wiesner RH, Ludwig J, Paya C. Recurrence of ductopenic rejection in liver allografts after retransplantation for vanishing bile duct syndrome. *Transplant Proc* 1991; **23,** 1442–1443.

16

Immunosuppression in liver transplantation

D White

Introduction

The acute immune destruction of an organ transplant represents a unique response of the immunologic repertoire. In this chapter the nature of that immune response will be discussed in detail and the way in which it applies to a liver transplant will be considered. The current protocols available for immunosuppressing a liver transplant will then be outlined with particular reference to the drugs now being tested in clinical trials.

The allogeneic effect

It has been known for many years that the T cell response to major histocompatibility antigens (MHC) in an organ allograft involves many more cell clones than the response to any other antigen.[1] This hyper-responsiveness has been termed the allogeneic effect and is responsible for acute allograft rejection. The reason for this effect lies in the immunologically pivotal role of the MHC in presenting antigen to T cells, the nature of self-tolerance and the inadvertent transfer of antigen presenting cells with the graft.

Tissue typing

Tissue matching developed during the 1960s in response to clinical demand for improved survival of kidney transplants. The principle upon which it was based was that if 'transplant antigens' could be matched identically between donor and recipient, rejection would be reduced.

This concept has been established beyond doubt both experimentally in inbred[2] and outbred[3] animals and in live donor sibling transplants in man.[4] However, the availability of an MHC identical sibling prepared to donate a liver for transplantation is limited. Thus, unrelated cadavers have become the main source of organ donors.

As the complexity of the MHC became apparent the probability of finding identity between donor and recipient decreased.[5] This has resulted in the organisation of national and international donor sharing schemes. Elusiveness of identity also generated the concept of 'best match'; thus, if one could not achieve identity, a mismatch for only one antigen should produce better survival than a mismatch for four antigens. However, data in support of this concept have never been convincing and in liver transplantation, contrary results have been reported. This lack of evidence for an association between tissue matching and liver graft survival has led to the establishment of a European multicentred trial of tissue typing in liver transplantation (L'Esprit). That such a trial should be undertaken in this manner suggests a lack of knowledge of the mechanisms underlying acute liver graft rejection.

MHC restricted self-tolerance

Most immune responses have as part of their regulatory processes an MHC restricted element.[6] Matzinger has proposed[7,8] that MHC restriction also applies to that poorly understood ontological process whereby tolerance to self-antigens is established.[9] Furthermore, both she[10] and others[11–13] have produced experimental data that support this concept. The classic experiments of Medawar and colleagues[14] demonstrate that, during ontogeny, a process of self-antigen recognition occurs within the thymus which results in the individual's ability to discriminate self from non-self. Matzinger suggests[7,8] that this self tolerising process acts not on self-antigens but upon the processed products of those self-antigens presented within the thymus by self-MHC, primarily class II. While such a process is eminently desirable considering the MHC restricted nature of immune recognition, this process causes an immunologic artifact when organs are transplanted. In order to prevent self-directed destruction the immune system has developed a complex antigen recognition process based upon the presentation of peptides bound within the MHC and presented by a specialised group of bone marrow derived antigen presenting cells. These antigen presenting cells are present in all organs of the body and are therefore transferred passively into a recipient with an organ transplant.[15,16] The result of this accidental transfer of antigen presenting cells has curious results. As an example, consider the consequences of a transplant between individuals who only differ by one class II incompatibility. The transplanted antigen presenting cell goes on presenting but now to the recipient T cell population. The vast majority of antigens presented will be self-antigens (both for the donor and recipient). The recipient will, of course, be tolerant of these recipient antigens but in the context of recipient MHC. Thus in the graft, a situation exists where self-antigens (probably many thousands of different peptide groups) are presented on an inappropriate MHC class II molecule. The recipient is not self-tolerant to this novel combination of self-peptide combined with non-self MHC. Thus a huge T cell response is induced as the result of a single MHC incompatibility and a subtle failure of the mechanism of self-tolerance. It is this overwhelming T cell response, sometimes called direct presentation, which is primarily responsible for acute graft rejection.

The MHC and acute rejection

The cell population performing direct presentation is bone marrow derived and has a relatively short life span. Thus these cells become replaced by those of recipient origin. Once this has occurred (probably within three months, see Figure 16.1) graft rejection can only occur as a result of these recipient antigen presenting cells presenting graft antigens. In such a case only anti-

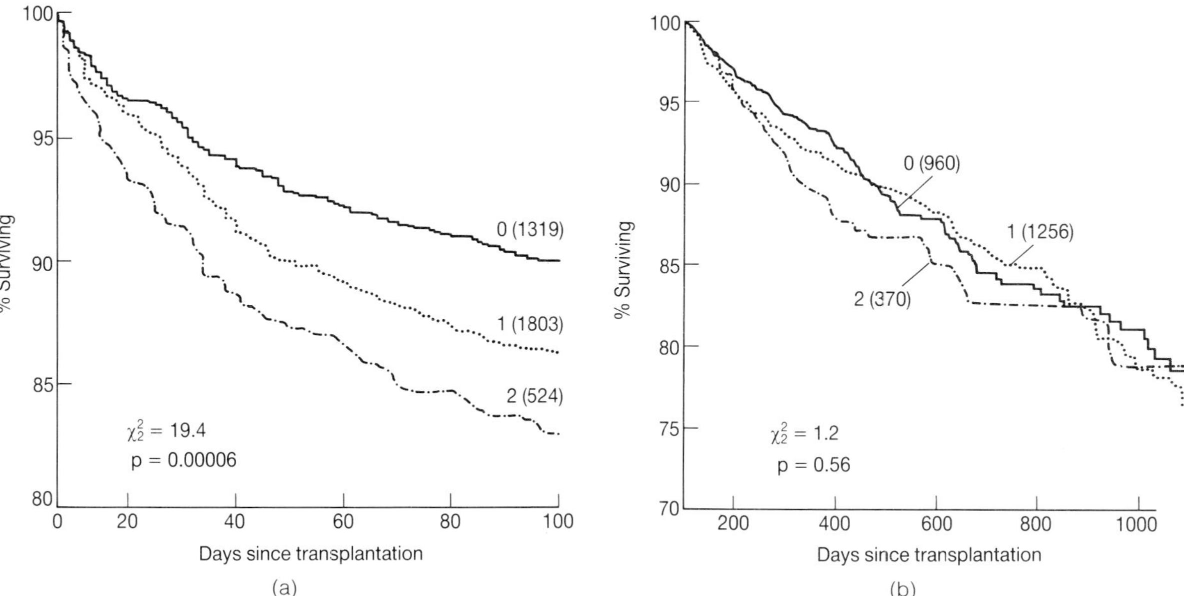

Fig. 16.1 (a) The effect on survival of kidney allografts of matching for DR days 7–100. This time scale was chosen to illustrate the effect of the presence of antigen presenting cells. (b) The complete loss of any benefit from matching for DR after day 100. All surviving grafts were normalised at 100% and survival effect over three years was investigated.

genic differences between donor and recipient will induce a response. This indirect presentation induces a response several orders of magnitude less than that achieved by direct presentation. Furthermore, the significance of the MHC in causing graft rejection is lost and it becomes reduced to the same status as any other antigenic incompatibility.

This phenomenon has been clearly demonstrated in kidney transplantation. Figure 16.1 illustrates the significance of MHC class II incompatibility to the survival of kidney transplants. The data are temporally subdivided into the first 100 days post-transplant (when direct presentation is taking place) and from day 101 to three years (indirect presentation). Analysis of the data in this fashion shows the overwhelming importance of a class II mismatch in the immediate post-transplant period with a subsequent total loss of the effect of matching once the donor antigen presenting cell has been replaced by those of the recipient. While a similar phenomenon has not been reported for liver grafts due to insufficient data, there is no reason to suppose that the principle of direct presentation does not apply to this organ also.

An understanding of the principles underlying allograft rejection is essential for the correct application of immunosuppressive protocols. It clarifies, for example, why it is possible to reduce the level of immunosuppression after the first few weeks post-transplant. Of necessity, immunosuppressive protocols have been designed to inhibit this direct presentation induced acute rejection episode. Little is known about how to control the effector mechanisms involved in chronic rejection and it may well be that current immunosuppressive protocols are not the most appropriate way of inhibiting this process. This is particularly important in liver transplantation where a substantial amount of data now exists to demonstrate that, uniquely for this organ, a consistent slow immunologic attrition does not take place.

Diagnosis of rejection

An analysis of the cause of death in liver transplantation reveals that rejection directly accounts for only a small percentage (10%) of these fatalities.[17] Perioperative mortality and systemic infection account for a far larger number of deaths.[18] The majority of liver transplant recipients, however, are treated for rejection in the first few weeks post-transplant. However, diagnosis of acute rejection on clinical features alone is unreliable.

Williams *et al.*,[19] in a study of 21 liver transplant recipients, reported 18 episodes of acute rejection diagnosed by clinical and biochemical criteria, only eight of which were confirmed histologically on biopsy. The remaining ten 'episodes' showed a histological picture of cholestasis and ballooning of hepatocytes. Furthermore, two of the 'biopsy proven' rejection episodes resolved spontaneously. An important consideration resolved by this study was the risk to the recipient of liver biopsy in the face of deteriorating hepatic function and decreased clotting ability. In a total series of 137 biopsies, there were only three complications, none of which resulted in death. Snover and colleagues reported similar findings. Of nine clinically diagnosed rejection episodes, only four were confirmed on histological examination. Thus it is an important tenet of any clinical management of immunosuppression that, before rejection is treated, it must be unequivocally diagnosed. Experience demonstrates that diagnosis on clinical criteria only is more often wrong than right.

Prophylactic immunosuppression

Cyclosporin

For the reasons described in the first section of this chapter, a liver graft will induce a substantial T cell driven rejection reaction. Over the years a number of prophylactic regimens have been developed with the aim of suppressing this response. Currently most of these are based upon the use of the drug cyclosporin.

Cyclosporin was first introduced into clinical practice by Calne *et al.*[20] Subsequently it has been shown to be effective in preventing clinical graft rejection in kidney, pancreas, heart and heart–lung transplantation as well as liver transplantation.[21] It has now become the immunosuppressive of choice in most transplant centres.

The use of this drug offers two major advantages in clinical practice. First, its mode of action is highly selective in that it restricts its effect to T cell function or immune responses requiring activation of T cells, particularly the CD4 helper T cell population.[22] This selectivity of action leaves the recipient of a liver graft with an intact myeloid system and an only partially restricted antibody responsiveness. This results in an improved capacity to resist opportunistic infections. The second advantage of using cyclosporin is corticosteroid sparing.

Initial studies on cyclosporin demonstrated that it could be used as the sole immunosuppressant in liver transplantation. Starzl[23] has, however, advocated its use in combination with low doses of steroids. There is no convincing clinical evidence that this combination confers any immunosuppressive benefit to the patient despite several clinical trials to test the effect of combined therapy. The availability of both azathioprine and prednisone do, however, offer an advantage of flexibility which is of great benefit in hepatic transplantation.

Of potential concern in liver transplantation is the hepatotoxicity of cyclosporin. Moreover, since the metabolism and primary route of excretion of the drug is via the liver, even low doses of the drug might prove hepatotoxic to the recipient of a liver graft. In view of the relatively mild rejection response induced by a liver allograft and the observation that experimentally very small doses of cyclosporin were sufficient to prevent rejection,[24] lower doses of cyclosporin tend to be used in liver transplants than for other grafts. Nephrotoxicity and failure to absorb the drug are both much more frequent complications than hepatotoxicity. Cyclosporin given orally in the first few days post-liver transplantation is poorly absorbed, probably due to lack of bile salts. Once the draining T tube is clamped and a normal bile flow established, most patients will absorb cyclosporin satisfactorily. In those patients whose primary disease was biliary atresia, oral cyclosporin absorption can be a particular problem. Such recipients are invariably children who metabolise and secrete the drug far more rapidly than adults. This is compounded by the Roux loop impairing the ability of these individuals to absorb the drug. Management of these recipients relies heavily on blood levels of cyclosporin and the children are often dosed four or more times a day. On occasions it has proved necessary to use doses in excess of 30 mg/kg to establish suitable blood levels.[25] One way to overcome this failure to absorb cyclosporin is by the use of intravenous cyclosporin. However, great care needs to be exercised with the use of this preparation if nephrotoxicity is to be avoided. In particular, IV cyclosporin should be given with great caution to an anuric recipient and should not be given in combination with nephrotoxic antibiotics.

Sequential immunosuppression

Because of these potential complications many groups have evolved a sequential immunosuppressive regime. This varies in detail from centre to centre but has the same common principles. Firstly azathioprine and steroids are given immediately post-transplant. If the recipient's renal function is satisfactory over the first 24 hours post-transplant, low dose (1–2 mg/kg bd) IV cyclosporin is started. Once the T tube is clamped, oral cyclosporin doses are added to the regime and when blood level determination provides evidence of oral absorption, the IV administration is stopped. This leaves the patient on triple therapy which many centres favour for long term immunosuppression. However, there are a number of groups who, over a period of months, will withdraw both the azathioprine and corticosteroids.

Liver transplantation has increased dramatically since the introduction of cyclosporin both in terms of success and in the numbers performed. Starzl[23] has ascribed this enhancement of survival to cyclosporin although it seems probable that improvement in immunosuppression was just one of many changes which have contributed to the current success rates in hepatic transplantation. Furthermore, the use of cyclosporin poses almost as many clinical management problems as it solves. Thus the search for better, less toxic immunosuppressives continues. Currently two new forms of immunosuppression are in various stages of clinical testing; these are FK506 and monoclonal antibodies.

FK506

FK506 is a novel macrolide first isolated from *Streptomyces tukubaesinsis* by Kino *et al.*[26] Extensive studies on cultured CD4+ (helper) T lymphocytes have shown that FK506 is approximately 100 times more potent on a weight for weight basis than CyA in selectively inhibiting the secretion of a variety of cytokines, in particular IL-2.[27,28] The precise degree of the potency of FK506 compared to CyA may be an important consideration in interpreting the *in vivo* data. From the very first *in vivo* studies on rats with cardiac grafts,[29] it became clear that the drug was a remarkably powerful immunosuppressive agent.

The uncertainty with FK506 lies in whether, and at what dose, side effects occur *in vivo*. In rats, Ochai *et al.*,[30] administering the drug at 0.32 mg/kg and 1 mg/kg, were able to achieve 100% heart graft survival. This was confirmed by Lim *et al.*[29] who also noted that, at 1 mg/kg, rats became emaciated and lost approximately 20% of their body weight during the 14 day treatment period. Nalesnik *et al.*,[31] in a formal toxicological study, found FK506 produced hyperglycaemia in rats given doses of 1–4 mg/kg. These data are in contrast to those of Takai *et al.*[32] who reported no weight loss seen in rats treated with 1 mg/kg FK506, although they did observe marked thymic changes.

Studies by Ochiai *et al.*.[33] and Collier *et al*[34] of FK506 in dogs with renal allografts revealed that the drug was immunosuppressive orally at a dose of 1 mg/kg. In the study reported by Collier *et al.*[34] animals suffered from nausea requiring treatment with metaclopramide and all animals surviving more than 84 days had histological evidence of acute vasculitis. Three of these animals died as a result of this vasculitis affecting the coronary arteries. At a dose of 0.5 mg/kg orally, FK506 did not prevent renal allograft rejection in the dog but vasculitis was still observed in this group. Todo *et al.*[35] also noted vasculitis in dogs treated with FK506. However, these workers subsequently claimed that such vasculitis could occur in untreated animals. Another paradox occurred in treatment of baboons with FK506. At a dose of 1 mg/kg and 0.5 mg/kg given intramuscularly, Collier *et al.* found that although immunosuppressive at these doses, many of the animals had elevated blood sugar levels. In the Pittsburgh primate studies, no significant side effects of the drug were noted.

Thus, animal studies show the drug to be a potent immunosuppressive at an oral dose of 0.5–1 mg/kg with a toxicity profile varying with species and probably route of administration. Armed with these data, Starzl *et al.*[36] initiated a clinical pilot study of the FK506 in liver transplant recipients who for a variety of reasons could no longer be treated with CyA. Initial drug administration was by IV infusion followed by oral dosing. The dose used was 0.15 mg/kg bd. This was substantially lower than the doses used in most of the experimental studies although, in his original rat study, Ochai[30] did report an immunosuppressive effect at 0.32 mg/kg. The dose chosen by Starzl is, however, entirely in keeping with the *in vitro* comparisons of FK506 with CyA. Shapiro *et al.*[37] reported that in 31 liver transplant recipients treated with oral FK506, 87% reported no side effects. Those side effects that were reported consisted for the most part of insomnia (16%) or headache (10%). There are currently several randomised clinical trials of FK506 in liver transplantation being undertaken. Preliminary results would suggest, however, that the experience reported by Shapiro is unusual. Most groups have experienced significant side effects in most patients receiving FK506. This may be resolved by an appropriate dose adjustment. However, FK506 will require more extensive use in a number of different centres before its real potential as an immunosuppressive in liver transplantation can be dispassionately assessed.

Monoclonal antibodies

Potentially one of the most important advances in the control of the immune system is the development of the therapeutic use of monoclonal antibodies. The concept of using antibodies directed against lymphocytes or lymphocyte subsets was developed many years ago. However, the practical problems of consistency of production severely limited the application of this approach. The development of hybridoma technology[38] has offered the clinician the option of using a well-defined product of known specificity and reproducible effect.

Several monoclonal antibodies which recognise human lymphocytes have been evaluated in clinical renal transplantation, but there is much less experience of their use in liver transplantation. Monoclonal antibodies may be used to prevent rejection following transplantation or to treat an acute rejection episode as it develops. In addition there is considerable interest in the preoperative perfusion of the graft with anti-leucocyte common antibodies to reduce its antigenicity by destroying antigen presenting cells (see Figure 16.1). As yet, experience with this technique is limited to kidney transplantation.[39] Hale and co-workers have used a rat IgM monoclonal antibody, Campath-1, prophylactically following liver transplantation in 36 patients.[40] This antibody recognises all mature T and B lymphocytes which it lyses by fixation of human complement.[41] Survival in this group was improved compared with controls. Esquivel *et al.*[42] carried out a trial of the use of OKT3 in the treatment of biopsy proven acute rejection of liver grafts in 52 patients. They demonstrated a significant improvement as a result of the monoclonal antibody therapy compared with steroid treatment in patients treated between ten and 90 days post-transplant. This study did not demonstrate the high incidence of recurrent rejection following the end of OKT3 treatment which has been reported in kidney transplantation.

Otto *et al.*,[43] in a pilot study of nine patients, reported that the prophylactic use of an anti-CD25 monoclonal antibody reduced the rejection rate in liver transplant recipients from a historical 80% to approximately 20%. This was an improvement on reported rejection rates for OKT3 in liver transplant recipients. In contrast, Friend *et al.*,[44] using a monoclonal against the IL-2 receptor, failed to demonstrate any significant benefit in liver transplant recipients. The IL-2 receptor is in principle a very attractive target for monoclonal antibody therapy because it appears on the surface of lymphocytes only on activation. Following organ transplantation only a minority of circulating lymphocytes express this receptor which becomes up-regulated at times of rejection. Thus treatment with an anti-IL-2 receptor monoclonal should in theory eliminate only those cells specifically committed to rejecting the graft and allow the remainder of the lymphocyte pool to respond unhindered once therapy with the monoclonal has finished. Experimental studies in rodents[45] and clinical trials in kidney transplant recipients[46] have suggested that such therapy should be successful for liver transplant recipients. It may be, however, that liver transplant recipients generate such high levels of soluble IL-2 receptor that they block the effect of the antibody.

One of the drawbacks of the use of monoclonal antibodies as immunosuppressive agents is their rodent origin. This results in most patients receiving monoclonal antibody therapy generating an antiglobulin response against the antibody. This effectively limits the duration of therapy to ten days and casts doubt upon the value of subsequent treatments. Recently, however, Winter and Milstein[47] have been able to genetically engineer a human equivalent of the rodent Campath-1 in which only a small portion of the idiotype remains of rat origin. Preliminary studies have suggested that prolonged therapy with this 'humanised' reagent does not result in the generation of an antiglobulin nor anti-idiotype reaction. If this observation can be confirmed and extended then it would seem probable that the use of monoclonal antibodies in immunosuppression will become much more extensive than at present.

References

1. Swain SL, Panfili PR, Duton RW, Lefkovits I. Frequency to allogeneic helper T cells responding to whole H2 differences and to an H-2K difference alone. *J Immunol* 1979; **123,** 1062.
2. Snell GD. The Homograft reaction *Ann Rev Microbiol* 1957; **11,** 339–458.
3. White DJG, Bradley BA, Calne RY, Binns RM. The relationship of the histocompatability locus in the pig to allograft survival. *Transplant Proc* 1973; **5,** 317–320.
4. Thorsby E. Present state of histocompatability typing and matching in renal transplantation: an introduction *Transplant Proc* 1982; **14,** 173–177.
5. Kountz S. Clinical transplantation – an overview. *Transplant Proc.* 1973; **6,** 59–65.
6. Zinkernagel RM, Doherty PC. Restriction of in vitro T–cell mediated cytotoxcity in lymphocytic choriomeningitis within syngenic or semi-allogeneic system. *Nature* 1974; **248,** 701–702.
7. Matzinger P. A one receptor view of T-cell behaviour. *Nature* 1981; **292,** 497–501
8. Matzinger P, Waterfield JJ. Is self-tolerance H-2 restricted. *Nature* 1980; **285,** 492–494.
9. Kappler JW, Roehm N, Marrack P. T-cell tolerance by clonal elimination in the thymus. *Cell* 1987; **49,** 273–280.
10. Matzinger P, Zamoyska R, Waldmann H. Self tolerance in H-2-restricted mice. *Nature* 1984; **308,** 738–741.
11. Rammensee HG, Bevan MJ. Evidence from in vitro studies that tolerance to self antigens is MHC restricted. *Nature* 1984; **308,** 741–749.
12. Desquenne-Clark L, Kimura H, Silvers WK. Evidence that major histocompatability complex restriction of foreign transplantation antigens occurs when tolerance is induced in neonatal mice and rats. *Proc Nat Acad Sci* 1985; **82,** 6265–6267.
13. Kimura H, Desquenne-Clark L, Miyamoto M, Silvers WK. Major histocompatability complex (MHC) restriction of foreign transplantation antigens in rats rendered tolerant at birth. *J Exp Med* 1986, **164,** 2031–2037.
14. Billingham RE, Brent L, Medawar BP. Actively

acquired tolerance of foreign cells. *Nature* 1953; **172,** 603–606.
15. Steinmuller D, Hart E. Passenger leukocytes and induction of allograft immunity. *Transplant Proc* 1971; **3,** 673.
16. Stuart FP, Bastien E, Holter A, Fitch FW, Elkins WL. Role of passenger leukocytes in the rejection of renal allografts. *Transplant Proc* 1971; **3,** 461–464.
17. Starzl TE, Weil R, Koep J, McCalmon RT, Terasaki P, Irraki Y *et al.* Fifteen years of clinical transplantation. *Gastroenterology* 1979; **77,** 375–378.
18. Starzl TE, Weil R, Lawrence J. Thoracic duct fistula and renal transplantation. *Ann Surg* 1979; **190,** 474–486.
19. Williams JW, Peters TG, Vera SR. Biopsy directed immuno-suppression following hepatic transplantation in man. *Transplantation* 1985; **39**(6), 589–596.
20. Calne RY, White DJG, Rolles K *et al.* Cyclosporin A initially as the only immunosuppressant in 34 recipients of cadaveric organs : 32 kidneys, 2 pancreases and 2 livers. *Lancet* 1979; **ii,** 1033–1036.
21. White DJG, Calne RY. The use of Cylosporin A immunosuppression in organ grafting. *Immunol Rev* 1987; **65,** 115–131.
22. White DJG, Plumb A, Calne RY. The immune status of transplant recipients immunosuppressed with cyclosporin A. *Transplant Proc* 1981; **13,** 1666–1668.
23. Starzl TE. Evolution of liver transplantation. *Hepatology*, 1982; **2,** 614. Gartner JC, Zitelli J, Malataell JJ *et al.*
24. Zimmermann FA, White DJG, Gokel JM, Calne RY. In: *Orthotopic liver transplants in rats* 339–344.
25. Land W, Castro LA, White DJG *et al.* In: *Ciclosporin*, Borel JF (ed). Basel: Karger, 1986.
26. Kino T, Hatanaka H, Hashimoto M, Nishiyama M, Goto T *et al.* FK506, a novel immunosuppresant isolated from a streptomyces I. Fermentation, isolation and physico-chemical and biological characteristics. *J Antibiotics* 1987; **40,** 1249–1261.
27. Yoshimura N, Matsui S, Hamashima T. Effect of new immunosuppressive agent, FK506, on human lymphocyte responses in vitro. *Transplantation* 1989; **47,** 351–356.
28. Tocci MJ, Matkovitch DA, Collier KA. The immunosuppressant FK506 selectivity inhibits expression of early T cell activation genes. *J Immunol* 1989; **143,** 718–726.
29. Lim SML, Thiru S, White DJG. Heterotropic heart transplantation in rat receiving FK506. *Transplant Proc* 1987; **19,** 68–70.
30. Ochai T, Nakajima K, Susuki T *et al.* Effect of a new immunosuppressive agent, FK506, on heterotopic cardiac allotransplantation in the rat. *Transplant Proc* 1987; **19,** 1284–1287.
31. Nalesnik MA, Todo S, Murase N *et al.* Toxicology of FK506 in the Lewis rat. *Transplant Proc* 1987; **19,** 89–93.
32. Takai K, Jojima K, Sakatoku J, Fukumoto T. Effect of FK506 on rat thymus: time course analysis by immunoperoxidase technique and flow cytometry. *Clin Exp Immunol* 1990; **82,** 445–451.
33. Ochiai T, Nagata M, Nakajima K *et al.* Studies of the effects of FK506 on renal allografting in the beagle dog. *Transplantation* 1987; **44,** 729–735.
34. Collier DStJ, Calne RY, Thiru S, Friend PJ, Lim SML, White DJG. FK506 in experimental renal allografts in dogs and primates. *Transplant Proc* 1988; **20,** 226–230.
35. Todo S, Murase N, Ueda Y *et al.* Effect of FK506 in experimental organ transplantation. *Transplant Proc* 1988; **20,** 215–217.
36. Starzl TE, Todo S, Fung J *et al.* FK506 for liver, kidney and pancreas transplantation. *Lancet* 1989; **ii,** 1000–1003.
37. Shapiro R, Fung JJ, Jain A. The side-effects of FK506 in humans. *Transplant Proc* 1990; **22,** 35–36.
38. Kohler G, Milstein C. Continuous cultures of fused cells secreting antibody of predefined specificity. *Nature* 1975; **256,** 495–497.
39. Oei J, Terasaki PI, Hardiwijajas, Mendez R. Treatment of kidney graft rejection with CKAL and CBL1 monoclonal antibodies. *Transplant Proc* 1985; **17,** 2740–2743.
40. Hale G, Waldmann H, Friend PJ, Calne RY. Pilot study of Campath-1, a rat monoclonal antibody that fires human complement, as an immunosuppressant in organ transplantation. *Transplantation* 1986; **42,** 308–311.
41. Bindon CI, Hale G, Clark U, Waldmann H. Therapeutic potential of monoclonal antibodies to the leukocytes common antigen. *Transplantation* 1985; **40,** 538–544.
42. Esquivel CO, Fung JJ, Markus B *et al.* OKT3 in the reversal of acute hepatic allograft rejection. *Transplant Proc* 1987; **19,** 2443–2446.
43. Otto G, Thies J, Kabelitz D *et al.* Anti-CD25 monoclonal antibody prevents early rejection in liver transplantation – a pilot study. *Transplant Proc* 1991; **23,** 1387–1389.
44. Friend PJ, Waldman H, Cobbold S *et al.* The anti-ILZ receptor monoclonal antibody TTH-906 in liver transplantation. *Transplant Proc* 1991; **23,** 1390–1392.
45. Kupiec-Weglinski JW, Diamanstein T, Tilney NL. Interleukin 2 receptor-targeted therapy-rationale and applications in organ transplantation. *Transplantation* 1988; **46,** 785–791.

46. Soulillou JP, Cantarovitch D, Le Mauff B. Randomised controlled trial of monoclonal antibody against the interleukin-2 receptor (33 B3.1) as compared with rabbit anti-thymocyte globulin for prophylaxis against rejection of renal allografts. *N Eng J Med* 1990; **322,** 1175–1181.
47. Winter G, Milstein C. Man-made antibodies. *Nature* 1991; **349,** 293–299.

17

Management of immunosuppression

C Trey, G Trey, S Robson and R Jenkins

Introduction

Preservation of liver graft function depends on appropriate immunotherapy and clinical care of the patient. After liver transplantation, currently the patient is committed to this treatment for life. An ideal immunosuppressive agent should preserve the graft with only minimal side effects. There are no ideal agents and different sub-ideal therapeutic regimes have been proposed. The various immunological effects and agents with their actions and side effects have been discussed elsewhere. On review of the various possible protocols for the management of transplant immunosuppression regimes, it is apparent that there is no firm consensus on the detailed approach to the care of these patients. There is a fine balance between the dosages of medication that allow for immunosuppression and those that lead to life threatening infection. Approaches range from extreme initial immunosuppression with eventual tapering to moderate initial immunosuppression while monitoring closely for evidence of rejection.

We review appropriate alternate management plans and provide a guide to the practical medical management of the liver transplant patient.

Pretransplant immunotherapy

Once the patient has been referred for liver transplantation, their condition should be fully assessed and fitness for transplantation optimised. Hepatitis B, hepatitis C, CMV, EBV and HIV screening and nutritional assessment should have been performed. If time allows the patient should receive the hepatitis B vaccine and provision of optimal nutrition should be instituted. Hepatitis B hyperimmune globulin infusion of patients who are HBsAg and HBeAg positive is controversial but is probably not effective. Studies of interferon in hepatitis C and B should be done on experimental protocol as this is currently being studied, but this also appears ineffective in patients treated at this stage.[1] Anti-CMV globulin may be administered intravenously to CMV antibody negative patients who are transplanted with CMV positive donors. In a study from Nebraska, such patients who were given intravenous immune globulin (IgG, 0.5 g/kg) at weekly intervals for six weeks and acyclovir for three months had a 23.8% incidence of CMV disease compared to controls who had a 71.4% incidence ($p < 0.01$).[2] In these patients, Saliba *et al.* achieved a reduction of CMV infection from 85.7% to 26.6% with CMV-Ig intravenous infusions at doses of 250 mg/kg at day 0 and 125 mg/kg every ten days for three months.[3]

Since most infections developing in immunocompromised patients arise from endogenous aerobic bacteria and fungi, the rationale for using selective bowel decontamination rests on the elimination of gram-negative aerobic colonisers with preservation of the anaerobic flora. Some transplant units favour a preoperative regime of tobramycin and amphotericin to sterilise the bowel. The Mayo Clinic group uses gentamicin 80 mg, nystatin 2 million U and polymyxin E 100 mg combined in a 10 ml orally administered suspension given for three days before and 21 days after the operation.[4] These attempts at selective decontamination have been shown in uncontrolled trials to decrease bacterial counts in the bowel and to decrease infection.[5,6] Wiesner showed that of 145 patients who had a liver transplantation with selective bowel decontamination, only five experienced a gram-negative infection and only one patient developed a systemic candida infection.[4] However, the Mayo Clinic, which uses selective bowel decontamination, had an infection rate (including minor infections) of 75% of 53 patients, while the University of Pittsburgh which did not use selective bowel decontamination had an infection rate of 50% of 110 patients.[6] The role of selective bowel decontamination awaits a controlled trial; at present, we only decontaminate the bowel with nystatin prior to and after surgery. We administer trimethoprim and sulphamethoxazole for prolonged periods after transplantation to prevent pneumocystitis pneumonia. Other centres give low dose acyclovir prophylaxis. The question of donor blood transfusions has not yet been addressed though this is standard practice in kidney transplants.[7]

Peri-operative and post-operative immunotherapy

Appropriate immunotherapy involves the use of combinations of immunosuppressive agents both to minimise drug toxicity and prevent graft rejection. Glucocorticoids, potent blockers of the activation of the IL-1 and IL-6 genes and the most widely used suppressor of cellular immunity and inflammation, are the first agents used to maintain the graft. Methylprednisolone, the product after metabolisation of hydrocortisone by the liver, is commonly used; but studies have shown that hydrocortisone, which is metabolised by the liver, is also effective.[8] Protocol administration varies; some groups give a bolus intravenously prior to surgery, but we give 500 mg of methylprednisolone intravenously just prior to revascularisation of the allograft, followed by a dose of 200 mg in four divided doses the first day tapering by 40 mg daily until the maintenance dose of 20 mg daily is reached on post-operative day six. Comparative studies of different dosage regimens of corticosteroids have not been done.

Azathioprine, by interfering with purine synthesis, blocks the synthesis of nucleic acids and other cell products. Thus, it interferes with all rapidly dividing cells including those of the lymphoproliferative system. The drug is synergistic with steroids and thus has a steroid sparing effect. Initially 100 mg of azathioprine is given after operation and daily dosages of 1–2 mg/kg/day are given unless the white count is less than 5000 or the patient has an infection.

Cyclosporin, which specifically interferes with T cell activation and antigen presentation, has revolutionised immunosuppression since its introduction by Calne in 1979.[9] Once adequate urine output (30–50 ml/hr) has been established after surgery, most centres will give the 2–4 mg/kg/24 hours of cyclosporin as an intravenous continuous infusion or in divided doses. When gastrointestinal motility and function resume, oral or nasogastric cyclosporin is started in two divided dosages of about three times the intravenous dosage, with a 12 hour overlap with tapered intravenous infusion. In children, bile salts or vitamin E analogues are administered to promote absorption. Whole blood trough cyclosporin levels are monitored daily, and dosages altered to achieve levels between 250–400 ng/ml. However, the nephrotoxicity and hepatotoxicity of intravenous cyclosporin given immediately after transplantation has lead us to start dosing with 6 mg/kg oral cyclosporin, usually down the nasogastric tube, on post-operative day two. Concomitant use of furosemide with cyclosporin decreases cyclosporin induced renal injury.[10] Ketoconazole administration to inhibit cyclosporin metabolism is not recommended. Cyclosporin levels are altered by drugs which enhance or suppress cytochrome P-450; the specifics will be discussed later. If the patient does not have adequate urine output at this time, we use OKT3 in place of cyclosporin until renal function improves.[11] Steininger *et al.* found in a study of 95 consecutive patients that by substituting cyclosporin with OKT3 for the first eight days of immunosuppression, they noted fewer acute rejections, but more late viral infections.[12] Others have shown a greater incidence of lymphomas with the use of OKT3.[13] However, Steininger *et al.* found that a polyclonal antibody thymoglobulin (ATG) administered in a dose of 2.5 mg/kg/day intravenously for ten days with oral cyclosporin started on day eight post-operatively lead to both decreased rejection and infection when compared to both cyclosporin and OKT3. The incidence of rejection in the 64 patients who received cyclosporin was 67%; in the 32 patients who received OKT3 there was a 44% rejection rate; but acute rejection was seen in only 24% of the 49 patients who received ATG.[12] The use of ATG needs further study. The blood cyclosporin levels increase markedly when the T tube is clamped as there is an enterohepatic circulation of cyclosporin. Thus, during this time the levels should be taken 12 hourly.

OKT3, a monoclonal mouse antibody directed

against the CD3 membrane protein of human T cells, can be substituted for cyclosporin if the patient has pre-existent or post-operative renal impairment.[11,14] The dose of 5 mg intravenously over two minutes is preceded by administration of 200 mg of methyl-prednisolone before the initial dose and 650 mg of acetaminophen and 50 mg of Benadryl one half hour prior to administration of every dose to decrease the invariable response of fever, chills and diarrhoea associated with the massive release of tumour necrosis factor and interferon associated with OKT3 use.[15] If patients still have these reactions to OKT3, the dosage may be paradoxically tripled as this appears to stop these reactions by maximally depressing these T cell mediated responses. Before courses of OKT3 administration are repeated or if the drug appears ineffective, CD3+ T cell levels and anti-OKT3 antibodies should be measured.[16] Concomitant use of azathioprine and steroids during OKT3 administration may decrease the likelihood of an anti-OKT3 response.[17] However, OKT3 should not be used routinely in place of cyclosporin because of the increased cost, incidence of malignancy and the possible decrease of effectiveness in its subsequent use for episodes of rejection. Indeed, McDiarmid *et al.*, could not find any long term benefit in renal function or episodes of rejection with the use of OKT3 in place of cyclosporin. Graft survival was 63% for the 46 patients who received OKT3 and 73% for the 39 patient cyclosporin group. There was no difference in the serum creatinine at 12 months.[18] Routine use of OKT3 would add about 15,000 dollars (£8000) to the cost of every transplantation and offer little benefit.[19]

Recently FK506, which has been shown to block proliferation of T lymphocytes and the activation of the IL-4 gene, has been used in place of cyclosporin for initial immunosuppression.[20] It has been shown in some preliminary studies to have fewer side effects than cyclosporin and to be more efficacious. However, FK506 administration causes hyperkalaemia in 35% of patients, alters glucose metabolism, and infrequently results in aphasia and seizures. It can cause a similar alteration in renal function as cyclosporin.[21] In a recent study from Pittsburgh, first graft survival rates at one year in 57 patients receiving FK506 were 80.8% compared to 68.5% in 54 patients receiving cyclosporin ($p < 0.01$).[22] Cyclosporin and FK506 are not routinely used together because of additive toxicities, pharmacological antagonism, and a dramatic rise in cyclosporin levels with concomitant use of FK506.[23,24] In the early post-operative period, FK506 is usually infused intravenously twice daily at a dose of 0.075 mg/kg over four hours. Oral dosage is started, as soon as possible as this has fewer side effects, with 0.15 mg/kg taken twice daily.[25,26,27] To avoid nephrotoxicity, we usually do not use intravenous FK506 and start oral dosing on post-operative day two. It appears that the first pass effect in the liver results in the formation of hydrosoluble metabolites of FK506 which are readily eliminated by the kidney, while intravenous FK506 accumulates in the kidney resulting in greater toxicity.[25] FK506 levels need to be monitored and maintained in the 0.5–2 ng/ml range to prevent rejection and toxicity.[25] The liver graft function dramatically influences the doses and trough levels of FK506.[28] FK506 does not need to be administered with steroids and may offer some benefit when steroids must be avoided. The role of FK506 has not been completely defined, but it promises to be a mainstay of the immunosuppressive regime.

Problems encountered in the post-operative period

Liver transplant recipients are susceptible to a variety of complications that must be recognised and distinguished from rejection. Rejection often requires increasing immunosuppression while other problems may call for decreasing immunosuppression or other remedies. If in the first few hours following surgery, patients have marked elevations of serum transaminases, uncorrectable elevation of PT, deteriorating mental status and decline in renal function, the most likely diagnosis is primary graft non-function. If this is not severe it may be possible to provide for liver support and maintenance of coagulation with blood products till hepatic function improves. However, in most instances, the patient will need urgent retransplantation. Prostaglandin E_1 administration has been shown to be of benefit in some cases in which a replacement donor could not be found.[29]

Hepatic artery thrombosis, which occurs in about 7% of transplants, most often presents clinically between days nine to 33 as recurrent bacteraemia or delayed biliary leak.[30] If Doppler ultrasound fails to detect hepatic artery flow or CT reveals necrotic areas in the liver, angiography or MRI should be done as the problem may be

Table 17.1 Taper of immunosuppressive regime in the outpatient

	Steroids (methylprednisolone)	**Cyclosporin (Sandimmun)**	**Azathioprine**	**FK506**
Post-operatively	Adults 200 mg/day rapid wean by 40 mg/day to 20 mg/day Children ½ dose	Oral dosage* 4–10 mg/kg/day in two doses (blood levels 400–600 μg/ml)	1–1.5 mg/kg/day (WCC > 5,000)	0.3 mg/kg/day in two doses (blood levels 0.5–2 ng/ml)
First month	Adults 16–20 mg/day Children < 20 kg, 5 mg/day Children > 20 kg, 7.5 mg/day	Dose 3–8 mg/kg/day (blood levels 400–600 μg/ml)	1 mg/kg/day	(Blood levels 0.5–1 ng/ml)
Month 1–3	Adults 10–16 mg/day Children <20 kg, 2.5 mg/day Children >20 kg, 5 mg/day	Dose 3–5 mg/kg/day (blood levels 300–400 μg/ml)	1 mg/kg/day	(Blood levels 0.5–1 ng/ml)
Month 4–6	Adults 6–12 mg/day Children 2.5 mg alternate days to 5+mg/day (maximum dose)	(Blood levels 200–300 μg/ml)	0.5–1 mg/kg/day	(Blood levels 0.5–1 ng/ml)
Month 7–12	Adults 4–8 mg/day Children 2.5 to 5+mg alt days	(Blood levels 200–300 μg/ml)	0.5–1 mg/kg/day	(Blood levels 0.5–1 ng/ml)
After one year	Adults 4–6 mg/day Children 2.5 to 5 mg alt days	(Blood levels 200–300 μg/ml)	0.5–1 mg/kg Consider stopping drug	(Blood levels 0.5–1 ng/ml)

*Add ursodeoxycholic acid or bile salt preparation when required.

corrected surgically. Recurrent variceal haemorrhage, ascites, hepatic necrosis or prolonged prothrombin time are signs of possible portal vein thrombosis and early thrombectomy or shunting can be life-saving.[31] Rising serum bilirubin in the post-operative period or decreased bile flow through the T tube may indicate a biliary tract leak or stricture and mandates cholangiographic investigation.[32] However, Doppler ultrasound of the hepatic artery should be done to rule out hepatic vein thrombosis as a cause of the leak. While strictures and major leaks are best repaired surgically or by radiographic manipulations, minor leaks often close spontaneously. The transplant patient's poor overall condition, the hospital environment, the operative stress, the infusion of blood product and the use of immunosuppressive regimes predispose the patient to bacterial, fungal and viral infection. Development of fever, elevated white count, elevated liver injury tests, gastro-intestinal ulcers and respiratory problems can herald infection which is a major cause of morbidity and mortality. Since cytomegalovirus, herpes virus, Epstein-Barr (EB) virus and adenoviruses are treated by decrease of immunosuppression or by specific medications; these infections must be distinguished from rejection and treated appropriately. Untreated, all can result in hepatic necrosis. CMV usually occurs between three and eight weeks after transplantation. Prophylactic hyperimmune CMV globulin may prevent infection in patients without documented immunity. These viral infections are best diagnosed by liver biopsy, but viral culture and serological testing has been shown to be useful in early detection of CMV.[33]

Rejection and its management

The diagnosis of rejection, the most often encountered complication of liver transplantation, cannot be established accurately by non-invasive means. Clinical signs and biochemical tests can suggest the diagnosis, radiology can rule out other causes, but histology is the only way to confirm the diagnosis. Rejection is classified as hyperacute, acute or chronic.[34] Hyperacute rejection, which results from preformed antibodies, is almost never seen in liver transplant candidates.[35] Acute rejection, a cell mediated process, rarely occurs before the fourth post-operative day, occurs in up to 60–80% of patients and indeed most patients have an episode within the first three months.[36,37] The clinical presentation of acute rejection is non-specific, and in the first few weeks post-operatively may consist of fever, diminished quantity and quality of bile output through the T tube, tachycardia, malaise, confusion, myalgias, right upper quadrant tenderness, hepatosplenomegaly or ileus. Rapid increase of gamma-glutyl transpeptidase level is often followed by an increase in bilirubin, alkaline phosphatase, and slight rise of the AST and ALT to less than five to seven times normal. Cyclosporin levels usually decrease because rejection causes decreased bile production, resulting in diminished drug absorption and impaired enterohepatic circulation. Over the first four days after transplantation, patients should have a gradual normalisation of their liver function tests and improvement of their clinical status. After this period any worsening of their clinical or biochemical status should prompt an investigation into the possible cause, with liver biopsy always being considered (Figure 17.1). An unexplained rise in ALT and AST on day 3–5 post-transplant can be seen following the use of Belzer's Wisconsin preservation solution.[37]

The histological criteria of rejection and grading of rejection into mild, moderate and severe will be considered in the preceeding chapters. Once other causes of liver abnormalities have been ruled out and rejection confirmed by biopsy, episodes of rejection are treated by pulsed steroids, courses of OKT3 or ATG, changing or increasing dosages of immunosuppressive agents. If hepatic function does not improve after three days to a week of treatment for acute rejection, liver biopsy is repeated to gauge the response and rule out other causes for the ongoing abnormalities.

The first line therapy for acute rejection remains that of bolus corticosteroids, usually starting at 500 mg of methylprednisolone daily for three days with increases of the daily dose of prednisone to 30 or 40 mg. If the episode of rejection shows only partial resolution or mild relapse after a steroid bolus, the daily dose of prednisone can be increased to 200 mg daily in four divided doses, decreasing the daily dose by 40 mg daily until 20 mg daily is reached. If this does not result in clinical improvement, a course of OKT3, as previously described, should be started.[38] If a patient has previously received OKT3, the presence of blocking antibodies should be determined by ELISA.[39] During OKT3 therapy the patient can be monitored by determinations of percentage of CD3 T cells. If the percentage of CD3 cells is less than ten, the dose is maintained. If greater than 30% CD3+ cells are noted, another mode of therapy is considered, and if the CD3 cell count is in between, the dose is tripled.[40] During these treatments, we favour continuation of normal doses of cyclosporin and azathioprine. However, some centres will hold azathioprine until day 12 of OKT3 and decrease the cyclosporin levels by half until day ten of OKT3 use in an attempt to decrease the high incidence of infection associated with OKT3.[41] Many centres also use prophylactic ganciclovir when giving OKT3. Rebound rejection, a common phenomenon following cessation of OKT3, usually responds to steroid boluses and increase in prednisone dosages. In cases that do not respond to steroids, OKT3 can be repeated with CD3 cell levels used to evaluate proper dosing. Using steroids and OKT3 in this manner leads to successful treatment of acute rejection in 88.9% of cases.[38]

If these standard modes of treatment of acute rejection fail, are not favoured by the transplant team, or toxicities of cyclosporin develop, the patient can be switched from cyclosporin to FK506. Cyclosporin is usually discontinued 24 hours prior to the initial intravenous dose of 0.075 mg/kg of FK506 over four hours. Oral dosage of 0.30 mg/kg in divided doses is started as soon as possible and we prefer to start dosing orally. If within 48 hours after FK506 is started, a severe rejection episode is not improved, then one should consider adding OKT3 or a course of high dose steroids.[42] In a recent study done at our institution, 13 patients with continued acute rejection despite treatment with cyclosporin, azathioprine, OKT3 and high dose steroids were

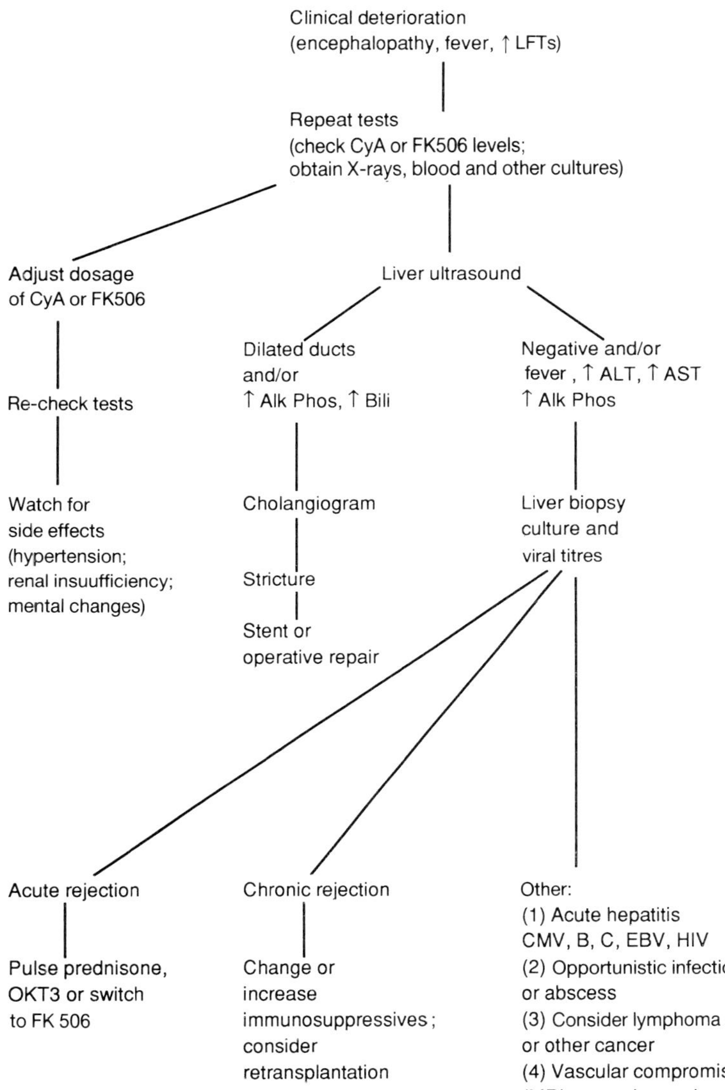

Fig. 17.1 Investigation and management of abnormal liver function tests after liver transplantation.

switched to FK506; five of the 13 had minimal evidence of rejection on liver biopsy and liver functions within two times normal at one month, six of 13 had partial response with improvement in histology but greater than minimal rejection, and with liver function tests greater than two times normal. Only two patients did not respond and were retransplanted. Overall 77% of these patients refractory to other treatments were salvaged with FK506.[43]

Hypertension is commonly encountered in patients in whom cyclosporin, FK506 or steroids are used. The initial treatment strategy is to decrease the immunosuppressive agents but this is not always possible as rejection must be considered. Hypertensive treatment is usually started with nifedipine or beta-blockers with addition of prazosin or captopril if needed. If possible diuretics should be avoided as they make the control of cyclosporin and FK506 more difficult. Prolonged use of cyclosporin and FK506 has been associated with renal function deterioration, but progression to chronic renal failure and the need for haemodialysis is rare. Patients with diabetes may be more predisposed to these complications.

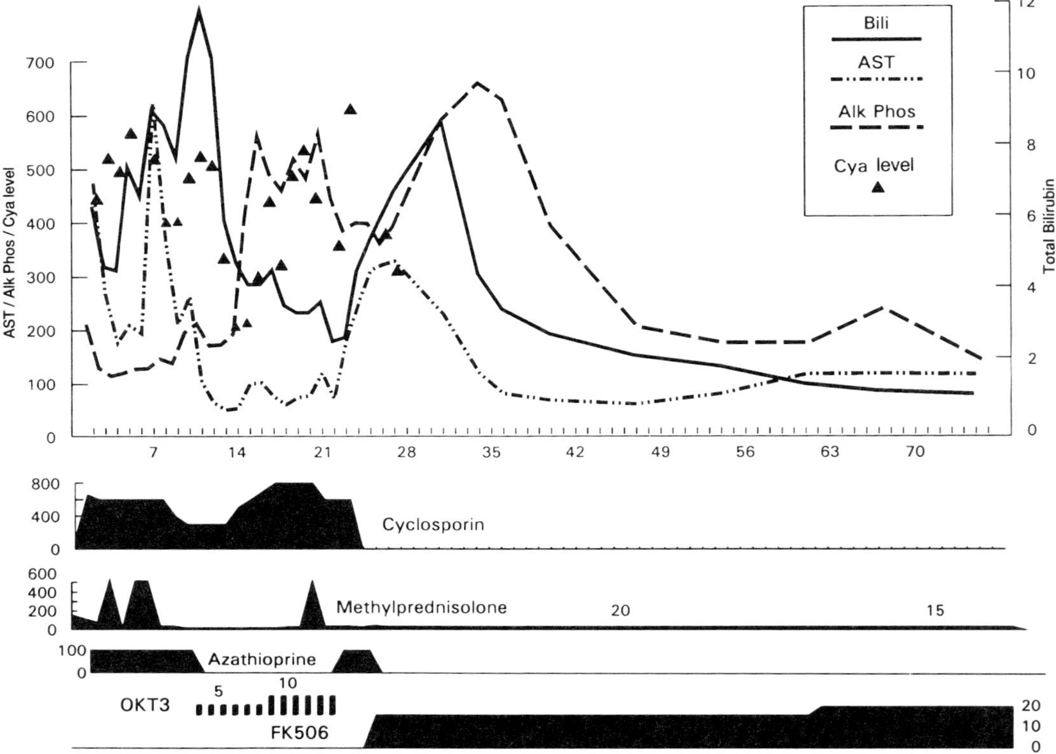

Fig. 17.2 Case history.

Case history

The use of multiple immunosuppressive agents and subsequent successful conversion of cyclosporin to FK506 is shown by the clinical course of a 49 year old female with primary biliary cirrhosis who had episodes of encephalopathy, ascites and variceal bleeding which required banding of the varices. She had progressive cholestasis and liver failure. She underwent an orthotopic liver transplantation and her post-operative course was complicated by multiple episodes of acute rejection as exemplified by fever, encephalopathy and fluctuating LFTs (Figure 17.2). There was no evidence of anastomotic breakdowns, thrombosis of grafted vessels or abscess formation. Post-operatively she was treated with methylprednisolone and cyclosporin intravenously. However, she had increased LFTs on day three which were treated with pulsed methylprednisolone. Azathioprine was introduced on day two and because of continued rejection as proved by liver biopsy, it was discontinued on day seven and a course of OKT3 introduced on day 11. The dose of OKT3 was doubled on post-operative day 16 because of encephalopathy and continued elevation of LFTs. On post-operative day 24, after the course of OKT3 and a steroid bolus, a biopsy revealed continued acute rejection (Figure 17.3). Thus, cyclosporin was stopped and 24 hours later FK506 was introduced. The AST and clinical condition improved. Liver biopsy done six days after introduction of the FK506 showed improvement. The patient continued to do well and liver biopsy at three months revealed significantly decreased inflammation (Figure 17.4). This case illustrates the strategies that can be employed in treating acute rejection.

Chronic rejection, the most common reason for late graft failure, may develop any-time after the first month post-operatively and may evolve from an episode of acute rejection unresponsive to therapy. Patients with chronic rejection experience a gradual rise in canalicular enzymes and

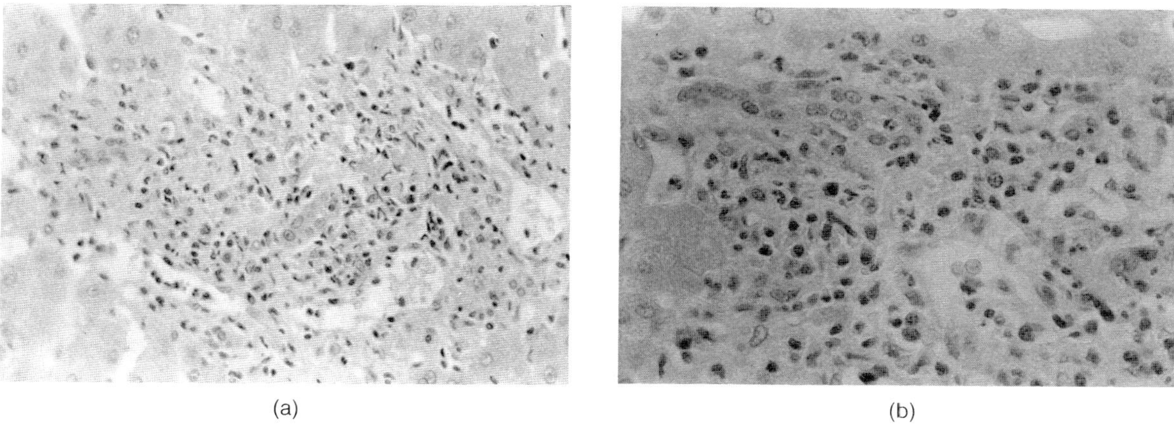

(a) (b)

Fig. 17.3 (a) Before FK506 treatment. The predominantly mononuclear portal infiltrate is seen to erode the limiting plate. Endothelialitis and bile duct damage are present. (b) High power.

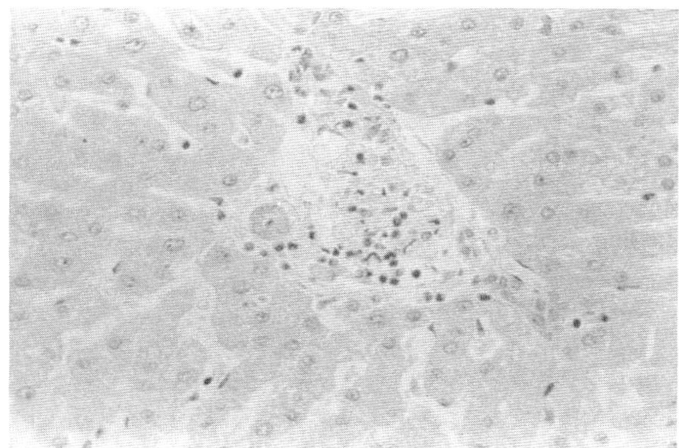

Fig. 17.4 After FK506 treatment. Significantly decreased portal inflammation with well preserved limiting plate and intact bile duct.

AST to about five times normal followed by jaundice. Two forms of chronic rejection can be distinguished on histology. Histology reveals bridging fibrosis, accumulation of foamy histiocytes and focal necrosis of the bile ducts. This syndrome may be tolerated for a prolonged period before retransplantation becomes necessary. The second form of rejection is the vanishing bile duct syndrome and this has a more rapid downhill course. Recently, FK506 has been shown to have some effectiveness in the treatment of early chronic rejection. In our experience, three out of five patients so treated had some improvement in liver function.[42]

Long term monitoring of patients

Patients are discharged from the hospital when hepatic function has stabilised, wounds are manageable, and infections are under control. At 10–12 weeks post-operatively the T tube is usually removed and patients are engaging in a relatively normal lifestyle. However, if the patient complains of pain or fever and there is a rise in the alkaline phosphatase or bilirubin, the patient should be hospitalised and bile duct leakage considered. ERCP or transhepatic cholangiogram should be done. Even after discharge from the hospital the patient must be closely followed with monitoring of liver tests, drug levels and clinical condition at regular intervals. The initial follow-up visits should be performed by the transplant team, until the patient is stabilised. This is judged by the liver function tests, creatinine clearance, white cell count and, above all, by the patient's clinical condition. These blood tests should all be within about two times the normal levels. The patient's immediate care can then be transferred to the referring physician or other physicians who are familiar with the management of post-transplant patients. To accomplish this, the patient's personal physician and the transplant team should be in close contact. All blood test results should be forwarded to the transplant team and close communication should be established. After the first three months following transplantation, most episodes of acute rejection are secondary to insufficient dosages of immunosuppression and can be treated with oral steroids and checking and correction of cyclosporin or FK506.

In our practice, for the first month after discharge the patient's blood tests and cyclosporin or FK506 levels are taken twice weekly, for the next month once weekly, for the first six months every month and thereafter every month or two depending on the patient's condition and previous problems in adjusting the dosages. If liver tests are found to deteriorate in the period two months after transplantation, the tests should be repeated immediately to insure against laboratory error. Whole blood cyclosporin trough levels should be taken 12 hours after oral dosing. The elevated liver tests may be secondary to high cyclosporin levels and reduction of dose may be all that is needed. However, it should noted that the cyclosporin levels are increased by the concomitant use of drugs that affect the hepatic microsomal enzymes such as erythromycin, ketoconazole, calcium channel blockers, cimetidine, methyltestosterone, oral contraceptives and others. Cyclosporin blood levels are decreased by inducers of cytochrome P-450 such as rifampicin, phenytoin, phenobarbital, IV trimethoprim and carbamazepine.[9] If the level is low, a temporary increase in the prednisone dosage along with correction of the cyclosporin dose will most probably be corrective. If the test shows a persistently greater than two-fold increase in liver function tests, it is best to do a full assessment including liver biopsy, with special attention to the possibility of CMV and EBV infection.

In the outpatient setting, mild episodes of rejection are usually treated with steroids, often initiating with 200 mg/day of prednisone and tapering by 40 mg daily. If episodes of rejection are more severe or unresponsive to oral steroids, the patient should be admitted for intravenous steroids or a change in the immunosuppressive regimen. A course of OKT3 can be considered unless contra-indicated by previous courses or reactions. Conversion from cyclosporin to FK506 or vice versa is another consideration, as illustrated in our case report. The long term use of FK506 has not yet been fully evaluated. The dosage to maintain immunosuppression of FK506 is titrated to maintain a trough level greater than 0.6 ng/ml. Toxicities and drug interactions are probably similar to those of cyclosporin. New immunosuppressive regimes such as rapamycin or 15-deoxyspergualin should be considered on compassionate protocols.[20]

Tapering of immunosuppressives helps to reduce long term morbidity. However, most of our patients are maintained on prednisone 5.0–10.0 mg/day depending on size and we do not attempt to wean beyond this. We also continue azathioprine at 1 mg/kg/day indefinitely, unless the white count is suppressed, and continue cyclosporin with levels in the 300–600 ng/ml range. More rapid tapering of steroids should be instituted if the patient has bone disease, especially aseptic necrosis of the femur, personality changes, frequent infections, cataracts, poor wound healing, steroid reactions or advanced age. Slower and lesser efforts at tapering should be pursued if the patient has frequent rejection episodes, has been retransplanted after rejection or has evidence of ongoing rejection. Azathioprine should be stopped if there are frequent episodes of infections as patients can be maintained long term without it.

The long term immunosuppressive regime is still being elaborated and different centres are using varying tapering regimes. Our approach to the patient relies on careful follow-up with use of a flow sheet documenting every post-operative blood test, drug, drug level, weight, blood pressure and clinical course. We have weekly meetings in which we review the flow sheets of every patient having a blood test done at our clinic or sent by the primary care givers to be reviewed at this meeting. The patient's subsequent treatment is then elaborated or adjusted and follow-up tests and appointments are made with us or scheduled with the primary care givers who routinely send us all blood test results.

If a specific clinical situation suggests a specific diagnostic test then the protocol can start with that test. For example, intermittent elevations of liver tests within six weeks of removing the T tube are often caused by strictures; cholangiography is an appropriate initial investigation. Changes in laboratory test or the patient's condition should always elicit a plan of action and close follow-up. In tapering immunosuppressive agents, the patient's clinical situation should be the guide. For example, if the patient has high blood pressure or renal impairment as exemplified by a high creatinine, then cyclosporin or FK506 should be tapered first if possible and other causes of renal diseases should also be considered and excluded by appropriate investigations. Steroids can be withdrawn completely if needed when FK506 is used but usually not with cyclosporin use.

The patient who develops a fever for over 24

hours needs prompt evaluation and treatment especially if the source is a bacterial pathogen. If no obvious cause is detected or the patient does not respond promptly to treatment of the suspected cause, it is probably best that they be referred to a transplant centre as their immunosuppressive medication may need to be adjusted. Patients with prolonged diarrhoeal illness are at risk for decreased absorption of immunosuppressives and should be monitored closely. The cause of the diarrhoeal illness may be directly related to the immunosuppression, such as CMV or other opportunistic infections.

The reported incidence of cancer in transplanted patients is 100 times greater than the general population matched for age. The risk of developing lymphoma is increased by as much as 350 times. It has been shown that immunosuppressive regimes, especially OKT3 in high doses, can significantly increase the appearance of these complications.[43,44] Early warning signs can be fever, a shift of the white cell population to relative lymphocytosis and leucopenia, the appearance of atypical lymphocytes in the blood or ascitic fluid, clinical pictures of rejection, bowel obstruction, renal failure or myocardial disease depending on the clinical presentation of the EB virus related lymphoma. The clinical presentation is affected by the age of the patient. In individuals under 40 years of age the course is similar to mononucleosis with lymphadenopathy, fevers and pharyngitis. In patients over 40, solid lymphomas and invasion of the liver, kidney, intestine, heart and lungs are usually seen. The clinical course can be slow or fulminant. In the slow evolution, the clinician has time to decrease the immunosuppressive regime or temporarily stop especially the cyclosporin and FK506 in an effort to decrease the stimulation of the EB virus related lymphoma. This can cause regression.[45,46] There have been reports of operative removal of a solid lymphoma in association with a decrease of immunosuppression leading to complete resolution of this complication.[47]

Transplant patients are usually required to take at least four and usually eight medications daily. This constant reminder of the need to maintain his graft as well as the other psychological effects of being a transplant recipient can lead to non-compliance. The physician needs to monitor and be sympathetic to the patient's psychological and social needs as early counselling could prevent more serious repercussions as well as detect early medical complications. The transplant patient maintains a difficult responsibility for his own health. The post-transplant patient can live a relatively normal life, but close follow-up is essential. This follow-up, after the first few months after the procedure, can be given by local physicians as long as close contact is kept with a transplant centre. This process can be emotionally and physically exacting for both the patient and physicians but is rewarded by great satisfaction in maintaining the health of the patient.

References

1. Todo S, Demetris AJ, van Thiel D, Teperman L, Fung JJ, Starzl TE. Orthotopic liver transplantation for patients with hepatitis B virus-related liver disease. *Hepatology*. 1991; **13**(4), 619–626.
2. Stratta RJ, Mark SS, Cushing KA *et al*. Successful prophylaxis of cytomegalovirus disease after primary CMV exposure in liver transplant recipients. *Transplantation* 1991; **51**(1), 90–97.
3. Salida F, Aruinaden JL, Gugenheim J *et al*. CMV hyperimmune globulin prophylaxis after liver transplantation: a prospective randomised controlled study. *Transplant Proc* 1989; **21**(1), 2260–2262.
4. Wiesner RH. Selective bowel decontamination for infection prophylaxis in liver transplantation patients. *Transplant Proc* 1991; **23**(3), 1927–1928.
5. Rosman C, Klompmaker IJ, Bonsel GJ, Bleichrodt RP, Arends JP, Slooff MJH. The efficacy of selective bowel decontamination as infection prevention after liver transplantation. *Transplant Proc* 1990; **22**(4), 1554–1555.
6. Martin M, Kusne S, Alessiani M, Simmons R, Starzl TE. Infections after liver transplantation: risk factors and prevention. *Transplant Proc* 1991; **23**(3), 1929–1930.
7. Langaaij P, Hennemann PH, Ruigrok M *et al*. Effect of one-HLA-DR-antigen matched and completely HLA-DR mismatched blood transfusions on survival of heart and kidney allografts. *N Eng J Med* 1989; **321**(11), 701–705.
8. Barron PT, Jamieson NV, Calne RV. Treatment of acute rejection following liver transplantation: a comparison between methylprednisolone and hydrocortisone. *Transplant Proc* 1991; **23**(4), 2266.
9. Kahan BD. Cyclosporine. *N Eng J Med* 1989; **321**(25), 1725–1738.
10. Driscoll DF, Pinson CW, Jenkins RL, Bistrian BR. Potential protective effects of furosemide against early cyclosporine-induced renal injury in hepatic transplantation. *Transplant Proc* 1989; **21**(3), 3549–3550.

11. Millis JM, Baquerizo A, Saleh S, Danovitch GM, Busuttil RW. Preservation of renal function using OKT3 in liver transplant patients. *Transplant Proc* 1989; **21,** 3551–3552.
12. Steininger R, Muhlbacher F, Hamilton G *et al.* Comparison of CyA, OKT3 and ATG immunoprophylaxis in human liver transplantation. *Transplant Proc* 1991; **23**(4), 2269–2271.
13. Swinnen LJ, Costanzo-Nordin MR, Fischer SG *et al.* Increased incidence of lymphoproliferative disorders after immunosuppression with monoclonal antibody OKT3 in cardiac transplant recipients. *N Eng J Med* 1990; **323,** 1723–1728.
14. Millis JM, McDiarmid SV, Hiatt JR *et al.* Randomised prospective trial of OKT3 for early prophylaxis of rejection after liver transplantation. *Transplantation* 1989; **47**(1), 82–88.
15. Chatenoud L, Ferrau C, Legendre C *et al.* Systemic reaction to the anti-T cell monoclonal antibody OKT3 in relation to serum levels of tumor necrosis factor and interferon alpha. *N Eng J Med* 1989; **320,** 1420–1426.
16. Chatenoud L, Ferran C, Bach JF. *In vivo* use of OKT3; main issues for the monitoring of treated patients. *Transplant Proc* 1990; **22**(6), 2605–2608.
17. Calliat-Zucman S, Blumenfold N, Legendre C *et al.* The OKT3 immunosuppressive effect. *Transplantation* 1990; **49,** 156–160.
18. McDiarmid SV, Busuttil RW, Patricia L, Millis JM, Terasaki PI, Ament ME. The long-term outcome of OKT3 compared with cyclosporin prophylaxis after liver transplantation. *Transplantation* 1991; **52**(1), 91–97.
19. Fung J, Starzl TE. Prophylactic use of OKT3 in liver transplantation: a review. *Digest Dis Sci* 1991; **36**(10), 1427–1430.
20. Simmons RL, Wang SC. New Horizons in immunosuppression. *Transplant Proc* 1991; **23**(4), 2152–2156.
21. Fung J. Clinical side effects of FK506. *FK506 First International Congress Abstracts 1991*; Abstract 65.
22. Fung J, Gordon R, Todo S *et al.* The use of FK506 in primary liver transplantation. *FK506 First International Congress Abstracts 1991*; Abstract 50.
23. Fung J, Todo S, Jain A *et al.* Conversion from cyclosporine to FK506 in liver allograft recipients with cyclosporine-related complications. *Transplant Proc* 1990; **22**(1), 6–12.
24. Vathsala A, Goto S, Yoshimura N, Stepkowski S, Chou TC, Kahan BD. The immunosuppressive antagonism of low doses of FK506 and cyclosporin. *Transplantation* 1991; **52,** 121–128.
25. Bonhomme P, Rucay P, Rudant E *et al.* Therapeutic monitoring of plasma FK506. *FK506 First International Congress Abstracts 1991*; Abstract p 43.
26. Abu-Elmagd K, Fung J, Alessiani M *et al.* The strategy of FK506 therapy in liver transplant patients: the effect of graft function. *FK506 First International Congress Abstracts 1991*; Abstract 16.
27. Todo S, Fung JJ, Starzl TE *et al.* Liver, kidney and thoracic organ transplantation under FK506. *Ann Surg* 1990; **212**(3), 295–231.
28. Abu-Elmagd K, Fung JJ, Alessiani M *et al.* The effect of graft function on FK506 plasma levels, dosages, and renal function, with particular reference to the liver. *Transplantation* 1991; **52**(1), 71–77.
29. Grieg PD, Woolf GM, Abecassis M *et al.* Prostaglandin El for primary nonfunction following liver transplantation. *Transplant Proc* 1989; **21,** 3360–3361.
30. Tzakis AG, Gordon RD, Shaw BW *et al.* Clinical presentation of hepatic artery thrombosis after liver transplantation in the cyclosporin era. *Hepatology* 1985; **40,** 667–671.
31. Koneru B, Esquivel CO, Bowen A *et al.* Early detection and management of portal vein thrombosis after hepatic transplantation. A case report. *Clin Transplant* 1988; **2,** 214–215.
32. Shaw BW Jr. Surgical and clinical aspects of liver transplantation and post-operative evaluation of complications. *Sem Int Radiol* 1986; **3,** 115–119.
33. Wood GL, Young A, Johnson A, Thield GM. Detection of cytomegalovirus by 24 well plate centrifugation assay using monoclonal antibody to an early antigen and by conversion cell culture. *J Viral Meth* 1987; **18,** 207–214.
34. Ludwig J. Classification and terminology of hepatic allograft rejection: whither bound? *Mayo Clinic Proc* 1989; **64,** 676–679.
35. Honto DW, Snover DC, Sibley RK *et al.* Hyperacute rejection of a human orthotopic liver allograft in a presensitized recipient. *Clin Transplant* 1987; **1,** 304–310.
36. Klintmalm GBG, Nery JR, Husberg BS. Rejection in liver transplantation. *Hepatology* 1989; **10,** 978–985.
37. Shaw BW, Stratta RJ, Donovan JP *et al.* Postoperative care after transplantation. *Sem Liver Dis* 1989; **9**(3), 202–230.
38. Klintmalm GB. Rejection therapies. *Digest Dis Sci* 1991; **36**(10), 1431–1433.
39. First MR, Schroeder TJ, Hurtubise PE *et al.* Successful retreatment of allograft rejection with OKT3. *Transplantation* 1989; **47**(1), 88–91.
40. Colonna JO, Millis JM, Martello J *et al.* The successful use of repeated courses of OKT3 for hepatic allograft rejection using % T3 cells to adjust dose. *Transplant Proc* 1989; **21**(1), 2247–2248.

41. Shaked A, Busuttil RW, Sher L, Makowka L. Case No. 6 – diagnosis and treatment of early rejection in liver transplantation. *Transplant Sci* 1991; **1**(1), 18–24.
42. Fung JJ, Demetris A, Todo S *et al.* Use of FK506 in the treatment of liver allograft rejection. *Transplant Sci* 1991; **1**(1), 50–54.
43. Lewis W, Jenkins R, Burke P *et al.* FK506 rescue therapy in liver transplant recipients with drug resistant rejection. *FK506 First International Congress Abstracts 1991*; Abstract CT105.
44. Trey C. Case study. *N Eng J Med* 1992 (in press).
45. Penn I. Cancer is a complication of severe immunosuppression. *Surg Gynecol Obstet* 1986; **162,** 603–610.
46. Starzl TE, Nalesnik MA, Porter KA *et al.* Reversibility of lymphomas and lymphoproliferative lesions developing under cyclosporin-steroid therapy. *Lancet* 1984; **1,** 583–587.
47. Cohen JI. Epstein-Barr virus lymphoproliferative disease associated with acquired immunodeficiency. *Medicine* 1991; **70**(2), 137–160.
48. Stieber AC, Boillot O, Scotti-Foglieni C *et al.* The surgical implications of post transplant lymphoproliferative disorders. *Transplant Proc* 1991; **23,** 1477–1479.

18

Newer immunosuppressive agents

J Neuberger and D Adams

Introduction

The increasing success of organ transplantation has drawn attention to the limitations of the drugs used for immunosuppression. Both in the short and longer term, side effects and complications include failure to prevent rejection, increased susceptibility to infection, progressive organ damage – notably renal – metabolic derangements and increased susceptibility to malignancy. As illustrated in the preceding chapter, the current main stays of immunosuppression, corticosteroids, azathioprine, cyclosporin, FK506 and OKT3, have their own additional complications. It is a sad reflection that there still remains a lack of properly controlled data to assess the relative role of each drug and there is little concordance as to the optimal immunosuppressive regime for the liver allograft recipient.

Over the past few years, the increasing understanding of the mechanisms of rejection and the application of the newer molecular biological techniques have contributed to the development of a wide variety of drugs with potential application to immunosuppression. Many of these drugs are still at a preclinical stage; the aim of this chapter is to review some of these newer agents. It is to be hoped that the role of these newer compounds will be evaluated much more carefully and rigorously than in the past.

Cyclosporin A (CyA)

The introduction of cyclosporin into clinical practice in the early 1980s was hailed as a major break through in immunosuppression. Most of the claims for the superiority of the drug were based on comparison with historical controls and there were few controlled studies. Nonetheless, the use of Cyclosporin A (CyA) has been associated with an explosion in the number of patients receiving allografts.

CyA is a neutral, lipophilic cyclic endecapeptide extracted from the fungus *Tolypocladium inflatum gams*. Early studies on the immunological activity of CyA were undertaken primarily by Borel.[84] Since then, the mode of action has been extensively investigated. Numerous studies have demonstrated that incubation of cytotoxic lymphocytes with CyA results in virtual abolition of IL-2 synthesis and release; this inhibitory effect can be overcome by the addition of extraneous IL-2. Subsequent work showed that CyA acts by inhibiting transcription of lymphokines and does not appear to block allo-antigen recognition. Thus studies, for example by Herold and colleagues,[85] showed that while CyA had no effect on the binding of clonotypic antibody against the TCR, mRNA transcription of IL-2, IL-3 and gamma-interferon was greatly inhibited. In contrast to the effect on CD4 lymphocytes, CyA appears to have a relatively weak effect on CD8 cells.[86] Thus, the main actions of CyA result in blocking activation of the IL-2 gene, inhibition of T lymphocyte proliferation, prevention of release of gamma-interferon and of B cell activation factors.

The mode of action of CyA is dependent on its binding to an intracellular protein termed cyclophilin.[87] The degree of binding is proportional to the *in vitro* effect on the MLR. Subsequent studies have shown that cyclophilin is a protein that is well conserved in all mammalian species; there are at least two isoforms, the major isoform is about 17 Kda. In a variety of cells, including hepatocytes and lymphocytes, cyclophilin is localised in the nucleus.[89]

The association between CyA binding to cyclophilin and its immunological effects was clarified when it was demonstrated that there was amino acid identity between cyclophilin and the enzyme cis-trans peptidyl-prolyl isomerase.[87,88] It was initially believed that CyA acted by inhibiting the rotamase action involved in the conformational changes that occur during peptide chain elongation or cell trafficking. As indicated below, it is now appreciated that the situation is more complex.

Orally administered CyA is absorbed in the distal ileum; because of the lipid solubility, bile is important for the efficient absorption of CyA so absorption is decreased in cholestasis. Some metabolism occurs within the enterocyte and so may explain, in part, some of the variability in dose requirements. Cyclosporin is metabolised primarily by the hepatic mixed function oxidase system, so metabolism is affected by enzyme inducing drugs (such as phenobarbitone or phenytoin) and enzyme inhibiting drugs (such as cimetidine). Side effects are common and may be dose dependent. Common side effects include nephrotoxicity, hepatotoxicity, headaches, hirsutism, hypertension, neurotoxicity, breast fibroadenosis and gingival hypertrophy.

FK506

FK506 is a macrolide lactone isolated from *Streptomyces tukabaesinsis*, with a molecular weight of 822.[90] Studies *in vitro* have shown that the immunosuppressive properties of FK506 are similar to CyA: the drug strongly inhibits the proliferative responses of lymphocytes to allo-antigen presentation, the generation of cytotoxic T cells and the production of T lymphocyte products including IL-2, IL-3 and gamma-interferon. FK506 also inhibits expression of the Tac antigen after stimulation with either specific antigen or alloantigen. However, on a weight for weight basis, FK506 is about 100 times more potent than CyA.

Animal studies have shown that FK506 can induce antigen specific tolerance in experimental glomerulonephritis and inhibits established lesions of collagen induced arthritis.[91] The sucess of the drug in a variety of animal transplant models encouraged its use in human heart, lung, kidney and liver transplantation.[92] These studies have all testified to the efficacy of the drug and many of the clinical applications are discussed elsewhere.

There seems a striking resemblance between the development of CyA and FK506. Both drugs were introduced without the benefit of controlled studies; it has taken some five years or longer for the physicians to learn how to give CyA, to establish a therapeutic range, determine the optimal methods of measuring the drug, understand the pharmacokinetics, drug interactions and side effects. Very similar considerations apply to FK506. Side effects are broadly similar to those seen with CyA, but neurotoxicity, nephrotoxicity and a tendency to diabetes seem more common with FK506. The results of prospective trials evaluating CyA with FK506 will allow for a balanced assessment of the place of these very powerful agents in the management of immunosuppression.

Despite the similar immunosuppressive effects of the two drugs, they bind to different proteins: FK506 binds to so-called FK binding proteins[93] which, like cyclophilins, are well conserved, abundant proteins and are active as peptidyl-prolyl cis-trans isomerases. It is now believed[81] that the drugs become active as a complex with their respective intracellular receptors by giving new properties to these receptors. This concept is supported by the observation that another immunosuppressive macrolide, rapamycin, also inhibits FK binding protein rotamase activity, although rapamycin does not block cytokine transcription at an early stage of T cell activation. McKeon[81] has suggested a unifying concept involving binding the drug/binding protein to calcineurin A (Fig 18.1). Calcineurin A is a highly conserved, calcium/calmodulin activated protein phosphatase with two subunits, which bind calmodulin and calcium.

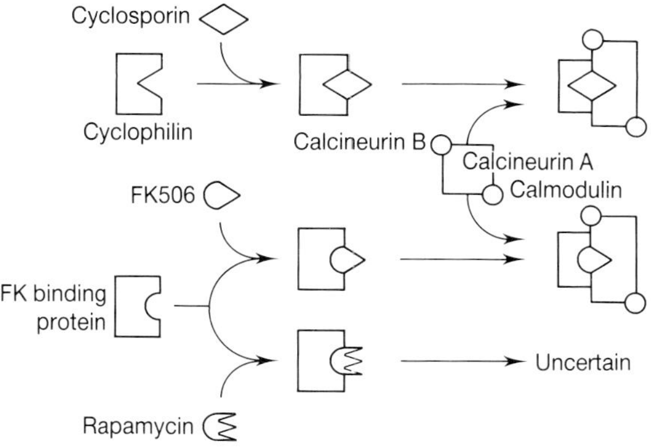

Fig. 18.1 Schematic mode of action of cyclosporin, FK506 and rapamycin (adapted from [81]).

Rapamycin

Rapamycin is a macrolide antibiotic produced by *Streptomyces hygrospicus*. Like cyclosporin and FK506, rapamycin is an antifungal antibiotic. Although these compounds are structurally unrelated, they are functionally similar. Both FK506 and rapamycin competitively inhibit the peptidyl-prolyl isomerase (PPIase) activity of immunophilin, the major binding protein for FK506.[1,2,81]

In vitro studies have shown that while rapamycin and FK506 have many similar effects on animal and human lymphocytes, there are a number of important differences.[3] For example, rapamycin inhibits T cell constitutive division, unlike FK506 which has no effect. Both drugs inhibit CD4 lymphocyte activation. Rapamycin, however, inhibits IL-2 and IL-4 dependent activation and calcium independent B and T cell activation whereas FK506 inhibits IL-2 expression. These observations may explain, in part, why rapamycin acts in synergy with cyclosporin but in antagonism with FK506.[3]

Rapamycin has been assessed in a number of animal models of rejection. The drug has been studied in mouse, rat, pig, dog and monkey using heart, kidney, skin, pancreas, small bowel and thymus.[4] Overall, the drug is effective in prolonging graft survival and suppressing graft versus host disease but appears to be less effective in xenografting.

In animal studies, the formulation is important: uneffective immunosuppression was achieved at a dose of 0.4 mg/kg/day using continuous intravenous infusions of rapamycin in a polyethylene glycol/polysorbate solution in a rat cardiac graft model.[5] Nevertheless, satisfactory immunosuppression can be achieved by oral or subcutaneous dosing. The effects can last long after the drug is discontinued.[6]

Rapamycin does not appear to cause renal dysfunction, hypotension or affect the response to infection. However, Whiting reported some evidence of mild–moderate focal myocardial necrosis in rats given rapamycin.[7] There appears to be a synergistic effect between rapamycin and cyclosporin.

Clinical trials of rapamycin are currently underway but as with other immunosuppressive agents, the benefit/toxicity ratio between rapamycin and cyclosporin has yet to be determined.

RS-61443

RS-61443 represents a 'designer drug' developed by Allison and Eugui.[8] RS-61443 is a morpholino ethyl ester of mycophenolic acid. Mycophenolic acid is a non-competitive inhibitor of inosine-5-monophosphate dehydrogenase (IMPDH), the enzyme that controls the rate of purine synthesis.[9,10] Mitogen and allo-antigens stimulated T and B cells have increased IMPDH activity and increased synthesis of guanine nucleotide; hence interference with the purine synthesis of lymphocytes will affect their function.

Mycophenolic acid was found to be effective in reducing T and B lymphocyte proliferative responses: a synthetic addition of a morpholino ethyl ester side chain increased bio-availability without affecting immunological function.[11] Hence the ester derivative rather than the parent compound is being increasingly used in clinical practice. Animal studies have shown that RS-61443 is highly effective in prolonging islet cell allograft function in mice, heart, allo- and xenografts in rats and canine renal allografts, amongst others.[12,13] Side effects are dose dependent;[14] gastro-intestinal complications appear the most significant, consisting of diarrhoea, often with bloody motions, anorexia and gastritis.

Clinical studies in man with a variety of different grafts, including renal, heart, liver and pancreas, have shown that RS-61443 is effective in doses greater than 2000 mg/day in preventing graft rejection without any apparent increase in susceptibility to infection.[15] Larger studies are underway to evaluate this promising new agent. The most recent,[66] using doses varying between 100 and 3500 mg/day, reported that RS-61443 was well tolerated; only one of 48 renal allograft recipients reported any adverse reaction (haemorrhagic gastritis). The drug was also effective in rescue treatment. Although there was a statistically significant correlation between dose and rejection, the authors did not recommend a therapeutic dose. Trials in liver transplantation are awaited with interest.

15-Deoxyspergualin

15-Deoxyspergualin (15-DSG) is a synthetically dehydroxylated form of spergualin (SG), the product of the *Bacillus lactosporos*.[16] *In vivo* and *in vitro* studies have shown both 15-DSG and SG have similar efficacy although 15-DSG is more potent.

Animal studies have shown that DSG is highly effective in controlling auto-immune disease and is effective not only in reducing the severity of rejection but also in the reversal of established acute rejection of kidney, liver, heart and skin.[17,18,19] In humans, 15-DSG has been evaluated in the treatment of severe allograft rejection with encouraging results.[20,21] Addition of high dose methylprednisolone appears to enhance its immunosuppressive effects.[22] However, one recently reported study[67] found that 15-DSG had very little effect on reversal of established renal allograft rejection and doses as low as 4 mg/kg were associated with significant side effects. These observations contrast with a report by the same group that 15-DSG was effective in treating liver allograft rejection.[68]

Toxic effects of 15-DSG are related to dose: bone marrow suppression, hypotension, anorexia and parasthesiae appear to be the most common. Bone marrow suppression usually responds rapidly to drug withdrawal.

The precise mode of action is unclear: *in vitro* studies have shown 15-DSG is effective in suppressing primary and secondary responses to thymic independent and dependent antigens. However, 15-DSG is thought to suppress rejection by suppression of IL-2 production and interferon production by CD4 cells,[16,19] by inhibition of the differentiation of B cells to plasma cells and by inhibiting clonal amplification of T cells. The former property makes the drug of potential value in xenografting.

Prostaglandins

Although there remains controversy as to the effects of prostaglandins on B cells, both PGE_1 and PGE_2 affect T cell functions through inhibition of IL-1 and IL-2 formation and class II antigen expression.[23,24,25] The development of two stable synthetic PGE_1 analogues, misoprostol and enisoprost, have allowed therapeutic studies of prostaglandins in prevention and treatment of allograft rejection. *In vitro* studies suggest that PGE_1 analogues suppress lymphocyte proliferative responses to allo-antigens and have an additive effect with both corticosteroids and cyclosporin. The effect can be counteracted by addition of recombinant IL-2.[26] A recent study in renal allografts suggested a marked beneficial effect;[27] however, a subsequent multicentre, prospective, randomised placebo controlled study in renal allografts found that enisoprost had no demonstrable effect on the incidence of acute rejection or renal dysfunction.[69] These findings are in agreement with a prospective randomised study in liver grafts carried out in the Liver Unit in Birmingham, which showed no effect of enisoprost on the incidence or severity of liver allograft rejection nor on cyclosporin associated nephrotoxicity (Ishmail, personal communication). It may be, however, that other prostaglandin analogues will be beneficial in allograft rejection.

Lipoxygenase inhibition has been reported to affect the immune response by enhancing arachidonic acid metabolism to prostaglandins or by inhibiting LTB4 production which stimulates CD8 function and increased IL-2 production. LTB4 may also increase cell mediated cytotoxicity. Preliminary *in vitro* studies[28] suggest that the combination of enisoprost and a 5-lipoxygenase inhibitor acts synergistically. Further work is required to assess the clinical relevance of such a combination.[70]

Thalidomide

The well-publicised teratogenic effects of thalidomide have resulted in the temporary lack of interest in this agent in medicine. The drug has been shown to be therapeutically effective in a variety of clinical situations, such as lepromatous leprosy, SLE, Behçet's syndrome and ulcerative colitis. Side effects include not only teratogenicity but neurotoxicity, vasculitis and myxoedema. Careful monitoring of blood levels appears to reduce these complications.[82]

However, it has become increasingly recognised that thalidomide may be of benefit in therapy of graft rejection. In animal studies, thalidomide is effective in bone marrow and renal transplantation.[29,30] It has a synergistic effect with cyclosporin in rat cardiac allografting and in the prophylaxis of graft versus host disease. *In vitro*, thalidomide inhibits mitogenic and allo-antigenic proliferation of lymphocytes but it does not appear in these studies to act synergistically with FK506.[31] Clinical trials do show a benefit with the drug in graft versus host disease[32] and may be of potential value in the treatment of patients following liver transplantation.

Ursodeoxycholic acid (UDCA)

UDCA is a hydrophilic bile acid which has been shown to be highly effective in improving the serum biochemistry in a wide variety of chronic cholestatic liver diseases. The drug has been best studied in patients with primary biliary cirrhosis, where patients in early disease have been reported to have improved symptoms and a reduction in serum bilirubin, alkaline phosphatase, immunoglobulins and antimitochondrial antibody titre. The mode of action is unclear, but it has been suggested that the agent may act by replacing the more hepatotoxic hydrophobic bile acids with less cytotoxic ones. *In vitro* hepatocyte MHC class I antigen expression, which appears to be increased in cholestasis of any cause, is reduced by UDCA[71] but it remains uncertain whether this observation could explain the mode of action of UDCA.

One study from Sweden suggested that UDCA may be effective in helping prevention of liver allograft rejection since biochemical values post-transplantation were lower compared with six historical controls.[72] This observation has some weight given to it by a subsequent study suggesting that administration of UDCA reduces acute rejection in the rat heart allograft model.[73] These rather surprising results need confirmation before UDCA can be included in the therapeutic armamentarium.

Brequinar

Brequinar is a potent anticancer drug that inhibits cell proliferation by reducing the activity of dihydro-oratate dehydrogenase and pyrimidine biosynthesis.[74] Clinically, the agent has been used for the treatment of metastatic cancer and some leukaemias. Brequinar has been shown to be more effective than cyclosporin in supressing rodent adjuvant arthritis.[75]

In rat allograft models of heart, liver and kidney transplantation, Brequinar was found to be highly effective in preventing rejection.[75] With respect to liver allografts, 50–90% liver grafts were permanently accepted after 30 days treatment with brequinar 12 mg/kg. Furthermore, challenge of long term liver graft survivors with donor cardiac grafts was associated with permanent acceptance of hearts of original, but not third party, strain; these observations suggest the drug may induce tolerance.

Whether these properties will be translated to the human model and whether side effects will be a problem is uncertain; nonetheless, this must remain a drug of great promise.

Other agents

There are many other drugs with potential application to liver allografting. These include SKF-105685, which is an azaspirane which induces suppressor cells and is effective in the rat cardiac allograft model.[76]

Platelet activating factor (PAF) antagonist, WEB 2170, improved the therapeutic efficacy of subtherapeutic doses of cyclosporin; in a renal allograft dog model, WEB 2170 given with cyclosporin was associated with an improvement in graft survival.[77]

Iron is an essential co-factor in many aspects of cell metabolism, including DNA synthesis and intracellular energy production. Pretreatment of rats with the oral iron chelator, desferrithiocin, was associated with improvement in cardiac allograft survival.[78] *In vivo* studies on monocytes showed that IL-2 and gamma-interferon production was suppressed but induction of IL-2R was unaffected. Clearly further work is required to determine the exact mode of action of this agent, but the approach lends itself to novel methods of immunosuppression.

One other approach which has shown success in animal models of allograft rejection is use of soluble class I antigen, which Kamada demonstrated improves survival of rat cardiac allografts. The effect was amplified by monoclonal anti-class I antibody. These observations are in line with the observations that serum from liver allografted rats can enhance graft survival and induce clonal deletion of alloreactive T cells (see Chapter 12).

Monoclonal antibodies

The increasing understanding of the mechanism of allograft rejection has allowed more specific intervention in both the prevention and treatment of allograft rejection. The development by Millstein and Kohler of techniques for generation of monoclonal antibodies has resulted in the possibility of therapeutic antibodies directed at specific epitopes on the leucocyte or target cells (Figure 18.2). In the last few years, an increasing number of such antibodies have been tested both in animal models and in humans for prevention and treatment of rejection. There have been suggestions that the response to monoclonal antibody therapy may vary between children and adults.[80]

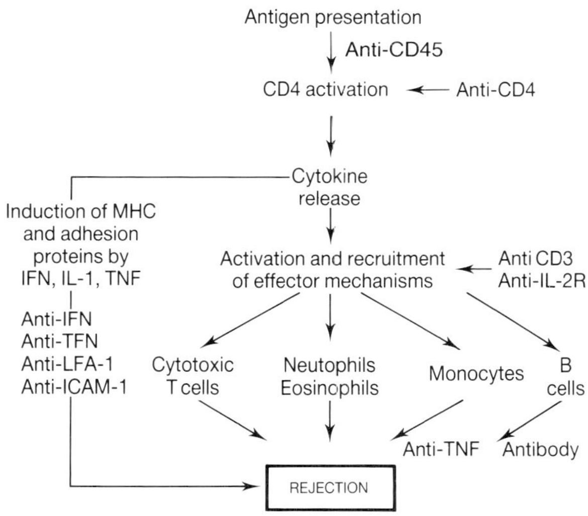

Fig. 18.2 Simplified scheme of rejection and sites of possible intervention with antibodies.

Anti-CD45 monoclonal antibody

As discussed elsewhere, dendritic cells in the allograft play an important role in stimulating the allograft response. Experimental studies have shown that depletion of dendritic cells from renal allografts by irradiation and cyclophosphamide prior to implantation results in prolonged survival of the graft.[33,34] Repletion with the dendritic cells abolishes this effect on improved graft survival. CD45 is an antigen present not only on dendritic cells but also on lymphocytes, so the antibody may act by depleting passenger leucocytes as well as blocking dendritic cells. A randomised controlled trial in renal allografts showed that the incidence of allograft rejection was reduced by pretreatment of the graft with antibody to CD45[35] although neither patient nor graft survival were improved.

Antibodies to lymphocyte antigens

Anti-CD5 monoclonal antibodies

The CD5 antigen is present on virtually all mature T lymphocytes and a small subpopulation of B lymphocytes which have been implicated in autoimmune diseases. One antibody, XMMLY-H-65-RTA, has been conjugated to ricin-A, which inhibits ribosomal protein synthesis,[36] and has been used in human graft versus host disease, some malignant diseases and auto-immune diseases. Furthermore, this antibody is associated with a beneficial effect in acute steroid resistant and in acute graft versus host disease.

Anti-CD7 monoclonal antibodies

The CD7 antigen is a 40 KDa surface antigen present on T cells, stem cells and CD16 natural killer cells. *In vitro* anti-CD7 antibodies partially inhibit allogeneic mixed lymphocyte responses and completely inhibit the autologous MLR.[37,38] CD7 is preferentially expressed on naive T cells and anti-CD7 preferentially inhibits alloresponses on naive T cells.[37,39] There is an additive effect of CD7 with cyclosporin. A chimeric mouse human CD7 antibody has been evaluated in patients following renal transplantation.[40] The chimeric antibody was well tolerated with little immunogenicity but apparently only delayed rather than prevented acute rejection.

Antibodies to the T cell receptor

As indicated in other chapters, the CD3 T cell receptor plays a crucial role in the immune process. A number of antibodies have been developed to interact with the TCR complex, of which the most widely used is OKT3. Use of this drug is discussed in greater detail elsewhere but there is no doubt this is a potent agent in both prevention and treatment of allograft rejection. One of the problems with OKT3 administration is the development of fever, diarrhoea and pulmonary oedema due to OKT3 induced release of tumour necrosis factor. A number of different approaches have been developed to overcome these side effects and include the use of anti-TNF,[41] pentoxifylline,[42] use of OKT3 F(Ab)2 fragments[43] or antibodies to CD3 of different isotypes.[44,45]

OKT3 is a murine IgG2A antibody; a number

of other monoclonal antibodies reacting with the CD3 TCR complex have been developed. These include BMA-031, a murine IgG 2b, T10B9.1A/31, a murine IgM kappa antibody, and WT32, a murine IgG 2a. These drugs are all potent and effective both in prevention and reversal of acute allograft rejection. At the moment there appears to be very little to choose between the various antibodies. However, a prospective randomised double blind trial comparing treatment of acute renal allograft rejection with either T10/B9.1A/31 and OKT3 suggested that T10B9.1A/31 reverses acute rejection earlier and more effectively than OKT3, with fewer severe side effects. Furthermore, this monoclonal antibody was associated with fewer side effects and potentially less infection.[46] Further studies are required to determine the role of these antibodies in treatment of acute allograft rejection.

Monoclonal antibodies to CD4

The CD4 antigen is present on the helper/inducer subset which is being increasingly recognised as playing a major role in the inflammatory responses associated with allograft rejection. *In vivo* administration of anti-CD4 antibodies is very effective in inhibiting antibody responses to thymic antigens and will deplete CD4 peripheral T cells.[47] Furthermore, in murine models this antibody induces tolerance to antigens administered during the period of anti-CD4 therapy.[48,49]

Anti-CD4 is effective in reducing the severity of inflammation in murine models of arthritis and SLE. The mechanism of action of CD4 monoclonal antibodies is complex: they prevent the interaction between T cells and antigen presenting cells, thus inhibiting T cell activation. Since CD4 antibodies may also inhibit T cell function in the absence of class II molecules, part of their mode of action may not be directly associated with the CD3 TCR interactions.[47] However, some other studies have indicated that these antibodies induce lymphocyte activation *in vitro* and may help regulate cell adhesion.

Anti-CD4 is effective in reducing the severity of rejection in mice, rats and monkeys given allografts of skin, heart, kidney and pancreatic islet cells.[50,51] Timing of the administration may be important since the antibody affects the afferent arm of the immune response.

A number of different anti-CD4 antibodies are available (YTS 191/1, GK 1.5, OK35, OK38, W3/25, BWH-4, OKT4, OKT4A, MT310, BL4, amongst others).

Experience in humans is limited. The first trial was by Herzog in 1987,[52] who showed that treatment of a small number of patients with rheumatoid arthritis was associated with a transient remission: the drug was well tolerated. However, other studies have shown there may be some adverse features such as fever, chills and urticaria. Humanised CD4 antibodies have been given to a limited number of patients, with good tolerance and successful immunosuppressive effect.[53]

A recent study of CD4 monoclonal antibodies in 12 renal transplants showed some reduction in the incidence of rejection.[53] Nonetheless, use of these antibodies remains at a preliminary stage. The reduction in peripheral CD4 cells has lead to concern about inducing an AIDS-like syndrome in these patients.

Antibodies to interleukin-2 receptor (CD25)

The interleukin-2 receptor consists of high and low affinity forms. Two distinct binding IL-2 products have been identified: the 55 KDa subunit (beta chain or Tac antigen in humans), and the 75KDa unit (alpha chain) which are expressed on a subset of activated T cells. Because of the central role of T cell activation in the inflammatory response, immunosuppressive protocols directed against the rejection cascade at this site are attractive. The development of therapeutic antibodies against the 55KDa unit of both mice and humans has allowed studies to be performed in this area.

Studies in mice and rats using a variety of different IL-2R antibodies have shown a beneficial effect of these antibodies in both prevention and treatment of rejection.[54]

In humans, anti-IL2 therapy prevented rejection in renal allograft recipients during the period of administration but some of these patients developed late acute rejection episodes subsequently, which responded well to OKT3 therapy.[55,56,57,58] In the clinical studies to date, no significant side effects have been noted. There appears to be synergism between cyclosporin and other immunosuppressive agents with anti-IL-2R.[59] It is likely that this approach will be used increasingly in liver allografts.

Modification of the chimeric IL-2 receptor antibody by combination with pseudomonas endotoxin has resulted in increased efficacy.[60] Studies in rat corneal and murine cardiac allografts shows that IL-2-PE40 is a very effective immunosuppressive agent. Other studies have confirmed its effect in other T cell mediated situations including experimental auto-immune uveoretinitis and adjuvant arthritis.

An alternative approach was adopted by Strom's group,[94,95] who used diphtheria toxin coupled to antibodies to the IL-2 receptor. When tested in delayed hypersensitivity and allograft models, antigen specific immunosuppression was observed.

Thus, monoclonal antibodies can be used effectively to deliver toxins with precision and may be more effective than the antibody alone.

Anti-cytokine antibodies

Prophylactic administration of anti-TNF alpha or anti-TNF beta prolongs graft survival in a rat heterotopic heart transplant model.[61,62] Other studies using antibodies against interferon-gamma and TNF in a monkey skin graft model have shown a beneficial effect.[63] The use of soluble TNF receptors or IL-1 antagonists may further increase the options of anti-cytokine therapy.

Anti-adhesion molecules

Therapeutic antibodies against adhesion molecules have been developed and are currently being evaluated in transplant recipients. To date, studies on anti-ICAM-I (CD-54) and anti-LFA-1 (CD-11/CD-18) have shown encouraging results.[64,65] Anti-LFA-1 has been shown to be effective not only in animal models, since, a prospective study in human kidney transplantation suggested that the anti-LFA-1 antibody was ineffective in controlling the course of acute rejection. These disappointing results in renal transplantation are at variance with the encouraging results seen in the treatment of steroid resistant severe acute graft versus host disease. A recent study demonstrated induction of long term tolerance in rat cardiac allografts using a combination of anti-LFA-1 and anti-ICAM-1.[83]

Antibodies to ICAM-1 are effective in both the prevention and treatment of monkey heart rejection. Preliminary studies in renal transplantation suggest a beneficial effect and current studies are underway in liver transplantation but the results are still awaited.

Conclusion

Recent years have seen the development of a wide variety of new agents which modify the immune response and may have a more specific effect on the prevention or treatment of allograft rejection and the induction of tolerance. The place of these newer agents is, as yet, uncertain; only the use of properly designed controlled studies will allow a more rational and logical approach to the prevention of allograft rejection.

References

1. Sigal NH, Sierkierka JJ, Dumont FH. Observations of the mechanism of action of FK506. *Biochem Pharmacol* 1990; **40**, 2201–2208.
2. Starzl T, Schreiber S, Alberts M *et al.* Hepatotrophic properties in dogs of human FKBP, the binding protein for FK506 and Rapamycin. *Transplantation* 1991; **52**, 751–753.
3. Morris RE. Rapamycin: FK506's fraternal twin or distant cousin? *Immunol Today* 1991; **12**, 137–140.
4. Kahan BD, Chang JY, Sehgal SN. Preclinical evaluation of a potent new immunosuppressive agent, rapamycin. *Transplantation* 1991; **52**, 185–191.
5. Stepkowski SM, Chen H, Daloze P, Kahan BD. Rapamycin, a potent immunosuppressive drug for vascularized heart, kidney and small bowel transplantation in the rat. *Transplantation* 1991; **51**, 22–26.
6. Morris RE, Wu J, Shorthouse R. A study of the contrasting effects of cyclosporine, FK 506 and rapamycin on the suppression of allograft rejection. *Transplant Proc* 1990; **22**, 1638–1641.
7. Whiting PH, Woo J, Adam BJ, Hasas NU, Davidson N, Thomson AW. Toxicity of rapamycin. *Transplantation* 1991; **52**, 203–208.
8. Platz KP, Sollinger HW, Hullett DA, Eckhoff, Eugui EM, Allison AC. RS-61443 – a new, potent immunosuppressive agent. *Transplantation* 1991; **51**, 27–31.
9. Sweeney MJ, Hoffman DH, Esterman MA. Metabolism and biochemistry of mycophenolic acid. *Cancer Res* 1972; **32**, 1803–1806.
10. Franklin TJ, Cook J. The inhibition of nucleic acid synthesis by mycophenolic acid. *Biochem J* 1969; **113**, 515–523.
11. Allison AC, Almquist SJ, Muller CD, Eugui E. *In vitro* immunosuppressive effects of mycophenolic

acid and an ester pro-drug RS-61443. *Transplant Proc* 1991; **23**, 10–12.

12. Hao L, Lafferty K, Allison AC, Eugui E. RS-61443 allows islet allografting and specific tolerance induction in adult mice. *Transplant Proc* 1990; **22**, 876–878.
13. Morris RE, Wang J, Blum JR *et al.* Immunosuppressive effects of morpholinoethyl ester of mycophenolic acid (RS-61443) in rat and nonhuman primate recipients of heart allografts. *Transplant Proc* 1991; **23**, 19–25.
14. Platz KP, Eckhoff DE, Hullett DA, Sollinger HW. RS-61443 studies: review and protocol. *Transplant Proc* 1991; **23**, 33–35.
15. Sollinger HW, Eugui E, Allison AC. RS-61443: mechanism of action, experimental and early clinical results. *Clin Transplant* (special issue) 1991; **5**, 523–526.
16. Morris RE. ±15-deoxyspergualin: a mystery wrapped within an enigma. *Clin Transplant* 1991; **5**, 530–533.
17. Reichenspurner H, Hildebrandt A, Hurman PA *et al.* 15-deoxyspergualin after cardiac and renal allotransplantation in primates. *Transplant Proc* 1990; **22**, 1618–1619.
18. Schorlemmer HU, Dickneite G, Seiler FR. Treatment of acute rejection episodes and induction of tolerance in rat skin allotransplantation by 15-deoxyspergualin. *Transplant Proc* 1990; **22**, 1626–1630.
19. Suzuki S, Hayashi R, Niiya S, Kenmochi T, Fukuoka T, Amemiya H. Remarkable recovery from rejection by treatment with deoxyspergualin and methylprednisolone on canine kidney allografts. *Transplant Proc* 1991; **23**, 545–546.
20. Waaga AM, Ulrichs K, Kryzmanski M *et al.* The immunosuppressive agent 15-deoxyspergualin induces tolerance and modulates MHC antigen expression and interleukin-1 production in the early phase of rat allograft responses. *Transplant Proc* 1990; **22**, 1613–1614.
21. Takahashi K, Ota K, Tanabe K *et al.* Effect of a novel immunosuppressive agent, deoxyspergualin, on rejection in kidney transplant recipients. *Transplant Proc* 1990; **22**, 1606–1612.
22. Amemiya H, Dohi K, Otsubo O *et al.* Markedly enhanced effect of deoxyspergualin on acute rejection when combined with methylprednisolone in kidney recipients. *Transplant Proc* 1991; **23**, 1087–1089.
23. Rapaport RS, Dodge GR. Prostaglandin E inhibits the production of interleukin 2. *J Exp Med* 1982: **155**, 943–950.
24. Chouaib S, Welte K, Mertelsmann R, Dupont B. Prostaglandin E1 acts on two distinct pathways of T-lymphocyte activation. *J Immunol* 1985; **135**, 1172–1175.
25. Walker C, Fristensen F, Bettens F, de Week AL. Lymphokine regulation of activated GI lymphocytes I. *J Immunol* 1983; **130**, 1770–1774.
26. Pollak R, Dumble LJ, Wiederkehr JC, Maddux M, Moran M. The immunosuppressive properties of new oral prostaglangin E1 analogues. *Transplantation* 1990; **50**, 834–838.
27. Moran M, Mozes MF, Maddux M *et al.* Prevention of acute graft rejection by the prostaglandin E1 analogue Misoprostol in renal transplant recipients treated with Cyclosporin and Prednisolone. *N Eng J Med* 1990; **322**, 1183–1185.
28. Weir MR, Li X-W, Gomolka D, Peppler R, O'Bryan-Tear G, Moran M. Immunosuppressive properties of enisoprost and a 5-lipoxygenase inhibitor (SC 45662). *Transplant Proc* 1991; **24**, 1074–1077.
29. Vogelsang GB, Wells MC, Santos GW, Chen T, Hess AD. Combination low-dose thalidomide and cyclosporine for acute graft versus host disease in a rat mismatched model *Transplant Proc* 1988; **20**, 226–228.
30. Tamura F, Vogelsang GB, Reitz BA, Baumgartner WA, Herskowitz A. Combination thalidomide and cyclosporine for cardiac allograft rejection. *Transplantation* 1990; **49**, 20–25.
31. Keenan RJ, Eiras G, Burckhart GJ *et al.* Immunosuppressive properties of thalidomide. *Transplantation* 1991; **52**, 980–910.
32. Vogelsang G, Hess AD, Gordon G, Brudette R, Santos GW. Thalidomide for treatment of graft versus host disease: a review. *Bone Marrow Transplant* 1988; **3**, 393–401.
33. McKenzie JL, Beard MEJ, Hart D. Depletion of donor kidney dendritic cells prolong graft survival. *Transplant Proc* 1984; **16**, 948–945.
34. Lechler RJ, Bachelor JR. Restoration of immunogenicity to passenger-cell depleted allografts by the addition of donor strain dendritic cells. *J Exp Med* 1982; **155**, 31–40.
35. Brewer Y, Palmer A, Taube D *et al.* Effect of graft perfusion with two CD45 monoclonal antibodies on incidence of kidney allograft rejection. *Lancet* 1989; **ii**, 935–937.
36. Lomen PL. Xoma Bone Marrow Transplantation Study Group. *Anti-CD5 Immunoconjugates in Acute Graft Versus Host Disease*. UCLA Symposium: New Strategies in Bone Marrow Transplantation, Keystone, 1990.
37. Akbar AN, Amlot P, Ivory K, Timms A, Janossy G. Inhibition of alloresponsive naive and memory T cells by CD7 and CD25 antibodies and by Cyclosporine. *Transplantation* 1990; **50**, 823–825.
38. Lazarovitz A, Karsh J. CD7 antibody inhibits proliferation in the mixed autologous mixed lymphocyte reaction. *Transplant Proc* 1989; **21**, 3235–3236.
39. Heinrich G, Gram H, Kocher HP *et al.* Characterization of a human T-cell specific chimeric anti-

body (CD7) with human constant and mouse variable regions. *J Immunol* 1989; **143,** 3589–3592.

40. Akbar A, Amlot P, Hawkins C *et al.* The effect of a chimeric mouse-human CD7 antibody on human T, natural killer and lymphokine-activated killer cell activity *in vitro*. *Transplantation* 1991; **52,** 325–330.
41. Ferran C, Sheehan K, Schreiber R, Bach JF, Chatenoud L. Anti-TNF abrogates the cytokine-related anti-CD3 induced syndrome. *Transplant Proc* 1991; **23,** 849–851.
42. Alegre M-L, Gastaldello K, Abramowicz D *et al.* Evidence that pentoxifylline reduces anti-CD3 monoclonal antibody induced cytokine release syndrome. *Transplantation* 1991; **52,** 674–679.
43. Woodle ES, Thistlethwaite JR, Ghobrial IA, Jolliffe LK, Stuart FP, Bluestone JA. OKT3 F (ab) 2 fragments – retention of the immunosuppressive properties of whole antibody with marked reduction in T cell activation and lymphokine release. *Transplantation* 1991; **52,** 354–360.
44. Rao P, Olini G, Kille J *et al.* OKT3E, an anti-CD3 antibody that does not elicit side effects or anti-idiotype responses in chimpanzees. *Transplantation* 1991; **52,** 691–697.
45. Woodle ES, Thistlethwaite JR, Jolliffe LK, Fucello AJ, Stuart FP, Bluestone JA. Anti-CD3 monoclonal antibody therapy. *Transplantation* 1991; **52,** 361–368.
46. Waid TH, Lucas BA, Thompson JS *et al.* Treatment of acute rejection with anti-T-cell antigen receptor complex alpha-beta (T10B9.1A-31) or anti-CD3 (OKT3) monoclonal antibody. *Transplant Proc* 1991; **23,** 1062–1065.
47. Sablinski T, Hancock WW, Tilney N, Kupiec-Weglinski JW. CD4 monoclonal antibodies in organ transplantation – a review of progress. *Transplantation* 1991; **52,** 579–589.
48. Shizuru JA, Seydal K, Flavin T *et al.* Induction of donor specific unresponsiveness to cardiac allografts in rats by pretransplant anti-CD4 monoclonal antibody therapy. *Transplantation* 1990; **50,** 366–371.
49. Cobbold SP, Martin G, Waldmann H. The induction of skin graft tolerance in MHC mismatched or primed recipients. *Eur J Immunol* 1990; **20,** 2747–2751.
50. Cosimi AB, Delmonico FL, Wright J *et al.* OKT4A monoclonal antibody therapy immunosuppression of cynomolgus renal allograft recipients. *Transplant Proc* 1991; **23,** 501–503.
51. Coulombe M, Hao L, Calcinaro F *et al.* Tolerance induction in adult animals. *Transplant Proc* 1991; **23,** 31–32.
52. Herzog CH, Walker C, Pichler W *et al.* Monoclonal anti-CD4 in arthritis. *Lancet* 1987; **2,** 1461–1463.
53. Morel P, Vincent C, Corgier G *et al.* Anti-CD4 monoclonal administration in renal transplanted patients. *Clin Immunol Immunopathol* 1990; **56,** 311–320.
54. Kupiec-Weglinski J, Diamantstein T, Tilney N. Interleukin 2 receptor-targeted therapy – rationale and applications in organ transplantation. *Transplantation* 1988; **46,** 785–792.
55. Cosimi AB, Delmonico L, Wright K *et al.* Prolonged survival of non-human primate renal allograft recipients treated only with anti-CD4 monoclonal antibody therapy. *Surgery* 1990; **108,** 406–415.
56. Kirkman R, Chapiro M, Carpenter C *et al.* A randomized trial of anti-Tac monoclonal antibody in human renal transplantation. *Transplantation* 1991; **51,** 107–112.
57. Soulillou JP, Cantarovich D, Le Mauff B *et al.* Randomised controlled trial of monoclonal antibody against the interleukin-2 receptor (33B3.1) as compared with rabbit anti-thymocyte globulin for prophylaxis against rejection of renal allografts. *N Eng J Med* 1990; **322,** 1175–1178.
58. Otto G, Thies J, Kabelitz D *et al.* Anti-CD25 monoclonal antibody prevents early rejection in liver transplantation – a pilot study. *Transplant Proc* 1991; **23,** 1387–1389.
59. Ueda H, Cheung YC, Masetti P *et al.* Synergy between cyclosporine and anti-IL2 receptor monoclonal antibodies in rats. *Transplantation* 1991; **52,** 437–442.
60. Herbort CP, de Smet M, Roberge F *et al.* Treatment of corneal allograft rejection with cytotoxin IL-2-PE40. *Transplantation* 1991; **52,** 470–474.
61. Imagawa DK, Millis JM, Olthoff KM *et al.* The role of tumor necrosis factor in allograft rejection. *Transplantation* 1990; **50,** 189–193.
62. Scheringa M, de Bruin R, Jeekel H, Marquet RL. Anti-tumor necrosis factor alpha serum prolongs heart allograft survival in rats. *Transplant Proc* 1991; **23,** 547–548.
63. Stevens H, van der Kwast T, van der Meide P *et al.* Synergistic immunosuppressive effects of monoclonal effects of interferon gamma and tumour necrosis factor alpha. *Transplantation* 1990; **50,** 856–860.
64. Flavin T, Ivens K, Rothlein R *et al.* Monoclonal antibodies against intercellular adhesion molecule 1 prolong cardiac allograft survival in Cynomolgus monkeys. *Transplant Proc* 1991; **23,** 533–534.
65. Le Mauff B, Hourmant M, Rougier JP *et al.* Effect of anti-LFA1 (CD11a) monoclonal antibodies in acute rejection in human kidney transplantation. *Transplantation* 1991; **52,** 291–296.
66. Sollinger HW, Deirhoi MH, Belzer FO, Diethelm AG, Kauffman RS. RS-61443 – a phase I clinical trial and pilot rescue study. *Transplantation* 1992; **53,** 428–432.

67. Ohlman S, Gannedahl G, Tyden G, Tufveson G, Groth G. Treatment of renal transplant rejection with 15-deoxyspergualin – a dose finding study in man. *Transplant Proc* 1992; **24,** 318–320.
68. Groth CG, Ohlman S, Ericzon BH, Barholt L, Reinholt FP. Deoxyspergualin for liver graft rejection. *Lancet* 1990; **336,** 626.
69. Adams MB and the Enisoprost Renal Transplant Study Group. Enisoprost in renal transplantation. *Transplantation* 1992; **53,** 338–345.
70. Weir MR, Li XW, Peppler R, O'Bryan-Tear CG, Moran M. The immunosuppressive properties of enisoprost and a 5-lipoxygenase inhibitor (SC-45662). *Transplantation* 1991; **52,** 1053–1057.
71. Calmus Y, Gane P, Rouger P *et al.* Hepatic expression of class I and class II major histocompatability complex molecules in primary biliary cirrhosis: effect of ursodeoxycholic acid. *Hepatology* 1990; **11,** 12–17.
72. Henriksson BA, Persson H, Friman S, Wangberg B, Svanvik J, Kariberg I. Adjuvant ursodeoxycholic acid prevents acute rejection in liver transplant recipients. *Transplant Proc* 1991; **23,** 1971.
73. Friman S, Mjornstedt L, Persson H, Karlberg I, Olausson M. Ursodeoxycholic acid reduces acute rejection in heart allografted rats. *Transplant Proc* 1992; **24,** 244–245.
74. Chen SF, Ruben RL, Dexter D. Mechanism of action of the novel anticancer agent 6-fluoro-2-(2'-fluoro-1, 1'-biphenyl-4-yl)-3-methyl-4-quinolone carboxylic acid sodium salt (NSC 368390): inhibition of *de novo* pyrimidine nucleotide biosynthesis. *Cancer Res* 1986; **46,** 5014–5020.
75. Cramer D, Chapman F, Jaffee BD *et al.* The effect of a new immunosuppressive drug, Brequinar sodium, on heart, liver and kidney allograft rejection in the rat. *Transplantation* 1992; **53,** 303–308.
76. Badger AM, Albright-Winslow CR, Kupiec-Weglinski JW. SKF 105685: a novel immunosuppressive compound with efficacy in animal models of autoimmunity and transplantation. *Transplant Proc* 1991; **23,** 194–198.
77. Metcalfe SM, Watson CJE, Collier D *et al.* Survival of renal allografted dogs after limited therapy with cyclosporine and the PAF antagonist WEB 2170. *Transplant Proc* 1991; **23,** 2219–2220.
78. Hancock WW, Whitley D, Kupiec-Weglinski JW, Tilney N. Oral iron chelator Desferrithiocin blocks allogeneic monocuclear cell activation and cytokine production *in vivo* and prolongs rat cardiac allograft survival. *Transplant Proc* 1992; **24,** 214–215.
79. Sumimoto R, Kamada N. Specific suppression of allograft rejection by soluble class I antigen and complexes with monoclonal antibody. *Transplantation* 1990; **50,** 678–662.
80. Panel Discussion. Monoclonal antibody therapy in paediatric transplantation. *Transplant Proc* 1992; **24,** 2–10.
81. McKeon F. When worlds collide, immunosuppressants meet protein phosphatases. *Cell* 1991; **66,** 823–826.
82. Koch HP. Thalidomide and congeners as anti-inflammatory agents. *Prog Med Chem* 1985; **22,** 165–241.
83. Isobe M, Yagita H, Okumurabe Y, Ihara A. Specific acceptance of cardiac allograft after treatment with antibodies to ICAM-1 and LFA-1. *Science* 1992; **255,** 1125–1127.
84. Borel J, Feurer C, Gubler H, Stahlein H. Biological effects of cyclosporin A. *Agents Actions* 1976; **6,** 468–476.
85. Herold K, Lancki DW, Moldwin RL, Fitch F. Immunosuppressive effects of cyclosporine A on cloned T-cells. *J Immunol* 1986; **136,** 1315–1321.
86. Hess AD, Tutscka PJ. Effect of cyclosporine A on human lymphocyte responses *in vitro* I. *J Immunol* 1980; **124,** 2601–2608.
87. Takahashi N, Hayano T, Suzuki M. Peptidyl-prolyl cis-trans isomerase is the cyclosporine A binding protein, cyclophilin. *Nature* 1989; **337,** 473–475.
88. Fischer G, Whitman B, Lang K *et al.* Cyclophilin and peptidylprolyl cis-trans isomerase are probably identical proteins. *Nature* 1989; **337,** 476–478.
89. Lorber MI. Cyclosporine: lessons learned – future strategies. *Clin Transplant* 1991; **5,** 505–516.
90. Kino T, Hatanaka H, Hashimoto M. FK506, a novel immunosuppressant isolated from a Streptomyces. II Immunosuppressive effects *in vitro*. *J Antibiotics* (Tokyo) 1987; **40,** 1256–1263.
91. White DJG. FK506: the promise and the paradox. *Clin Exp Immunol* 1991; **83,** 1–3.
92. Todo S, Fung JJ, Starzl TE *et al.* Liver, kidney and thoracic organ transplantation under FK506. *Ann Surg* 1990; **212,** 295–305.
93. Harding MW, Galat A, Uehling D, Schreiber S. A receptor for the immunosuppressant FK506 is a cis-trans peptidyl-prolyl isomerase. *Nature* 1989; **341,** 758–760.
94. Bacha P, Williams DP, Waters C *et al.* Interleukin-2 receptor-targeted toxicity: interleukin 2 receptor mediated action of a diphtheria toxin related interleukin 2 fusion protein. *J Exp Med* 1988; **167,** 612–621.
95. Murphy J, Kelley V, Storm T. Interleukin-2 toxin: a step towards selective immunomodulation. *Am J Kidney Dis* 1988; **11,** 159–162.

19

HLA/ABO matching

G Steinhoff

Introduction

Differences in histocompatibility antigens form the basis for the rejection of organ transplants. A number of polymorphic antigen systems have been defined. Of these, the human leucocyte antigens (HLA) coded by the major histocompatibility complex (MHC) and blood group antigen (ABO) systems have major importance for the induction of immunological reactivity after organ transplantation. The potential importance of other molecules in the generation of clinical rejection, however, has to be considered. At present, in clinical liver transplantation, matching of tissue antigens between donor and recipient is only practised for the main blood group antigens (ABO). Compatibility between other tissue antigens, such as the HLA system, occurs only by chance and lymphocyte crossmatching is not routinely used.[1]

The clinical importance of allo-antigen incompatibility depends on the cell type and organ transplanted. Differences in tissue expression and release of allo-antigens in response not only to rejection but also immune responses to virus, microbial antigens, auto-antigens and tumour cells have to be considered.

HLA incompatibility

In the early days of experimental and clinical liver transplantation, the liver was thought to be an organ of low immunogenicity.[2] This assumption was prompted by experimental and clinical observations of tolerance. The problem of tissue incompatibility was overshadowed by limited organ resources, short preservation time and technical problems. As in heart transplantation, the limited organ availability and short preservation time made prospective matching of HLA loci between donor and recipient impossible. Liver transplantation has now been established for a decade and rejection is still a clinical problem influencing long-term results. Although the treatment of acute rejection is usually successful, chronic rejection and hyperacute rejection in sensitised recipients have a major effect on graft survival. For this reason, it is important to re-assess the effect of matching tissue antigens in the face of wider organ availability and extended preservation time. The latter would be a requirement for prospective matching considering the time needed for tissue typing and organ transport. In the last 20 years the beneficial effect of prospective HLA matching[3] for the outcome of organ transplants has been documented in renal and bone marrow transplantation.[4,5] The question arises whether the same benefit in long-term graft survival would result from HLA matching in liver transplantation.

Clinical results

The large number of patients who have received liver or heart transplants has allowed retrospective analysis of the effect of HLA mismatches on rejection and graft outcome. In a multicentre study of heart transplants, a beneficial effect of matching of HLA-B and HLA-DR MHC antigens on graft outcome has been demonstrated.[6] These results resemble the effect seen in renal transplants.[5] In liver transplantation, however, the clinical results were different (Table 19.1). The largest series, analysed in Pittsburgh[7] compared the clinical outcome of 500 liver transplants to class I or class II HLA compatibility. A dualistic effect of HLA matching on liver transplant outcome was found. The overall transplant survival

Table 19.1 Studies of HLA/ABO matching after liver transplation

Authors	Centre	Patients (n)
HLA incompatibility		
Donaldson *et al.* 1987	Cambridge	62
Markus *et al.* 1988	Pittsburgh	574
O'Grady *et al.* 1988	Cambridge	101
Gubernatis *et al.* 1988	Hanover	81
Batts *et al.* 1988	Rochester	55
Superina *et al.* 1989	Toronto	41
Calmus *et al.* 1990	Paris	155
Saito *et al.* 1991	Nebraska	212
ABO incompatibility		
Ramsey *et al.* 1984	Pittsburgh	171
Gordon *et al.* 1987	Pittsburgh	745
White *et al.* 1987	Cambridge	220
Fischel *et al.* 1989	Minnesota	93
Gugenheim *et al.* 1990	Paris	234

was decreased in grafts matched for MHC class I (HLA-A) or class II (HLA-DR). Conversely, in 108 failed grafts requiring retransplantation, there was a higher incidence of failure due to rejection correlated with a lower degree of HLA compatibility particularly for HLA-DR. The incidence of graft failures due to primary non-function was significantly correlated with HLA-DR compatibility.

In other studies, similarly contradictory effects of HLA compatibility and incompatibility were reported. Patients developing chronic rejection with vanishing bile duct syndrome (VBDS) showed a pattern of HLA-A,B incompatibility together with HLA-DR compatibility.[8,9] Other groups[10] reported a relationship between the development of a VBDS and positive lymphocyte crossmatch as well as HLA-DR incompatibility. A similar observation was made by the Hanover group,[11] who concluded that rejection types with bile duct damage are correlated with HLA-DR incompatibility. Partial HLA compatibility had no influence on rejection incidence.

In a small series[12] a high incidence of severe rejection leading to retransplantation in DRw6+ recipients was reported. Other authors,[13] however, could not confirm this observation and found an equal risk in DRw6 positive and negative recipients irrespective of their individual HLA mismatch. Recently, Calmus *et al.*[14] found that hepatitis B recurrence with manifestation of hepatic lesions after transplantation was associated with HLA class I compatibility, but not with class II HLA-DR compatibility. The question arises as to whether these observations reflect the role of HLA antigens in different pathogeneic mechanisms leading to graft injury after transplantation (Table 19.2).

Table 19.2 Clinical complications of HLA/ABO incompatibility

Recipient sensitisation to:	
HLA	Acute/chronic cellular rejection (hyperacute/ humoral rejection)
ABO	Hyperacute/humoral rejection Severe acute/chronic rejection Vascular thrombosis Sclerosing cholangitis
Graft sensitisation to:	
HLA	Graft versus host disease (GvH) Thrombocytopenia
ABO	GvH Haemolytic anaemia

Donor/recipient immune reactivity and recurrence of disease

The prevalence and severity of rejection in the liver is comparable to that seen in other organs such as the kidney or the heart. For this reason it is conceivable that HLA identity between donor and recipient would reduce the severity of acute rejection and incidence of chronic rejection. However, late rejection after liver transplantation is less common than in kidney or heart grafts.

Whilst HLA matching may reduce immune reactivity to donor HLA, auto-immune or virus directed T cell cytolytic reactivity associated with the original liver disease may be enhanced. In addition, full HLA-DR compatibility may enhance the T cell response to viral or auto-immune antigens and to minor histocompatibility antigens. These immune reactions may mediate graft injury in addition to the anti-HLA rejection response and this could lead to recurrent liver disease (PBC or recurrent hepatitis), and also augment rejection by induction of donor HLA and secondary sensitisation to allo-antigens (Table 19.3).

The transplantation of immune competent donor cells with the liver has a number of consequences: HLA allo-immunisation against host antigens (graft versus host reaction – GvH) is possible (see Table 19.2). Lethal GvH disease has been reported in liver transplant recipients,[15,16] as well as minor clinical complications such as

Table 19.3 Dualistic effect of HLA matching in human liver transplantation

Compatible
- Recipient sensitisation to minor (non-HLA) transplantation antigens
- Enhancement of antiviral immune response to the graft (HBV,HCV,CMV,EBV)
- Persistence and recurrence of auto-immune T cell reactivity (PBC,PSC)
- Persistence of donor lymphocytes and development of GvH activity (minor transplantation and blood group antigens)

Incompatible
- Acute and chronic rejection response of the recipient
- GvH activity of transplanted donor lymphocytes
- Tolerance phenomena (soluble donor HLA antigens, 'veto' cells)

thrombocytopenia. It is possible that immune cells transplanted with the graft acting as 'veto' cells induce specific tolerance across certain HLA barriers.[17] Furthermore, parenchymal liver cells may influence immune reactivity and even induce tolerance by the secretion of soluble HLA class I antigens of donor type.[18]

Blood group (ABO) incompatibility

Even in the early days of organ transplantation, the beneficial effect of ABO bloodgroup compatibility was noted.[19] In the presence of ABO incompatibility, hyperacute humoral rejection was observed in renal transplants.[20] This was directly related to the extent of anti-A and/or anti-B antibody titres present in the recipients prior to transplantation[19] and due to the fact that the ABO antigens were widely distributed thoughout human tissues and organs.[21,22]

In emergency situations such as acute hepatic failure, liver transplantation across ABO barriers may be necessary (see Table 19.4). For many years it had been thought that the liver is resistant to hyperacute rejection.[2] In recent years, however, it has become clear that ABO incompatible liver transplantation in sensitised recipients may lead to humoral and hyperacute rejection with graft loss.[23,24] Unlike renal or heart transplantation, however, liver transplantation across ABO barriers can still be successfully performed in urgent clinical situations.[25]

Clinical results

The analysis of ABO compatibility and liver transplant outcome in larger clinical series showed a significant advantage of ABO identity between donor and recipient.[26,27] Figure 19.1 shows the results of one such study. The outcome of grafts with ABO compatibility (O donor to A, B, or AB recipient) was associated with a slightly reduced survival compared with ABO identical (O to O, A to A, etc.) grafts.[24,26,27] Many of the ABO non-identical grafts were done as an emergency.[24,26] However, even when only emergency grafts are considered, survival of ABO incompatible grafts is less than compatible ones.[24] This difference is due to a high incidence of hyperacute/severe rejection and vascular thrombosis.

Hyperacute/humoral rejection

With increasing numbers of ABO incompatible grafts transplanted in emergency cases, a clinical syndrome of antibody mediated rejection has been described in liver transplants.[23] A number of groups reported cases of graft loss due to hyperacute rejection in presensitised (ABO incompatible) recipients. Studies suggest that the rejection was mediated by iso-agglutinins causing endothelial damage, vessel thrombosis and haemorrhagic necrosis of the graft.[23] The risk of hyperacute rejection may be diminished in sensitised recipients with pre-operative plasma exchange, splenectomy and post-operative ALG treatment.[25] Late humoral rejection after transplantation is rare. It may be diagnosed by an increase in titres to blood group antigens and may

Table 19.4 Liver transplantation across ABO barriers

ABO mismatch*	Donor	Recipient	Therapeutic regimen
Compatible	0	A,B,AB	Standard immunosuppression (0-RBC transfusion)
Incompatible	A,B,AB	0,A,B	Antilymphocyte globulin, plasmapheresis, splenectomy, 0-RBC transfusion

*Identical match: 0 to 0, A to A, etc.

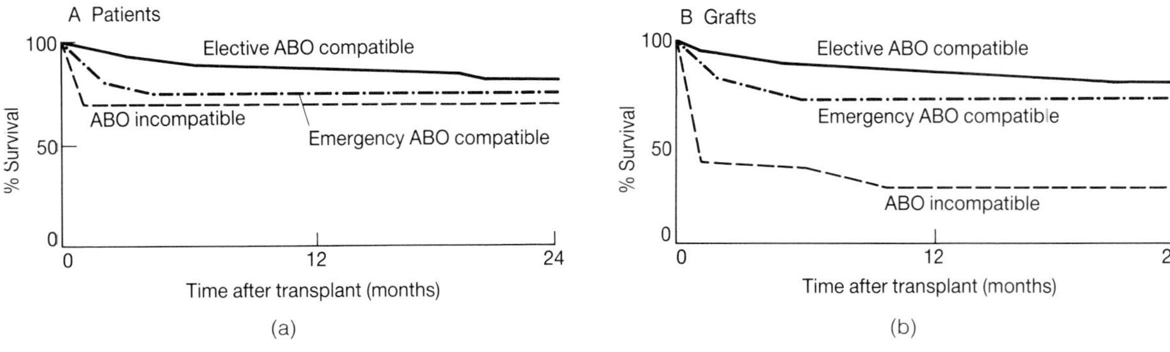

Fig. 19.1 Patient (a) and graft (b) survival in patients receiving A,B,O compatible grafts in elective and in emergency situations (taken from [24] with kind permission from *The Lancet*).

be treated by plasma exchange and increased immunosuppression.[25]

Graft versus host reactivity

Ramsey *et al.* first reported the finding of isohaemagglutinins of graft origin directed to incompatible recipient blood group antigens after liver transplantation.[28] They observed haemolysis in the majority of these patients. Most probably, the antibodies were produced by persisting donor B lymphocytes transplanted with the graft. Clinical observations of non-ABO related graft versus host disease in liver graft recipients have also been reported.[15,16] It has to be assumed that lymphoid cells transplanted with the graft have a limited life span and that GvH reactivity therefore usually occurs only in the first weeks after transplantation and ceases with the elimination of donor cells. Although full blown GvH disease is rare, in ABO non-identical transplantation, temporary GvH activity leading to haemolysis occurs more often. Haemolytic anaemia caused by anti-A,B or AB directed graft versus host reactions is treated by repeated transfusion of red cells, plasmapheresis and a reduction in immunosuppression to allow the elimination of donor immune cells. Only in critical exacerbations are steroid and ALG treatments necessary.

Clinical indication and management of ABO mismatched transplantation

Liver transplantation across ABO barriers should be restricted to cases of acute hepatic failure since the long-term prognosis of incompatible grafts is inferior to that of compatible ones. Bile duct complications, severe rejection and an increased risk of portal and hepatic artery thrombosis have been reported to occur. Therefore, ABO incompatible grafts are now usually used as a bridge until a compatible graft is available. To circumvent the threat of hyperacute rejection, presensitised recipients should undergo plasmapheresis. Splenectomy and post-operative ALG[25] treatment to prevent additional recipient sensitisation to donor blood group antigens have been recommended. Patients with non-identical and incompatible grafts should be regularly monitored for isohaemagglutinin titres. Rising titres may require treatment with plasmapheresis.

Clinical importance of other allo-antigenic systems

The importance of sensitisation to minor blood group and minor transplantation antigens is not clear in human liver transplantation. Sensitisation to minor blood group antigens such as rhesus factor and Lewis has been reported by Ramsey *et al.*[29,30] but did not result in decreased graft survival. Haemolysis, increased blood requirement during transplantation and thrombocytopenia, however, may result from sensitisation to minor blood group antigens. The polymorphism of complement factors that are produced in the liver may also lead to recipient sensitisation.[31] The role of these and additional soluble and membrane bound polymorphic molecules as targets for the rejection response[32] or inducers of tolerance still has to be clarified.

References

1. Iwatsuki S, Rabin BS, Shaw BW Jr, Starzl TE. Liver transplantation against T cell-positive warm crossmatches. *Transplant Proc* 1984; **16,** 1427–1429.
2. Starzl TE, Ishikawa M, Putnam CW *et al.* Progress in and deterrents to orthotopic liver transplantation, with special reference to survival, resistance to hyperacute rejection, and biliary duct reconstruction. *Transplant Proc* 1974; **6,** 129–139.
3. Terasaki PI, Mickey MR, Singal DP, Mittal KK, Patel R. Serotyping for homotransplantation. Selection of recipients for cadaver donor transplants. *N Eng J Med* 1968; **279,** 1101–1103.
4. O'Reilly RJ. Current developments in marrow transplantation. *Transplant Proc* 1987; **19**(1), 92–102.
5. Opelz G. Effect of HLA matching in 10,000 cyclosporine treated cadaver kidney transplants. *Transplant Proc* 1987; **19,** 641–646.
6. Opelz G for the Collaborative Heart Transplant Study. Effect of HLA matching in heart transplantation. *Transplant Proc* 1989; **21**(1), 794–796.
7. Markus BH, Duquesnoy RJ, Gordon RD *et al.* Histocompatibility and liver transplant outcome. Does HLA exert a dualistic effect? *Transplantation* 1988; **46,** 372–377.
8. Donaldson PT, Alexander GJM, O'Grady JG *et al.* Evidence for an immune response to HLA class I antigens in the vanishing bile duct syndrome after liver transplantation. *Lancet* 1987; **1,** 945–951.
9. O'Grady JG, Alexander GJ, Sutherland S *et al.* Cytomegalovirus infection and donor/recipient HLA-antigens: interdependent co-factors in pathogenesis of vanishing bile-duct syndrome after liver transplantation. *Lancet* 1988; **2,** 302–305.
10. Batts KP, Moore SB, Perkins JD, Wiesner RH, Grambsch PM, Krom RF. Influence of positive lymphocyte crossmatch and HLA-mismatching on vanishing bile duct syndrome in human liver allografts. *Transplantation* 1988; **45,** 376–379.
11. Gubernatis G, Kemnitz J, Tusch G, Pichlmayr R. HLA compatibility and different features of liver allograft rejection. *Transplant Int* 1988; **1,** 155–160.
12. Superina RA, Pearl RH, Greig PD, Levy G, Falk J, Langer B. Effect of DRw6 antigen in recipients and donors on survival after liver transplant. *Transplant Proc* 1989; **21,** 786–788.
13. Saito S, Stratta RJ, Grazi GL *et al.* Effect of the HLA-DRw6 antigen in liver transplantation. *Transplant Proc* 1991; **23,** 1430–1431.
14. Calmus Y, Hannoun L, Dousset B *et al.* HLA class I matching is responsible for the hepatic lesions in recurrent viral hepatitis B after liver transplantation. *Transplant Proc* 1990; **22,** 2311–2313.
15. Burdick JF, Vogelsang GB, Smith WJ *et al.* Severe graft-versus-host disease in a liver-transplant recipient. *N Eng J Med* 1988; **318,** 689–691.
16. Marubayashi S, Matsuzaka C, Takeda A *et al.* Fatal generalized acute graft-versus-host disease in a liver transplant recipient. *Transplantation* 1990; **50,** 709–711.
17. Thomas JM, Carver FM, Cunningham PRG, Olson LC, Thomas FT. Kidney allograft tolerance in primates without chronic immunosuppression – the role of veto cells. *Transplantation* 1991; **51,** 198–207.
18. Davies HS, Pollard SG, Calne RY. Soluble HLA antigens in the circulation of liver graft recipients. *Transplantation* 1989; **47,** 524–7.
19. Starzl TE, Tzakis A, Makowka L *et al.* The definition of ABO factors in transplantation: relation to other humoral antibody states. *Transplant Proc* 1987; **19,** 4492–4497.
20. Starzl TE, Marchioro TL, Holmes JH *et al.* Renal homografts in patients with major donor-recipient blood group incompatibilities. *Surgery* 1964; **55,** 195–200.
21. Szulman AD. The histological distribution of blood group substances A and B in man. *J Exp Med* 1960; **111,** 785–800.
22. Breimer ME, Samuelsson BE. The specific distribution of glycolipid based blood group A antigens in human kidney related to A1/A2, Lewis, and secretor status of single individuals: a possible molecular explanation for the successful transplantation of A2 kidneys into O recipients. *Transplantation* 1986; **42,** 88–91.
23. Demetris AJ, Jaffe R, Tzakis A *et al.* Antibody mediated rejection of human liver allografts: transplantation across ABO blood group barriers. *Transplant Proc* 1989; **21,** 2217–2220.
24. Gugenheim J, Samuel D, Reynes M, Bismuth H. Liver transplantation across ABO blood group barriers. *Lancet* 1990; **336,** 519–523.
25. Fischel RJ, Ascher NL, Payne WD *et al.* Pediatric liver transplantation across ABO blood group barriers. *Transplant Proc* 1989; **21,** 2221–2222.
26. Gordon RD, Iwatsuki S, Esquivel CO, Tsakis A, Todo S, Starzl TE. Liver transplantation across ABO blood groups. *Surgery* 1986; **100,** 342–348.
27. White DJ, Gore SM, Barroso E, Calne RY. The significance of ABO blood groups in liver transplantation. *Transplant Proc* 1987; **19,** 4571–4574.
28. Ramsey G, Nusbacher J, Starzl TE, Lindsay GD. Isohemagglutinins of graft origin after ABO-unmatched liver transplantation. *N Eng J Med* 1984; **311,** 1167–1170.
29. Ramsey G, Wolford J, Boczkowski DJ, Cornell FQ, Larson P, Starzl TE. The Lewis blood group

system in liver transplantation. *Transplant Proc* 1987; **19,** 4591–4594.

30. Ramsey G, Hahn LF, Cornell FW *et al*. Low rate of Rhesus immunization from Rh-incompatible blood transfusions during liver and heart transplant surgery. *Transplantation* 1989; **47,** 993–995.
31. Woelpl A, Robin-Winn M, Pichlmayr R, Goldmann SG. Fourth component of complement (C4) polymorphism in human orthotopic liver transplantation. *Transplantation* 1985; **40,** 154–157.
32. Van Els C, Bueger MH, Kempenaar J, Donec M, Goulmy E. Susceptibility of human male keratinocytes to MHC-restricted H-Y specific lysis. *J Exp Med* 1989; **170,** 1469–1474.

20

Liver preservation and rejection

LH Toledo-Pereyra, J Lopez-Ranger, R Xavier and A Chousleb

Introduction

Current advances in hepatic transplantation are in part dependent on the development of effective preservation solutions and the use of better immunosuppressive regimens for the treatment of rejection.

The liver has been one of the most difficult solid organs to preserve. Researchers have attempted to improve liver viability by maintenance or inhibition of its cellular metabolism. Hypothermia is the principal method used for inhibition of cellular metabolism and decrease in oxygen requirements.[1] To maintain the liver metabolic demands, the use of high energy compounds or appropriate nutrients is needed.

Historical developments of preservation

The liver is especially sensitive to anoxia,[2] a property which results in a lack of tolerance to the various methods of preservation. In 1960, the first long term survival of a transplanted dog liver was reported. The donor dog was immersed in an ice bath, to reduce the body temperature to 30° and 15° C, and the liver was perfused through the portal vein with cold Ringer's lactate solution (4–7° C).[3] The first human orthotopic liver transplant was performed in 1963.[4]

In 1969, the works of Collins *et al.*[5] on kidneys and Schalm *et al.*[6] on the liver suggested that a crystalloid solution with a composition comparable to the intracellular environment should be used to supplement the effect of core cooling and hypothermia, allowing for longer preservation periods of 30 hours for the kidney and just over two hours for the liver.

In 1970, the utilisation of hypothermia and low flow perfusion with cryoprecipitated plasma permitted the preservation of porcine livers for up to ten hours, but when the duration of preservation was extended, most of the animals died because of a bleeding diathesis.[7] The use of a balanced electrolyte solution with low molecular weight dextran for the initial flush and reconstituted frozen plasma and hyperbaric oxygen at 3 atm improved the storage time to 12 hours.[8]

In 1975, Toledo-Pereyra *et al.* obtained better results with a silica gel fraction of plasma (SGF) (Table 20.1), with the addition of KCl, dextran and albumin.[9] They also demonstrated the protective effect of allopurinol in ischaemic livers.[10] Four years later, the same authors obtained longer survival after auxiliary liver transplantation of organs preserved with Sacks solution instead of Ringer's lactate. The silica gel fraction of plasma proved to be superior to Collins and Sacks sol-

Table 20.1 Composition of the silica gel fraction solutions (SGF-I and SGF-III)

SGF-I		SGF-III	
Plasma SGF	400 ml	Plasma SGF	400 ml
25% Albumin	100 ml	25% Albumin	100 ml
$MgSO_4$	8 mEq/l	$MgSO_4$	8 mEq/L
KCl	20 mEq/l	KCl	20 mEq/L
Solu-Medrol	250 mg	Solu-Medrol	250 mg
Dextrose	5 gm	Dextrose (50%)	10 gm
		Ampicillin	250 mg
Osmolarity	430 mOsm/l	Osmolarity	420 mOsm/l

utions because of its colloidal properties, with less damage to endothelial cells.[11,12]

Preservation solutions

Organ viability is directly dependent on the quality of the harvested organ, the preservation time and the preservation solution utilised. These solutions can be colloidal or crystalloid, hypertonic or isotonic, with different electrolyte concentrations and with the possible addition of various drugs.

The efficacy of these solutions depends on the composition, warm ischaemia time and length of preservation.

UW solution

In 1987 Belzer and his associates introduced a new solution (University of Wisconsin solution) for experimental pancreatic preservation,[13] based on lactobionate and raffinose for the suppression of oedema, hydroxyethyl starch to diminish the shift of electrolytes to the extracellular space and water to the interstitial space, and other compounds that modify the xanthine oxidase pathway (allopurinol), stimulate the build-up of high energy compounds (adenosine) and glutathione, an inhibitor of lipid peroxidation. Successful hepatic preservation was achieved in dogs for 30 hours with this solution.[14] Since then, the UW solution has been routinely used for liver preservation in clinical transplantation[15] (Figure 20.1).

Comparison of UW with other solutions

Comparative studies between UW and Collins solutions for hepatic preservation showed better results with the UW solution,[16,17,18,19] with longer graft survival with a lower incidence of primary graft non-function, less hepatic artery thrombosis and extended preservation times.[20,21,22,23,24] Patient survival was 79% for UW solution compared with 63% for the Collins solution.[25] (See Figure 20.1)[26]

The introduction of the UW solution into clinical transplantation has revolutionised many clinical aspects of liver transplantation. Today, the majority of liver transplants can be scheduled as semi-elective procedures, unless the patient's medical condition dictates otherwise. Studies,

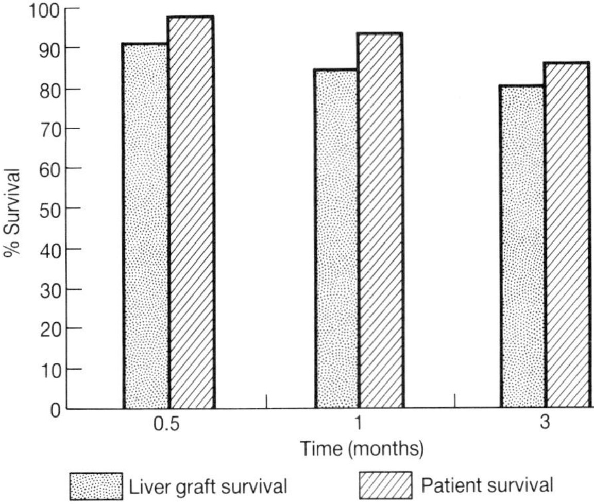

Fig. 20.1 Patient and graft survival of human livers subjected to various periods of hypothermic storage with UW solution. Although consistently high results were observed, patient and graft survival diminished somewhat by the third month (modified from Olthoff *et al.*[23]).

between UW and a modified silica get fraction of plasma to which lactobionate has been added provided improved liver protection in dogs (26)

Essential components of UW solution

Studies that systematically assessed the components of the UW solution (Table 20.2) showed that the omission of hydroxyethyl starch,[27,28,29] adenosine, allopurinol, buffer phosphate or $MgSO_4$ did not alter graft survival.[27] The elimination of lactobionate, glutathione and dexamethasone resulted in decreased survival,[27,30] whereas the elimination of insulin increased survival.[27] Other work using perfused rabbit liver

Table 20.2 UW solution for preservation

K+ -Lactobionate	100 mmol
KH_2PO_4	25 mmol
$MgSO_4$	5 mmol
Raffinose	30 mmol
Adenosine	5 mmol
Glutathione	3 mmol
Insulin	100 U
Bactrim	0.5 ml
Dexamethasone	8 mg
Allopurinol	1 mM
Hydroxyethyl starch	50 g

demonstrated that only lactobionate, raffinose and glutathione were essential components of the UW solution.[31]

Drugs used in liver preservation

Pretreatment of the donor with chlorpromazine improved the quality of organs preserved with UW, probably due to its vaso-active or calcium channel blocking effects and its membrane stabilising properties.[32] Compounds that inhibit free radical production or modify the xanthine oxidase pathway, such as catalase,[33] allopurinol[34,35] and superoxide dismutase,[34,35,36] have had a protective effect in liver preservation.

Drugs that block calcium channels (such as nisoldipine) have been shown experimentally to improve hepatic microcirculation.[37] This is consistent with the hypothesis that Kupffer cells are activated early in the sequence of events, leading to endothelial cell mediated alterations in the microcirculation[37] early in the microcirculation and graft failure.[37]

Recently, the pretreatment of donors with an experimental platelet activating factor antagonist, such as SRI 63–441, has been shown to further reduce the cold ischaemic injury.[38]

Development of new solutions

Modifications of the UW solution by reducing the potassium concentration from 120 mM to 9±4 mM and increasing the sodium concentration from 30 mM to 140±5 mM produce results similar to the original UW solution, without the endothelial damage or risk of cardiac arrest in the recipient produced by high potassium concentrations.[39]

New solutions, like the Carolina rinse solution, contain electrolytes at concentrations similar to those in plasma, oncotic support against interstitial oedema (modified hydroxyethyl starch), anti-oxidants against oxygen radicals (allopurinol, desferroxamine and glutathione), vasodilators to improve microcirculation (nicardipine and adenosine), substrates to regenerate ATP (fructose and glucose plus insulin), and mildly acidic pH. These solutions have produced effective results in extending the preservation time of livers in animals.[40]

Recently, the HTK or Bretschneider's solution has been used for successful liver preservation for 24 hours.[41]

Liver rejection

Rejection was not considered to be a major problem when human liver transplantation began in the 1960s.[42] The major difficulties were ischaemia, poor preservation of the donor liver, technical complications of the vascular and biliary anastomoses, and infections.[43] It is now recognised that hyperacute rejection, as described in renal transplantation (induced by humoral immune mechanisms), is rare in liver transplantation[44,45,46] but other patterns of rejection occur.

The increased experience with liver transplantation since 1983 has modified understanding about the appearance and consquences of rejection. In part, this has resulted from the use of liver biopsies in most centres for the histological diagnosis of rejection.[47,48] Furthermore, improvements in operative techniques, treatment of infections, and the intensive care of these patients has reduced the incidence of non-immunological complications, so that rejection has become a major clinical problem occupying in up to 77% of patients.[43] In one study from Pittsburgh 16% of patients required retransplantation because of liver failure due to rejection.[49]

Mechanisms of liver allograft rejection

Brief observations

A variety of mechanisms for allograft rejection have been identified (see other chapters of this book). It is well recognized now that the rejection response which is generated against transplant organs by normal and genetically dissimilar recipients is mainly a cell-mediated immune process.[42,50] However, an important role can also be assigned to humoral antibodies in bringing about tissue destruction under some circumstances.[44,51]

The process of induction of specific immunological unresponsiveness by transplanted organs in respect to their own antigens is of great interest. The distribution of class I and II Major Histocompatibility Complex (MHC) antigens in the liver appears to be important during rejection.[52,53] Class I antigens are in the hepatocytes, and the

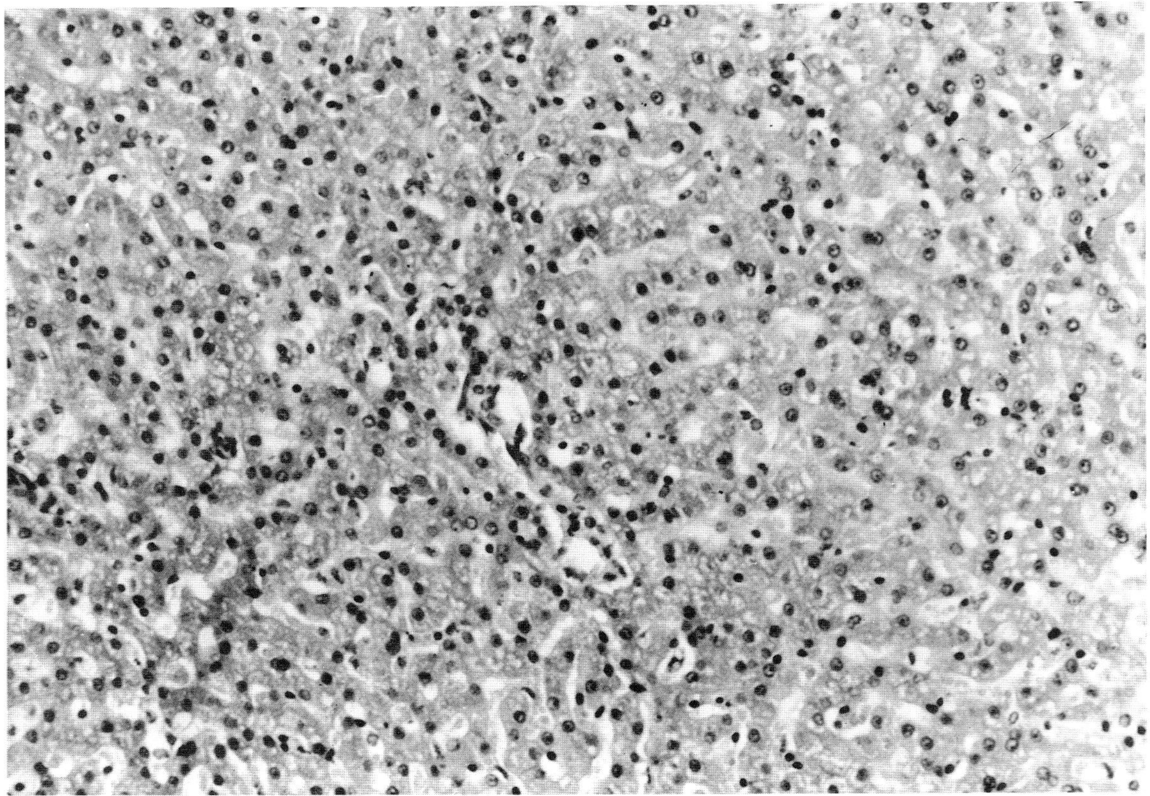

Fig. 20.2 Mild chronic passive congestion was noted after 40 minutes of ischaemic damage in canine livers protected with allopurinol (50 mg/l) intravenously ten minutes before the ischaemic insult. Reactive hepatocytes were quite prominent. Microvacuolisation was noted in some of the hepatocytes (haematoxylin and eosin ×40).

class II antigens are rarely expressed.[54,55,56] In contrast, the bile duct epithelium and central vein endothelium are rich in both class I and class II expression antigens. An important expression of the MHC occurs in these sites when the liver develops acute rejection.

Careful observations have demonstrated that early in the acute rejection lymphocytic infiltration occurs in portal tracts and in the walls of central veins due to damage in the bile duct epithelium and central vein endothelium.[43,50,57,58] Furthermore, an increase in the expression of class I antigens on hepatocytes was shown during acute rejection.[59]

Previous experience with liver transplants has shown that these grafts survive better than kidneys or hearts, perhaps because the liver mass was too great to be destroyed quickly by the antibody.[43,50] Another explanation for this lack of response from preformed cytolytic antibodies is the dilution effect that frequently accompanies liver transplantation. Blood loss and replacement translates to one or several volume exchanges in many patients. This lowers antibody titres and may also deplete the host of circulating lymphocytes that amplify the antibody response.[43]

Ischaemia, organ preservation and rejection

It has been demonstrated in renal transplantation that ischaemia and preservation injury can modify the immunogenicity of the graft.[60,61,62] In the liver, there are a few isolated studies[70,71] that have reviewed such findings. The main reason, until recently had to do with the lack of appropriate presentation solutions. In fact, Howard and associates[70] and Furukawa and his group[71] demonstrated that preservation injury by prolonged

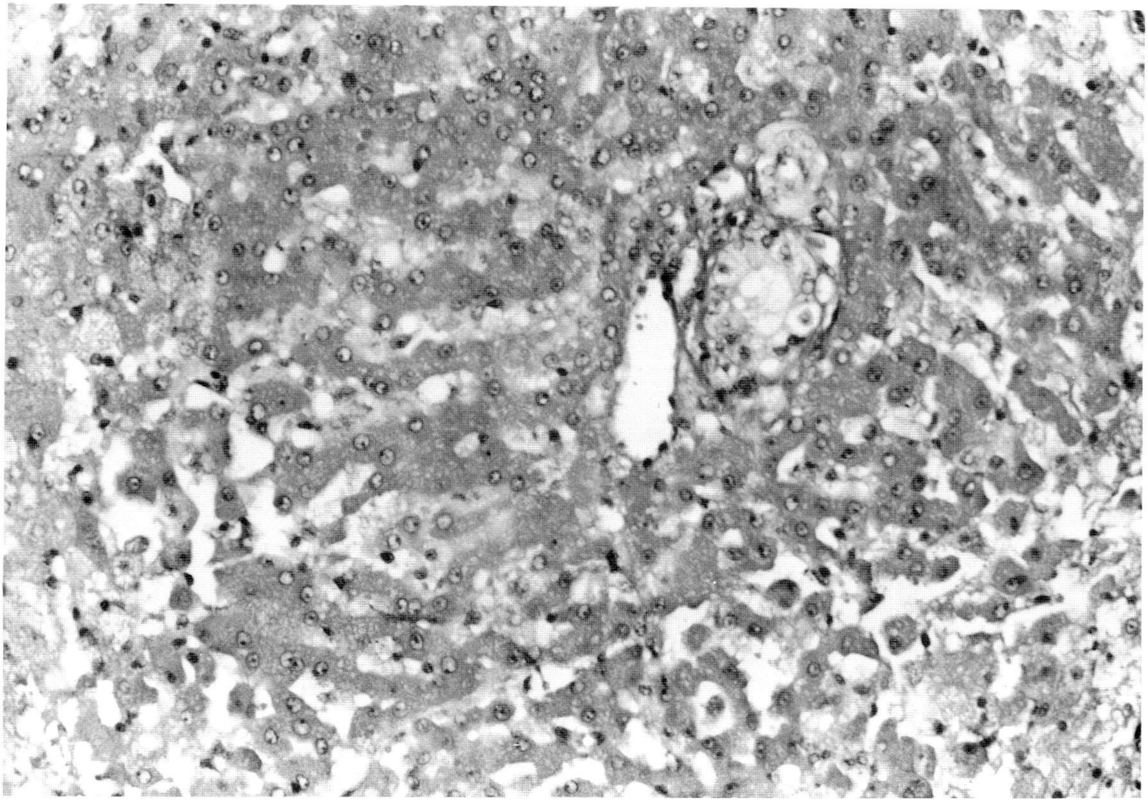

Fig. 20.3 Moderate chronic passive congestion was noted after 12 hours of canine liver intermittent non-pulsatile hypothermic perfusion with modified silica gel fraction of plasma (MSGF). No ischaemia was applied. The sinusoids are dilated and empty. The portal triad is in the right upper centre (haematoxylin and eosin ×40).

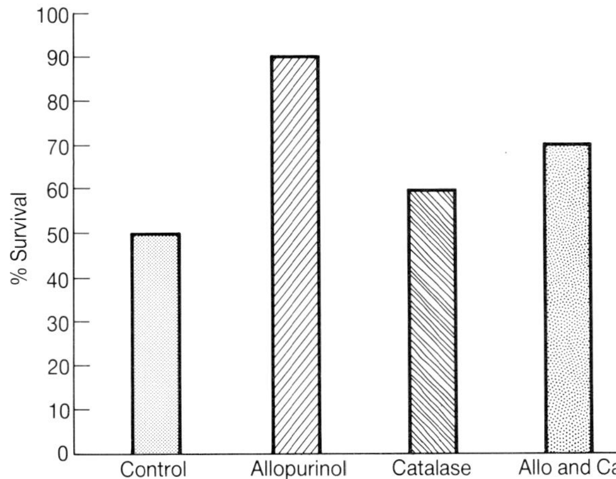

Fig. 20.4 A significant improvement in survival was noted after allopurinol (Allo) administration, alone or with catalase (Cat), in rats subjected to haemorrhagic shock prior to harvesting (modified from Cederna *et al.*[69]).

preservation times produced lower graft survival rates, unless modified by retransplantation of the failing liver. It is probable that the same events that modify the response of the kidney[60,61,62] and possibly the pancreas[63] might also occur in the liver. The liver appears to be very sensitive to ischaemia and preservation, and the immunogenicity of the liver might change after prolonged periods of ischaemia and/or preservation (Figures 20.2 and 20.3).

Reperfusion injury

The term 'reperfusion injury' has been recognised in recent years as a well defined clinical and pathological entity which occurs early during revascularisation.[64] The multitude of factors involved in the production of this lesion has made it difficult to determine the exact mechanism and site of revascularisation injury observed after liver transplantation.

The role of microvascular injury in the development of cellular damage after transplantation has recently occupied the interest of a great number of researchers.[65,66] During liver ischaemia or preservation injury, the production of free radicals, probably from the xanthine dehydrogenase/oxidase system, plays an important role in producing liver damage.[67,68] Drug therapy aimed at reducing free radical production might be the key to further reducing the damage seen after transplantation. Oxygen free radical scavengers or inhibitors of the xanthine oxidase pathway have been used before. Since 1975 we have utilised adenosine and allopurinol, among other substances, to protect ischaemically damaged liver allografts.[67,68] The results indicated some evidence of protection in the immediately transplanted livers.

In recent years, the protective effect of allopurinol, either alone or with catalase, on animals suffering from haemorrhagic shock has been established (Figure 20.4). The potential implication of these changes to multiple organ harvests is evident.[69] Further studies will be necessary, however, to extend the meaning of this finding to other species.

Recently, it has been demonstrated[40] that damage induced after storage and reperfusion, was specific for endothelial cells. The use of a solution containing concentration of electrolytes similar to plasma, with oncotic support based on hydroxyethyl starch, anti-oxidants such as allopurinol, desferroxamine and glutathione, vasodilators to improve microcirculation such as nicardipine and adenosine, substrates to regenerate adenosine triphosphate (ATP) such as fructose, and mildly acidic pH, has prevented some of the damage that occurs to sinusoidal endothelial cells with the alteration of the microcirculation due to reperfusion injury.[40] This protective effect should be taken into consideration when studying the immediate response of liver allograft recipients.

Conclusions

Advances in preservation have allowed for improved liver transplantation results. The limit of successful clinical liver preservation has remained at less than 24 hours. It is possible that further refining of the composition of the current solutions and better understanding of reperfusion injury will allow for improved preservation time and results after transplantation.

At present it is not possible to recognise, with any degree of certainty, the role that ischaemia and preservation might play in the modification of liver allograft survival. Only the comparison of prolonged preservation times would clarify the effect of this method on the immunological response of hepatic transplants.

References

1. Toledo-Pereyra LH. Kidney harvesting and preservation. In: *Kidney Transplantation*, Toledo-Pereyra LH (ed). Philadelphia: FA Davis Company, 1988.
2. Lambotte L. Liver preservation. In: *Basic Concepts in Organ Procurement, Perfusion and Preservation for Transplantation*, Toledo-Pereyra LH (ed). New York: Academic Press, 1982.
3. Starzl TE, Kaupp AH, Brock DR *et al.* Reconstructive problems in canine livers homotransplantation with special reference to the post-operative role of hepatic venous flow. *Surg Gynecol Obstet* 1960; **111,** 733.
4. Starzl TE, Marchioro TL, von Krauffa KN *et al.* Homotransplantation of the liver in humans. *Surg Gynecol Obstet* 1963; **117,** 659.
5. Collins GH, Bravo-Shugarman MB, Terasaki PI. Kidney preservation for transplantation. Initial perfusion and 30 hour ice storage. *Lancet* 1969; **2,** 1219.
6. Schalm SW, Terpstra JL, Drayer B *et al.* A simple method for short-term preservation of a liver homograft. *Transplantation* 1969; **8,** 887.
7. Belzer FO, May R, Berry MN. Short term preservation of porcine livers. *J Surg Res* 1970; **10,** 55.
8. Spilg H, Uys CJ, Hickman R *et al.* 12 hour liver preservation in the pig using hypothermic and hyperbaric oxygen. *Br J Surg* 1972; **59,** 273.
9. Toledo-Pereyra LH, Beselmeier TJ, Najarian JS. Protective effect of modified silica gel fraction (MSGF) on storage of canine livers for transplantation. *Trans Am Soc Artif Intern Organs* 1975; **21,** 79.
10. Toledo-Pereyra LH, Simmons RL, Najarian JS. Effect of allopurinol on preservation of ischemic kidneys perfused with plasma or plasma substitutes. *Ann Surg* 1975; **181,** 289.
11. Toledo-Pereyra LH, Chee M, Lillehei RC *et al.* Liver preservation by storage with hyperosmolar solutions for twenty-four hours. *Cryobiology* 1979; **16,** 43.
12. Toledo-Pereyra LH, MacKenzie GH, Baughman RD. Comparative results of prolonged hypo-

thermic storage of canine kidneys preserved with hyperosmolar colloid (TP-II) or crystalloid (Eurocollins) solution. *J Urol* 1983; **129,** 166.
13. Ploeg RJ, Goossens D, Belzer O *et al.* Successful 72-hour cold storage of dog kidneys with UW solution. *Transplantation* 1988; **46,** 191.
14. Jamieson NV, Sundberg R, Lindell S *et al.* Successful 24 to 30 hour preservation of the canine liver: a preliminary report. *Transplant Proc* 1988; **120,** 945.
15. Kalayoglu M, Sollinger HW, Stratta R *et al.* Extended preservation of the liver for clinical transplantation. *Lancet* 1988; **1,** 617.
16. Todo S, Nery J *et al.* Extended preservation of human liver grafts with UW solution. *J Am Med Assoc* 1989; **261,** 711.
17. Belzer FO. Clinical organ preservation with UW solution. *Transplantation* 1989; **47,** 1097.
18. Belzer FO, Kalayoglu M, D'Alessandro AM *et al.* Organ preservation: experience with University of Wisconsin solution and plans for the future. *Transplantation* 1990; **4,** 73.
19. D'Alessandro AM, Kalayoglu HW, Sollinger RM *et al.* Experience with Belzer UW cold storage solution in human liver transplantation. *Transplant Proc* 1990; **2,** 474.
20. Cooper J, Rettke J, Ludwig J *et al.* UW solution improves duration and quality of clinical liver preservation. *Transplant Proc* 1990; **2,** 477.
21. Todo S, Tzakis A, Starzl TE. Preservation of livers with UW or Eurocollins solution. *Transplantation* 1988; **46,** 925.
22. Cofer JB, Klintmalm GB, Howard TK *et al.* A comparison of UW with Eurocollins preservation solution in liver transplantation. *Transplantation* 1990; **49,** 1088.
23. Olthoff KM, Millis JM, Imagawa DK *et al.* Comparison of UW solution and Euro-Collins solutions for cold preservation of human liver grafts. *Transplantation* 1990; **49,** 284.
24. Stratta RJ, Wood RP, Langnas AN *et al.* Effect of extended preservation and reduced-size grafting on organ availability in pediatric liver transplantation. *Transplant Proc* 1990; **2,** 482.
25. Ferla G, Colledan M, Fassati LR *et al.* Liver cold storage using UW solution: clinical results in 23 consecutive transplants. *Transplant Proc* 1990; **2,** 480.
26. Toledo-Pereyra LH, Finkelstein I *et al.* Comparative analysis of colloid solutions for liver preservation: a bimodal distribution of solution on its protective effect. *Transplant Proc* 1990; **2,** 516.
27. Yu W, Coddington D, Bitter-Suermann H. Rat liver preservation. The components of UW that are essential to its success. *Transplantation* 1990; **49,** 1060.
28. Howden BO, Jablonski P, Thomas AC *et al.* Liver preservation with UW solution. Evidence that hydroxyethyl starch is not essential. *Transplantation* 1990; **49,** 869.
29. Nedelec JF, Capron-Laudereau M, Adam R *et al.* Mouse liver metabolism after 24-hour cold preservation using UW hydroxyethyl starch-free UW, and Euro-Collins solutions: a 31P, 13C NMR spectroscopy and biochemical analysis. *Transplant Proc* 1990; **2,** 492.
30. Boudjema K, van Gulik TM, Lindell SL *et al.* Effect of oxidized and reduced glutathione in liver preservation. *Transplantation* 1990; **50,** 948.
31. Jamieson NV, Lindell S, Sundberg R *et al.* An analysis of the components in UW using the isolated perfused rabbit liver. *Transplantation* 1988; **46,** 512.
32. Sundberg R, Ar'Rajab A, Ahren B. Improved liver preservation with UW solution by chlorpromazine donor pretreatment. *Transplant Proc* 1990; **2,** 508.
33. Toledo-Pereyra LH, Cederna J. Protection of liver allografts from ischemic damage prior to transplantation using insulin and catalase. In: *Oxygen Free Radicals in Shock*, Novelli GP and Ursini F, (eds). Florence: Krager 1985.
34. Castillo M, Toledo-Pereyra LH, Shapiro E *et al.* Protective effect of allopurinol, catalase, or superoxide dismutase in ischemic rat liver. *Transplant Proc* 1990; **2,** 490.
35. Toledo-Pereyra LH. Liver preservation: experimental and clinical observations. *Transplant Proc* 1988; **20,** 965.
36. Olson LM, Klintmalm GB, Husberg BS *et al.* Superoxide dismutase improves organ preservation in liver transplantation. *Transplant Proc* 1988; **20** (suppl 1), 961.
37. Takei Y, Marzi I, Kauffman FC *et al.* Increase in survival time of liver transplants by protease inhibitors and a calcium channel blocker, nisoldipine. *Transplantation* 1990; **50,** 14.
38. Ontell SJ, Makowka L, Ove P, Starzl TE. Improved hepatic function in the 24-hour preserved rat liver with UW-lactobionate solution and SRI 63–441. *Gastroenterology* 1988; **95,** 1617.
39. Moen J, Claesson K, Pienaar H, *et al.* Preservation of dog liver, kidney, and pancreas using the Belzer UW solution with a high-sodium and low-potassium content. *Transplantation* 1989; **47,** 940.
40. Currin R, Toole JG, Thurman RG, Lemasters JJ. Evidence that Carolina rinse solution protects sinusoidal endothelial cells against reperfusion injury after cold ischemic storage of rat liver. *Transplantation* 1990; **50,** 1076.
41. Lamesch P, Raygrotzki S, Kehrer G *et al.* Preservation of the liver with the HTK solution. *Transplant Proc* 1990; **2,** 518.
42. Calne RY, Williams R. Liver Transplantation. In:

Current Problems in Surgery, Ravitch MM (ed). Chicago: 1979.

43. Ascher NL, Freese DK, Paradis K *et al.* Rejection of the transplanted liver. In: *Transplantation of the Liver*, Maddrey WC (ed). New York: Elsevier, 1988.
44. Williams GM, Hume DM, Huson RP. 'Hyperacute' renal homograft rejection in man. *N Eng J Med* 1968; **279,** 611.
45. Hayry P Immunobiology of transplant rejection. *Ann Clin Res* 1981; **13,** 172.
46. Iwatsuki S, Iwaki Y, Kano T *et al.* Successful liver transplantation from crossmatch-positive donors. *Transplant Proc* 1981; **13,** 286.
47. Snover DC, Sibley RK, Freese DK *et al.* Orthotopic liver transplantation: a pathological study of 63 serial liver biopsies from 17 patients with specific reference to the diagnostic features and natural history of rejection. *Hepatology* 1984; **4,** 1212.
48. Snover DC, Freese DK, Sharp HL *et al.* Liver allograft rejection: an analysis of the use of biopsy in determining the outcome of rejection. *Am J Surg Pathol* 1987; **11,** 1.
49. Demetris AJ, Lasky S, van Thiel DH *et al.* Pathology of hepatic transplantation. A review of 62 adult allograft recipients immunosuppressed with a cyclosporine/steroid regimen. *Am J Pathol* 1985; **118,** 151.
50. Russell PS. Some immunological considerations in liver transplantation. *Hepatology* 1984; **4,** 76S.
51. Winn HJ, Baldamus CA, Jooste SV *et al.* Acute destruction by humoral antibody of rat skin grafted to mice. *J Exp Med* 1973; **137,** 893.
52. Demetris AJ, Lasey S, van Thiel DH *et al.* Induction of DR/Ia antigen in human liver allografts. *Transplantation* 1985; **40,** 504.
53. Takais L, Szend B, Monostari E *et al.* Expression of HLA-DR antigens in bile ducts of rejection liver transplants. *Lancet* 1985; **2,** 8365.
54. So SKS, Platt JL, Luckes LM *et al.* Cytolytic T lymphocyte-mediated injury of cultured hepatocytes as H-2 restricted. *Hepatology* 1985; **5,** 1017.
55. Davies H, Taylor JE, Daniel MR *et al.* Differences between pig tissues in the expression of major transplantation antigens: possible relevance for organ transplants. *J Exp Med* 1976; **143,** 987.
56. Davies H, Kamada N, Roser BJ. Mechanisms of donor-specific unresponsiveness induced by liver grafting. *Transplant Proc* 1983; **15,** 831.
57. Starzl TE. *Experience in hepatic transplantation.* Philadelphia: W.B. Saunders, 1969.
58. Starzl TE, Iwatsuki S, van Thiel DH *et al.* Evolution of liver transplantation. *Hepatology* 1982; **2,** 614.
59. So SKS, Platt JL, Ascher NL *et al.* Increased expression of class I major histocompatibility complex antigens on hepatocytes in rejecting human liver allografts. *Transplantation* 1987; **43,** 79.
60. Payne WD, Michels LD, Toledo-Pereyra LH *et al.* Effects of pulsatile perfusion on the immunogenicity of renal allograft. *J Surg Res* 1977; **22,** 380.
61. Toledo-Pereyra LH, Simmons RL, Moberg AW *et al.* Organ preservation in success of cadaver transplants. *Arch Surg* 1975; **110,** 1031.
62. Toledo-Pereyra LH, Simmons RL, Olson LC *et al.* Perfusion time and the survival of cadaver transplants. *Surgery* 1976; **79,** 377.
63. Sutherland DER, Moundry-Munns KC and Gillingham K. Results of pancreas transplantation in the UNOS Registry. In: *Clinical Transplantation*, Terasaki P (ed). Los Angeles: UCLA, 1989.
64. Toledo-Pereyra LH. Liver transplantation reperfusion injury. Factors in its development and avenues for treatment. *Klinische Woshenschrift* (in press).
65. McKeown CMB, Edwards V, Phillips MJ *et al.* Sinusoidal lining cell damage: the critical injury in cold preservation of liver allografts in the rat. *Transplantation* 1988; **46,** 178.
66. Toledo-Pereyra LH. The role of allopurinol and oxygen free radical scavengers in liver preservation. In: *Oxygen Radicals in Biology and Medicine*, Simic MG (ed). New York: Plenum Publishing Corp., 1989.
67. Toledo-Pereyra LH, Simmons RL, Najarian JS. Protection of the ischemic liver by donor pretreatment before transplantation. *Am J Surg* 1975; **129,** 513.
68. Toledo-Pereyra LH, Cederna J, Choudhury S. Oxygen free radicals, allopurinol and the xanthine oxidase pathway during liver ischemia. *Surg Res Comm* 1989; **5,** 297.
69. Cederna J, Bandlien K, Toledo-Pereyra LH *et al.* Effect of allopurinol and/or catalase on hemorrhagic shock and their potential application to multiple organ harvesting. *Transplant Proc* 1990; **22,** 444.
70. Howard TK, Kluitmalm CBC, Cofer JB, *et al.* The influence of preservation injury on rejection in the hepatic transplant recipient. *Transplantation*, 1990; **49,** 103.
71. Furukawa H, Todo S, Imventarza O, *et al.* Effect of cold ischemia time on the early outcome of human hepatic allografts preserved with UW solution. *Transplantation*, 1991; **51,** 1000.

21

Viral and opportunistic infection

J O'Grady, R Williams and S Sutherland

Introduction

The pharmacologically induced state of immunosuppression that is required to prevent rejection of the transplanted liver facilitates the development of a wide range of infections, ranging from nosocomial to true opportunistic infections. In addition, viral infections which caused or were associated with the original liver disease may recur after transplantation and the expression of these re-infections may be significantly altered by the immunosuppressive therapy. There is some evidence that the pattern and severity of these infections are, in part, influenced by the level of immunosuppression used, and in particular by the need to use the monoclonal antibody OKT3.[1-3]

Hepatitis viruses

Hepatitis A

Acute liver failure following hepatitis A is rare but increasing in some Western countries as a consequence of the delayed exposure to the virus,[4] and a number of such patients have undergone liver transplantation.[5-8] The data on recurrent disease are limited, but one study using both monoclonal antibody and *in situ* hybridisation techniques demonstrated the presence of HAV in liver tissue as early as seven days, and up to two and seven months after liver transplantation.[9] One of the cases described had a mild self-resolving hepatitis at two months that was attributed to hepatitis A on the basis of concurrent excretion of the virus in faeces. The second patient had evidence of persistent hepatitis A virus in the liver tissue until the graft was lost to chronic rejection at six months, but no clearcut episode of graft dysfunction could be attributed to it.

Hepatitis B and D

Infection from these viruses is a frequent indication for liver transplantation, either because of acute liver failure or more commonly because of end-stage chronic liver disease or hepatocellular carcinoma. Recurrence of the viral hepatitis B infection after transplantation has been shown to worsen the outcome, and two studies have shown significantly lower survival rates between one and five years after transplantation in these patients.[10,11] In cases of fulminant hepatic failure, studies suggest that in the majority of patients the virus has ceased to replicate by the time of admission to hospital. In two studies, HBeAg was detected in serum in 12% and 37% of patients, while in the latter only 9% of cases were seropositive for HBV DNA.[12,13] This would appear to suggest that, in theory, most patients with fulminant hepatitis B should not carry a risk of recurrent infection, although one study has documented re-infection in 87.5% of such cases after liver transplantation.[14]

Recurrence of HBV infection is a more predictable problem after transplantation in chronic carriers. The natural history of such re-infection was studied in 29 patients transplanted in the Cambridge and King's College Hospital joint programme between 1975 and April 1989, who did not receive systematic immunoprophylactic therapy.[11] The analysis was confined to patients who survived at least two months after transplantation. Of this cohort, 82% reverted to being chronic HBsAg carriers after liver transplantation, an identical figure to that observed in another single centre study of 45 patients, 39 of whom received aggressive immunoprophylaxis, with or without treatment with interferon, for up to six weeks after transplantation.[14] Four of the five patients who cleared HBsAg from serum did not have any evidence of HBV recurrence, while the fifth seroconverted after an acute hepatitic illness. None of these patients had any evidence of HBV replication (HBeAg and HBV DNA seronegative) at the time of transplantation. In contrast, 58% of those who re-infected with HBV had serological evidence of viral replication at the time of transplantation, and this increased to 88% after transplantation. Furthermore, the rate of HBV replication increased dramatically after transplantation in those patients who did not have a co-existing hepatitis D infection, with HBV DNA levels rising to >800 pg/40 µl serum in all but one case, as compared to the maximum observed level of 131 pg/40 µl serum prior to transplantation (Table 21.1). This is presumed to be a consequence of immunosuppressive therapy, especially the corticosteroid component.

The early reports of liver transplantation in patients with co-existing hepatitis D infection were inconsistent.[15–18] Two of the seven patients in the original description developed fulminant hepatic failure following liver transplantation,[15] but a later paper reported more favourable results when patients were maintained on low doses of HBIg.[17] Comparative data are now available from three series; in two, hepatitis D was associated with a better intermediate term prognosis with respect to HBV re-infection whether or not immunoprophylaxis was used,[19,11] while the third, in which immunoprophylaxis was used, found no significant difference between those with hepatitis B alone and those with hepatitis B and D infections.[14] Interestingly, the HBV DNA levels in serum after transplantation were found to be lower in patients with co-existing hepatitis D (range 8–797 pg/40 µl serum) than in a comparable group of patients with HBV infection alone (>800 pg/40 µl serum), suggesting that the hepatitis D virus is acting as a natural suppressor of HBV replication.[11]

Of the strategies that have been attempted to prevent HBV re-infection after liver transplantation, passive immunoprophylaxis with anti-HBs (HBIg) holds most promise. This was first described in 1975 in a 29 year old man with HBV infection and hepatocellular carcinoma who remains well with no evidence of recurrence of either condition 17 years later.[20] A total dose of 1100 ml of solution containing 10 g protein/100 ml was administered during the anhepatic phase of the transplant and again on the sixth postoperative day. Subsequently, passive immunoprophylaxis was widely used by other groups with diverse regimens and varying degrees of success.[14–17,21,22] The amounts of HBIg administered intra-operatively ranged from 500–128,000 units and the duration of therapy ranged up to one year. Some groups also used adjuvant active vaccination[14,15,22] or interferon therapy.[14] A recent report of 110 patients receiving high dose passive immunoprophylaxis showed an overall actuarial recurrence rate of 29% over a two year period.[19] However, the equivalent figures for three subgroups indicated that most failures occurred in patients with chronic HBV infection (59% recurrence), as compared to patients with hepatitis B and D chronic infection (13%) or fulminant hepatic failure (0%). Within the former group, recurrence of HBV infection was almost universal (96%) in those patients who had HBV DNA detectable in serum at the time of transplantation, as compared to 29% in the HBV DNA seronegative cohort.[19] The cost/benefit ratio for passive immunoprophylaxis suggests its administration

Table 21.1 Recurrence of hepatitis B virus (HBV) after liver transplantation in the King's College Hospital and Cambridge series without the use of long term HBIg

Category	Number	Pretransplant HBV DNA	Post-transplant HBV DNA	HBV recurrence	Graft loss to HBV
Hepatitis B alone – without replication	9	0	130 → 800	7 (77.8%)	4 (44.4%)
Hepatitis B alone – with replication	11	10–131	>800	11 (100%)	7 (63.6%)
Hepatitis B and D	9	0–15	0–797	7 (77.8%)	1 (11.1%)

should be confined to patients who are HBV DNA seronegative at the time of transplantation, although an amelioration of the pathological sequelae of HBV recurrence in the remaining patients cannot be excluded at this time. No clear role for other antiviral agents has yet been defined post-transplantation. Interferon has been used in a small number of cases but the available data are insufficient to justify a conclusion as to its efficacy.[23,24]

The impact of HBV replication on graft function is variable and a wide range of histological patterns of disease have been described. A minority of patients have no biochemical or histological evidence of liver disease secondary to hepatitis B over periods ranging up to six years.[11,25] About half of the patients develop an acute hepatitis after re-infection, which is indistinguishable histologically from acute hepatitis B in immunocompetent patients, apart from a possible reduction in the intensity of the inflammatory infiltrate.[25] This hepatitic illness is self-limiting in most cases, although a small number develop fulminant hepatic failure leading to death or retransplantation.[11,25] Those patients who have been retransplanted in this situation have shown an even earlier recurrence of fulminant hepatic failure.[14] Chronic disease in the graft related to hepatitis B ranges from chronic persistent or active hepatitis to a rapid progression to cirrhosis.[25,26] A case of *de novo* development of a hepatocellular carcinoma in association with cirrhosis four years after transplantation has recently been described.[27] However, the most fascinating pattern of disease is a unique clinical and histological syndrome termed fibrosing cholestatic hepatitis (FCH). The clinical features are of progressive jaundice in association with a rapidly rising prothrombin time and loss of the graft within 4–6 weeks of clinical presentation.[11] The abnormalities seen in the liver enzyme profile are remarkably mild considering the severity of the disease process; in particular, a marked increase in serum transaminase levels is unusual. The histological features are of extensive serpiginous periportal fibrosis, canalicular and cellular cholestasis with prominent cytoplasmic HBsAg and HBeAg expression.[26] High level expression of intracellular HBsAg and HBcAg has been documented in these cases,[28] and a direct cytopathic role for the virus has been proposed.[25,28] The only possible treatment for this manifestation of HBV infection is retransplantation, but to date the results have been very poor because of high early post-operative mortality or aggressive recurrence of FCH.

Non-A, non-B hepatitis and hepatitis C

The new serological tests for hepatitis C indicate that this represents a subset of the condition previously described as presumed non-A, non-B viral hepatitis. In an American study of patients with acute presumed non-A, non-B viral hepatitis, antibodies to hepatitis C were found in 61% of intravenous drug abusers, 33% of post-transfusion cases and 22% of sporadic infections.[29] The detection rate was higher in chronic infection, being 89%, 71% and 27% in the respective groups.[29] The vast majority of patients with acute hepatic failure attributed to presumed non-A, non-B hepatitis are sporadic cases and most are seronegative for hepatitis C.[30,31]

The emerging data with respect to the frequency and impact of recurrent hepatitis C infection after liver transplantation are somewhat conflicting, although the problem is considerably less than with hepatitis B. In one study of six patients who were seropositive at the time of transplantation, two developed clinically significant graft dysfunction attributed to viral re-infection, and one of these lost two grafts through the rapid development of cirrhosis.[32] Another study of 44 patients with post-hepatitis cirrhosis detected antibodies to hepatitis C in 91% and there was associated graft dysfunction in 48% of cases.[33] When the more sensitive polymerase chain reaction (PCR) technique was used in a further study to detect HCV RNA after transplantation, 65% were found to be positive and 73% of these were judged to have a related histological hepatitis.[34] The estimates for the *de novo* acquisition of hepatitis C infection during the transplant range from 0–40%, and in the latter study 75% of these cases developed clinical disease.[32,34]

A toga-like virus was isolated from the liver of one patient with fulminant hepatic failure attributed to presumed non-A, non-B hepatitis, and was also in two grafts explanted at two and ten days.[35] The first graft was removed because of size related mechanical problems, but the second was removed as a result of graft failure with the clinical and histological characteristics of non-thrombotic graft infarction. Similar viruslike particles were identified in another patient with a similar clinical course, but this case was complicated by the co-existence of severe gram-negative sepsis at the time of graft loss.[36] It has yet to be proven that these apparent viral particles represent another cause of non-A, non-B hepatitis.

Other viral infections

Cytomegalovirus (CMV)

This is recognised as the single most important pathogen following liver transplantation. The outcome for the patient with an active CMV infection depends not only on the severity of the infection and the degree of endogenous immunosuppression it may induce, but also on many other factors such as the intensity of pharmacological immunosuppression, the number and severity of rejection episodes, the donor–recipient HLA match, the type and timing of anti-CMV therapy and the other opportunistic infections that may co-exist.

CMV infections may be acquired from an exogenous source or result from re-activation of latent endogenous virus. The donor organ and transfused blood are recognised sources, especially posing a problem for the seronegative recipient but also potentially a source of re-infection for seropositive recipients. The seroprevalence in donors and recipients varies with age, socio-economic status, ethnic, geographic and cultural characteristics. In Europe and North America about 50–70% of adults and about 20% of paediatric recipients will be seropositive pretransplant.

Infections may be symptomatic or asymptomatic, though in general primary infections are more likely than secondary infections to show clinical manifestations – 88% compared with 32%.[2] The incidence of CMV infections following liver transplantation, between 45% and 78%,[2,37,38] is similar to that seen in kidney and heart recipients (32% and 34%), but the rate of symptomatic infections in liver and heart recipients (32% and 34%) is much greater than in renal recipients (8%) on the same immunosuppressive regimen.[39] Asymptomatic infections are detected by culturing virus from urine or by demonstrating rising antibody titres in serum. The severity of symptomatic infections ranges from a febrile illness to disseminated life-threatening multiple organ involvement. The fever is characteristically a high swinging fever with a median onset at 28 days and duration of 2–3 weeks. It may be accompanied by muscle aches particularly of the back and thighs. Less frequently, arthralgia or thrombocytopenic purpura may be present.[39] Clinical disease may manifest as involvement of a single solid organ, most commonly the liver.[40] More severe infections show widespread dissemination with additional involvement of the lungs, gastro-intestinal tract and bone marrow. Pneumonitis is the life-threatening complication which requires early detection if it is to be successfully treated. Chorioretinitis has been documented, but is a late feature usually presenting six or more months after transplantation,[41] while rare manifestations include skin lesions, endometritis and encephalopathy.[42–44] Laboratory investigations reflect the pattern of disease and the abnormalities include leucopenia, atypical lymphocytosis, thrombocytopenia and a cholestatic pattern of liver enzymes. Radiological evidence of pneumonitis with scattered areas of consolidation on chest X-ray is a relatively late finding, and patients with primary infections are best monitored using blood gas analysis to detect hypoxaemia and so identify the earliest phase of this complication. Such patients should always be subjected to broncho-alveolar lavage to establish the diagnosis and to screen for co-existing opportunistic pathogens which are especially common in this situation. The classical histological evidence of CMV hepatitis on liver biopsy is the identification of inclusion bodies, but these are seen in only a minority of cases. More frequently the sentinel finding of a small cluster of neutrophils in the lobular parenchyma is observed. However, most cases of CMV hepatitis are diagnosed by using immunohistochemistry or *in situ* hybridisation techniques.[45,46]

The mortality from CMV infection prior to the introduction of ganciclovir ranged from none in one study,[1] to accounting for two-thirds of post-transplant deaths in another series of 26 paediatric liver transplant recipients.[47] In the latter study the overall incidence of CMV infection was similar to that seen in adults, 54%, but six of the 14 children with CMV infection died in spite of treatment with ganciclovir and immunoglobulins or foscarnet. All had received livers from seropositive donors, and had been treated with either ALG or OKT3. The high mortality rate may reflect the delay in commencing specific antiviral therapy until tissue confirmation of the diagnosis of CMV pneumonitis was established. However, in a larger series of 84 children, the incidence of CMV disease was found to be lower than in adults, 27.4% versus 39.4% although a significantly higher risk for children being transplanted for post-necrotic cirrhosis as compared to metabolic disease was identified.[40] A similar trend was not evident amongst the adult patients in the same series.

The effect of immunosuppression on CMV infections differs depending on the immunosuppressive drugs used.[48] Some, such as OKT3, tend to re-activate latent infection, while others like cyclosporin, by preventing the normal controlling response, allow widespread dissemination of either primary or secondary infections. Some studies have suggested that the benefits of OKT3 prophylaxis were achieved at the expense of a significant increase in viral infections,[49] but others were unable to detect a significant difference in CMV infection rates comparing OKT3 with cyclosporin induced immunosuppression.[50]

The conventional ways of diagnosing CMV infection by isolating virus in tissue culture, detecting seroconversion or rising antibody titres are not satisfactory for giving rapid laboratory confirmation, since the virus is slow growing and antibodies may not be detectable for ten days to two weeks after onset of symptoms of an active CMV infection. Several other techniques have been developed in recent years but are not universally available. The combination of culture with detection of immediate early antigens by specific monoclonal antibodies can give a rapid answer within 24–48 hours and is the most widely available of the rapid methods (Figure 21.1). It is excellent for detecting CMV in bronchial washings or urine and can be used with blood samples though less successfully. One of the earliest markers of an active CMV infection is the detection of antigenaemia; however this method is extremely labour intensive, gives problems in interpretation and false negatives are frequent if specimen processing is delayed even for a few hours. Gene amplification

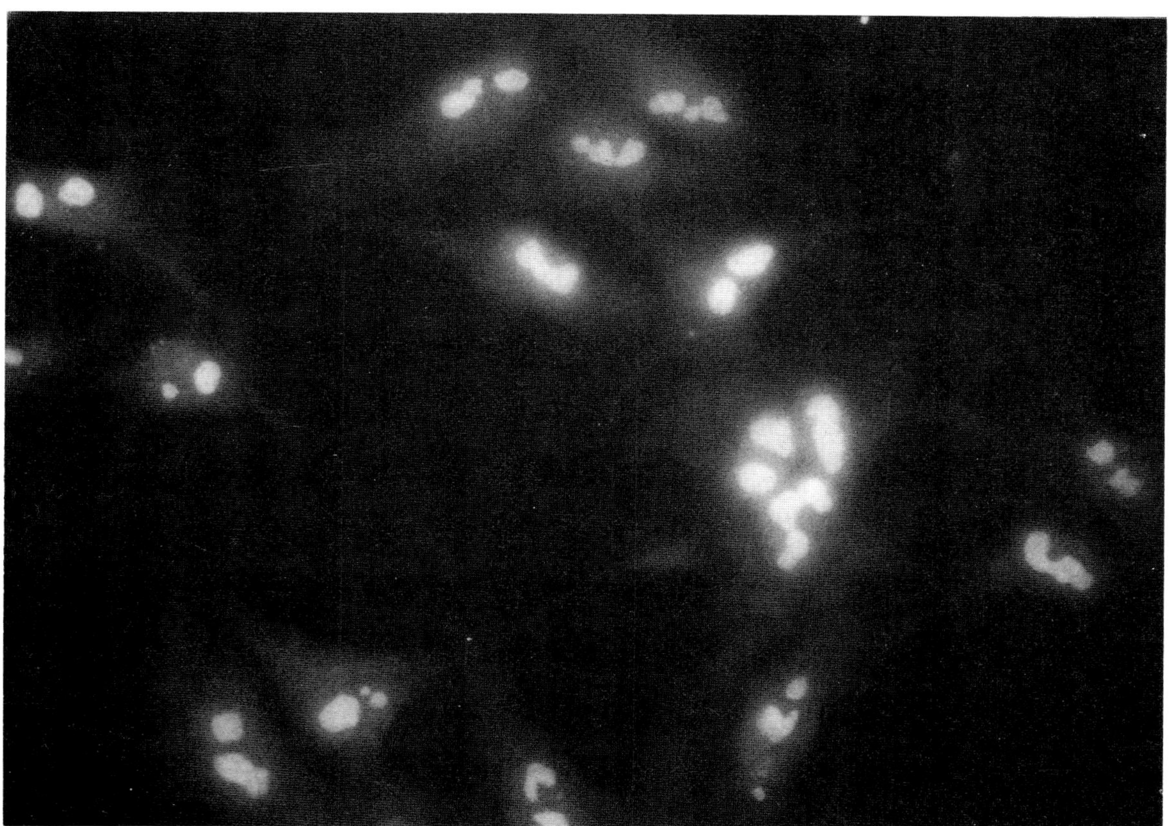

Fig. 21.1 Rapid CMV diagnosis – early nuclear fluorescence detected following culture of broncho-alveolar washings for 48 hours using CMV specific mononuclear antibody.

organs and saliva of relatives, friends and staff are all likely sources.

In one large study, 92% of 1214 adults and 50% of 253 children were EBV antibody positive at transplant.[66] Following transplant, 33% of seropositive adults and 48% of seropositive children had serological evidence of re-activation, while primary infections developed in 82% and 77% of seronegative adults and children respectively. In the children receiving liver transplants, the mean incubation time for primary infections was 66 days and for re-activations 61 days post-transplant.[67] Only two of the children with primary infections had symptoms attributable to EBV. However, another series identified seroconversion in 12 of 19 (63.3%) seronegative paediatric liver recipients 2–3 months after transplantation, and 11 (91%) of these had clinical signs.[68] These included pharyngitis or tonsillits 5, splenomegaly 4, lymphadenopathy 3, hepatomegaly 3, fever 2 and purpura 1. EBV re-activation is generally asymptomatic.

EBV associated lymphoproliferation was described in 19 renal transplant recipients in 1983, with an overall incidence of 1.2%.[69] The risk of a post-transplant patient developing lymphoma was assessed at 350 times greater than in immunocompetent subjects. Serological studies indicated that only two of these patients had primary infections, about half had re-activations and the remainder had markers of past infection. Three patterns of lymphoproliferation have been identified:

1. Diffuse polymorphic B cell hyperplasia with no evidence of cytogenetic abnormalities which presents clinically as EBV mononucleosis;
2. A polymorphic B cell tumour which progresses from polyclonality to monoclonality with cytogenetic abnormalities; and
3. Single extranodal malignant tumours which tend to involve the central nervous system or intestine.[66,69]

A later study reported 20 cases of the lymphoproliferative syndrome in 1467 patients transplanted between 1981 and 1985.[66] This gave an incidence of 0.8% in adults and 4% in children, with ten of 11 lymphoproliferative syndrome cases in children following primary EBV infections. Three later studies have identified an increased risk of post-transplant lymphoproliferative syndrome associated with the use of OKT3 for treatment of rejection in renal, cardiac and paediatric liver transplant recipients, respectively.[70–2] The risk of lymphoproliferative syndrome in 124 paediatric liver recipients transplanted between 1984 and 1989 and who received OKT3 for rejection was quantified at 14% (five of 36), compared to 4.5% (four of 88) when OKT3 was not given.[72] Three of the five patients in the OKT3 group with the lymphoproliferative syndrome had primary EBV infection, as compared to only two of 31 in the OKT3 group without LPS. Thus, the combination of a primary EBV infection with OKT3 led to a significantly increased risk of lymphoproliferative syndrome in paediatric liver transplant recipients.

The diagnosis of primary EBV infection is made serologically by detection of heterophile antibody, EBV viral capsid (VCA) IgM or a seroconversion to EBV VCA IgG. Two other markers may be helpful in assessing the EBV status, particularly in patients whose EBV IgM has become undetectable. These are the antibodies to early antigen (EA) and to nuclear antigen (EBNA). After primary and persistent infections EA antibodies appear late. High persistent EA and EBNA antibodies are present in re-activated infection, while in recent primary or chronic persistent EBV infections, the EBNA antibodies are absent or low. An inactive past EBV infection is characterised by low or absent EA antibodies, while EBNA is detectable.[66]

Biopsies from EBV related tumours are classified in several ways by the use of histology, immunologic cell typing, cytogenetic studies, EBV markers and cell adhesion markers.[69,73,74] A range of tumour types may be detected from polyclonal B cell proliferation to monoclonal B cell lymphomas. Those tumours showing polyclonal B cell proliferation may be subdivided into those with no detectable cytogenetic abnormalities and those which, in spite of having polyclonal immunological markers, also show monoclonal expansion of cells with malignant features.[66,69,75] In the majority of post-transplant tumours EBV markers are present. EBV genome can be detected by hybridisation or gene amplification techniques and the antigens characteristic of a latent infection, EBNA 1 and 2 and latent membrane protein (LMP), are usually present while the lytic cycle markers, early antigen and membrane antigen are absent. This differs markedly from the pattern of markers detected in Burkitt's lymphoma where only EBNA 1 and no LMP is expressed.[73]

The prognosis and response to treatment relates closely to the type of presentation. In most primary EBV infections no treatment will be necessary. Resolution of the lymphoproliferative syndrome has been reported after reduction in immunosuppression[72] and consequently this is now considered mandatory in all symptomatic cases. In addition, intravenous acyclovir appears to be useful, especially in those cases with polyclonal proliferation.[69] Surgery may be sufficient in some patients with extranodal malignant tumours. In those where the tumour did not regress, chemotherapy or radiotherapy for lymphoma was not found to be useful.[76]

Human immunodeficiency virus (HIV)

HIV infection may be latent at the time of transplantation, or may be acquired during transplantation through the donor organ or unscreened blood products.[77–82] The experience at centres who have knowingly or unknowingly transplanted livers to HIV positive recipients has been that AIDS-free survival following transplant correlated directly with the CD4 count at the time of transplantation, and inversely with age.[82] Haemophiliacs appeared to survive for shorter periods than other HIV positive recipients, but this may simply reflect a longer seropositive period pre transplant.[82,83] One adult HIV positive liver recipient transplanted in 1982 has remained AIDS free for over eight years[84] and several children have remained AIDS-free for 5–6 years.[83] The best available long term survival data currently available relate to 25 transplant patients, including 15 liver recipients, seven of whom were HIV positive at transplant and eight were seronegative but seroconverted following transplantation.[83] Both survival and the time to development of AIDS was similar in these two groups up to five years post-transplant. At 4.5 years post-transplant, 47% of the 15 were alive and well. When the HIV positive group were compared with liver transplants overall, there was no difference in survival at one year but by five years survival was 53% in the HIV positive group compared with 63% overall. Survival was better in those who did not develop rejection, while children were less likely than adults to die from an AIDS related disease. In at least one liver transplant case with AIDS, cessation of immunosuppression did not lead to rejection of the liver.[85]

It is obviously important that all organ donors should be screened for HIV antibody and that individuals with high risk behaviour who may be HIV infected but have not seroconverted should not be blood or organ donors. Since it is not always possible to identify risk status in a donor, there remains a small risk of HIV transmission.

Miscellaneous viruses

Other viruses that cause latent infections, such as adenoviruses, polyomaviruses (wart virus and papovaviruses), JC and BK, can re-activate following transplantation due to the long term immunosuppression. The papovavirus JC causes progressive multifocal leuco-encephalopathy (PML) in chronically immunosuppressed individuals and is a potential problem in the long term. Similarly, anxieties raised in women with AIDS about increased risk from carcinoma of the cervix due to re-activation of wart virus might justify more frequent cervical screening in the transplant recipient.[86]

Most cases of adenoviral hepatitis reported in transplanted patients have died.[87] The majority were children with congenital immunodeficiencies who manifested such features of acute liver failure as coagulopathy, encephalopathy and gastrointestinal tract bleeding. Adenovirus induced liver failure has also been seen in children after liver transplantion.[87,88] Adenoviral infections, usually caused by serotypes 1 and 2, developed in 22 of 262 paediatric liver transplant recipients in one series. Most of the children recovered uneventfully, but five cases developed hepatitis and the virus isolated in each instance was serotype 5. A later study reported that ten of 393 (2.5%) paediatric liver transplants developed adenoviral hepatitis during a seven month period, with a 30% case fatality rate.[88] Once again, the predominant serotype was adenovirus 5. This serotype was also isolated from blood, stool, urine, lungs and liver of a child who died five days after retransplantation, necessitated by massive acute rejection of the first liver which was retrieved from a donor who died following surgery for intussusception.[89] Adenovirus antigens were detected in the first and second transplanted livers but not in the patient's original liver. Since adenovirus is known to be associated with intussusception, it is likely that the virus was transmitted to the patient with the first liver transplanted and then infected the liver transplanted 12 days later.

In another case of disseminated adenovirus infection, the virus, probably the child's own, was also transmitted to both the first and second transplants, causing failure in both livers.[90] In this report it was suggested that, since the adenovirus 7 isolate was found in retrospect to be sensitive *in vitro* to ganciclovir, treatment with this agent should be considered in future cases.[90]

Fungal and other opportunistic infections

Opportunist fungal and protozoal infections present a major hazard after liver transplantation. The commonest fungal infections are with *Candida* spp and *Aspergillus* spp. Liver transplant recipients have been reported to have a higher incidence of invasive fungal infection than other transplant recipients,[91] and the risk is greatest in those patients transplanted for acute liver failure, patients with chronic rejection and those who have required aggressive anti-rejection therapy. *Aspergillus* is a particularly common co-existing pathogen in patients with CMV pneumonitis. The incidence of fungal infection has been reported to be as high as 48%, with *Aspergillus fumigatus* being isolated in eight of 46 (17%) liver recipients in one series.[92] Three of the eight survived following treatment with either intravenous amphotericin B or itraconazole. The remainder died and at autopsy *Aspergillus* was identified in the lungs of all, the brain in two and the thyroid and abdominal cavity of one. However, another study found evidence of cerebral *Aspergillus* in 90% of the cases with *Aspergillus pneumonitis*, and highlighted a seasonal predisposition during the winter and spring months.[93] The former study identified *Candida albicans* colonisation in 23 (50%) of their patients and invasive yeast infections in seven (15%).[92] A more recent report identified disseminated fungal infections in 38% with a mortality rate of 73%.[94]

Candida infections are commonest in the first month after transplant, and were identified in 63% of liver transplant patients in one series.[1] Disseminated *Candida* infections were detected in 14% of the children during the first month after transplant and a further 23% showed colonisation at the time. Although 40% of the adults had colonisation, none developed dissemination in the first four weeks. These authors concluded that rates of infection were higher in those patients who required treatment with ALG or OKT3. *Candida albicans* colonisation can be detected by culture from routinely collected throat swabs, sputum, faeces, urine, bile and drain effluent. *Candida* oesophagitis commonly presents as odinophagia, despite the use of prophylactic antifungals. Culture from blood or vascular cannulae, or from two of the above sites, requires systemic treatment in most instances, while single site infections are usually treated with topical antifungals.

The pattern of infection with other mycoses differs with geographical susceptibility, and in some parts of the United States *coccidiomycosis, blastomycosis* and *histoplasmosis* are reasonably frequently encountered. *Nocardia asteroides* can be difficult to diagnose because of the usual absence of a fever, and the main sites involved are lungs, brain and skin.[95] *Listeria monocytogenes* may present with an acute meningitis or focal lesions within the brain, while *Cryptococcus neoformans* causes a subacute or chronic meningitis. The incidence of *Pneumocystis carinii* infections is considered sufficient by some centres to justify prophylactic therapy with co-trimoxazole after liver transplantation, although most confine this practice to the cohort that required treatment with OKT3. *Legionella* spp outbreaks have been reported amongst immunosuppressed patients in hospital, and have been traced to shower heads in wards and to water cooling towers of air conditioning systems.[96] Mycobacterial, including atypical, infections occur with increased frequency in liver transplant recipients and manifestations include pulmonary infection, peritonitis, meningitis, bone infections and chronic cryptic miliary tuberculosis. The choice of antitubercular drugs is sometimes complicated by the presence of impaired graft function or consideration of interactions with elements of the immunosuppression regimen, but in most instances streptomycin, isoniazid and ethambutol is a reasonable first line approach.

References

1. Ascher NL, Stock PG, Bumgardner GL, Payne WD, Najarian JS. Infection and rejection of primary hepatic transplant in 93 consecutive patients treated with triple immunosuppressive therapy. *Surg Gynec Obstet* 1988; **167,** 474–484.

2. Singh N, Dummer JS, Kusne S *et al.* Infections with cytomegalovirus and other herpesviruses in 121 liver transplant recipients: transmission by donated organ and the effect of OKT3 antibodies. *J Inf Dis* 1988; **158,** 124–131.
3. Shaw BW, Wood RP, Stratta RJ, Pillen TJ, Langnas AN. Stratifying the causes of death in liver transplant recipients: an approach to improving survival. *Arch Surg* 1989; **124,** 895–900.
4. Forbes A, Williams R. Increasing age – an important adverse prognostic factor in hepatitis A virus infection. *J Roy Coll Phys* 1988; **22,** 237–239.
5. Bismuth H, Samuel D, Gugenheim J *et al.* Emergency liver transplantation for fulminant hepatitis. *Ann Intern Med* 1987; **107,** 337–341.
6. O'Grady JG, Alexander GJM, Thick M, Potter D, Calne RY, Williams R. Outcome of orthotopic liver transplantation in the aetiological and clinical variants of acute liver failure. *Quart J Med* 1988; **69,** 817–824.
7. Schafer DF, Shaw BW. Fulminant hepatic failure and orthotopic liver transplantation. *Sem Liver Dis* 1989; **9,** 189–194.
8. Brems JJ, Hiatt JR, Ramming KP *et al.* Fulminant hepatic failure: the role of liver transplantation as primary therapy. *Am J Surg* 1987; **154,** 137–141.
9. Fagan E, Yousef G, Brahm J *et al.* Persistence of hepatitis A virus in fulminant hepatitis and after liver transplantation. *J Med Virol* 1990; **30,** 131–136.
10. Iwatsuki S, Starzl TE, Todo S *et al.* Experience in 1000 liver transplants under cyclosporine-steroid therapy: a survival report. *Transplant Proc* 1988; **20,** 498–504.
11. O'Grady JG, Smith HM, Davies SE *et al.* Hepatitis B virus reinfection after orthotopic liver transplantation: serological and clinical implications. *J Hepatol* 1992; **14,** 104–111.
12. Gimson AES, Tedder RS, White YS, Eddleston ALWF, Williams R. Serological markers in fulminant hepatitis B. *Gut* 1983; **24,** 615–617.
13. Brechot C, Bernuau J, Thiers V *et al.* Multiplication of hepatitis B virus in fulminant hepatitis B. *Br Med J* 1984; **288,** 270–271.
14. Todo S, Demetris AJ, van Thiel D, Teperman L, Fung JJ, Starzl TE. Orthotopic liver transplantation for patients with hepatitis B virus-related liver disease. *Hepatology* 1991: **13,** 619–626.
15. Rizzetto M, Macagno S, Chiaberge E *et al.* Liver transplantation in hepatitis delta virus disease. *Lancet* 1987; **ii,** 469–471.
16. Reynes M, Zignego L, Samuel D *et al.* Graft hepatitis delta virus reinfection after orthotopic liver transplantation in HDV cirrhosis. *Transplant Proc* 1989; **21,** 2424–2425.
17. Colledan M, Grendele M, Gridelli B *et al.* Long-term results after liver transplantation in B and delta hepatitis. *Transplant Proc* 1989; **21,** 2421–2423.
18. Agnes S, Avolio AW, Magalini SC *et al.* Results of liver transplantation for hepatitis delta disease without immunoprophylaxis. *Transplant Proc* 1989; **21,** 2426–2428.
19. Samuel D, Bismuth A, Mathieu D *et al.* Passive immunoprophylaxis after liver transplantation in HBsAg-positive patients. *Lancet* 1991; **337,** 813–815.
20. Johnson PJ, Wansbcrough-Jones MH, Portmann B *et al.* Familial HBsAg-positive hepatoma: treatment with orthotopic liver transplantation and specific immunoglobulin. *Br Med J* 1978; **i,** 216.
21. Demetris AJ, Jaffe R, Sheahan DG *et al.* Recurrent hepatitis B in liver allograft recipients: differentiation between viral hepatitis B and rejection. *Am J Pathol* 1986; **125,** 161–172.
22. Lauchart W, Muller R, Pichlmayr R. Immunoprophylaxis of hepatitis B virus reinfection in recipients of human liver allografts. *Transplant Proc* 1987; **19,** 2387–2389.
23. Rakela J, Wooten RS, Batts KP, Perkins JD, Taswell HF, Krom RAF. Failure of interferon to prevent recurrent hepatitis B infection in hepatic allograft. *Mayo Clin Proc* 1989; **64,** 429–432.
24. Mancini C, Gaeta A, Lorino G *et al.* Alpha interferon therapy in patients with hepatitis infection undergoing organ transplantation. *Transplant Proc* 1989; **21,** 2429–2430.
25. Demetris AJ, Todo S, van Thiel DH *et al.* Evolution of hepatitis B virus liver disease after hepatic replacement: practical and theoretical considerations. *Am J Pathol* 1990; **137,** 667–676.
26. Davies S, Portmann B, O'Grady JG *et al.* Hepatic histological findings after transplantation for chronic hepatitis B virus infection, including a unique pattern of fibrosing cholestatic hepatitis. *Hepatology* 1991; **13,** 150–157.
27. Luketic V, Shiffman ML, McCall JB, Posner MP, Mills AS, Carithers RL. Primary hepatocellular carcinoma after orthotopic liver transplantation for chronic hepatitis B infection. *Ann Int Med* 1991; **114,** 212–213.
28. Lau JYN, Bain VG, Davies SE *et al.* High level expression of hepatitis B viral antigens in fibrosing cholestastic hepatitis: evidence that HBV may be cytopathic in liver grafts. *Gastroenterology* (in press).
29. McHutchinson JG, Kuo G, Houghton M, Choo QL, Redeker AG. Hepatitis C virus antibodies in acute icteric and chronic non-A, non-B hepatitis. *Gastroenterology* 1991; **101,** 1117–1119.
30. Wright T, Hsu H, Donegan E *et al.* Hepatitis C virus not found in fulminant non-A, non-B hepatitis. *Ann Int Med* 1991; **115,** 111–113.
31. O'Grady JG, Smith HM, Sutherland S, Sheron N, Williams R. Low detection of hepatitis C anti-

bodies in serum after liver transplantation (abstract). *J Hepatol* 1990; **11,** S47.

32. Martin P, Munoz SJ, di Bisceglie AM *et al.* Recurrence of hepatitis C virus infection after liver transplantation. *Hepatology* 1991; **13,** 719–721.
33. Samuel D, David MF, Gigou M, Ait-Arkoub Z, Reynes M, Bismuth H. Liver transplantation for post-hepatitis cirrhosis (abstract). *Hepatology* 1991; **14,** 53A.
34. Wright TL, Ferrell L, Donegan E *et al.* Impact of hepatitis C viral (HCV) infection on the allograft following liver transplantation (abstract). *Hepatology* 1991; **14,** 51A.
35. Fagan EA, Ellis DS, Tovey GM *et al.* Toga-like virus as a cause of fulminant hepatitis attributed to sporadic non-A, non-B. *J Med Virol* 1989; **28,** 150–155.
36. Fagan EA, Ellis DS, Portmann B, Tovey GM, Williams R, Zuckerman AJ. Microbial structures in a patient with sporadic non-A, non-B fulminant hepatitis treated by liver transplantation. *J Med Virol* 1987; **22,** 189–198.
37. Rakela J, Wiesner RH, Taswell HF *et al.* Incidence of cytomegalovirus infection and its relationship to donor-recipient serologic status in liver transplantation. *Transplant Proc* 1987; **19,** 2399–2402.
38. Paya CV, Herman PE, Wiesner RH *et al.* Cytomegalovirus hepatitis in liver transplantation: Prospective analysis of 93 consecutive orthotopic liver transplantations. *J Inf Dis* 1989; **160,** 752–758.
39. Dummer JS. Cytomegalovirus infection after liver transplantation: clinical manifestations and strategies for prevention. *Rev Inf Dis* 1990; **12,** S767–775.
40. Stratta RJ, Shaefer MS, Markin RS *et al.* Clinical patterns of cytomegalovirus disease after liver transplantation. *Arch Surg* 1989; **124,** 1443–1450.
41. Rubin RH. The indirect effects of cytomegalovirus infection on the outcome of organ transplantation. *J Am Med Assoc* 1989; **261,** 3607–3609.
42. Elenitsas R, Cohen BA. Generalised eruption in a liver transplant patient. *Arch Dermatol* 1990; **126,** 1497–1502.
43. Sayage L, Gunby R, Gonwa T, Husberg B, Goldstein R, Klintmalm G. Cytomegalovirus and endometritis after liver transplantation. *Transplantation* 1990; **49,** 815–817.
44. Power C, Poland SD, Kassim KH, Kaufmann JC, Rice GP. Encephalopathy in liver transplantation: neuropathology and CMV infection. *Can J Neurol Sci* 1990; **17,** 378–381.
45. Naoumov NV, Alexander GJM, O'Grady JG, Aldis P, Portmann BC, Williams R. Rapid diagnosis of cytomegalovirus infection by *in situ* hybridisation in the liver graft. *Lancet* 1988; **i,** 1361–1364.
46. Paya CV, Holley KE, Wiesner RH *et al.* Early diagnosis of cytomegalovirus hepatitis in liver transplant recipients: role of immunostaining, DNA hybridization and culture of hepatic tissue. *Hepatology* 1990; **12,** 19–26.
47. King SM, Petric M, Superina R, Graham N, Roberts EA. Cytomegalovirus infections in paediatric liver transplantations. *Am J Dis Child* 1990; **144,** 1307–1310.
48. Rubin RH. Impact of cytomegalovirus infection on organ transplant recipients. *Rev Inf Dis* 1990; **12,** S754–766.
49. Cosimi AB, Jenkins RL, Rohner RJ, Delmonico FL, Hoffman M, Monaco AP. A randomised clinical trial of prophylactic OKT3 monoclonal antibody in liver allograft recipients. *Arch Surg* 1990; **125,** 781–785.
50. Muhlbacher F, Steininger R, Lange F *et al.* Prophylaxis with OKT3 for liver transplantation. *Transplant Proc* 1989; **21,** 2253–2254.
51. Sutherland S, Bracken P, Wreghitt TG, O'Grady J, Williams R. The donated organ as a source of cytomegalovirus in orthotopic liver transplantation. *J Med Virol* (in press).
52. Ho M. Circulating cytomegalovirus and Epstein-Barr virus-infected cells and transfusions. *Transplant Proc* 1988; **20,** 1118–1120.
53. Plotkin SA, Smiley MC, Friedman HM *et al.* Towne-vaccine-induced prevention of cytomegalovirus disease after renal transplants. *Lancet* 1984; **i,** 528–530.
54. Winston DJ, Ho WG, Li CH *et al.* Intravenous immunoglobulin for prevention of cytomegalovirus infection and interstitial pneumonia after bone marrow transplantation. *Ann Int Med* 1987; **106,** 12–18.
55. Syndman DR, Werner BG, Heinze-Lacey B *et al.* Use of cytomegalovirus immune globulin to prevent cytomegalovirus disease in renal transplant recipients. *N Eng J Med* 1987; **317,** 1049–1054.
56. Saliba F, Arulnaden JL, Gugenheim J *et al.* CMV hyperimmune globulin prophylaxis after liver transplantation· a prospective randomised controlled study. *Transplant Proc* 1989; **21**(1), 2260–2262.
57. Cohen AT, O'Grady JG, Sutherland S, Sallie R, Tan K-C, Williams R. Controlled trial of prophylactic versus therapeutic use of ganciclovir after liver transplantation in adults. *J. Med Virol* (in press).
58. Haagsma EB, Klompmaker IJ, Grond J *et al.* Herpes virus infections after orthotopic liver transplantation. *Transplant Proc* 1987; **19,** 4054–4056.
59. Kusne S, Schwatz M, Breinig MK *et al.* Herpes simplex virus hepatitis after solid organ transplantation in adults. *J Inf Dis* 1991; **63,** 1001–1007.
60. Ward KN, Gray JJ, Efstathiou S. Primary human herpesvirus 6 infection in a patient following liver

transplantation from a seropositive donor. *J Virol* 1989; **28,** 69–72.

61. Sutherland S, Christofinis G, O'Grady J, Williams R. A serological investigation of human herpesvirus 6 infection in liver transplant recipients and the detection of cross-reacting antibodies to cytomegalovirus. *J Med Virol* 1991; **33,** 172–176.
62. Briggs M, Fox J, Tedder RS. Age prevalence of antibody to human herpesvirus 6. *Lancet* 1988; **i,** 1058–1059.
63. McGregor RS, Zitelli BJ, Urbach AH, Malatack JJ, Gartner JC. Varicella in pediatric orthotopic liver transplant recipients. *Pediatrics* 1989; **83,** 256–261.
64. Alonso EM, Fox AS, Franklin WA, Whittington PF. Postnecrotic cirrhosis following varicella hepatitis in a liver transplant patient. *Transplantation* 1990; **49,** 650–653.
65. Yao QY, Rickinson AB, Epstein MA. A re-examination of the Epstein-Barr virus carrier state in healthy seropositive individuals. *Int J Can* 1985; **35,** 43–49.
66. Ho M, Jaffe R, Miller G *et al.* The frequency of Epstein-Barr virus infection and associated lymphoproliferative syndrome after transplantation and its manifestations in children. *Transplantation* 1989; **45,** 719–727.
67. Breinig MK, Zitelli B, Starzl TE, Ho M. Epstein-Barr virus, cytomegalovirus and other viral infections in children after liver transplantations. *J Inf Dis* 1987; **156,** 273–279.
68. Lamy ME, Favart AM, Cornu C *et al.* Epstein-Barr virus infection in 59 orthotopic liver transplant patients. *Med Micro Immunol* 1990; **179,** 137–144.
69. Hanto DW, Gajl-Peczalska KJ, Frizzera G *et al.* Epstein-Barr virus (EBV) induced polyclonal and monoclonal B cell lymphoproliferative diseases occurring after renal transplantation. *Ann Surg* 1983; **198,** 356–369.
70. Cockfield SM, Preiksaitis J, Harvey E *et al.* Is sequential use of ALG and OKT3 in renal transplants associated with an increased incidence of fulminant post-transplant lymphoproliferative disorder? *Transplant Proc* 1991; **23,** 1106–1107.
71. Swinnen LJ, Constanzo-Nordin MR, Fisher SG *et al.* Increased incidence of lymphoproliferative disorder after immunosuppression with the monoclonal antibody OKT3 in cardiac-transplant recipients. *N Eng J Med* 1990; **323,** 1723–1728.
72. Renard T, Andrews W. Relationship between OKT3 administration, EBV seroconversion and the lymphoproliferative syndrome in pediatric liver transplant recipients. *Transplant Proc* 1991; **23,** 1473–1476.
73. Thomas JA, Hotchin NA, Allday MJ *et al.* Immunohistology of Epstein-Barr virus-associated antigens in B cell disorders from immunocompromised individuals. *Transplantation* 1990; **49,** 944–953.
74. Patton DF, Wilkowski CW, Hanson CA *et al.* Epstein-Barr virus-determined clonality in post transplant, lymphoproliferative disease. *Transplantation* 1990; **49,** 1080–1084.
75. Editorial. Lymphoma in organ transplant recipients. *Lancet* 1984; **i,** 601–603.
76. Starzl TE, Nalesnik MA, Porter KA *et al.* Reversibility of lymphomas and lymphoproliferative lesions developing under cyclosporin-steroid therapy. *Lancet* 1984; **i,** 583–587.
77. Prompt CA, Reis MM, Grillo FM *et al.* Transmission of AIDS virus at renal transplantation. *Lancet* 1985; **ii,** 672.
78. L'Age-Stehr J, Schwartz A, Offerman G *et al.* HTLV III infection in kidney transplant recipients. *Lancet* 1985; **ii,** 1361–1362.
79. Rubin HR, Jenkins RL, Shaw BW *et al.* The acquired immunodeficiency syndrome and transplantation. *Transplantation* 1987; **44,** 1–4.
80. Kumar P, Pearson JE, Martin DH *et al.* Transmission of human immunodeficiency virus by transplantation of a renal allograft with development of the Acquired Immunodeficiency Syndrome. *Ann Int Med* 1987; **106,** 244–245.
81. Dummer JS, Erb S, Breinig MK *et al.* Infection with human immunodeficiency virus in the Pittsburgh transplantation population: a study of 583 donors and 1043 recipients 1981–86. *Transplantation* 1989; **47,** 134–140.
82. Ragni MV, Bontempo FA, Lewis JH. Organ transplantation in HIV-positive patients with hemophilia. *N Eng J Med* 1990; **322,** 1886–1887.
83. Tzakis AG, Cooper MH, Dummer JS, Ragni M, Ward JW, Starzl TE. Transplantation in HIV+ patients. *Transplantation* 1990; **49,** 354–358.
84. Jacobson SK, Calne RY, Wreghitt TG. Outcome of HIV infection in transplant patients on cyclosporin. *Lancet* 1991; **i,** 794.
85. Vanhems P, Bresson-Hadni S, Vicitton DA *et al.* Long term survival without immunosuppression in HIV-positive liver-graft recipients. *Lancet* 1991; **337,** 126.
86. Gentile G, Formelli G, Selva S. Atypical picture of cervico-vaginal condylomatosis in a patient submitted to hepatic transplant. *Clin Exp Obstet Gynecol* 1990; **17,** 155–157.
87. Koneru B, Jaffe R, Esquivel CO *et al.* Adenoviral infections in pediatric liver transplant recipients. *J Am Med Assoc* 1987; **258,** 489–492.
88. Koneru B, Atchison R, Jaffe R, Cassavilla A, van Thiel DH, Starzl TE. Serological studies of adenoviral hepatitis following pediatric liver transplantation. *Transplant Proc* 1990; **22,** 1547–1548.
89. Varki NM, Bhuta S, Drake T, Porter DD. Adenovirus hepatitis in two successive liver trans-

plants in a child. *Arch Path Lab Med* 1990; **114,** 106–109.

90. Wreghitt TG, Gray JJ, Ward KN *et al.* Disseminated adenovirus infection after liver transplantation and its possible treatment with ganciclovir. *J Infect* 1989; **19,** 88–89.
91. Dummer JS, Hardy A, Poorsattar A, Ho M. Early infections in kidney, heart and liver transplant recipients on cyclosporine. *Transplantation* 1983; **36,** 259–267.
92. Rossi G, Tortorano A, Viviani MA *et al.* Aspergillus fumigatus infections in liver transplant patients. *Transplant Proc* 1989; **21,** 2268–2270.
93. Boon AP, Adams DH, Buckels J, McMaster P. Cerebral aspergillosis in liver transplantation. *J Clin Pathol* 1990; **43,** 114–118.
94. Tollemar J, Ericzon BG, Holmberg K, Anderssen J. The incidence and diagnosis of invasive fungal infections in liver transplant recipients. *Transplant Proc* 1990; **22,** 242–244.
95. Forbes GM, Harvey FAH, Philpott-Howard JN *et al.* Nocardiosis in liver transplantation: variation in presentation, diagnosis and therapy. *J Infect* 1990; **20,** 11–19.
96. Tobin JO, Beare J, Dunnill MS *et al.* Legionnaire's disease in a transplant unit: isolation of the causative agent from shower baths. *Lancet* 1980; **ii,** 118–121.

Appendix

Characteristics of CD Antigens

CD	Sub Group	MW KD	Comments
CD1	CD1a	49	early cortical thyomyocytes, interdigitating
	CD1b	45	cells foetal B cells and Langerhans cells
	CD1c	43	Associated with B_2 microglobulin
CD2 (T11 antigen)		50	T cells. Antigen receptor for sheep red blood cells. Binds to CD58, involved in cell adherence
CD3 (T3 antigen)		16–28	T cells. Associated with T cell receptor. Consists of 5 chains. Involved in signalling after antigen binding
CD4 (T4 antigen)		59	T cells, especially helper/inducer, monocytes, macrophages. Binds to class II MHC molecules
CD5 (T1 antigen)		67	Most T cells. Some B cells
CD6 (T12 antigen)		100	Most T cells. Some B cells
CD7		40	Mostly T cells. Probable FC receptor for IgM
CD8 (T8 antigen)		32	T cells, especially cytotoxic/suppressor and spleen sinusoidal lining cells. Binds to class I molecules on antigen presenting cells
CD9		24	Pre B-cells, granulocytes, platelets, monocytes, endothelium
CD10		100	Stem cells, pre-B cells, fibroblasts, bile canaliculi. An enkephalinase
CD11	CD11a	180	Leucocytes. The alpha chain of leucocyte function associated antigen-1 (LFA-1); binds ICAM-1, ICAM-2 and ICAM-3
	CD11b	165	Granulocytes, monocytes, weakly on T cells, NK cells. The Alpha chain of MAC-1a

CD	Sub Group	MW KD	Comments
	CD11c	150	Granulocytes, monocytes, NK cells, weakly on T and B cells, alpha chain of P150
CD12		90–120	Monocyte and macrophages
CD13		150	Granulocytes, monocytes and some macrophages. Aminopeptidase-N
CD14		55	Monocytes, some granulocytes and macrophages, and dendritic cells
CD15			Neutrophil secondary granules. Hapten X
CD16			Granulocytes, NK cells. Involved in ADCC
CD17w			Granulocytes, some monocytes and platelets
CD18		95	Leucocytes. Integrin chain non covalently linked to CD11a, b, c; involved in adhesion
CD19		95	B cells until plasma cell stage
CD20		35	B cells
CD21		140	Dendritic cells, B cells. Receptor for EBV, C3d
CD22		130	Mature B cells and in cytoplasm of pre-B cells. Homology with CD56
CD23		45	Mature B cells, activated B cells and monocytes. Possible receptor for B cell growth factor and low affinity IgE receptor
CD24		41	B cells
CD25 (Tac antigen)			Activated T + B cells and macrophages. Low affinity receptor (α subunit) for IL2 which associates with TSRD β subunit
CD26		120	Activated T + B cells, macrophages, bile canaliculi. A dipeptidylpeptidase IV
CD27		110	T cells transformed B cells
CD28		88	Subpopulation of T cells and activated B cells
CD29		130	Widely distributed. β1 integrin chains, common β subunit of VLA 1–6. Involved in adhesion and signalling

CD	Sub Group	MW KD	Comments
CD30		105	Activated T + B cells, some lymphoma cells
CD31		140	Granulocytes, platelets, T cell subsets and endothelial cells. Also known as platelet endothelial adhesion cell molecule (PECAM)
CD32w		400	Granulocytes, B cells, monocytes, platelets
CD33		67	Myeloid cells, monocytes and some leukaemias
CD34		105	Immature haemopoetic cells and endothelial cells
CD35		160–250	Various cell types including red cell, B cells, monocytes, granulocytes, some NK cells. The complement receptor for C3B
CD36		90	Monocytes, macrophages, platelets, some endothelial cells and B cells known as gpiv and gpiiiB. Receptor for thrombospondin and collagen. Endothelial receptor for red cells infected with plasmodium falciparum
CD37		40	B cells and weakly on macrophages, neutrophils, monocytes and activated T cells
CD38		45	Plasma cells, pre-B cells, immature and activated T cells. Involved in T cell activation
CD39		80	B cells, monocyte, macrophages, vascular endothelium. Activated T cells
CD40		44	Peripheral blood and tonsillar B cells. Weakly on monocytes and interdigitating cells, known gp50
CD41			Platelets, megakaryocytes. Associated with CD 61. Receptor for fibrinogen. Binds Von Willebrand factor, fibronectin and collagen
CD42	CD42a	23	Megakaryocytes and platelets. Equivalent to glycoprotein ix. Receptor for Von Willebrand factor
	CD42b		Platelets and megakaryocyte. Complexes with CD 42a

CD	Sub Group	MW KD	Comments
CD43		95	Leucocytes, T cells, erythrocytes. Binds to ICAM-1
CD44		80–95	Widely distributed on leukocytes: monocytes, neutrophils and T cells. Also endothelium red cells, platelets and epithelium. Role in T cell endothelial binding. Receptor for hyaluronate.
CD45			Leucocyte common antigen. Exists in several isoforms due to alternative splicing and differential glycosylation
CD45RO		180	T cells, some B cells and macrophages. High expression on 'memory' T cells associated with memory cells
CD45ra		220	B cells and monocytes, some B cells. High expression associated with 'naive' T cells
CD45rb		190–220	B cells, some T cells, monocytes and granulocytes. High expression on 'naive' T cells
CD46		56–66	Widely distributed
CD47		47–52	Widely distributed
CD48			Widely distributed
CD49			The alpha chains of the β_1 integrins which associate with the β chain CD29. Also known as the very late activation antigens (VLA)1–6
	CD49a	130–210	VLA-1. Activated T cells and endothelium. Collagen and laminin receptor
	CD49b	170	VLA-2. Activated T cells, platelets, endothelium. Collagen receptor on T cells
	CD49c	135	VLA-3. Activated T cells, some endothelial cells. Receptor for collagen laminin and fibronectin
	CD49d	150	VLA-4. Resting T cells (increases with activation), B cells, monocytes. Receptor for fibronectin, and VCAM-1

41. Shaked A, Busuttil RW, Sher L, Makowka L. Case No. 6 – diagnosis and treatment of early rejection in liver transplantation. *Transplant Sci* 1991; **1**(1), 18–24.
42. Fung JJ, Demetris A, Todo S *et al.* Use of FK506 in the treatment of liver allograft rejection. *Transplant Sci* 1991; **1**(1), 50–54.
43. Lewis W, Jenkins R, Burke P *et al.* FK506 rescue therapy in liver transplant recipients with drug resistant rejection. *FK506 First International Congress Abstracts 1991*; Abstract CT105.
44. Trey C. Case study. *N Eng J Med* 1992 (in press).
45. Penn I. Cancer is a complication of severe immunosuppression. *Surg Gynecol Obstet* 1986; **162,** 603–610.
46. Starzl TE, Nalesnik MA, Porter KA *et al.* Reversibility of lymphomas and lymphoproliferative lesions developing under cyclosporin-steroid therapy. *Lancet* 1984; **1,** 583–587.
47. Cohen JI. Epstein-Barr virus lymphoproliferative disease associated with acquired immunodeficiency. *Medicine* 1991; **70**(2), 137–160.
48. Stieber AC, Boillot O, Scotti-Foglieni C *et al.* The surgical implications of post transplant lymphoproliferative disorders. *Transplant Proc* 1991; **23,** 1477–1479.

18

Newer immunosuppressive agents

J Neuberger and D Adams

Introduction

The increasing success of organ transplantation has drawn attention to the limitations of the drugs used for immunosuppression. Both in the short and longer term, side effects and complications include failure to prevent rejection, increased susceptibility to infection, progressive organ damage – notably renal – metabolic derangements and increased susceptibility to malignancy. As illustrated in the preceding chapter, the current main stays of immunosuppression, corticosteroids, azathioprine, cyclosporin, FK506 and OKT3, have their own additional complications. It is a sad reflection that there still remains a lack of properly controlled data to assess the relative role of each drug and there is little concordance as to the optimal immunosuppressive regime for the liver allograft recipient.

Over the past few years, the increasing understanding of the mechanisms of rejection and the application of the newer molecular biological techniques have contributed to the development of a wide variety of drugs with potential application to immunosuppression. Many of these drugs are still at a preclinical stage; the aim of this chapter is to review some of these newer agents. It is to be hoped that the role of these newer compounds will be evaluated much more carefully and rigorously than in the past.

Cyclosporin A (CyA)

The introduction of cyclosporin into clinical practice in the early 1980s was hailed as a major break through in immunosuppression. Most of the claims for the superiority of the drug were based on comparison with historical controls and there were few controlled studies. Nonetheless, the use of Cyclosporin A (CyA) has been associated with an explosion in the number of patients receiving allografts.

CyA is a neutral, lipophilic cyclic endecapeptide extracted from the fungus *Tolypocladium inflatum gams*. Early studies on the immunological activity of CyA were undertaken primarily by Borel.[84] Since then, the mode of action has been extensively investigated. Numerous studies have demonstrated that incubation of cytotoxic lymphocytes with CyA results in virtual abolition of IL-2 synthesis and release; this inhibitory effect can be overcome by the addition of extraneous IL-2. Subsequent work showed that CyA acts by inhibiting transcription of lymphokines and does not appear to block allo-antigen recognition. Thus studies, for example by Herold and colleagues,[85] showed that while CyA had no effect on the binding of clonotypic antibody against the TCR, mRNA transcription of IL-2, IL-3 and gamma-interferon was greatly inhibited. In contrast to the effect on CD4 lymphocytes, CyA appears to have a relatively weak effect on CD8 cells.[86] Thus, the main actions of CyA result in blocking activation of the IL-2 gene, inhibition of T lymphocyte proliferation, prevention of release of gamma-interferon and of B cell activation factors.

The mode of action of CyA is dependent on its binding to an intracellular protein termed cyclophilin.[87] The degree of binding is proportional to the *in vitro* effect on the MLR. Subsequent studies have shown that cyclophilin is a protein that is well conserved in all mammalian species; there are at least two isoforms, the major isoform is about 17 Kda. In a variety of cells, including hepatocytes and lymphocytes, cyclophilin is localised in the nucleus.[89]

The association between CyA binding to cyclophilin and its immunological effects was clarified when it was demonstrated that there was amino acid identity between cyclophilin and the enzyme cis-trans peptidyl-prolyl isomerase.[87,88] It was initially believed that CyA acted by inhibiting the rotamase action involved in the conformational changes that occur during peptide chain elongation or cell trafficking. As indicated below, it is now appreciated that the situation is more complex.

Orally administered CyA is absorbed in the distal ileum; because of the lipid solubility, bile is important for the efficient absorption of CyA so absorption is decreased in cholestasis. Some metabolism occurs within the enterocyte and so may explain, in part, some of the variability in dose requirements. Cyclosporin is metabolised primarily by the hepatic mixed function oxidase system, so metabolism is affected by enzyme inducing drugs (such as phenobarbitone or phenytoin) and enzyme inhibiting drugs (such as cimetidine). Side effects are common and may be dose dependent. Common side effects include nephrotoxicity, hepatotoxicity, headaches, hirsutism, hypertension, neurotoxicity, breast fibroadenosis and gingival hypertrophy.

FK506

FK506 is a macrolide lactone isolated from *Streptomyces tukabaesinsis*, with a molecular weight of 822.[90] Studies *in vitro* have shown that the immunosuppressive properties of FK506 are similar to CyA: the drug strongly inhibits the proliferative responses of lymphocytes to allo-antigen presentation, the generation of cytotoxic T cells and the production of T lymphocyte products including IL-2, IL-3 and gamma-interferon. FK506 also inhibits expression of the Tac antigen after stimulation with either specific antigen or allo-antigen. However, on a weight for weight basis, FK506 is about 100 times more potent than CyA.

Animal studies have shown that FK506 can induce antigen specific tolerance in experimental glomerulonephritis and inhibits established lesions of collagen induced arthritis.[91] The sucess of the drug in a variety of animal transplant models encouraged its use in human heart, lung, kidney and liver transplantation.[92] These studies have all testified to the efficacy of the drug and many of the clinical applications are discussed elsewhere.

There seems a striking resemblance between the development of CyA and FK506. Both drugs were introduced without the benefit of controlled studies; it has taken some five years or longer for the physicians to learn how to give CyA, to establish a therapeutic range, determine the optimal methods of measuring the drug, understand the pharmacokinetics, drug interactions and side effects. Very similar considerations apply to FK506. Side effects are broadly similar to those seen with CyA, but neurotoxicity, nephrotoxicity and a tendency to diabetes seem more common with FK506. The results of prospective trials evaluating CyA with FK506 will allow for a balanced assessment of the place of these very powerful agents in the management of immunosuppression.

Despite the similar immunosuppressive effects of the two drugs, they bind to different proteins: FK506 binds to so-called FK binding proteins[93] which, like cyclophilins, are well conserved, abundant proteins and are active as peptidyl-prolyl cis-trans isomerases. It is now believed[81] that the drugs become active as a complex with their respective intracellular receptors by giving new properties to these receptors. This concept is supported by the observation that another immunosuppressive macrolide, rapamycin, also inhibits FK binding protein rotamase activity, although rapamycin does not block cytokine transcription at an early stage of T cell activation. McKeon[81] has suggested a unifying concept involving binding the drug/binding protein to calcineurin A (Fig 18.1). Calcineurin A is a highly conserved, calcium/calmodulin activated protein phosphatase with two subunits, which bind calmodulin and calcium.

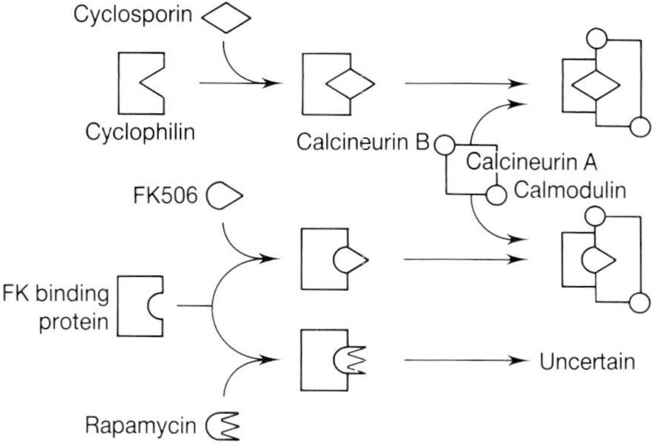

Fig. 18.1 Schematic mode of action of cyclosporin, FK506 and rapamycin (adapted from [81]).

Rapamycin

Rapamycin is a macrolide antibiotic produced by *Streptomyces hygrospicus*. Like cyclosporin and FK506, rapamycin is an antifungal antibiotic. Although these compounds are structurally unrelated, they are functionally similar. Both FK506 and rapamycin competitively inhibit the peptidyl-prolyl isomerase (PPIase) activity of immunophilin, the major binding protein for FK506.[1,2,81]

In vitro studies have shown that while rapamycin and FK506 have many similar effects on animal and human lymphocytes, there are a number of important differences.[3] For example, rapamycin inhibits T cell constitutive division, unlike FK506 which has no effect. Both drugs inhibit CD4 lymphocyte activation. Rapamycin, however, inhibits IL-2 and IL-4 dependent activation and calcium independent B and T cell activation whereas FK506 inhibits IL-2 expression. These observations may explain, in part, why rapamycin acts in synergy with cyclosporin but in antagonism with FK506.[3]

Rapamycin has been assessed in a number of animal models of rejection. The drug has been studied in mouse, rat, pig, dog and monkey using heart, kidney, skin, pancreas, small bowel and thymus.[4] Overall, the drug is effective in prolonging graft survival and suppressing graft versus host disease but appears to be less effective in xenografting.

In animal studies, the formulation is important: uneffective immunosuppression was achieved at a dose of 0.4 mg/kg/day using continuous intravenous infusions of rapamycin in a polyethylene glycol/polysorbate solution in a rat cardiac graft model.[5] Nevertheless, satisfactory immunosuppression can be achieved by oral or subcutaneous dosing. The effects can last long after the drug is discontinued.[6]

Rapamycin does not appear to cause renal dysfunction, hypotension or affect the response to infection. However, Whiting reported some evidence of mild–moderate focal myocardial necrosis in rats given rapamycin.[7] There appears to be a synergistic effect between rapamycin and cyclosporin.

Clinical trials of rapamycin are currently underway but as with other immunosuppressive agents, the benefit/toxicity ratio between rapamycin and cyclosporin has yet to be determined.

RS-61443

RS-61443 represents a 'designer drug' developed by Allison and Eugui.[8] RS-61443 is a morpholino ethyl ester of mycophenolic acid. Mycophenolic acid is a non-competitive inhibitor of inosine-5-monophosphate dehydrogenase (IMPDH), the enzyme that controls the rate of purine synthesis.[9,10] Mitogen and allo-antigens stimulated T and B cells have increased IMPDH activity and increased synthesis of guanine nucleotide; hence interference with the purine synthesis of lymphocytes will affect their function.

Mycophenolic acid was found to be effective in reducing T and B lymphocyte proliferative responses: a synthetic addition of a morpholino ethyl ester side chain increased bio-availability without affecting immunological function.[11] Hence the ester derivative rather than the parent compound is being increasingly used in clinical practice. Animal studies have shown that RS-61443 is highly effective in prolonging islet cell allograft function in mice, heart, allo- and xenografts in rats and canine renal allografts, amongst others.[12,13] Side effects are dose dependent;[14] gastro-intestinal complications appear the most significant, consisting of diarrhoea, often with bloody motions, anorexia and gastritis.

Clinical studies in man with a variety of different grafts, including renal, heart, liver and pancreas, have shown that RS-61443 is effective in doses greater than 2000 mg/day in preventing graft rejection without any apparent increase in susceptibility to infection.[15] Larger studies are underway to evaluate this promising new agent. The most recent,[66] using doses varying between 100 and 3500 mg/day, reported that RS-61443 was well tolerated; only one of 48 renal allograft recipients reported any adverse reaction (haemorrhagic gastritis). The drug was also effective in rescue treatment. Although there was a statistically significant correlation between dose and rejection, the authors did not recommend a therapeutic dose. Trials in liver transplantation are awaited with interest.

15-Deoxyspergualin

15-Deoxyspergualin (15-DSG) is a synthetically dehydroxylated form of spergualin (SG), the product of the *Bacillus lactosporos*.[16] *In vivo* and *in vitro* studies have shown both 15-DSG and SG have similar efficacy although 15-DSG is more potent.

Animal studies have shown that DSG is highly effective in controlling auto-immune disease and is effective not only in reducing the severity of rejection but also in the reversal of established acute rejection of kidney, liver, heart and skin.[17,18,19] In humans, 15-DSG has been evaluated in the treatment of severe allograft rejection with encouraging results.[20,21] Addition of high dose methylprednisolone appears to enhance its immunosuppressive effects.[22] However, one recently reported study[67] found that 15-DSG had very little effect on reversal of established renal allograft rejection and doses as low as 4 mg/kg were associated with significant side effects. These observations contrast with a report by the same group that 15-DSG was effective in treating liver allograft rejection.[68]

Toxic effects of 15-DSG are related to dose: bone marrow suppression, hypotension, anorexia and parasthesiae appear to be the most common. Bone marrow suppression usually responds rapidly to drug withdrawal.

The precise mode of action is unclear: *in vitro* studies have shown 15-DSG is effective in suppressing primary and secondary responses to thymic independent and dependent antigens. However, 15-DSG is thought to suppress rejection by suppression of IL-2 production and interferon production by CD4 cells,[16,19] by inhibition of the differentiation of B cells to plasma cells and by inhibiting clonal amplification of T cells. The former property makes the drug of potential value in xenografting.

Prostaglandins

Although there remains controversy as to the effects of prostaglandins on B cells, both PGE_1 and PGE_2 affect T cell functions through inhibition of IL-1 and IL-2 formation and class II antigen expression.[23,24,25] The development of two stable synthetic PGE_1 analogues, misoprostol and enisoprost, have allowed therapeutic studies of prostaglandins in prevention and treatment of allograft rejection. *In vitro* studies suggest that PGE_1 analogues suppress lymphocyte proliferative responses to allo-antigens and have an additive effect with both corticosteroids and cyclosporin. The effect can be counteracted by addition of recombinant IL-2.[26] A recent study in renal allografts suggested a marked beneficial effect;[27] however, a subsequent multicentre, prospective, randomised placebo controlled study in renal allografts found that enisoprost had no demonstrable effect on the incidence of acute rejection or renal dysfunction.[69] These findings are in agreement with a prospective randomised study in liver grafts carried out in the Liver Unit in Birmingham, which showed no effect of enisoprost on the incidence or severity of liver allograft rejection nor on cyclosporin associated nephrotoxicity (Ishmail, personal communication). It may be, however, that other prostaglandin analogues will be beneficial in allograft rejection.

Lipoxygenase inhibition has been reported to affect the immune response by enhancing arachidonic acid metabolism to prostaglandins or by inhibiting LTB4 production which stimulates CD8 function and increased IL-2 production. LTB4 may also increase cell mediated cytotoxicity. Preliminary *in vitro* studies[28] suggest that the combination of enisoprost and a 5-lipoxygenase inhibitor acts synergistically. Further work is required to assess the clinical relevance of such a combination.[70]

Thalidomide

The well-publicised teratogenic effects of thalidomide have resulted in the temporary lack of interest in this agent in medicine. The drug has been shown to be therapeutically effective in a variety of clinical situations, such as lepromatous leprosy, SLE, Behçet's syndrome and ulcerative colitis. Side effects include not only teratogenicity but neurotoxicity, vasculitis and myxoedema. Careful monitoring of blood levels appears to reduce these complications.[82]

However, it has become increasingly recognised that thalidomide may be of benefit in therapy of graft rejection. In animal studies, thalidomide is effective in bone marrow and renal transplantation.[29,30] It has a synergistic effect with cyclosporin in rat cardiac allografting and in the prophylaxis of graft versus host disease. *In vitro*, thalidomide inhibits mitogenic and allo-antigenic proliferation of lymphocytes but it does not appear in these studies to act synergistically with FK506.[31] Clinical trials do show a benefit with the drug in graft versus host disease[32] and may be of potential value in the treatment of patients following liver transplantation.

Ursodeoxycholic acid (UDCA)

UDCA is a hydrophilic bile acid which has been shown to be highly effective in improving the serum biochemistry in a wide variety of chronic cholestatic liver diseases. The drug has been best studied in patients with primary biliary cirrhosis, where patients in early disease have been reported to have improved symptoms and a reduction in serum bilirubin, alkaline phosphatase, immunoglobulins and antimitochondrial antibody titre. The mode of action is unclear, but it has been suggested that the agent may act by replacing the more hepatotoxic hydrophobic bile acids with less cytotoxic ones. *In vitro* hepatocyte MHC class I antigen expression, which appears to be increased in cholestasis of any cause, is reduced by UDCA[71] but it remains uncertain whether this observation could explain the mode of action of UDCA.

One study from Sweden suggested that UDCA may be effective in helping prevention of liver allograft rejection since biochemical values post-transplantation were lower compared with six historical controls.[72] This observation has some weight given to it by a subsequent study suggesting that administration of UDCA reduces acute rejection in the rat heart allograft model.[73] These rather surprising results need confirmation before UDCA can be included in the therapeutic armamentarium.

Brequinar

Brequinar is a potent anticancer drug that inhibits cell proliferation by reducing the activity of dihydro-oratate dehydrogenase and pyrimidine biosynthesis.[74] Clinically, the agent has been used for the treatment of metastatic cancer and some leukaemias. Brequinar has been shown to be more effective than cyclosporin in supressing rodent adjuvant arthritis.[75]

In rat allograft models of heart, liver and kidney transplantation, Brequinar was found to be highly effective in preventing rejection.[75] With respect to liver allografts, 50–90% liver grafts were permanently accepted after 30 days treatment with brequinar 12 mg/kg. Furthermore, challenge of long term liver graft survivors with donor cardiac grafts was associated with permanent acceptance of hearts of original, but not third party, strain; these observations suggest the drug may induce tolerance.

Whether these properties will be translated to the human model and whether side effects will be a problem is uncertain; nonetheless, this must remain a drug of great promise.

Other agents

There are many other drugs with potential application to liver allografting. These include SKF-105685, which is an azaspirane which induces suppressor cells and is effective in the rat cardiac allograft model.[76]

Platelet activating factor (PAF) antagonist, WEB 2170, improved the therapeutic efficacy of subtherapeutic doses of cyclosporin; in a renal allograft dog model, WEB 2170 given with cyclosporin was associated with an improvement in graft survival.[77]

Iron is an essential co-factor in many aspects of cell metabolism, including DNA synthesis and intracellular energy production. Pretreatment of rats with the oral iron chelator, desferrithiocin, was associated with improvement in cardiac allograft survival.[78] *In vivo* studies on monocytes showed that IL-2 and gamma-interferon production was suppressed but induction of IL-2R was unaffected. Clearly further work is required to determine the exact mode of action of this agent, but the approach lends itself to novel methods of immunosuppression.

One other approach which has shown success in animal models of allograft rejection is use of soluble class I antigen, which Kamada demonstrated improves survival of rat cardiac allografts. The effect was amplified by monoclonal anti-class I antibody. These observations are in line with the observations that serum from liver allografted rats can enhance graft survival and induce clonal deletion of alloreactive T cells (see Chapter 12).

Monoclonal antibodies

The increasing understanding of the mechanism of allograft rejection has allowed more specific intervention in both the prevention and treatment of allograft rejection. The development by Millstein and Kohler of techniques for generation of monoclonal antibodies has resulted in the possibility of therapeutic antibodies directed at specific epitopes on the leucocyte or target cells (Figure 18.2). In the last few years, an increasing number of such antibodies have been tested both in animal models and in humans for prevention and treatment of rejection. There have been suggestions that the response to monoclonal antibody therapy may vary between children and adults.[80]

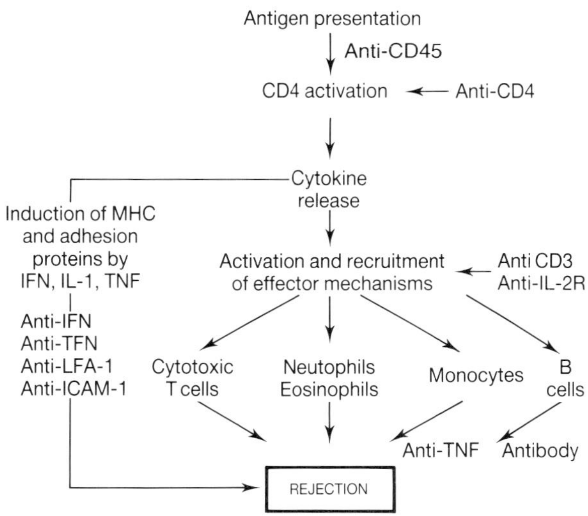

Fig. 18.2 Simplified scheme of rejection and sites of possible intervention with antibodies.

Anti-CD45 monoclonal antibody

As discussed elsewhere, dendritic cells in the allograft play an important role in stimulating the allograft response. Experimental studies have shown that depletion of dendritic cells from renal allografts by irradiation and cyclophosphamide prior to implantation results in prolonged survival of the graft.[33,34] Repletion with the dendritic cells abolishes this effect on improved graft survival. CD45 is an antigen present not only on dendritic cells but also on lymphocytes, so the antibody may act by depleting passenger leucocytes as well as blocking dendritic cells. A randomised controlled trial in renal allografts showed that the incidence of allograft rejection was reduced by pretreatment of the graft with antibody to CD45[35] although neither patient nor graft survival were improved.

Antibodies to lymphocyte antigens

Anti-CD5 monoclonal antibodies

The CD5 antigen is present on virtually all mature T lymphocytes and a small subpopulation of B lymphocytes which have been implicated in auto-immune diseases. One antibody, XMMLY-H-65-RTA, has been conjugated to ricin-A, which inhibits ribosomal protein synthesis,[36] and has been used in human graft versus host disease, some malignant diseases and auto-immune diseases. Furthermore, this antibody is associated with a beneficial effect in acute steroid resistant and in acute graft versus host disease.

Anti-CD7 monoclonal antibodies

The CD7 antigen is a 40 KDa surface antigen present on T cells, stem cells and CD16 natural killer cells. *In vitro* anti-CD7 antibodies partially inhibit allogeneic mixed lymphocyte responses and completely inhibit the autologous MLR.[37,38] CD7 is preferentially expressed on naive T cells and anti-CD7 preferentially inhibits alloresponses on naive T cells.[37,39] There is an additive effect of CD7 with cyclosporin. A chimeric mouse human CD7 antibody has been evaluated in patients following renal transplantation.[40] The chimeric antibody was well tolerated with little immunogenicity but apparently only delayed rather than prevented acute rejection.

Antibodies to the T cell receptor

As indicated in other chapters, the CD3 T cell receptor plays a crucial role in the immune process. A number of antibodies have been developed to interact with the TCR complex, of which the most widely used is OKT3. Use of this drug is discussed in greater detail elsewhere but there is no doubt this is a potent agent in both prevention and treatment of allograft rejection. One of the problems with OKT3 administration is the development of fever, diarrhoea and pulmonary oedema due to OKT3 induced release of tumour necrosis factor. A number of different approaches have been developed to overcome these side effects and include the use of anti-TNF,[41] pentoxifylline,[42] use of OKT3 F(Ab)2 fragments[43] or antibodies to CD3 of different isotypes.[44,45]

OKT3 is a murine IgG2A antibody; a number

of other monoclonal antibodies reacting with the CD3 TCR complex have been developed. These include BMA-031, a murine IgG 2b, T10B9.1A/31, a murine IgM kappa antibody, and WT32, a murine IgG 2a. These drugs are all potent and effective both in prevention and reversal of acute allograft rejection. At the moment there appears to be very little to choose between the various antibodies. However, a prospective randomised double blind trial comparing treatment of acute renal allograft rejection with either T10/B9.1A/31 and OKT3 suggested that T10B9.1A/31 reverses acute rejection earlier and more effectively than OKT3, with fewer severe side effects. Furthermore, this monoclonal antibody was associated with fewer side effects and potentially less infection.[46] Further studies are required to determine the role of these antibodies in treatment of acute allograft rejection.

Monoclonal antibodies to CD4

The CD4 antigen is present on the helper/inducer subset which is being increasingly recognised as playing a major role in the inflammatory responses associated with allograft rejection. *In vivo* administration of anti-CD4 antibodies is very effective in inhibiting antibody responses to thymic antigens and will deplete CD4 peripheral T cells.[47] Furthermore, in murine models this antibody induces tolerance to antigens administered during the period of anti-CD4 therapy.[48,49]

Anti-CD4 is effective in reducing the severity of inflammation in murine models of arthritis and SLE. The mechanism of action of CD4 monoclonal antibodies is complex: they prevent the interaction between T cells and antigen presenting cells, thus inhibiting T cell activation. Since CD4 antibodies may also inhibit T cell function in the absence of class II molecules, part of their mode of action may not be directly associated with the CD3 TCR interactions.[47] However, some other studies have indicated that these antibodies induce lymphocyte activation *in vitro* and may help regulate cell adhesion.

Anti-CD4 is effective in reducing the severity of rejection in mice, rats and monkeys given allografts of skin, heart, kidney and pancreatic islet cells.[50,51] Timing of the administration may be important since the antibody affects the afferent arm of the immune response.

A number of different anti-CD4 antibodies are available (YTS 191/1, GK 1.5, OK35, OK38, W3/25, BWH-4, OKT4, OKT4A, MT310, BL4, amongst others).

Experience in humans is limited. The first trial was by Herzog in 1987,[52] who showed that treatment of a small number of patients with rheumatoid arthritis was associated with a transient remission: the drug was well tolerated. However, other studies have shown there may be some adverse features such as fever, chills and urticaria. Humanised CD4 antibodies have been given to a limited number of patients, with good tolerance and successful immunosuppressive effect.[53]

A recent study of CD4 monoclonal antibodies in 12 renal transplants showed some reduction in the incidence of rejection.[53] Nonetheless, use of these antibodies remains at a preliminary stage. The reduction in peripheral CD4 cells has lead to concern about inducing an AIDS-like syndrome in these patients.

Antibodies to interleukin-2 receptor (CD25)

The interleukin-2 receptor consists of high and low affinity forms. Two distinct binding IL-2 products have been identified: the 55 KDa subunit (beta chain or Tac antigen in humans), and the 75KDa unit (alpha chain) which are expressed on a subset of activated T cells. Because of the central role of T cell activation in the inflammatory response, immunosuppressive protocols directed against the rejection cascade at this site are attractive. The development of therapeutic antibodies against the 55KDa unit of both mice and humans has allowed studies to be performed in this area.

Studies in mice and rats using a variety of different IL-2R antibodies have shown a beneficial effect of these antibodies in both prevention and treatment of rejection.[54]

In humans, anti-IL2 therapy prevented rejection in renal allograft recipients during the period of administration but some of these patients developed late acute rejection episodes subsequently, which responded well to OKT3 therapy.[55,56,57,58] In the clinical studies to date, no significant side effects have been noted. There appears to be synergism between cyclosporin and other immunosuppressive agents with anti-IL-2R.[59] It is likely that this approach will be used increasingly in liver allografts.

Modification of the chimeric IL-2 receptor antibody by combination with pseudomonas endo-

body (CD7) with human constant and mouse variable regions. *J Immunol* 1989; **143,** 3589–3592.
40. Akbar A, Amlot P, Hawkins C *et al.* The effect of a chimeric mouse-human CD7 antibody on human T, natural killer and lymphokine-activated killer cell activity *in vitro*. *Transplantation* 1991; **52,** 325–330.
41. Ferran C, Sheehan K, Schreiber R, Bach JF, Chatenoud L. Anti-TNF abrogates the cytokine-related anti-CD3 induced syndrome. *Transplant Proc* 1991; **23,** 849–851.
42. Alegre M-L, Gastaldello K, Abramowicz D *et al.* Evidence that pentoxifylline reduces anti-CD3 monoclonal antibody induced cytokine release syndrome. *Transplantation* 1991; **52,** 674–679.
43. Woodle ES, Thistlethwaite JR, Ghobrial IA, Jolliffe LK, Stuart FP, Bluestone JA. OKT3 F (ab) 2 fragments – retention of the immunosuppressive properties of whole antibody with marked reduction in T cell activation and lymphokine release. *Transplantation* 1991; **52,** 354–360.
44. Rao P, Olini G, Kille J *et al.* OKT3E, an anti-CD3 antibody that does not elicit side effects or anti-idiotype responses in chimpanzees. *Transplantation* 1991; **52,** 691–697.
45. Woodle ES, Thistlethwaite JR, Jolliffe LK, Fucello AJ, Stuart FP, Bluestone JA. Anti-CD3 monoclonal antibody therapy. *Transplantation* 1991; **52,** 361–368.
46. Waid TH, Lucas BA, Thompson JS *et al.* Treatment of acute rejection with anti-T-cell antigen receptor complex alpha-beta (T10B9.1A-31) or anti-CD3 (OKT3) monoclonal antibody. *Transplant Proc* 1991; **23,** 1062–1065.
47. Sablinski T, Hancock WW, Tilney N, Kupiec-Weglinski JW. CD4 monoclonal antibodies in organ transplantation – a review of progress. *Transplantation* 1991; **52,** 579–589.
48. Shizuru JA, Seydal K, Flavin T *et al.* Induction of donor specific unresponsiveness to cardiac allografts in rats by pretransplant anti-CD4 monoclonal antibody therapy. *Transplantation* 1990; **50,** 366–371.
49. Cobbold SP, Martin G, Waldmann H. The induction of skin graft tolerance in MHC mismatched or primed recipients. *Eur J Immunol* 1990; **20,** 2747–2751.
50. Cosimi AB, Delmonico FL, Wright J *et al.* OKT4A monoclonal antibody therapy immunosuppression of cynomolgus renal allograft recipients. *Transplant Proc* 1991; **23,** 501–503.
51. Coulombe M, Hao L, Calcinaro F *et al.* Tolerance induction in adult animals. *Transplant Proc* 1991; **23,** 31–32.
52. Herzog CH, Walker C, Pichler W *et al.* Monoclonal anti-CD4 in arthritis. *Lancet* 1987; **2,** 1461–1463.
53. Morel P, Vincent C, Corgier G *et al.* Anti-CD4 monoclonal administration in renal transplanted patients. *Clin Immunol Immunopathol* 1990; **56,** 311–320.
54. Kupiec-Weglinski J, Diamantstein T, Tilney N. Interleukin 2 receptor-targeted therapy – rationale and applications in organ transplantation. *Transplantation* 1988; **46,** 785–792.
55. Cosimi AB, Delmonico L, Wright K *et al.* Prolonged survival of non-human primate renal allograft recipients treated only with anti-CD4 monoclonal antibody therapy. *Surgery* 1990; **108,** 406–415.
56. Kirkman R, Chapiro M, Carpenter C *et al.* A randomized trial of anti-Tac monoclonal antibody in human renal transplantation. *Transplantation* 1991; **51,** 107–112.
57. Soulillou JP, Cantarovich D, Le Mauff B *et al.* Randomised controlled trial of monoclonal antibody against the interleukin-2 receptor (33B3.1) as compared with rabbit anti-thymocyte globulin for prophylaxis against rejection of renal allografts. *N Eng J Med* 1990; **322,** 1175–1178.
58. Otto G, Thies J, Kabelitz D *et al.* Anti-CD25 monoclonal antibody prevents early rejection in liver transplantation – a pilot study. *Transplant Proc* 1991; **23,** 1387–1389.
59. Ueda H, Cheung YC, Masetti P *et al.* Synergy between cyclosporine and anti-IL2 receptor monoclonal antibodies in rats. *Transplantation* 1991; **52,** 437–442.
60. Herbort CP, de Smet M, Roberge F *et al.* Treatment of corneal allograft rejection with cytotoxin IL-2-PE40. *Transplantation* 1991; **52,** 470–474.
61. Imagawa DK, Millis JM, Olthoff KM *et al.* The role of tumor necrosis factor in allograft rejection. *Transplantation* 1990; **50,** 189–193.
62. Scheringa M, de Bruin R, Jeekel H, Marquet RL. Anti-tumor necrosis factor alpha serum prolongs heart allograft survival in rats. *Transplant Proc* 1991; **23,** 547–548.
63. Stevens H, van der Kwast T, van der Meide P *et al.* Synergistic immunosuppressive effects of monoclonal effects of interferon gamma and tumour necrosis factor alpha. *Transplantation* 1990; **50,** 856–860.
64. Flavin T, Ivens K, Rothlein R *et al.* Monoclonal antibodies against intercellular adhesion molecule 1 prolong cardiac allograft survival in Cynomolgus monkeys. *Transplant Proc* 1991; **23,** 533–534.
65. Le Mauff B, Hourmant M, Rougier JP *et al.* Effect of anti-LFA1 (CD11a) monoclonal antibodies in acute rejection in human kidney transplantation. *Transplantation* 1991; **52,** 291–296.
66. Sollinger HW, Deirhoi MH, Belzer FO, Diethelm AG, Kauffman RS. RS-61443 – a phase I clinical trial and pilot rescue study. *Transplantation* 1992; **53,** 428–432.

67. Ohlman S, Gannedahl G, Tyden G, Tufveson G, Groth G. Treatment of renal transplant rejection with 15-deoxyspergualin – a dose finding study in man. *Transplant Proc* 1992; **24,** 318–320.
68. Groth CG, Ohlman S, Ericzon BH, Barholt L, Reinholt FP. Deoxyspergualin for liver graft rejection. *Lancet* 1990; **336,** 626.
69. Adams MB and the Enisoprost Renal Transplant Study Group. Enisoprost in renal transplantation. *Transplantation* 1992; **53,** 338–345.
70. Weir MR, Li XW, Peppler R, O'Bryan-Tear CG, Moran M. The immunosuppressive properties of enisoprost and a 5-lipoxygenase inhibitor (SC-45662). *Transplantation* 1991; **52,** 1053–1057.
71. Calmus Y, Gane P, Rouger P *et al.* Hepatic expression of class I and class II major histocompatability complex molecules in primary biliary cirrhosis: effect of ursodeoxycholic acid. *Hepatology* 1990; **11,** 12–17.
72. Henriksson BA, Persson H, Friman S, Wangberg B, Svanvik J, Kariberg I. Adjuvant ursodeoxycholic acid prevents acute rejection in liver transplant recipients. *Transplant Proc* 1991; **23,** 1971.
73. Friman S, Mjornstedt L, Persson H, Karlberg I, Olausson M. Ursodeoxycholic acid reduces acute rejection in heart allografted rats. *Transplant Proc* 1992; **24,** 244–245.
74. Chen SF, Ruben RL, Dexter D. Mechanism of action of the novel anticancer agent 6-fluoro-2-(2'-fluoro-1, 1'-biphenyl-4-yl)-3-methyl-4-quinolone carboxylic acid sodium salt (NSC 368390): inhibition of *de novo* pyrimidine nucleotide biosynthesis. *Cancer Res* 1986; **46,** 5014–5020.
75. Cramer D, Chapman F, Jaffee BD *et al.* The effect of a new immunosuppressive drug, Brequinar sodium, on heart, liver and kidney allograft rejection in the rat. *Transplantation* 1992; **53,** 303–308.
76. Badger AM, Albright-Winslow CR, Kupiec-Weglinski JW. SKF 105685: a novel immunosuppressive compound with efficacy in animal models of autoimmunity and transplantation. *Transplant Proc* 1991; **23,** 194–198.
77. Metcalfe SM, Watson CJE, Collier D *et al.* Survival of renal allografted dogs after limited therapy with cyclosporine and the PAF antagonist WEB 2170. *Transplant Proc* 1991; **23,** 2219–2220.
78. Hancock WW, Whitley D, Kupiec-Weglinski JW, Tilney N. Oral iron chelator Desferrithiocin blocks allogeneic monocuclear cell activation and cytokine production *in vivo* and prolongs rat cardiac allograft survival. *Transplant Proc* 1992; **24,** 214–215.
79. Sumimoto R, Kamada N. Specific suppression of allograft rejection by soluble class I antigen and complexes with monoclonal antibody. *Transplantation* 1990; **50,** 678–662.
80. Panel Discussion. Monoclonal antibody therapy in paediatric transplantation. *Transplant Proc* 1992; **24,** 2–10.
81. McKeon F. When worlds collide, immunosuppressants meet protein phosphatases. *Cell* 1991; **66,** 823–826.
82. Koch HP. Thalidomide and congeners as anti-inflammatory agents. *Prog Med Chem* 1985; **22,** 165–241.
83. Isobe M, Yagita H, Okumurabe Y, Ihara A. Specific acceptance of cardiac allograft after treatment with antibodies to ICAM-1 and LFA-1. *Science* 1992; **255,** 1125–1127.
84. Borel J, Feurer C, Gubler H, Stahlein H. Biological effects of cyclosporin A. *Agents Actions* 1976; **6,** 468–476.
85. Herold K, Lancki DW, Moldwin RL, Fitch F. Immunosuppressive effects of cyclosporine A on cloned T-cells. *J Immunol* 1986; **136,** 1315–1321.
86. Hess AD, Tutscka PJ. Effect of cyclosporine A on human lymphocyte responses *in vitro* I. *J Immunol* 1980; **124,** 2601–2608.
87. Takahashi N, Hayano T, Suzuki M. Peptidyl-prolyl cis-trans isomerase is the cyclosporine A binding protein, cyclophilin. *Nature* 1989; **337,** 473–475.
88. Fischer G, Whitman B, Lang K *et al.* Cyclophilin and peptidylprolyl cis-trans isomerase are probably identical proteins. *Nature* 1989; **337,** 476–478.
89. Lorber MI. Cyclosporine: lessons learned – future strategies. *Clin Transplant* 1991; **5,** 505–516.
90. Kino T, Hatanaka H, Hashimoto M. FK506, a novel immunosuppressant isolated from a Streptomyces. II Immunosuppressive effects *in vitro*. *J Antibiotics* (Tokyo) 1987; **40,** 1256–1263.
91. White DJG. FK506: the promise and the paradox. *Clin Exp Immunol* 1991; **83,** 1–3.
92. Todo S, Fung JJ, Starzl TE *et al.* Liver, kidney and thoracic organ transplantation under FK506. *Ann Surg* 1990; **212,** 295–305.
93. Harding MW, Galat A, Uehling D, Schreiber S. A receptor for the immunosuppressant FK506 is a cis-trans peptidyl-prolyl isomerase. *Nature* 1989; **341,** 758–760.
94. Bacha P, Williams DP, Waters C *et al.* Interleukin-2 receptor-targeted toxicity: interleukin 2 receptor mediated action of a diphtheria toxin related interleukin 2 fusion protein. *J Exp Med* 1988; **167,** 612–621.
95. Murphy J, Kelley V, Storm T. Interleukin-2 toxin: a step towards selective immunomodulation. *Am J Kidney Dis* 1988; **11,** 159–162.

19

HLA/ABO matching

G Steinhoff

Introduction

Differences in histocompatibility antigens form the basis for the rejection of organ transplants. A number of polymorphic antigen systems have been defined. Of these, the human leucocyte antigens (HLA) coded by the major histocompatibility complex (MHC) and blood group antigen (ABO) systems have major importance for the induction of immunological reactivity after organ transplantation. The potential importance of other molecules in the generation of clinical rejection, however, has to be considered. At present, in clinical liver transplantation, matching of tissue antigens between donor and recipient is only practised for the main blood group antigens (ABO). Compatibility between other tissue antigens, such as the HLA system, occurs only by chance and lymphocyte crossmatching is not routinely used.[1]

The clinical importance of allo-antigen incompatibility depends on the cell type and organ transplanted. Differences in tissue expression and release of allo-antigens in response not only to rejection but also immune responses to virus, microbial antigens, auto-antigens and tumour cells have to be considered.

HLA incompatibility

In the early days of experimental and clinical liver transplantation, the liver was thought to be an organ of low immunogenicity.[2] This assumption was prompted by experimental and clinical observations of tolerance. The problem of tissue incompatibility was overshadowed by limited organ resources, short preservation time and technical problems. As in heart transplantation, the limited organ availability and short preservation time made prospective matching of HLA loci between donor and recipient impossible. Liver transplantation has now been established for a decade and rejection is still a clinical problem influencing long-term results. Although the treatment of acute rejection is usually successful, chronic rejection and hyperacute rejection in sensitised recipients have a major effect on graft survival. For this reason, it is important to re-assess the effect of matching tissue antigens in the face of wider organ availability and extended preservation time. The latter would be a requirement for prospective matching considering the time needed for tissue typing and organ transport. In the last 20 years the beneficial effect of prospective HLA matching[3] for the outcome of organ transplants has been documented in renal and bone marrow transplantation.[4,5] The question arises whether the same benefit in long-term graft survival would result from HLA matching in liver transplantation.

Clinical results

The large number of patients who have received liver or heart transplants has allowed retrospective analysis of the effect of HLA mismatches on rejection and graft outcome. In a multicentre study of heart transplants, a beneficial effect of matching of HLA-B and HLA-DR MHC antigens on graft outcome has been demonstrated.[6] These results resemble the effect seen in renal transplants.[5] In liver transplantation, however, the clinical results were different (Table 19.1). The largest series, analysed in Pittsburgh[7] compared the clinical outcome of 500 liver transplants to class I or class II HLA compatibility. A dualistic effect of HLA matching on liver transplant outcome was found. The overall transplant survival

Table 19.1 Studies of HLA/ABO matching after liver transplation

Authors	Centre	Patients (n)
HLA incompatibility		
Donaldson *et al.* 1987	Cambridge	62
Markus *et al.* 1988	Pittsburgh	574
O'Grady *et al.* 1988	Cambridge	101
Gubernatis *et al.* 1988	Hanover	81
Batts *et al.* 1988	Rochester	55
Superina *et al.* 1989	Toronto	41
Calmus *et al.* 1990	Paris	155
Saito *et al.* 1991	Nebraska	212
ABO incompatibility		
Ramsey *et al.* 1984	Pittsburgh	171
Gordon *et al.* 1987	Pittsburgh	745
White *et al.* 1987	Cambridge	220
Fischel *et al.* 1989	Minnesota	93
Gugenheim *et al.* 1990	Paris	234

was decreased in grafts matched for MHC class I (HLA-A) or class II (HLA-DR). Conversely, in 108 failed grafts requiring retransplantation, there was a higher incidence of failure due to rejection correlated with a lower degree of HLA compatibility particularly for HLA-DR. The incidence of graft failures due to primary non-function was significantly correlated with HLA-DR compatibility.

In other studies, similarly contradictory effects of HLA compatibility and incompatibility were reported. Patients developing chronic rejection with vanishing bile duct syndrome (VBDS) showed a pattern of HLA-A,B incompatibility together with HLA-DR compatibility.[8,9] Other groups[10] reported a relationship between the development of a VBDS and positive lymphocyte crossmatch as well as HLA-DR incompatibility. A similar observation was made by the Hanover group,[11] who concluded that rejection types with bile duct damage are correlated with HLA-DR incompatibility. Partial HLA compatibility had no influence on rejection incidence.

In a small series[12] a high incidence of severe rejection leading to retransplantation in DRw6+ recipients was reported. Other authors,[13] however, could not confirm this observation and found an equal risk in DRw6 positive and negative recipients irrespective of their individual HLA mismatch. Recently, Calmus *et al.*[14] found that hepatitis B recurrence with manifestation of hepatic lesions after transplantation was associated with HLA class I compatibility, but not with class II HLA-DR compatibility. The question arises as

Table 19.2 Clinical complications of HLA/ABO incompatibility

Recipient sensitisation to:	
HLA	Acute/chronic cellular rejection (hyperacute/ humoral rejection)
ABO	Hyperacute/humoral rejection Severe acute/chronic rejection Vascular thrombosis Sclerosing cholangitis
Graft sensitisation to:	
HLA	Graft versus host disease (GvH) Thrombocytopenia
ABO	GvH Haemolytic anaemia

to whether these observations reflect the role of HLA antigens in different pathogeneic mechanisms leading to graft injury after transplantation (Table 19.2).

Donor/recipient immune reactivity and recurrence of disease

The prevalence and severity of rejection in the liver is comparable to that seen in other organs such as the kidney or the heart. For this reason it is conceivable that HLA identity between donor and recipient would reduce the severity of acute rejection and incidence of chronic rejection. However, late rejection after liver transplantation is less common than in kidney or heart grafts.

Whilst HLA matching may reduce immune reactivity to donor HLA, auto-immune or virus directed T cell cytolytic reactivity associated with the original liver disease may be enhanced. In addition, full HLA-DR compatibility may enhance the T cell response to viral or auto-immune antigens and to minor histocompatibility antigens. These immune reactions may mediate graft injury in addition to the anti-HLA rejection response and this could lead to recurrent liver disease (PBC or recurrent hepatitis), and also augment rejection by induction of donor HLA and secondary sensitisation to allo-antigens (Table 19.3).

The transplantation of immune competent donor cells with the liver has a number of consequences: HLA allo-immunisation against host antigens (graft versus host reaction – GvH) is possible (see Table 19.2). Lethal GvH disease has been reported in liver transplant recipients,[15,16] as well as minor clinical complications such as

Table 19.3 Dualistic effect of HLA matching in human liver transplantation

Compatible
- Recipient sensitisation to minor (non-HLA) transplantation antigens
- Enhancement of antiviral immune response to the graft (HBV,HCV,CMV,EBV)
- Persistence and recurrence of auto-immune T cell reactivity (PBC,PSC)
- Persistence of donor lymphocytes and development of GvH activity (minor transplantation and blood group antigens)

Incompatible
- Acute and chronic rejection response of the recipient
- GvH activity of transplanted donor lymphocytes
- Tolerance phenomena (soluble donor HLA antigens, 'veto' cells)

thrombocytopenia. It is possible that immune cells transplanted with the graft acting as 'veto' cells induce specific tolerance across certain HLA barriers.[17] Furthermore, parenchymal liver cells may influence immune reactivity and even induce tolerance by the secretion of soluble HLA class I antigens of donor type.[18]

Blood group (ABO) incompatibility

Even in the early days of organ transplantation, the beneficial effect of ABO bloodgroup compatibility was noted.[19] In the presence of ABO incompatibility, hyperacute humoral rejection was observed in renal transplants.[20] This was directly related to the extent of anti-A and/or anti-B antibody titres present in the recipients prior to transplantation[19] and due to the fact that the ABO antigens were widely distributed thoughout human tissues and organs.[21,22]

In emergency situations such as acute hepatic failure, liver transplantation across ABO barriers may be necessary (see Table 19.4). For many years it had been thought that the liver is resistant to hyperacute rejection.[2] In recent years, however, it has become clear that ABO incompatible liver transplantation in sensitised recipients may lead to humoral and hyperacute rejection with graft loss.[23,24] Unlike renal or heart transplantation, however, liver transplantation across ABO barriers can still be successfully performed in urgent clinical situations.[25]

Clinical results

The analysis of ABO compatibility and liver transplant outcome in larger clinical series showed a significant advantage of ABO identity between donor and recipient.[26,27] Figure 19.1 shows the results of one such study. The outcome of grafts with ABO compatibility (O donor to A, B, or AB recipient) was associated with a slightly reduced survival compared with ABO identical (O to O, A to A, etc.) grafts.[24,26,27] Many of the ABO nonidentical grafts were done as an emergency.[24,26] However, even when only emergency grafts are considered, survival of ABO incompatible grafts is less than compatible ones.[24] This difference is due to a high incidence of hyperacute/severe rejection and vascular thrombosis.

Hyperacute/humoral rejection

With increasing numbers of ABO incompatible grafts transplanted in emergency cases, a clinical syndrome of antibody mediated rejection has been described in liver transplants.[23] A number of groups reported cases of graft loss due to hyperacute rejection in presensitised (ABO incompatible) recipients. Studies suggest that the rejection was mediated by iso-agglutinins causing endothelial damage, vessel thrombosis and haemorrhagic necrosis of the graft.[23] The risk of hyperacute rejection may be diminished in sensitised recipients with pre-operative plasma exchange, splenectomy and post-operative ALG treatment.[25] Late humoral rejection after transplantation is rare. It may be diagnosed by an increase in titres to blood group antigens and may

Table 19.4 Liver transplantation across ABO barriers

ABO mismatch*	Donor	Recipient	Therapeutic regimen
Compatible	0	A,B,AB	Standard immunosuppression (0-RBC transfusion)
Incompatible	A,B,AB	0,A,B	Antilymphocyte globulin, plasmapheresis, splenectomy, 0-RBC transfusion

*Identical match: 0 to 0, A to A, etc.

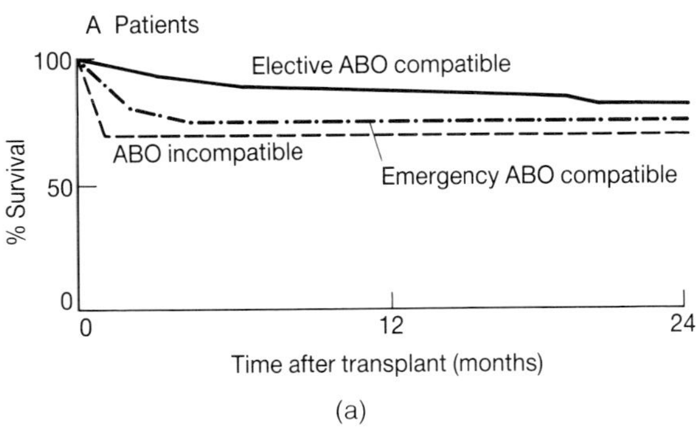

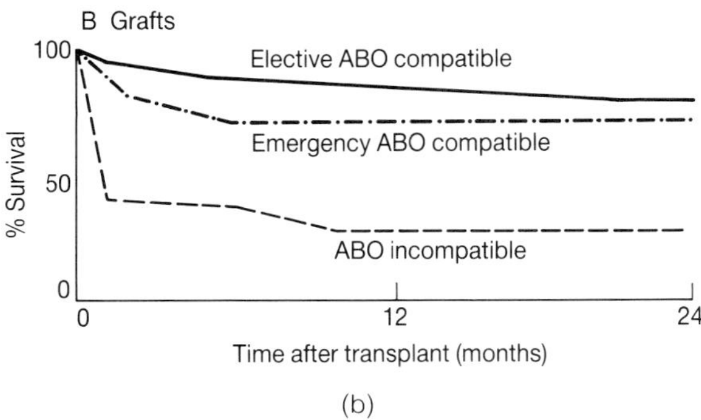

Fig. 19.1 Patient (a) and graft (b) survival in patients receiving A,B,O compatible grafts in elective and in emergency situations (taken from [24] with kind permission from *The Lancet*).

be treated by plasma exchange and increased immunosuppression.[25]

Graft versus host reactivity

Ramsey *et al.* first reported the finding of isohaemagglutinins of graft origin directed to incompatible recipient blood group antigens after liver transplantation.[28] They observed haemolysis in the majority of these patients. Most probably, the antibodies were produced by persisting donor B lymphocytes transplanted with the graft. Clinical observations of non-ABO related graft versus host disease in liver graft recipients have also been reported.[15,16] It has to be assumed that lymphoid cells transplanted with the graft have a limited life span and that GvH reactivity therefore usually occurs only in the first weeks after transplantation and ceases with the elimination of donor cells. Although full blown GvH disease is rare, in ABO non-identical transplantation, temporary GvH activity leading to haemolysis occurs more often. Haemolytic anaemia caused by anti-A,B or AB directed graft versus host reactions is treated by repeated transfusion of red cells, plasmapheresis and a reduction in immunosuppression to allow the elimination of donor immune cells. Only in critical exacerbations are steroid and ALG treatments necessary.

Clinical indication and management of ABO mismatched transplantation

Liver transplantation across ABO barriers should be restricted to cases of acute hepatic failure since the long-term prognosis of incompatible grafts is inferior to that of compatible ones. Bile duct complications, severe rejection and an increased risk of portal and hepatic artery thrombosis have been reported to occur. Therefore, ABO incompatible grafts are now usually used as a bridge until a compatible graft is available. To circumvent the threat of hyperacute rejection, presensitised recipients should undergo plasmapheresis. Splenectomy and post-operative ALG[25] treatment to prevent additional recipient sensitisation to donor blood group antigens have been recommended. Patients with non-identical and incompatible grafts should be regularly monitored for isohaemagglutinin titres. Rising titres may require treatment with plasmapheresis.

Clinical importance of other allo-antigenic systems

The importance of sensitisation to minor blood group and minor transplantation antigens is not clear in human liver transplantation. Sensitisation to minor blood group antigens such as rhesus factor and Lewis has been reported by Ramsey *et al.*[29,30] but did not result in decreased graft survival. Haemolysis, increased blood requirement during transplantation and thrombocytopenia, however, may result from sensitisation to minor blood group antigens. The polymorphism of complement factors that are produced in the liver may also lead to recipient sensitisation.[31] The role of these and additional soluble and membrane bound polymorphic molecules as targets for the rejection response[32] or inducers of tolerance still has to be clarified.

References

1. Iwatsuki S, Rabin BS, Shaw BW Jr, Starzl TE. Liver transplantation against T cell-positive warm crossmatches. *Transplant Proc* 1984; **16,** 1427–1429.
2. Starzl TE, Ishikawa M, Putnam CW *et al.* Progress in and deterrents to orthotopic liver transplantation, with special reference to survival, resistance to hyperacute rejection, and biliary duct reconstruction. *Transplant Proc* 1974; **6,** 129–139.
3. Terasaki PI, Mickey MR, Singal DP, Mittal KK, Patel R. Serotyping for homotransplantation. Selection of recipients for cadaver donor transplants. *N Eng J Med* 1968; **279,** 1101–1103.
4. O'Reilly RJ. Current developments in marrow transplantation. *Transplant Proc* 1987; **19**(1), 92–102.
5. Opelz G. Effect of HLA matching in 10,000 cyclosporine treated cadaver kidney transplants. *Transplant Proc* 1987; **19,** 641–646.
6. Opelz G for the Collaborative Heart Transplant Study. Effect of HLA matching in heart transplantation. *Transplant Proc* 1989; **21**(1), 794–796.
7. Markus BH, Duquesnoy RJ, Gordon RD *et al.* Histocompatibility and liver transplant outcome. Does HLA exert a dualistic effect? *Transplantation* 1988; **46,** 372–377.
8. Donaldson PT, Alexander GJM, O'Grady JG *et al.* Evidence for an immune response to HLA class I antigens in the vanishing bile duct syndrome after liver transplantation. *Lancet* 1987; **1,** 945–951.
9. O'Grady JG, Alexander GJ, Sutherland S *et al.* Cytomegalovirus infection and donor/recipient HLA-antigens: interdependent co-factors in pathogenesis of vanishing bile-duct syndrome after liver transplantation. *Lancet* 1988; **2,** 302–305.
10. Batts KP, Moore SB, Perkins JD, Wiesner RH, Grambsch PM, Krom RF. Influence of positive lymphocyte crossmatch and HLA-mismatching on vanishing bile duct syndrome in human liver allografts. *Transplantation* 1988; **45,** 376–379.
11. Gubernatis G, Kemnitz J, Tusch G, Pichlmayr R. HLA compatibility and different features of liver allograft rejection. *Transplant Int* 1988; **1,** 155–160.
12. Superina RA, Pearl RH, Greig PD, Levy G, Falk J, Langer B. Effect of DRw6 antigen in recipients and donors on survival after liver transplant. *Transplant Proc* 1989; **21,** 786–788.
13. Saito S, Stratta RJ, Grazi GL *et al.* Effect of the HLA-DRw6 antigen in liver transplantation. *Transplant Proc* 1991; **23,** 1430–1431.
14. Calmus Y, Hannoun L, Dousset B *et al.* HLA class I matching is responsible for the hepatic lesions in recurrent viral hepatitis B after liver transplantation. *Transplant Proc* 1990; **22,** 2311–2313.
15. Burdick JF, Vogelsang GB, Smith WJ *et al.* Severe graft-versus-host disease in a liver-transplant recipient. *N Eng J Med* 1988; **318,** 689–691.
16. Marubayashi S, Matsuzaka C, Takeda A *et al.* Fatal generalized acute graft-versus-host disease in a liver transplant recipient. *Transplantation* 1990; **50,** 709–711.
17. Thomas JM, Carver FM, Cunningham PRG, Olson LC, Thomas FT. Kidney allograft tolerance in primates without chronic immunosuppression – the role of veto cells. *Transplantation* 1991; **51,** 198–207.
18. Davies HS, Pollard SG, Calne RY. Soluble HLA antigens in the circulation of liver graft recipients. *Transplantation* 1989; **47,** 524–7.
19. Starzl TE, Tzakis A, Makowka L *et al.* The definition of ABO factors in transplantation: relation to other humoral antibody states. *Transplant Proc* 1987; **19,** 4492–4497.
20. Starzl TE, Marchioro TL, Holmes JH *et al.* Renal homografts in patients with major donor-recipient blood group incompatibilities. *Surgery* 1964; **55,** 195–200.
21. Szulman AD. The histological distribution of blood group substances A and B in man. *J Exp Med* 1960; **111,** 785–800.
22. Breimer ME, Samuelsson BE. The specific distribution of glycolipid based blood group A antigens in human kidney related to A1/A2, Lewis, and secretor status of single individuals: a possible molecular explanation for the successful transplantation of A2 kidneys into O recipients. *Transplantation* 1986; **42,** 88–91.
23. Demetris AJ, Jaffe R, Tzakis A *et al.* Antibody mediated rejection of human liver allografts: transplantation across ABO blood group barriers. *Transplant Proc* 1989; **21,** 2217–2220.
24. Gugenheim J, Samuel D, Reynes M, Bismuth H. Liver transplantation across ABO blood group barriers. *Lancet* 1990; **336,** 519–523.
25. Fischel RJ, Ascher NL, Payne WD *et al.* Pediatric liver transplantation across ABO blood group barriers. *Transplant Proc* 1989; **21,** 2221–2222.
26. Gordon RD, Iwatsuki S, Esquivel CO, Tsakis A, Todo S, Starzl TE. Liver transplantation across ABO blood groups. *Surgery* 1986; **100,** 342–348.
27. White DJ, Gore SM, Barroso E, Calne RY. The significance of ABO blood groups in liver transplantation. *Transplant Proc* 1987; **19,** 4571–4574.
28. Ramsey G, Nusbacher J, Starzl TE, Lindsay GD. Isohemagglutinins of graft origin after ABO-unmatched liver transplantation. *N Eng J Med* 1984; **311,** 1167–1170.
29. Ramsey G, Wolford J, Boczkowski DJ, Cornell FQ, Larson P, Starzl TE. The Lewis blood group

system in liver transplantation. *Transplant Proc* 1987; **19,** 4591–4594.
30. Ramsey G, Hahn LF, Cornell FW *et al.* Low rate of Rhesus immunization from Rh-incompatible blood transfusions during liver and heart transplant surgery. *Transplantation* 1989; **47,** 993–995.
31. Woelpl A, Robin-Winn M, Pichlmayr R, Goldmann SG. Fourth component of complement (C4) polymorphism in human orthotopic liver transplantation. *Transplantation* 1985; **40,** 154–157.
32. Van Els C, Bueger MH, Kempenaar J, Donec M, Goulmy E. Susceptibility of human male keratinocytes to MHC-restricted H-Y specific lysis. *J Exp Med* 1989; **170,** 1469–1474.

20

Liver preservation and rejection

LH Toledo-Pereyra, J Lopez-Ranger, R Xavier and A Chousleb

Introduction

Current advances in hepatic transplantation are in part dependent on the development of effective preservation solutions and the use of better immunosuppressive regimens for the treatment of rejection.

The liver has been one of the most difficult solid organs to preserve. Researchers have attempted to improve liver viability by maintenance or inhibition of its cellular metabolism. Hypothermia is the principal method used for inhibition of cellular metabolism and decrease in oxygen requirements.[1] To maintain the liver metabolic demands, the use of high energy compounds or appropriate nutrients is needed.

Historical developments of preservation

The liver is especially sensitive to anoxia,[2] a property which results in a lack of tolerance to the various methods of preservation. In 1960, the first long term survival of a transplanted dog liver was reported. The donor dog was immersed in an ice bath, to reduce the body temperature to 30° and 15° C, and the liver was perfused through the portal vein with cold Ringer's lactate solution (4–7° C).[3] The first human orthotopic liver transplant was performed in 1963.[4]

In 1969, the works of Collins *et al.*[5] on kidneys and Schalm *et al.*[6] on the liver suggested that a crystalloid solution with a composition comparable to the intracellular environment should be used to supplement the effect of core cooling and hypothermia, allowing for longer preservation periods of 30 hours for the kidney and just over two hours for the liver.

In 1970, the utilisation of hypothermia and low flow perfusion with cryoprecipitated plasma permitted the preservation of porcine livers for up to ten hours, but when the duration of preservation was extended, most of the animals died because of a bleeding diathesis.[7] The use of a balanced electrolyte solution with low molecular weight dextran for the initial flush and reconstituted frozen plasma and hyperbaric oxygen at 3 atm improved the storage time to 12 hours.[8]

In 1975, Toledo-Pereyra *et al.* obtained better results with a silica gel fraction of plasma (SGF) (Table 20.1), with the addition of KCl, dextran and albumin.[9] They also demonstrated the protective effect of allopurinol in ischaemic livers.[10] Four years later, the same authors obtained longer survival after auxiliary liver transplantation of organs preserved with Sacks solution instead of Ringer's lactate. The silica gel fraction of plasma proved to be superior to Collins and Sacks sol-

Table 20.1 Composition of the silica gel fraction solutions (SGF-I and SGF-III)

SGF-I		SGF-III	
Plasma SGF	400 ml	Plasma SGF	400 ml
25% Albumin	100 ml	25% Albumin	100 ml
$MgSO_4$	8 mEq/l	$MgSO_4$	8 mEq/L
KCl	20 mEq/l	KCl	20 mEq/L
Solu-Medrol	250 mg	Solu-Medrol	250 mg
Dextrose	5 gm	Dextrose (50%)	10 gm
		Ampicillin	250 mg
Osmolarity	430 mOsm/l	Osmolarity	420 mOsm/l

utions because of its colloidal properties, with less damage to endothelial cells.[11,12]

Preservation solutions

Organ viability is directly dependent on the quality of the harvested organ, the preservation time and the preservation solution utilised. These solutions can be colloidal or crystalloid, hypertonic or isotonic, with different electrolyte concentrations and with the possible addition of various drugs.

The efficacy of these solutions depends on the composition, warm ischaemia time and length of preservation.

UW solution

In 1987 Belzer and his associates introduced a new solution (University of Wisconsin solution) for experimental pancreatic preservation,[13] based on lactobionate and raffinose for the suppression of oedema, hydroxyethyl starch to diminish the shift of electrolytes to the extracellular space and water to the interstitial space, and other compounds that modify the xanthine oxidase pathway (allopurinol), stimulate the build-up of high energy compounds (adenosine) and glutathione, an inhibitor of lipid peroxidation. Successful hepatic preservation was achieved in dogs for 30 hours with this solution.[14] Since then, the UW solution has been routinely used for liver preservation in clinical transplantation[15] (Figure 20.1).

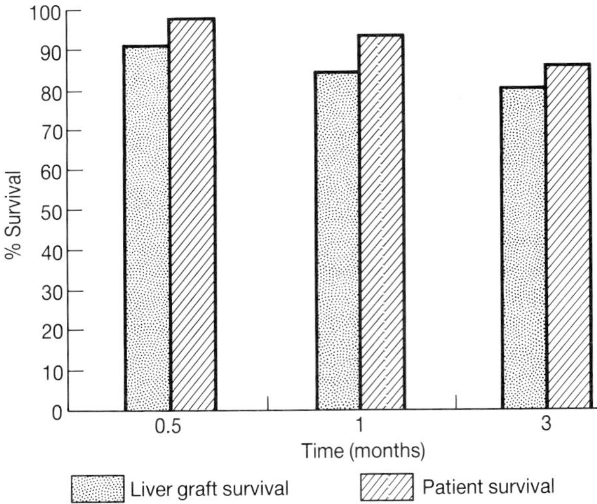

Fig. 20.1 Patient and graft survival of human livers subjected to various periods of hypothermic storage with UW solution. Although consistently high results were observed, patient and graft survival diminished somewhat by the third month (modified from Olthoff *et al.*[23]).

Comparison of UW with other solutions

Comparative studies between UW and Collins solutions for hepatic preservation showed better results with the UW solution,[16,17,18,19] with longer graft survival with a lower incidence of primary graft non-function, less hepatic artery thrombosis and extended preservation times.[20,21,22,23,24] Patient survival was 79% for UW solution compared with 63% for the Collins solution.[25] (See Figure 20.1)[26]

The introduction of the UW solution into clinical transplantation has revolutionised many clinical aspects of liver transplantation. Today, the majority of liver transplants can be scheduled as semi-elective procedures, unless the patient's medical condition dictates otherwise. Studies, between UW and a modified silica get fraction of plasma to which lactobionate has been added provided improved liver protection in dogs (26)

Essential components of UW solution

Studies that systematically assessed the components of the UW solution (Table 20.2) showed that the omission of hydroxyethyl starch,[27,28,29] adenosine, allopurinol, buffer phosphate or $MgSO_4$ did not alter graft survival.[27] The elimination of lactobionate, glutathione and dexamethasone resulted in decreased survival,[27,30] whereas the elimination of insulin increased survival.[27] Other work using perfused rabbit liver

Table 20.2 UW solution for preservation

K+ -Lactobionate	100 mmol
KH_2PO_4	25 mmol
$MgSO_4$	5 mmol
Raffinose	30 mmol
Adenosine	5 mmol
Glutathione	3 mmol
Insulin	100 U
Bactrim	0.5 ml
Dexamethasone	8 mg
Allopurinol	1 mM
Hydroxyethyl starch	50 g

demonstrated that only lactobionate, raffinose and glutathione were essential components of the UW solution.[31]

Drugs used in liver preservation

Pretreatment of the donor with chlorpromazine improved the quality of organs preserved with UW, probably due to its vaso-active or calcium channel blocking effects and its membrane stabilising properties.[32] Compounds that inhibit free radical production or modify the xanthine oxidase pathway, such as catalase,[33] allopurinol[34,35] and superoxide dismutase,[34,35,36] have had a protective effect in liver preservation.

Drugs that block calcium channels (such as nisoldipine) have been shown experimentally to improve hepatic microcirculation.[37] This is consistent with the hypothesis that Kupffer cells are activated early in the sequence of events, leading to endothelial cell mediated alterations in the microcirculation[37] early in the microcirculation and graft failure.[37]

Recently, the pretreatment of donors with an experimental platelet activating factor antagonist, such as SRI 63–441, has been shown to further reduce the cold ischaemic injury.[38]

Development of new solutions

Modifications of the UW solution by reducing the potassium concentration from 120 mM to 9±4 mM and increasing the sodium concentration from 30 mM to 140±5 mM produce results similar to the original UW solution, without the endothelial damage or risk of cardiac arrest in the recipient produced by high potassium concentrations.[39]

New solutions, like the Carolina rinse solution, contain electrolytes at concentrations similar to those in plasma, oncotic support against interstitial oedema (modified hydroxyethyl starch), anti-oxidants against oxygen radicals (allopurinol, desferroxamine and glutathione), vasodilators to improve microcirculation (nicardipine and adenosine), substrates to regenerate ATP (fructose and glucose plus insulin), and mildly acidic pH. These solutions have produced effective results in extending the preservation time of livers in animals.[40]

Recently, the HTK or Bretschneider's solution has been used for successful liver preservation for 24 hours.[41]

Liver rejection

Rejection was not considered to be a major problem when human liver transplantation began in the 1960s.[42] The major difficulties were ischaemia, poor preservation of the donor liver, technical complications of the vascular and biliary anastomoses, and infections.[43] It is now recognised that hyperacute rejection, as described in renal transplantation (induced by humoral immune mechanisms), is rare in liver transplantation[44,45,46] but other patterns of rejection occur.

The increased experience with liver transplantation since 1983 has modified understanding about the appearance and consquences of rejection. In part, this has resulted from the use of liver biopsies in most centres for the histological diagnosis of rejection.[47,48] Furthermore, improvements in operative techniques, treatment of infections, and the intensive care of these patients has reduced the incidence of non-immunological complications, so that rejection has become a major clinical problem occupying in up to 77% of patients.[43] In one study from Pittsburgh 16% of patients required retransplantation because of liver failure due to rejection.[49]

Mechanisms of liver allograft rejection

Brief observations

A variety of mechanisms for allograft rejection have been identified (see other chapters of this book). It is well recognized now that the rejection response which is generated against transplant organs by normal and genetically dissimilar recipients is mainly a cell-mediated immune process.[42,50] However, an important role can also be assigned to humoral antibodies in bringing about tissue destruction under some circumstances.[44,51]

The process of induction of specific immunological unresponsiveness by transplanted organs in respect to their own antigens is of great interest. The distribution of class I and II Major Histocompatibility Complex (MHC) antigens in the liver appears to be important during rejection.[52,53] Class I antigens are in the hepatocytes, and the

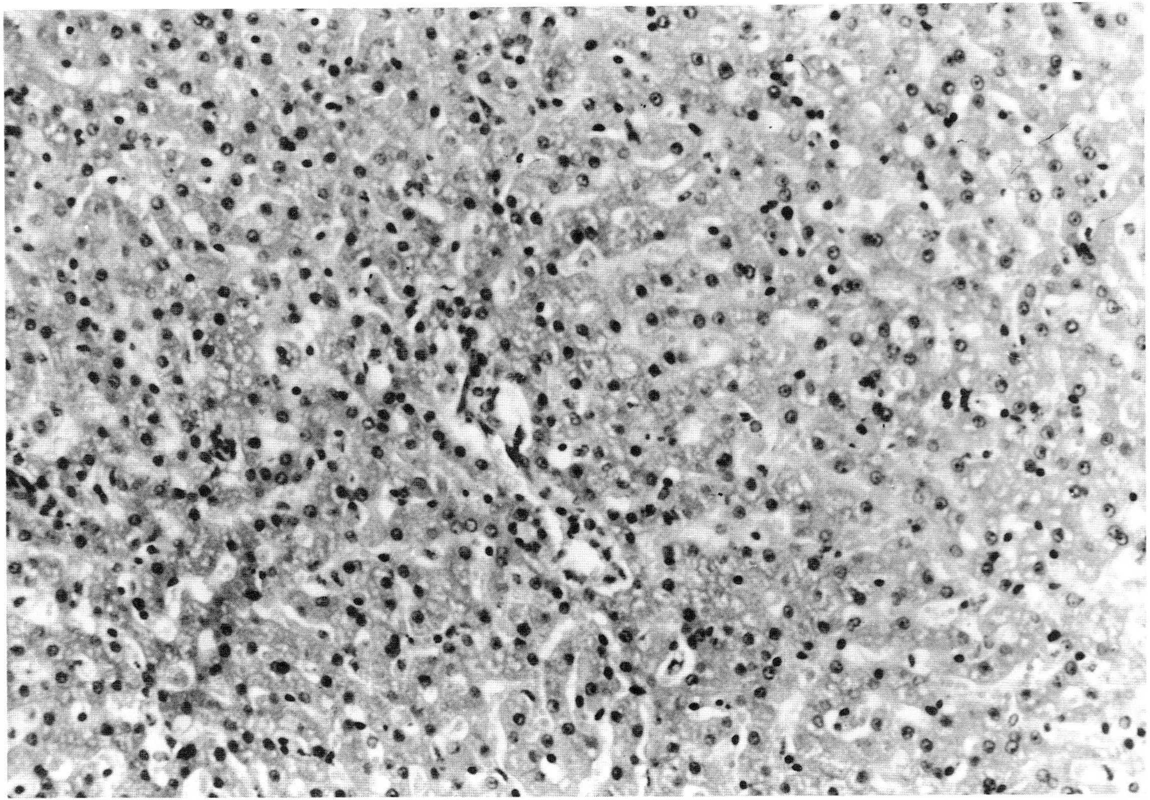

Fig. 20.2 Mild chronic passive congestion was noted after 40 minutes of ischaemic damage in canine livers protected with allopurinol (50 mg/l) intravenously ten minutes before the ischaemic insult. Reactive hepatocytes were quite prominent. Microvacuolisation was noted in some of the hepatocytes (haematoxylin and eosin ×40).

class II antigens are rarely expressed.[54,55,56] In contrast, the bile duct epithelium and central vein endothelium are rich in both class I and class II expression antigens. An important expression of the MHC occurs in these sites when the liver develops acute rejection.

Careful observations have demonstrated that early in the acute rejection lymphocytic infiltration occurs in portal tracts and in the walls of central veins due to damage in the bile duct epithelium and central vein endothelium.[43,50,57,58] Furthermore, an increase in the expression of class I antigens on hepatocytes was shown during acute rejection.[59]

Previous experience with liver transplants has shown that these grafts survive better than kidneys or hearts, perhaps because the liver mass was too great to be destroyed quickly by the antibody.[43,50] Another explanation for this lack of response from preformed cytolytic antibodies is the dilution effect that frequently accompanies liver transplantation. Blood loss and replacement translates to one or several volume exchanges in many patients. This lowers antibody titres and may also deplete the host of circulating lymphocytes that amplify the antibody response.[43]

Ischaemia, organ preservation and rejection

It has been demonstrated in renal transplantation that ischaemia and preservation injury can modify the immunogenicity of the graft.[60,61,62] In the liver, there are a few isolated studies[70,71] that have reviewed such findings. The main reason, until recently had to do with the lack of appropriate presentation solutions. In fact, Howard and associates[70] and Furukawa and his group[71] demonstrated that preservation injury by prolonged

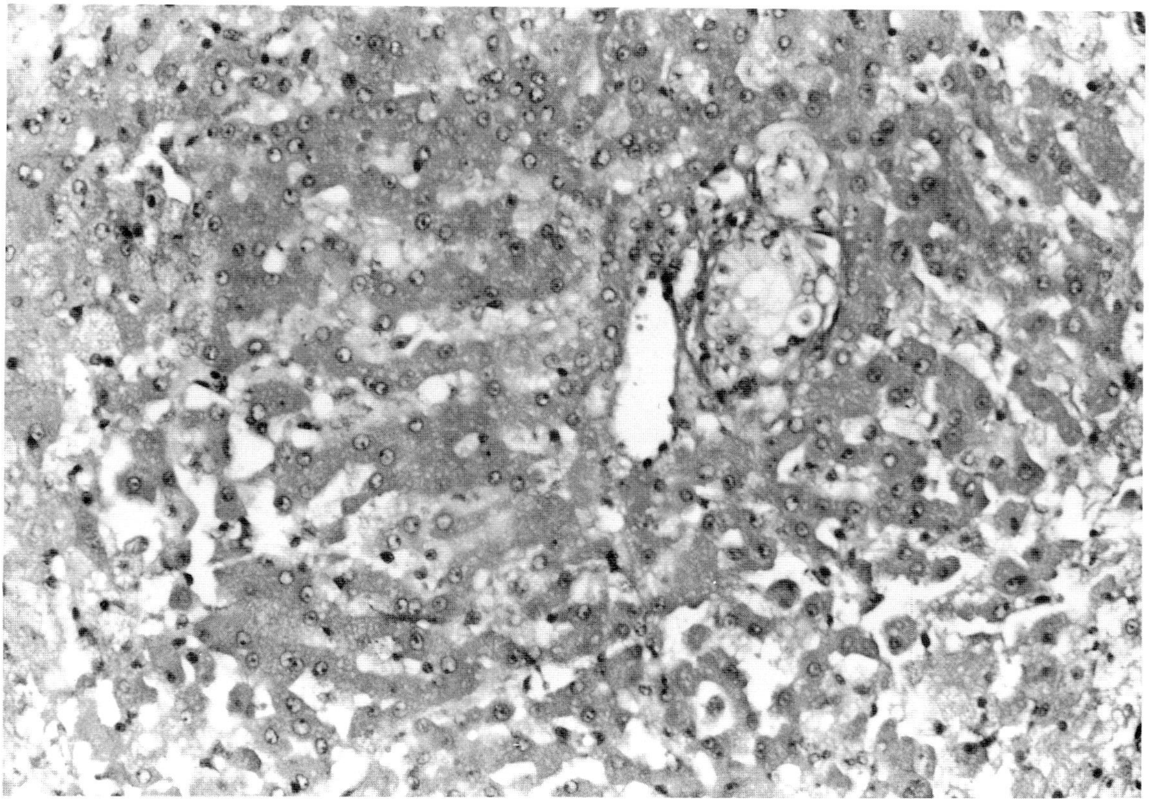

Fig. 20.3 Moderate chronic passive congestion was noted after 12 hours of canine liver intermittent non-pulsatile hypothermic perfusion with modified silica gel fraction of plasma (MSGF). No ischaemia was applied. The sinusoids are dilated and empty. The portal triad is in the right upper centre (haematoxylin and eosin ×40).

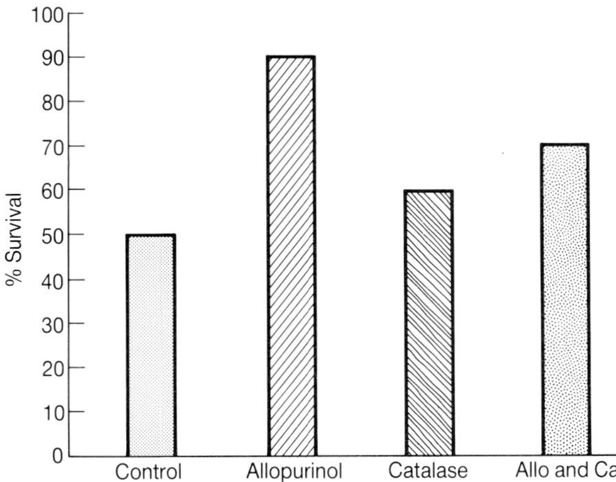

Fig. 20.4 A significant improvement in survival was noted after allopurinol (Allo) administration, alone or with catalase (Cat), in rats subjected to haemorrhagic shock prior to harvesting (modified from Cederna *et al.*[69]).

preservation times produced lower graft survival rates, unless modified by retransplantation of the failing liver. It is probable that the same events that modify the response of the kidney[60,61,62] and possibly the pancreas[63] might also occur in the liver. The liver appears to be very sensitive to ischaemia and preservation, and the immunogenicity of the liver might change after prolonged periods of ischaemia and/or preservation (Figures 20.2 and 20.3).

Reperfusion injury

The term 'reperfusion injury' has been recognised in recent years as a well defined clinical and pathological entity which occurs early during revascularisation.[64] The multitude of factors involved in the production of this lesion has made it difficult to determine the exact mechanism and site of revascularisation injury observed after liver transplantation.

The role of microvascular injury in the development of cellular damage after transplantation has recently occupied the interest of a great number of researchers.[65,66] During liver ischaemia or preservation injury, the production of free radicals, probably from the xanthine dehydrogenase/oxidase system, plays an important role in producing liver damage.[67,68] Drug therapy aimed at reducing free radical production might be the key to further reducing the damage seen after transplantation. Oxygen free radical scavengers or inhibitors of the xanthine oxidase pathway have been used before. Since 1975 we have utilised adenosine and allopurinol, among other substances, to protect ischaemically damaged liver allografts.[67,68] The results indicated some evidence of protection in the immediately transplanted livers.

In recent years, the protective effect of allopurinol, either alone or with catalase, on animals suffering from haemorrhagic shock has been established (Figure 20.4). The potential implication of these changes to multiple organ harvests is evident.[69] Further studies will be necessary, however, to extend the meaning of this finding to other species.

Recently, it has been demonstrated[40] that damage induced after storage and reperfusion, was specific for endothelial cells. The use of a solution containing concentration of electrolytes similar to plasma, with oncotic support based on hydroxyethyl starch, anti-oxidants such as allopurinol, desferroxamine and glutathione, vasodilators to improve microcirculation such as nicardipine and adenosine, substrates to regenerate adenosine triphosphate (ATP) such as fructose, and mildly acidic pH, has prevented some of the damage that occurs to sinusoidal endothelial cells with the alteration of the microcirculation due to reperfusion injury.[40] This protective effect should be taken into consideration when studying the immediate response of liver allograft recipients.

Conclusions

Advances in preservation have allowed for improved liver transplantation results. The limit of successful clinical liver preservation has remained at less than 24 hours. It is possible that further refining of the composition of the current solutions and better understanding of reperfusion injury will allow for improved preservation time and results after transplantation.

At present it is not possible to recognise, with any degree of certainty, the role that ischaemia and preservation might play in the modification of liver allograft survival. Only the comparison of prolonged preservation times would clarify the effect of this method on the immunological response of hepatic transplants.

References

1. Toledo-Pereyra LH. Kidney harvesting and preservation. In: *Kidney Transplantation*, Toledo-Pereyra LH (ed). Philadelphia: FA Davis Company, 1988.
2. Lambotte L. Liver preservation. In: *Basic Concepts in Organ Procurement, Perfusion and Preservation for Transplantation*, Toledo-Pereyra LH (ed). New York: Academic Press, 1982.
3. Starzl TE, Kaupp AH, Brock DR *et al.* Reconstructive problems in canine livers homotransplantation with special reference to the post-operative role of hepatic venous flow. *Surg Gynecol Obstet* 1960; **111,** 733.
4. Starzl TE, Marchioro TL, von Krauffa KN *et al.* Homotransplantation of the liver in humans. *Surg Gynecol Obstet* 1963; **117,** 659.
5. Collins GH, Bravo-Shugarman MB, Terasaki PI. Kidney preservation for transplantation. Initial perfusion and 30 hour ice storage. *Lancet* 1969; **2,** 1219.
6. Schalm SW, Terpstra JL, Drayer B *et al.* A simple method for short-term preservation of a liver homograft. *Transplantation* 1969; **8,** 887.
7. Belzer FO, May R, Berry MN. Short term preservation of porcine livers. *J Surg Res* 1970; **10,** 55.
8. Spilg H, Uys CJ, Hickman R *et al.* 12 hour liver preservation in the pig using hypothermic and hyperbaric oxygen. *Br J Surg* 1972; **59,** 273.
9. Toledo-Pereyra LH, Beselmeier TJ, Najarian JS. Protective effect of modified silica gel fraction (MSGF) on storage of canine livers for transplantation. *Trans Am Soc Artif Intern Organs* 1975; **21,** 79.
10. Toledo-Pereyra LH, Simmons RL, Najarian JS. Effect of allopurinol on preservation of ischemic kidneys perfused with plasma or plasma substitutes. *Ann Surg* 1975; **181,** 289.
11. Toledo-Pereyra LH, Chee M, Lillehei RC *et al.* Liver preservation by storage with hyperosmolar solutions for twenty-four hours. *Cryobiology* 1979; **16,** 43.
12. Toledo-Pereyra LH, MacKenzie GH, Baughman RD. Comparative results of prolonged hypo-

thermic storage of canine kidneys preserved with hyperosmolar colloid (TP-II) or crystalloid (Euro-collins) solution. *J Urol* 1983; **129,** 166.

13. Ploeg RJ, Goossens D, Belzer O *et al.* Successful 72-hour cold storage of dog kidneys with UW solution. *Transplantation* 1988; **46,** 191.
14. Jamieson NV, Sundberg R, Lindell S *et al.* Successful 24 to 30 hour preservation of the canine liver: a preliminary report. *Transplant Proc* 1988; **120,** 945.
15. Kalayoglu M, Sollinger HW, Stratta R *et al.* Extended preservation of the liver for clinical transplantation. *Lancet* 1988; **1,** 617.
16. Todo S, Nery J *et al.* Extended preservation of human liver grafts with UW solution. *J Am Med Assoc* 1989; **261,** 711.
17. Belzer FO. Clinical organ preservation with UW solution. *Transplantation* 1989; **47,** 1097.
18. Belzer FO, Kalayoglu M, D'Alessandro AM *et al.* Organ preservation: experience with University of Wisconsin solution and plans for the future. *Transplantation* 1990; **4,** 73.
19. D'Alessandro AM, Kalayoglu HW, Sollinger RM *et al.* Experience with Belzer UW cold storage solution in human liver transplantation. *Transplant Proc* 1990; **2,** 474.
20. Cooper J, Rettke J, Ludwig J *et al.* UW solution improves duration and quality of clinical liver preservation. *Transplant Proc* 1990; **2,** 477.
21. Todo S, Tzakis A, Starzl TE. Preservation of livers with UW or Eurocollins solution. *Transplantation* 1988; **46,** 925.
22. Cofer JB, Klintmalm GB, Howard TK *et al.* A comparison of UW with Eurocollins preservation solution in liver transplantation. *Transplantation* 1990; **49,** 1088.
23. Olthoff KM, Millis JM, Imagawa DK *et al.* Comparison of UW solution and Euro-Collins solutions for cold preservation of human liver grafts. *Transplantation* 1990; **49,** 284.
24. Stratta RJ, Wood RP, Langnas AN *et al.* Effect of extended preservation and reduced-size grafting on organ availability in pediatric liver transplantation. *Transplant Proc* 1990; **2,** 482.
25. Ferla G, Colledan M, Fassati LR *et al.* Liver cold storage using UW solution: clinical results in 23 consecutive transplants. *Transplant Proc* 1990; **2,** 480.
26. Toledo-Pereyra LH, Finkelstein I *et al.* Comparative analysis of colloid solutions for liver preservation: a bimodal distribution of solution on its protective effect. *Transplant Proc* 1990; **2,** 516.
27. Yu W, Coddington D, Bitter-Suermann H. Rat liver preservation. The components of UW that are essential to its success. *Transplantation* 1990; **49,** 1060.
28. Howden BO, Jablonski P, Thomas AC *et al.* Liver preservation with UW solution. Evidence that hydroxyethyl starch is not essential. *Transplantation* 1990; **49,** 869.
29. Nedelec JF, Capron-Laudereau M, Adam R *et al.* Mouse liver metabolism after 24-hour cold preservation using UW hydroxyethyl starch-free UW, and Euro-Collins solutions: a 31P, 13C NMR spectroscopy and biochemical analysis. *Transplant Proc* 1990; **2,** 492.
30. Boudjema K, van Gulik TM, Lindell SL *et al.* Effect of oxidized and reduced glutathione in liver preservation. *Transplantation* 1990; **50,** 948.
31. Jamieson NV, Lindell S, Sundberg R *et al.* An analysis of the components in UW using the isolated perfused rabbit liver. *Transplantation* 1988; **46,** 512.
32. Sundberg R, Ar'Rajab A, Ahren B. Improved liver preservation with UW solution by chlorpromazine donor pretreatment. *Transplant Proc* 1990; **2,** 508.
33. Toledo-Pereyra LH, Cederna J. Protection of liver allografts from ischemic damage prior to transplantation using insulin and catalase. In: *Oxygen Free Radicals in Shock*, Novelli GP and Ursini F, (eds). Florence: Krager 1985.
34. Castillo M, Toledo-Pereyra LH, Shapiro E *et al.* Protective effect of allopurinol, catalase, or superoxide dismutase in ischemic rat liver. *Transplant Proc* 1990; **2,** 490.
35. Toledo-Pereyra LH. Liver preservation: experimental and clinical observations. *Transplant Proc* 1988; **20,** 965.
36. Olson LM, Klintmalm GB, Husberg BS *et al.* Superoxide dismutase improves organ preservation in liver transplantation. *Transplant Proc* 1988; **20** (suppl 1), 961.
37. Takei Y, Marzi I, Kauffman FC *et al.* Increase in survival time of liver transplants by protease inhibitors and a calcium channel blocker, nisoldipine. *Transplantation* 1990; **50,** 14.
38. Ontell SJ, Makowka L, Ove P, Starzl TE. Improved hepatic function in the 24-hour preserved rat liver with UW-lactobionate solution and SRI 63–441. *Gastroenterology* 1988; **95,** 1617.
39. Moen J, Claesson K, Pienaar H, *et al.* Preservation of dog liver, kidney, and pancreas using the Belzer UW solution with a high-sodium and low-potassium content. *Transplantation* 1989; **47,** 940.
40. Currin R, Toole JG, Thurman RG, Lemasters JJ. Evidence that Carolina rinse solution protects sinusoidal endothelial cells against reperfusion injury after cold ischemic storage of rat liver. *Transplantation* 1990; **50,** 1076.
41. Lamesch P, Raygrotzki S, Kehrer G *et al.* Preservation of the liver with the HTK solution. *Transplant Proc* 1990; **2,** 518.
42. Calne RY, Williams R. Liver Transplantation. In:

Current Problems in Surgery, Ravitch MM (ed). Chicago: 1979.
43. Ascher NL, Freese DK, Paradis K *et al.* Rejection of the transplanted liver. In: *Transplantation of the Liver*, Maddrey WC (ed). New York: Elsevier, 1988.
44. Williams GM, Hume DM, Huson RP. 'Hyperacute' renal homograft rejection in man. *N Eng J Med* 1968; **279,** 611.
45. Hayry P Immunobiology of transplant rejection. *Ann Clin Res* 1981; **13,** 172.
46. Iwatsuki S, Iwaki Y, Kano T *et al.* Successful liver transplantation from crossmatch-positive donors. *Transplant Proc* 1981; **13,** 286.
47. Snover DC, Sibley RK, Freese DK *et al.* Orthotopic liver transplantation: a pathological study of 63 serial liver biopsies from 17 patients with specific reference to the diagnostic features and natural history of rejection. *Hepatology* 1984; **4,** 1212.
48. Snover DC, Freese DK, Sharp HL *et al.* Liver allograft rejection: an analysis of the use of biopsy in determining the outcome of rejection. *Am J Surg Pathol* 1987; **11,** 1.
49. Demetris AJ, Lasky S, van Thiel DH *et al.* Pathology of hepatic transplantation. A review of 62 adult allograft recipients immunosuppressed with a cyclosporine/steroid regimen. *Am J Pathol* 1985; **118,** 151.
50. Russell PS. Some immunological considerations in liver transplantation. *Hepatology* 1984; **4,** 76S.
51. Winn HJ, Baldamus CA, Jooste SV *et al.* Acute destruction by humoral antibody of rat skin grafted to mice. *J Exp Med* 1973; **137,** 893.
52. Demetris AJ, Lasey S, van Thiel DH *et al.* Induction of DR/Ia antigen in human liver allografts. *Transplantation* 1985; **40,** 504.
53. Takais L, Szend B, Monostari E *et al.* Expression of HLA-DR antigens in bile ducts of rejection liver transplants. *Lancet* 1985; **2,** 8365.
54. So SKS, Platt JL, Luckes LM *et al.* Cytolytic T lymphocyte-mediated injury of cultured hepatocytes as H-2 restricted. *Hepatology* 1985; **5,** 1017.
55. Davies H, Taylor JE, Daniel MR *et al.* Differences between pig tissues in the expression of major transplantation antigens: possible relevance for organ transplants. *J Exp Med* 1976; **143,** 987.
56. Davies H, Kamada N, Roser BJ. Mechanisms of donor-specific unresponsiveness induced by liver grafting. *Transplant Proc* 1983; **15,** 831.
57. Starzl TE. *Experience in hepatic transplantation.* Philadelphia: W.B. Saunders, 1969.
58. Starzl TE, Iwatsuki S, van Thiel DH *et al.* Evolution of liver transplantation. *Hepatology* 1982; **2,** 614.
59. So SKS, Platt JL, Ascher NL *et al.* Increased expression of class I major histocompatibility complex antigens on hepatocytes in rejecting human liver allografts. *Transplantation* 1987; **43,** 79.
60. Payne WD, Michels LD, Toledo-Pereyra LH *et al.* Effects of pulsatile perfusion on the immunogenicity of renal allograft. *J Surg Res* 1977; **22,** 380.
61. Toledo-Pereyra LH, Simmons RL, Moberg AW *et al.* Organ preservation in success of cadaver transplants. *Arch Surg* 1975; **110,** 1031.
62. Toledo-Pereyra LH, Simmons RL, Olson LC *et al.* Perfusion time and the survival of cadaver transplants. *Surgery* 1976; **79,** 377.
63. Sutherland DER, Moundry-Munns KC and Gillingham K. Results of pancreas transplantation in the UNOS Registry. In: *Clinical Transplantation*, Terasaki P (ed). Los Angeles: UCLA, 1989.
64. Toledo-Pereyra LH. Liver transplantation reperfusion injury. Factors in its development and avenues for treatment. *Klinische Woshenschrift* (in press).
65. McKeown CMB, Edwards V, Phillips MJ *et al.* Sinusoidal lining cell damage: the critical injury in cold preservation of liver allografts in the rat. *Transplantation* 1988; **46,** 178.
66. Toledo-Pereyra LH. The role of allopurinol and oxygen free radical scavengers in liver preservation. In: *Oxygen Radicals in Biology and Medicine*, Simic MG (ed). New York: Plenum Publishing Corp., 1989.
67. Toledo-Pereyra LH, Simmons RL, Najarian JS. Protection of the ischemic liver by donor pretreatment before transplantation. *Am J Surg* 1975; **129,** 513.
68. Toledo-Pereyra LH, Cederna J, Choudhury S. Oxygen free radicals, allopurinol and the xanthine oxidase pathway during liver ischemia. *Surg Res Comm* 1989; **5,** 297.
69. Cederna J, Bandlien K, Toledo-Pereyra LH *et al.* Effect of allopurinol and/or catalase on hemorrhagic shock and their potential application to multiple organ harvesting. *Transplant Proc* 1990; **22,** 444.
70. Howard TK, Kluitmalm CBC, Cofer JB, *et al.* The influence of preservation injury on rejection in the hepatic transplant recipient. *Transplantation*, 1990; **49,** 103.
71. Furukawa H, Todo S, Imventarza O, *et al.* Effect of cold ischemia time on the early outcome of human hepatic allografts preserved with UW solution. *Transplantation*, 1991; **51,** 1000.

21

Viral and opportunistic infection

J O'Grady, R Williams and S Sutherland

Introduction

The pharmacologically induced state of immunosuppression that is required to prevent rejection of the transplanted liver facilitates the development of a wide range of infections, ranging from nosocomial to true opportunistic infections. In addition, viral infections which caused or were associated with the original liver disease may recur after transplantation and the expression of these re-infections may be significantly altered by the immunosuppressive therapy. There is some evidence that the pattern and severity of these infections are, in part, influenced by the level of immunosuppression used, and in particular by the need to use the monoclonal antibody OKT3.[1-3]

Hepatitis viruses

Hepatitis A

Acute liver failure following hepatitis A is rare but increasing in some Western countries as a consequence of the delayed exposure to the virus,[4] and a number of such patients have undergone liver transplantation.[5-8] The data on recurrent disease are limited, but one study using both monoclonal antibody and *in situ* hybridisation techniques demonstrated the presence of HAV in liver tissue as early as seven days, and up to two and seven months after liver transplantation.[9] One of the cases described had a mild self-resolving hepatitis at two months that was attributed to hepatitis A on the basis of concurrent excretion of the virus in faeces. The second patient had evidence of persistent hepatitis A virus in the liver tissue until the graft was lost to chronic rejection at six months, but no clearcut episode of graft dysfunction could be attributed to it.

Hepatitis B and D

Infection from these viruses is a frequent indication for liver transplantation, either because of acute liver failure or more commonly because of end-stage chronic liver disease or hepatocellular carcinoma. Recurrence of the viral hepatitis B infection after transplantation has been shown to worsen the outcome, and two studies have shown significantly lower survival rates between one and five years after transplantation in these patients.[10,11] In cases of fulminant hepatic failure, studies suggest that in the majority of patients the virus has ceased to replicate by the time of admission to hospital. In two studies, HBeAg was detected in serum in 12% and 37% of patients, while in the latter only 9% of cases were seropositive for HBV DNA.[12,13] This would appear to suggest that, in theory, most patients with fulminant hepatitis B should not carry a risk of recurrent infection, although one study has documented re-infection in 87.5% of such cases after liver transplantation.[14]

Recurrence of HBV infection is a more predictable problem after transplantation in chronic carriers. The natural history of such re-infection was studied in 29 patients transplanted in the Cambridge and King's College Hospital joint programme between 1975 and April 1989, who did not receive systematic immunoprophylactic therapy.[11] The analysis was confined to patients who survived at least two months after transplantation. Of this cohort, 82% reverted to being chronic HBsAg carriers after liver transplantation, an identical figure to that observed in another single centre study of 45 patients, 39 of whom received aggressive immunoprophylaxis, with or without treatment with interferon, for up to six weeks after transplantation.[14] Four of the five patients who cleared HBsAg from serum did not have any evidence of HBV recurrence, while the fifth seroconverted after an acute hepatitic illness. None of these patients had any evidence of HBV replication (HBeAg and HBV DNA seronegative) at the time of transplantation. In contrast, 58% of those who re-infected with HBV had serological evidence of viral replication at the time of transplantation, and this increased to 88% after transplantation. Furthermore, the rate of HBV replication increased dramatically after transplantation in those patients who did not have a co-existing hepatitis D infection, with HBV DNA levels rising to >800 pg/40 μl serum in all but one case, as compared to the maximum observed level of 131 pg/40 μl serum prior to transplantation (Table 21.1). This is presumed to be a consequence of immunosuppressive therapy, especially the corticosteroid component.

The early reports of liver transplantation in patients with co-existing hepatitis D infection were inconsistent.[15–18] Two of the seven patients in the original description developed fulminant hepatic failure following liver transplantation,[15] but a later paper reported more favourable results when patients were maintained on low doses of HBIg.[17] Comparative data are now available from three series; in two, hepatitis D was associated with a better intermediate term prognosis with respect to HBV re-infection whether or not immunoprophylaxis was used,[19,11] while the third, in which immunoprophylaxis was used, found no significant difference between those with hepatitis B alone and those with hepatitis B and D infections.[14] Interestingly, the HBV DNA levels in serum after transplantation were found to be lower in patients with co-existing hepatitis D (range 8–797 pg/40 μl serum) than in a comparable group of patients with HBV infection alone (>800 pg/40 μl serum), suggesting that the hepatitis D virus is acting as a natural suppressor of HBV replication.[11]

Of the strategies that have been attempted to prevent HBV re-infection after liver transplantation, passive immunoprophylaxis with anti-HBs (HBIg) holds most promise. This was first described in 1975 in a 29 year old man with HBV infection and hepatocellular carcinoma who remains well with no evidence of recurrence of either condition 17 years later.[20] A total dose of 1100 ml of solution containing 10 g protein/100 ml was administered during the anhepatic phase of the transplant and again on the sixth postoperative day. Subsequently, passive immunoprophylaxis was widely used by other groups with diverse regimens and varying degrees of success.[14–17,21,22] The amounts of HBIg administered intra-operatively ranged from 500–128,000 units and the duration of therapy ranged up to one year. Some groups also used adjuvant active vaccination[14,15,22] or interferon therapy.[14] A recent report of 110 patients receiving high dose passive immunoprophylaxis showed an overall actuarial recurrence rate of 29% over a two year period.[19] However, the equivalent figures for three subgroups indicated that most failures occurred in patients with chronic HBV infection (59% recurrence), as compared to patients with hepatitis B and D chronic infection (13%) or fulminant hepatic failure (0%). Within the former group, recurrence of HBV infection was almost universal (96%) in those patients who had HBV DNA detectable in serum at the time of transplantation, as compared to 29% in the HBV DNA seronegative cohort.[19] The cost/benefit ratio for passive immunoprophylaxis suggests its administration

Table 21.1 Recurrence of hepatitis B virus (HBV) after liver transplantation in the King's College Hospital and Cambridge series without the use of long term HBIg

Category	Number	Pretransplant HBV DNA	Post-transplant HBV DNA	HBV recurrence	Graft loss to HBV
Hepatitis B alone – without replication	9	0	130 → 800	7 (77.8%)	4 (44.4%)
Hepatitis B alone – with replication	11	10–131	>800	11 (100%)	7 (63.6%)
Hepatitis B and D	9	0–15	0–797	7 (77.8%)	1 (11.1%)

should be confined to patients who are HBV DNA seronegative at the time of transplantation, although an amelioration of the pathological sequelae of HBV recurrence in the remaining patients cannot be excluded at this time. No clear role for other antiviral agents has yet been defined post-transplantation. Interferon has been used in a small number of cases but the available data are insufficient to justify a conclusion as to its efficacy.[23,24]

The impact of HBV replication on graft function is variable and a wide range of histological patterns of disease have been described. A minority of patients have no biochemical or histological evidence of liver disease secondary to hepatitis B over periods ranging up to six years.[11,25] About half of the patients develop an acute hepatitis after re-infection, which is indistinguishable histologically from acute hepatitis B in immunocompetent patients, apart from a possible reduction in the intensity of the inflammatory infiltrate.[25] This hepatitic illness is self-limiting in most cases, although a small number develop fulminant hepatic failure leading to death or retransplantation.[11,25] Those patients who have been retransplanted in this situation have shown an even earlier recurrence of fulminant hepatic failure.[14] Chronic disease in the graft related to hepatitis B ranges from chronic persistent or active hepatitis to a rapid progression to cirrhosis.[25,26] A case of *de novo* development of a hepatocellular carcinoma in association with cirrhosis four years after transplantation has recently been described.[27] However, the most fascinating pattern of disease is a unique clinical and histological syndrome termed fibrosing cholestatic hepatitis (FCH). The clinical features are of progressive jaundice in association with a rapidly rising prothrombin time and loss of the graft within 4–6 weeks of clinical presentation.[11] The abnormalities seen in the liver enzyme profile are remarkably mild considering the severity of the disease process; in particular, a marked increase in serum transaminase levels is unusual. The histological features are of extensive serpiginous periportal fibrosis, canalicular and cellular cholestasis with prominent cytoplasmic HBsAg and HBeAg expression.[26] High level expression of intracellular HBsAg and HBcAg has been documented in these cases,[28] and a direct cytopathic role for the virus has been proposed.[25,28] The only possible treatment for this manifestation of HBV infection is retransplantation, but to date the results have been very poor because of high early post-operative mortality or aggressive recurrence of FCH.

Non-A, non-B hepatitis and hepatitis C

The new serological tests for hepatitis C indicate that this represents a subset of the condition previously described as presumed non-A, non-B viral hepatitis. In an American study of patients with acute presumed non-A, non-B viral hepatitis, antibodies to hepatitis C were found in 61% of intravenous drug abusers, 33% of post-transfusion cases and 22% of sporadic infections.[29] The detection rate was higher in chronic infection, being 89%, 71% and 27% in the respective groups.[29] The vast majority of patients with acute hepatic failure attributed to presumed non-A, non-B hepatitis are sporadic cases and most are seronegative for hepatitis C.[30,31]

The emerging data with respect to the frequency and impact of recurrent hepatitis C infection after liver transplantation are somewhat conflicting, although the problem is considerably less than with hepatitis B. In one study of six patients who were seropositive at the time of transplantation, two developed clinically significant graft dysfunction attributed to viral reinfection, and one of these lost two grafts through the rapid development of cirrhosis.[32] Another study of 44 patients with post-hepatitis cirrhosis detected antibodies to hepatitis C in 91% and there was associated graft dysfunction in 48% of cases.[33] When the more sensitive polymerase chain reaction (PCR) technique was used in a further study to detect HCV RNA after transplantation, 65% were found to be positive and 73% of these were judged to have a related histological hepatitis.[34] The estimates for the *de novo* acquisition of hepatitis C infection during the transplant range from 0–40%, and in the latter study 75% of these cases developed clinical disease.[32,34]

A toga-like virus was isolated from the liver of one patient with fulminant hepatic failure attributed to presumed non-A, non-B hepatitis, and was also in two grafts explanted at two and ten days.[35] The first graft was removed because of size related mechanical problems, but the second was removed as a result of graft failure with the clinical and histological characteristics of non-thrombotic graft infarction. Similar viruslike particles were identified in another patient with a similar clinical course, but this case was complicated by the co-existence of severe gram-negative sepsis at the time of graft loss.[36] It has yet to be proven that these apparent viral particles represent another cause of non-A, non-B hepatitis.

Other viral infections

Cytomegalovirus (CMV)

This is recognised as the single most important pathogen following liver transplantation. The outcome for the patient with an active CMV infection depends not only on the severity of the infection and the degree of endogenous immunosuppression it may induce, but also on many other factors such as the intensity of pharmacological immunosuppression, the number and severity of rejection episodes, the donor–recipient HLA match, the type and timing of anti-CMV therapy and the other opportunistic infections that may co-exist.

CMV infections may be acquired from an exogenous source or result from re-activation of latent endogenous virus. The donor organ and transfused blood are recognised sources, especially posing a problem for the seronegative recipient but also potentially a source of re-infection for seropositive recipients. The seroprevalence in donors and recipients varies with age, socio-economic status, ethnic, geographic and cultural characteristics. In Europe and North America about 50–70% of adults and about 20% of paediatric recipients will be seropositive pretransplant.

Infections may be symptomatic or asymptomatic, though in general primary infections are more likely than secondary infections to show clinical manifestations – 88% compared with 32%.[2] The incidence of CMV infections following liver transplantation, between 45% and 78%,[2,37,38] is similar to that seen in kidney and heart recipients (32% and 34%), but the rate of symptomatic infections in liver and heart recipients (32% and 34%) is much greater than in renal recipients (8%) on the same immunosuppressive regimen.[39] Asymptomatic infections are detected by culturing virus from urine or by demonstrating rising antibody titres in serum. The severity of symptomatic infections ranges from a febrile illness to disseminated life-threatening multiple organ involvement. The fever is characteristically a high swinging fever with a median onset at 28 days and duration of 2–3 weeks. It may be accompanied by muscle aches particularly of the back and thighs. Less frequently, arthralgia or thrombocytopenic purpura may be present.[39] Clinical disease may manifest as involvement of a single solid organ, most commonly the liver.[40] More severe infections show widespread dissemination with additional involvement of the lungs, gastro-intestinal tract and bone marrow. Pneumonitis is the life-threatening complication which requires early detection if it is to be successfully treated. Chorioretinitis has been documented, but is a late feature usually presenting six or more months after transplantation,[41] while rare manifestations include skin lesions, endometritis and encephalopathy.[42–44] Laboratory investigations reflect the pattern of disease and the abnormalities include leucopenia, atypical lymphocytosis, thrombocytopenia and a cholestatic pattern of liver enzymes. Radiological evidence of pneumonitis with scattered areas of consolidation on chest X-ray is a relatively late finding, and patients with primary infections are best monitored using blood gas analysis to detect hypoxaemia and so identify the earliest phase of this complication. Such patients should always be subjected to broncho-alveolar lavage to establish the diagnosis and to screen for co-existing opportunistic pathogens which are especially common in this situation. The classical histological evidence of CMV hepatitis on liver biopsy is the identification of inclusion bodies, but these are seen in only a minority of cases. More frequently the sentinel finding of a small cluster of neutrophils in the lobular parenchyma is observed. However, most cases of CMV hepatitis are diagnosed by using immunohistochemistry or *in situ* hybridisation techniques.[45,46]

The mortality from CMV infection prior to the introduction of ganciclovir ranged from none in one study,[1] to accounting for two-thirds of post-transplant deaths in another series of 26 paediatric liver transplant recipients.[47] In the latter study the overall incidence of CMV infection was similar to that seen in adults, 54%, but six of the 14 children with CMV infection died in spite of treatment with ganciclovir and immunoglobulins or foscarnet. All had received livers from seropositive donors, and had been treated with either ALG or OKT3. The high mortality rate may reflect the delay in commencing specific antiviral therapy until tissue confirmation of the diagnosis of CMV pneumonitis was established. However, in a larger series of 84 children, the incidence of CMV